Fitness
for College and Life

Fitness
for College and Life

William E. Prentice, PhD, PT, AT, C

Professor, Coordinator of the Sports Medicine Specialization,
Department of Physical Education, Exercise, and Sport Science;

Clinical Professor, Division of Physical Therapy,
Department of Medical Allied Health Professions;

Associate Professor, Department of Orthopaedics, School of Medicine,
The University of North Carolina at Chapel Hill

Director, Sports Medicine Education and Fellowship Program,
HEALTHSOUTH Corporation,
Birmingham, Alabama

FIFTH EDITION

with 263 illustrations

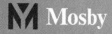 Mosby

St. Louis   Baltimore   Boston   Carlsbad   Chicago   Naples   New York   Philadelphia   Portland
London   Madrid   Mexico City   Singapore   Sydney   Tokyo   Toronto   Wiesbaden

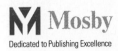

Mosby
Dedicated to Publishing Excellence

A Times Mirror
Company

Vice President and Publisher: James M. Smith
Senior Acquisitions Editor: Vicki Malinee
Developmental Editor: Brian Morovitz
Project Manager: John Rogers
Senior Production Editor: Lavon Wirch Peters
Composition Specialist: Joan Herron
Designers: Sheilah Barrett, Yael Kats, Liz Young
Manufacturing Manager: Theresa Fuchs
Cover Art: © John Clausen/Mountain Stock

FIFTH EDITION

Printed in the United States of America

Composition by Mosby Electronic Production
Lithography/color film by The Arthur Morgan Company
Printing/binding by Von Hoffmann Press

Mosby–Year Book, Inc.
11830 Westline Industrial Drive
St. Louis, Missouri 63146

Library of Congress Cataloging in Publication Data
Prentice, William E.
    Fitness for college and life / William E. Prentice. -- 5th ed.
        p.   cm.
    Includes bibliographical references and index.
    ISBN 0-8151-8452-2
    1. Physical fitness.   I. Title.
GV481.P77   1997
613.7--dc20   96-17738
                                                       CIP

96 97 98 99 00 / 9 8 7 6 5 4 3 2 1

Preface

PHYSICAL FITNESS

In many respects, *physical fitness* appears to be an integral part of the American lifestyle. It is virtually impossible to go through a day without being exposed to something involving physical fitness. We are bombarded by images that suggest the importance of being physically fit and healthy. We hear about fitness on TV, on the radio, and in videos. We read about fitness in magazines, books, and newspapers. The image of the attractive, healthy, physically fit person is used to sell everything from foods, nutrient supplements, clothing, and sports equipment to memberships in health and fitness clubs. Even our friends and co-workers are willing to give opinions on the best way to work out or to get "in shape."

If you believed what you hear, see, and read in the media you would think that every person in America has become a "fitness junkie." It is true that millions of people do exercise in some way, shape, or form on a somewhat consistent basis, but the fact is that for most people the thought of going out and "exercising" never even crosses their minds.

The "modern lifestyle" with all of its technology and labor-saving devices is essentially sedentary. Fortunately, people seem to be realizing that there really is a reason to pay attention to living a healthy lifestyle and incorporate regular exercise of some type into their everyday life.

Perhaps nowhere is this interest in physical activity more evident than on college or university campuses. On any given day, summer or winter, the campuses and recreation centers are crowded with people jogging, walking, bicycling, doing aerobics, lifting weights, and playing sports. In many cases college students are establishing patterns of living that may well affect their long-term health and leisure pursuits.

WHY IS *FITNESS FOR COLLEGE AND LIFE* A USEFUL RESOURCE?

The fifth edition of *Fitness for College and Life* provides a comprehensive, readable text for use in general fitness classes that are designed to acquaint college students with the nature and scope of fitness. The text emphasizes the value of establishing lifelong patterns of fitness. It provides facts and principles that provide the basis for motivating people to incorporate some form of physical activity into their daily lives. The text also identifies the exercises, activities, resources, and assessment instruments that can be used in developing an individualized, well-rounded fitness program. Although there are many different approaches that will ultimately lead to physical fitness, following certain principles and guidelines makes the pursuit of physical fitness safer and more effective.

Working to Develop a Healthy Lifestyle

In recognizing the importance of today's trend toward living a more healthy lifestyle, this text concentrates on the importance of the health-related aspects of physical fitness in addition to stressing aspects of performance or motor skill–related fitness. Health-related fitness is concerned with developing the components necessary to function efficiently and achieve or maintain a healthy lifestyle. Physical fitness is viewed as one very important part of the whole picture of an individual's well-being.

As people of all ages become more aware of the importance of being physically fit and trying to achieve a more healthful style of living, a need arises to present information dealing with a wide variety of topics regarding strength training, cardiorespiratory endurance, flexibility, weight control, nutrition, injury prevention, and stress management. The public's interest in becoming more physically fit has created a multi–billion dollar industry that does not always promote items or services that are safe, effective, or necessary. Self-proclaimed fitness "experts" unfortunately disseminate a great deal of misinformation. Thus consumers of fitness products need a source of reliable information. A college fitness class can provide not only the instruction about proper exercises but also information about how to become a more careful consumer.

Building Upon a Scientific Base of Knowledge

This text discusses various concepts, principles, and theories that are supported by scientific research to the extent that is reasonable for this audience. Sources of information are from disciplines such as exercise physiology, nutrition, athletic training, biomechanics, and physical therapy. It is important for anyone involved in a physical activity program to have at least a basic understanding of why it is more efficient to make use of a specific technique to maximize results. Therefore this text deals not only with principles but also with specific activities and recommendations for applications.

WHAT DOES THIS TEXT COVER?

Fitness for College and Life has long been perceived as a superior text in this market due to its accuracy and thoroughness of content. The fifth edition continues to focus on the importance of the individual taking responsibility for his or her fitness and health.

The text covers all of the important elements of fitness for the college student. An examination of the table of contents provides the student with an appreciation for the comprehensive nature of the text. Diverse and important topics, such as tips for exercising in extreme weather conditions or during pregnancy, are included. In addition, information about purchasing exercise equipment and fitness club memberships is both timely and practical. A discussion about causes and treatments of common fitness injuries is extremely valuable for anyone involved in exercise. In this fifth edition, as in the past, fitness principles blend with practical examples, enabling students to evaluate their physical condition and apply information.

Wellness Approach to Health and Fitness

Various other aspects of healthful living are presented as part of the wellness approach to health and fitness. The first half of the book describes fitness and health-related principles. Facts about the development of cardiorespiratory endurance, muscular strength and endurance, and flexibility are included. Deterrents to fitness, such as substance abuse and sedentary lifestyle, are described. The second half introduces facts about fitness-related topics such as body composition determination, weight management, nutritious food selection, and injury prevention and management. Because the management of stress is an important aspect of any fitness program, this subject is also discussed, along with practical suggestions and techniques for learning how to cope with stress. Furthermore, a series of lifetime fitness activities suitable for personalizing anyone's fitness program is described. General discussions of the various fitness-related topics are followed by more than 50 individual Lab Activities that include assessments, inventories, worksheets, and specific activities to which the principles are applied. The text concludes with a chapter on consumer information relative to purchasing and using fitness products. Fitness is a fascinating subject, and I have tried to communicate my enthusiasm for it throughout the book.

WHAT IS NEW AND DIFFERENT IN THIS FIFTH EDITION?

College instructors who are teaching courses in fitness, wellness, and exercise physiology reviewed the fourth edition of *Fitness for College and Life*. Reviewers were asked to determine what health information is necessary for a comprehensive fitness text. In addition, experts in the fields of nutrition and stress management provided technical reviews necessary to update chapter content. After careful consideration, these suggestions have been incorporated into the fifth edition of this text. This research provides the assurance that the content is up-to-date, accurate, practical, and relevant to today's college students and adults in general.

NEW AND SUCCESSFUL FEATURES

This edition of *Fitness for College and Life* presents topics in a more readable style, with organization geared to the general college student's level of understanding and background. Descriptions of anatomical structures, techniques for assessing specific fitness components, and suggestions for specific training are clearly explained so that the student can comprehend and apply what is being discussed. Color photographs and diagrams illustrate the correct way to exercise and explain more abstract concepts. The text pages are perforated so that Lab Activities and related worksheets can be completed and turned in for assignments.

- The fifth edition has a new four-color format with completely new photographs and revised artwork.
- Chapter 3, Overcoming Behaviors That Interfere With Health and Fitness, is a new chapter that focuses on lifestyle habits that are deterrents to healthful living. Included are discussions on drug, alcohol, and tobacco abuse as well as sexually transmitted diseases, particularly HIV.

- Chapter 9, Eating Healthy, has been updated with information from the newest edition of *Nutrition and Your Health: Dietary Guidelines for Americans* (1995).
- Chapter 13, Buying Fitness Products, focuses on fitness and consumer issues. New guidelines for the consumer of health and fitness products are set forth for those individuals who wish to be more careful of how their resources are spent to get the most from their fitness plan.
- A new feature has been added at the beginning of each chapter to incorporate *Healthy People 2000* and how it relates to the content throughout the text. This feature is meant to inspire and inform as well as warn the reader about personal health choices. As continuing research establishes the link between select physical activity and increased levels of physical health, educated individuals will be able to choose activities that are ideally suited to address their individual health risks.
- Additional learning aids including *Safe Tips, Health Links,* and *Fit Lists* are presented in individual chapters.
- New *Get Moving* boxes highlight behavior change and motivational strategies throughout the text.
- *Your Personal Trainer* boxes address common fitness questions and misconceptions and offer case-study scenarios for successful fitness programs.
- *Margin definitions* appear throughout the text as key terms are introduced, helping to expand the working vocabulary of the reader.
- Additional headings throughout the text break the narrative into smaller sections, making content easily manageable.
- A new appendix lists various health and fitness resources available on many college and university campuses.
- Mosby's NutriTrac software and an accompanying Diet Fitness Log is available as a package with this text to enable students to fully integrate a successful exercise and weight-management program.
- A comprehensive ViewStudy™ presentation has been created to include art from several related health and fitness texts.

PEDAGOGICAL FEATURES

This text includes numerous pedagogical aids to facilitate its use by students and instructors:
- **Health Goals 2000** boxes stress the importance of physical fitness in everyone's life and relate *Healthy People 2000* goals with the content of each chapter.
- **Chapter Objectives** introduce to students the important concepts in the chapter. Mastering knowledge of the objectives indicates fulfillment of the chapter's intent.
- Each chapter begins with **Key Terms** that list the most important terms for students to become familiar with while reading the chapter. The terms are defined in margin boxes where they appear in the text.
- **Fit Lists, Safe Tips,** and **Health Links** summarize important health and fitness concerns throughout the text.
- **Get Moving** boxes provide behavior change and motivational strategies to increase adherence to an individual's fitness program.
- **Your Personal Trainer** boxes detail scenarios for effecting successful fitness programs.
- Each chapter has a **Summary** outlining and reinforcing the major points covered.
- **References** have been expanded and include the most up-to-date documentation for the student who wishes to further research topics being discussed.
- **Suggested Readings** with annotations present additional resources for further information.
- More than 50 **Lab Activities** help the student apply the theoretical information presented in the text. These pages are perforated for easy removal upon completion of the assignment.
- Appendixes: **Appendix A** provides recommendations for the available health and fitness resources on college and university campuses. **Appendix B** is a food composition table compatible with Mosby's NutriTrac™ software. It lists nutritional information on commonly eaten foods and foods from popular fast food restaurants.

SUPPLEMENTS
Instructor's Manual with Test Bank

An Instructor's Manual containing 700 test items is also available. It provides suggestions on how to use the text to its fullest potential. The manual includes chapter overviews, learning objectives, key terms, and a topical teaching outline. A test bank of true/false, multiple-choice, and discussion questions for each chapter is a useful resource. Extensive lists of additional readings and annotated media and software resources are included. For convenience, directories of addresses and telephone numbers for resources are also provided.

There are 54 transparency masters from lists and illustrations in the text and several that summarize content. Perforated for easy removal, these have been included to help explain more difficult concepts and to facilitate classroom and laboratory instruction.

Valuable resources for the instructor are the two instructional plans outlining suggested activities that can be used in a 10-week (four sessions a week) and a 14-week (three sessions a week) college class pattern. Activities will include such things as lectures, physical activities, testing, and demonstrations. Instructors will be able to use the instructional plans as outlined for their classes, or they can adapt them in a way that will better fit into their own pattern of instruction.

Transparency Acetates

Available to qualified adopters, 54 four-color transparency acetates illustrate and summarize important concepts in the text.

Computerized Test Bank

ESATEST Computerized Test Bank with 700 multiple choice, true/false, fill-in-the-blank, and short essay questions is available in IBM Windows and Macintosh formats to qualified adopters of this text.

NutriTrac™ Software and Diet/Fitness Log

Available for Windows and Macintosh, this nutrient-analysis software allows you and your students to analyze diets easily, using an icon-based interface and on-screen help features. Foods for breakfast, lunch, dinner, and snacks may be selected from more than 2250 items in the database. Records may be kept for any number of days. The program can provide intake analyses for individual foods, meals, days, or for an entire intake period. Intake analyses can compare nutrient values to RDA or RNI values and to the USDA Food Guide Pyramid and can provide breakdowns of fat and calorie sources. An accompanying diet and fitness log motivates students to keep track of their progress. This package is available for a nominal fee with the text.

ViewStudy™ Presentation Software

This CD-ROM, compatible with either Windows or Macintosh, contains key illustrations from Mosby's health and fitness texts. A slide show tool allows selection of prearranged images. Illustrations can also be printed full size for use as acetates and may be exported for use with other programs and applications, such as the computerized test bank. This software is available to qualified adopters.

Laboratory Activity Software

Available in IBM DOS, this convenient program contains more than 100 fitness and health activities and assessments for students to complete and print out. The software is available to qualified adopters and can be purchased with the text for a nominal fee.

ACKNOWLEDGMENTS

The preparation of a manuscript for a textbook involves a collective, coordinated effort on the part of many individuals. The quality of the text is generally reflective of many special talents, as well as the dedication and commitment to the project of all those involved. My developmental editor for this text, Brian Morovitz, deserves tremendous credit and sincere gratitude for his diligence, his creativity, and his invaluable input and considerable expertise in the completion of this revision.

Particular credit is due Michael J. Keenan, PhD, Associate Professor in Human Nutrition and Food, Louisiana State University, for updating Chapter 9 with the most current information on nutrition and the recently revised USDA dietary guidelines.

Our photographer, Missy Bello, and our models, Meleata Smalls, Jonathon Raynor, Lina Patel, Angela Deal, Liz Roede, Douglas Horlick, John White, Jose Dominguez, David Carter, and Connie Regnerus did a professional and artistic job, and I respect and again appreciate their contribution.

In addition, my thanks must also be expressed to the following reviewers whose recommendations and suggestions have helped to focus the direction and influence the evolution of this edition.

David A. Cameron	Cameron University
Jennie Gilbert	California State University, San Bernardino
Paul S. Krebs	Kansas State University
George Matthews	Santa Fe Community College
Ronald J. Schick	Tyler Junior College
Randle S. Williams	Missouri Western State College

Finally, my wife Tena and our two sons, Brian and Zachary, provide inspiration and support in every project I choose to pursue.

William E. Prentice

Contents

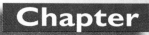

Chapter 1

Getting Fit—What It's All About

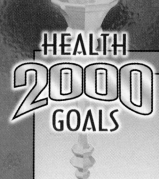

HEALTH 2000 GOALS

- **Physical Activity and Fitness.** Increase to at least 40% the proportion of people age 6 and older who regularly perform physical activities that enhance and maintain muscular strength, muscular endurance, and flexibility.
- **Risk-Reduction Objectives.** Increase to at least 30% the proportion of people age 6 and older who engage regularly, preferably daily, in light to moderate physical activity for at least 30 minutes per day. In 1985, 22% of people age 18 and older were active for at least 30 minutes five or more times per week, and 12% were active seven or more times per week in 1985. *Midpoint Update: headed in the right direction with current statistic of 24%.*
- **Lifelong Health Habits.** As students leave the school setting they lose their physical and social support system and incur time constraints that can result in decreased levels of physical activity.

OBJECTIVES

After completing this chapter, you will be able to do the following:

- Describe the nature and scope of fitness as it exists today.
- Discuss recommendations relative to the quality and quantity of exercise.
- Explain the role of physical activity in achieving an optimal state of well-being.
- Define the terms *fitness, physical fitness, health-related fitness,* and *motor skill–related fitness.*

- List the component parts of physical fitness.
- Describe the relationship between the body systems and fitness.
- Explain the importance of physical fitness to college students.
- Explain the importance of regularly engaging in a physical activity program.
- Determine your present level of physical fitness.
- Explain the importance of finding methods of motivation in an exercise program.

KEY TERMS

While reading this chapter, you will become familiar with the following terms:

- fitness
- physical fitness
- health-related fitness
- motor skill–related fitness

- cardiorespiratory endurance
- flexibility
- muscular strength

- muscular endurance
- body composition
- speed
- power
- agility

- neuromuscular coordination
- balance
- reaction time

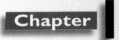

EXERCISE TRENDS

Enthusiasm for exercise and fitness in the United States is at an unprecedented level, with millions of people spending countless hours and billions of dollars on sport and exercise. This interest in fitness, initially perceived by some as a fad or a short-lived phenomenon, grew steadily throughout the 1970s and 1980s but seems to have reached a plateau in the last few years.

Surveys indicate that virtually all adults believe that exercise is important to health and fitness and that regular physical activity is essential for themselves and for their children. Still, despite this increased interest in exercise and fitness, the U.S. Department of Health and Human Services reports that only 24% of adults participate in a minimum of 30 minutes of light-to-moderate exercise at least five times per week and only 12% are active seven times per week. Approximately 54% of the population is somewhat active but fails to achieve exercise intensity levels necessary for improving cardiorespiratory endurance. Unfortunately, approximately 24% of American adults are essentially sedentary and do not engage in any type of leisure-time physical activity.

Who Is Most Likely to Exercise?

In the general population of Americans, men are more likely to engage in some form of physical activity, intense exercise, or sport than are women. Nevertheless, more women are now choosing to become involved in exercise. Fortunately, many of the long-standing historical prejudices and misconceptions regarding women and fitness are disappearing, and the "feminine image" for the 1990s has been redefined. Women are becoming physically active at a much higher rate than are their male counterparts, participating in both recreational and competitive activities. Men engage in a wider range of sports and fitness activities than do women, but women engage more in calisthenics/aerobics than do men.

Children and teenagers in the United States are alarmingly inactive. Children often lack fitness because more time is spent watching television than engaging in any type of physical activity. Teenagers tend to become less active after they finish elementary school. The result is a youthful population lacking in physical fitness.

The amount of time spent engaging in physical activity steadily decreases with increasing age. This tendency to accept a more sedentary lifestyle as we become older is detrimental to good health. Of those adults over age 65, more than twice as many are inactive compared to adults under age 30. As our society ages, this becomes an increasing concern.

Those adults who have been educated about fitness and exercise are more likely to participate in regular physical activity during their lifetime. They realize the potential health benefits of incorporating regular physical activity into the daily routine.

Geographically, persons who live in the western part of the country are more physically active than those who live in other sections of the nation. The next most active inhabitants are in the Midwest, South, and Northeast, in that order.

Sports and activities with the greatest number of participants are walking/jogging, swimming, bicycling, calisthenics/aerobics, use of exercise machines, golf, bowling, tennis, baseball/softball, soccer, hiking/backpacking, pool/billiards, and squash/racquetball.

How Do Americans Perceive Their Level of Fitness?

Fifty-eight percent of Americans feel they are in "excellent" or "good" physical condition. The rest of the population say they are in "fair" or "poor" physical condition. But how realistic are their estimations of their level of fitness? Age and education influence the way Americans rate themselves. Those in the 18- to 34-year age bracket rate themselves higher than do those in the 50-year and older age group, and of those who did not graduate from high school most feel they are in "fair" or "poor" condition.

It is interesting to note that most Americans put considerable emphasis on their weight in rating their physical condition. If they feel their weight is right, they are more likely to rate themselves as being in "excellent" physical condition. However, if they are overweight, they are more likely to rate themselves as being in "fair" or "poor" shape.

One of every two Americans feels he or she is overweight, but only 1 of every 12 feels he or she is underweight. The rest say they are satisfied with what the scales indicate. Being overweight is perceived to be a greater problem for women than for men. At the same time, although being overweight is a problem affecting all ages, it is more evident in the 35- to 64-year age range.

What Has Prompted This Interest in Fitness?

Concern About Appearance

A number of factors have prompted this interest in fitness. Many individuals choose to become involved in a physical activity program because of the potential for changing both the way others see them and the way they see themselves. Certainly weight is associated with appearance. The images of the thin, "hardbody," picture-perfect people created by the advertising media have contributed to this obsession with weight. Chapter 8 examines issues relating to weight control and maintenance of body composition.

Fitness Contributes to a Healthy Lifestyle

Increased leisure time and the desire for youthfulness and self-improvement have prompted some to exercise. The growing realization that exercise and fitness are integral components of a healthy lifestyle has also contributed to the interest in fitness. The positive effects of remaining active throughout one's life have encouraged many to continue their participation in activities or to start regular exercise programs such as walking, jogging, or swimming. One of the most obvious reasons for becoming physically fit is the benefit derived from a healthy lifestyle that includes proper exercise and nutrition.

The concept of physical fitness is not new. Primitive humans relied primarily on speed, agility, and strength in the fight for survival. Life was a constant struggle that could be met only through physical prowess. Without knowing the scientific benefits of fitness, primitive humans existed, adapted to a variety of environmental conditions, and lived vigorous lives.

In contrast, we now rely largely on our intellect in coping with problems of survival. Whereas cognitive activity is essential for many work-related skills, little physical effort is required in most activities of our modern society. In fact, the modern lifestyle fosters a lack of physical fitness. Technological advances such as the automobile, television, elevators, escalators, and moving sidewalks eliminate the need for physical exertion and contribute to a sedentary lifestyle. Too often our society is so concerned with developing superiority of the intellect that there is a danger of neglecting the development of the whole person. Engaging in physical activity may enhance problem solving, reasoning, and perhaps even memory. Physical fitness affects the total person: his or her intellect, emotional stability, and physical conditioning.

In addition, our society is characterized by a fast-paced lifestyle, with obligations and stresses that affect our physical and emotional fitness. A common misconception among college students is that daily living incorporates enough exercise to maintain an adequate level of fitness. Walking leisurely back and forth to class or working at a part-time job provides a limited amount of physical exertion, which in most cases is not adequate to improve fitness or health.

Escalating Cost of Health Care

The escalating cost of health care has also served as an impetus for individuals and corporations to become increasingly aware of the benefits gained from health promotion efforts (see Chapter 2). Spiraling health care costs and the realization of the benefits of participation in health and fitness programs have prompted many individuals to become more involved in fitness activities. Corporations have also found that in an economic sense fitness is good business. It is fairly well documented that health care costs for organizations that offer prevention and health promotion programs show an approximate 20% savings in the cost of health care per employee per year. Certainly, many corporations are using existing fitness and health programs as recruitment incentives for potential employees.

A physical activity program should be initiated and followed on a regular basis to overcome inactivity and maintain an optimal level of fitness. Furthermore, such things as an adequate amount of rest, social and emotional outlets, and proper diet are also required for an appropriate level of fitness.

How Should You Exercise?

It has been well documented that engaging in regular, moderate-intensity physical activity will result in substantial health benefits. Based on this concept, it is recommended that everyone should try to engage in a minimum of 30 minutes of physical activity on most days—ideally, every day. This 30-minute total does not have to consist solely of what has traditionally been considered exercise (i.e., walking, swimming, cycling, etc.). It can involve a series of short bouts of physical activity that collectively accumulate to a total of at least 30 minutes of moderate-intensity physical exercise and that may include more intermittent activities such as walking up or down stairs, doing lawnwork or gardening, and cleaning the house. Table 1-1 shows examples of the relative intensities of various activities.

This most recent recommendation relative to the quantity and quality of exercise is substantially less formal than what has been recommended in the past. An exercise period of 30 to 60 minutes' duration at an intensity of 60% to 90% of maximum heart rate performed three or more times per week was, for years, the recommended standard for promoting good health and preventing disease. Recent research has

TABLE 1-1. Examples of Common Physical Activities for Healthy Adults by Intensity of Effort

Light	Moderate	Hard/Vigorous
Walking: slowly (strolling) (1-2 mph)	Walking: briskly (3-4 mph)	Walking: briskly uphill or with a load
Cycling: stationary (<50 W)	Cycling: for pleasure or transportation (≤10 mph)	Cycling: fast or racing (>10 mph)
Swimming: slow treading	Swimming: moderate effort	Swimming: fast treading or crawl
Conditioning exercise: light stretching	Conditioning exercise: general calisthenics	Conditioning exercise: stair ergometer, ski machine
—	Racket sports: table tennis	Racket sports: singles tennis, racquetball
Golf: power cart	Golf: pulling cart or carrying clubs	—
Bowling	—	—
Fishing: sitting	Fishing: standing/casting	Fishing: in stream
Boating: power	Canoeing: leisurely (2.0-3.9 mph)	Canoeing: rapidly (≥4 mph)
Home care: carpet sweeping	Home care: general cleaning	Moving furniture
Mowing lawn: riding mower	Mowing lawn: power mower	Mowing lawn: hand mower
Home repair: carpentry	Home repair: painting	

Modified from Pate R, Pratt M, Blair S, et al: Physical activity and public health: a recommendation from the Centers for Disease Control and Prevention and the American College of Sports Medicine, *JAMA* 273(5):402-407, 1995.
Data from Ainsworth et al, Leon, and McArdle et al.

indicated that many health benefits can be achieved by engaging in moderate-intensity physical activities not typically associated with formal exercise. The total amount of activity appears to be more critical to improving health than the specific manner in which the activity is performed.

The total amount of activity can be measured either in minutes of physical activity performed or in the number of calories expended. Moderate-intensity activity means that about 200 calories would be expended during 30 minutes of exercise performed periodically throughout the course of a day. The intensity of the activities should correspond to walking at a pace of 3 to 4 mph. Any type of activity that meets this moderate intensity level, regardless of whether it involves formal exercise, can be added to the daily total.

It has been estimated that the majority of Americans do not meet this minimum standard for daily physical actitivity. Thus it is recommended that everyone make an effort to gradually incorporate brief periods of physical activity into his or her daily routine, eventually increasing to a minimum total of 30 minutes on a regular, consistent basis.

WHAT IS PHYSICAL FITNESS?

Fitness is a broad term that means different things to different people. Consequently, establishing a precise definition of physical fitness is difficult. Physical fitness means that the various systems of the body are healthy and function efficiently so as to enable the fit person to engage in activities of daily living, as well as in recreational pursuits and leisure activities, without unreasonable fatigue. Beyond physical development, muscular strength, and stamina, physical fitness implies efficient performance in exercise or work and a reasonable measure of motor skill in the performance of selected physical activities. (The terms *exercise* and *physical activities* will be used interchangeably throughout this text.)

Being physically fit is critical to our overall health and well-being. Physical fitness is an important component of *wellness* (see Chapter 2). Being physically fit can help you satisfy your needs regarding mental and emotional stability, social consciousness and adaptability, spiritual and moral fiber, and physical health consistent with your heredity.

The same degree of physical fitness is not essential for everyone. However, everyone needs a minimal amount of fitness to be healthy, and everyone is capable of achieving minimal fitness levels. The level of fitness necessary depends on factors such as the tasks you must perform and your potential for physical effort. Physical fitness varies with the individual and with the demands and requirements of a specific task. The college athlete must constantly work to improve his or her strength, endurance, flexiblity, speed, and cardiorespiratory efficiency, whereas the nonathlete student who cycles to class requires less effort to maintain his or her level of physical fitness. The weekend golfer needs a different level of physical fitness than the mountain climber or wheelchair athlete.

Physical fitness varies according to the circumstances of a person at different times in his or her life. Because no set standard of physical fitness applies to all people, an optimal level of fitness depends on your age, sex, body type, vocation, and physical limitations such as those associated with diabetes or asthma.

Physical fitness is not entirely dependent on exercise. Desirable health practices also play an important role. Physical fitness affects the total person: intellect, emotional stability, physical conditioning, and stress levels. The road to physical fitness includes proper medical care, the right kinds of food in the right amounts, good oral hygiene, appropriate physical activity that is adapted to individual needs and physical limitations, satisfying work and study, healthy play and recreation, and proper amounts of rest and relaxation.

There are varying degrees of physical fitness. Practically anyone can improve his or her fitness status, and physical activity is essential to achieving physical fitness. Physical fitness cannot be stored up; it requires daily attention. The person who plays tennis all summer and then gives up all physical activity when autumn starts will not remain physically fit. The sprinter who fails to run after the track season ends will backslide in respect to his or her physical fitness level.

HEALTH-RELATED VERSUS MOTOR SKILL–RELATED COMPONENTS OF FITNESS

The American Alliance of Health, Physical Education, Recreation, and Dance (AAHPERD) has classified the components of fitness into two categories: health-related components and motor skill–related components. The health-related fitness components concern the development of qualities necessary to function efficiently and maintain a healthy lifestyle. These components include muscular strength, muscular endurance, cardiorespiratory endurance, flexibility, and body composition. Motor skill–related fitness includes qualities such as speed, power, balance, agility, reaction time, and coordination that are conducive to better performance in sports and other physical activities.

The components of health-related and motor skill–related fitness overlap. For example, cardiorespiratory endurance, muscular strength, muscular endurance, flexibility, and body composition are essential for healthy living; they are also important in skillful motor performance. However, the degree of

development each requires varies according to the type of physical activity. A more extensive development of these components may be required to achieve an appropriate level of motor skill–related fitness, which is often associated with sport. For example, athletes may need to develop speed and power to a greater degree than most individuals who are interested solely in improving and maintaining health-related fitness.

When designing an individualized physical fitness program, you must first decide what it is you are trying to accomplish and then select those specific components of fitness that ultimately will help you reach your goal. For example, the goals of fitness improvement for a 55-year-old person would probably differ considerably from those of a 20-year-old college student who is preparing to compete in varsity gymnastics. The 55-year-old person would be more concerned with fitness components such as cardiorespiratory endurance, flexibility, muscular endurance, and body composition. Improvement in these four specific areas would enhance performance in daily tasks without undue fatigue, as stated in the definition of physical fitness. On the other hand, the 20-year-old gymnast must be concerned not only with the previously mentioned components but also with components such as strength, speed, power, balance, and agility. If he or she does not include activities in the training regimen that specifically address these various skill-related fitness components, chances are that he or she will be unsuccessful in a competitive situation.

A number of different factors collectively contribute to an individual's physical fitness. Although a complete consensus on the components of physical fitness does not exist, most authorities agree on the following basic elements.

---

fitness broad term denoting dynamic qualities that allow one to satisfy needs regarding mental and emotional stability, social consciousness and adaptability, spirituality, and physical health

physical fitness healthy and efficient functioning of various body systems that allows one to engage in activities of daily living, recreation, and leisure

health-related fitness pertains to the development of qualities necessary to function efficiently and maintain a healthy lifestyle—including muscular strength, muscular endurance, cardiorespiratory endurance, flexibility, and body composition

motor skill–related fitness includes qualities such as speed, power, balance, agility, reaction time, and coordination that can be developed to better performance in sports and other physical activities

HEALTH-RELATED COMPONENTS OF FITNESS
Cardiorespiratory Endurance

Cardiorespiratory endurance is the ability to persist in a physical activity requiring oxygen for physical exertion without experiencing undue fatigue (Figure 1-1). The student who runs 2 miles or swims 2000 yards is displaying cardiorespiratory endurance. The functioning of the heart, lungs, and blood vessels is essential for distribution of oxygen and nutrients and removal of wastes from the body. For performance of vigorous activities, efficient functioning of the heart and lungs is necessary. The more efficiently they function, the easier it will be to walk, run, study, and concentrate for longer periods of time. A more efficient student will be able to maintain effort for a longer time.

Cardiorespiratory endurance is characterized by moderate contractions of large muscle groups for a relatively long time, during which adjustments of the cardiorespiratory system to the activity are necessary, as in distance running or swimming. Exercise of this nature involves the heart, the vessels supplying blood to all parts of the body, and the oxygen-carrying capacity of the blood. Cardiorespiratory endurance may be assessed by using a number of tests that measure or predict the maximum rate at which oxygen can be used during exercise. These tests are often taken during a resting state and then again after exercise.

Flexibility

Flexibility is the ability to move freely throughout a full, nonrestricted, pain-free range of motion about a joint or series of joints (Figure 1-2). It may be improved by engaging in consistent stretching. Flexibility is important for performance in most active sports; it is also important for maintaining good posture. Furthermore, it is essential in carrying on many daily activities and can help to prevent muscle strain and orthopedic problems such as backaches.

Muscular Strength

Muscular strength is the ability or capacity of a muscle or muscle group to exert a one-time maximal force against resistance through a full range of motion (Figure 1-3). Strength is needed in all kinds of work and physical activity. Strength is also an important element of athletic activity. Strong muscles provide better protection of body joints, resulting in fewer sprains, strains, and muscular difficulties. Furthermore, muscle strength helps in maintaining proper posture and provides greater endurance, power, and resistance to fatigue. In many cases, the lack of strength of abdominal muscles is a primary cause of recurrent low back problems. Weak abdominal muscles and inflexible posterior thigh muscles allow the pelvis to tip forward, thereby causing an abnormal arch in the lower back that results in low back pain. By overemphasizing strenthening of a particular muscle group, postural abnormalities may also develop. For optimal performance it is critical to develop a balance in strength between various muscle groups.

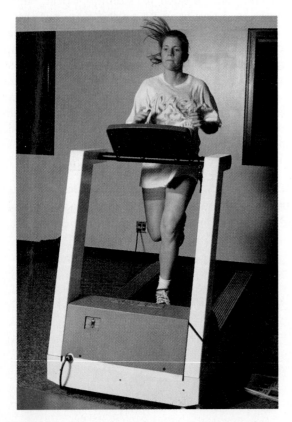

FIGURE I-I. Cardiorespiratory Endurance.
Perhaps the most essential fitness component for both good health and athletic performance.

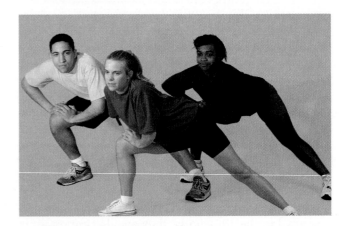

FIGURE I-2. Flexibility.
The ability to move freely through a range of motion.

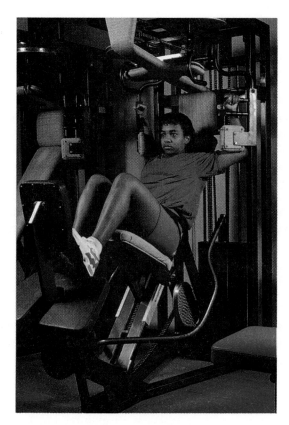

FIGURE 1-3. **Muscular Strength.**
The ability to generate force against resistance.

Muscular Endurance

Muscular endurance is the ability of a muscle or muscle group to perform or sustain a submaximal muscle contraction repeatedly over a period of time (Figure 1-4). Muscular endurance is closely related to muscular strength. An individual who is strong will be less resistant to fatigue, because relatively less effort will be required to produce repeated muscular contractions.

Body Composition

Body composition relates to the makeup of the body in terms of muscle, bone, fat, and other elements (Figure 1-5). With respect to physical fitness, the term particularly refers to the percentage of fat in the body relative to the fat-free content. An excess of fat in the body is unhealthy, because it requires more energy for movement and may reflect a diet high in saturated fat. The demand on the cardiorespiratory system is greater when the percentage of body fat is high. Furthermore, it is believed that obesity contributes to degenerative diseases such as high blood pressure and atherosclerosis. Obesity can also result in psychological maladjustments and may shorten life. A balance between caloric intake and caloric expenditure is necessary to maintain proper body-fat content. Adequate exercise, therefore, is effective in controlling body fat.

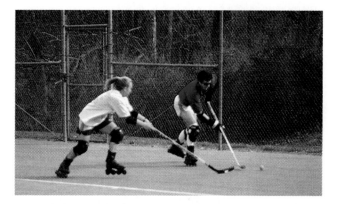

FIGURE 1-4. **Muscular Endurance.**
The ability to perform muscular contractions repeatedly over a period of time.

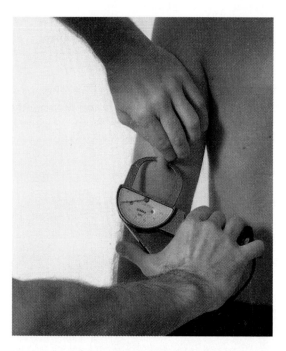

FIGURE 1-5. **Altering Body Composition.**
Aerobic exercise reduces the percentage of total body weight that is fat tissue.

cardiorespiratory endurance ability to persist in a physical activity requiring oxygen for physical exertion without experiencing undue fatigue
flexibility ability to move freely throughout a full, unrestricted, pain-free range of motion about a joint or series of joints
muscular strength capacity of a muscle or muscle group to exert a one-time maximal force against resistance throughout a full range of motion
muscular endurance ability of a muscle or muscle group to perform or sustain a submaximal contraction repeatedly over a period of time
body composition relates to the makeup of the body in terms of muscle, bone, fat, and other elements

MOTOR SKILL–RELATED COMPONENTS OF FITNESS

Speed

Speed is the ability to perform a particular movement very rapidly (Figure 1-6). It is a function of distance and time. It is an important component for successful performance in many competitive athletic situations. Lab Activity 1-1 will help you assess your speed.

Power

Power is the ability to generate great amounts of force against a certain resistance in a short period of time (Figure 1-7). Power is a function of both strength and speed. The ability to drive a golf ball, hit a softball, or kick a soccer ball a long distance requires some element of power. Lab Activity 1-2 will help you assess your ability to generate power.

Agility

Agility is the ability to change or alter, quickly and accurately, the direction of body movement during activity (Figure 1-8). Agility is to a large extent dependent on neuromuscular coordination and reaction time. Agility may be improved with increased flexibility and muscular strength. Lab Activity 1-3 will help you measure your agility in moving in different directions.

Neuromuscular Coordination

Neuromuscular coordination is the ability to integrate the senses—visual, auditory, and proprioceptive (knowing the position of your body in space)—with motor function to produce smooth, accurate, and skilled movement (Figure 1-9).

Balance

Balance is the ability to maintain some degree of equilibrium while moving or standing still (Figure 1-10). Lab Activity 1-4 will help you determine your balance capabilities.

Reaction Time (Movement Time)

Reaction time is the time required to produce an appropriate and accurate physiological or mechanical response to some external stimulus (Figure 1-11). Lab Activity 1-5 will help you assess your ability to react to a stimulus and then to move quickly and accurately.

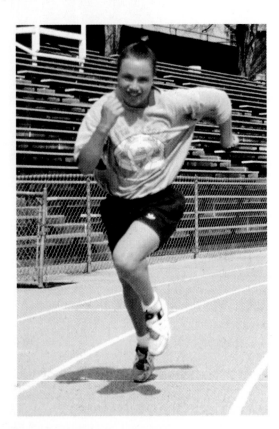

FIGURE 1-6. Speed.
An important component in many competitive athletic situations.

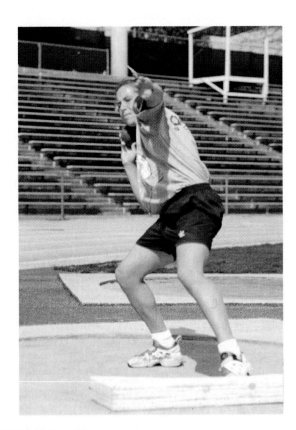

FIGURE 1-7. Power.
The ability to generate large amounts of force rapidly.

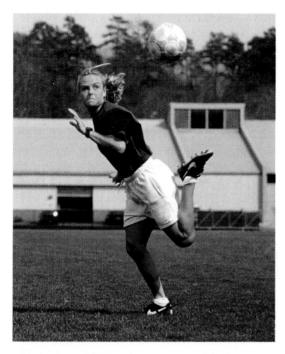

FIGURE 1-8. Agility.
The ability to change direction of movement quickly and accurately.

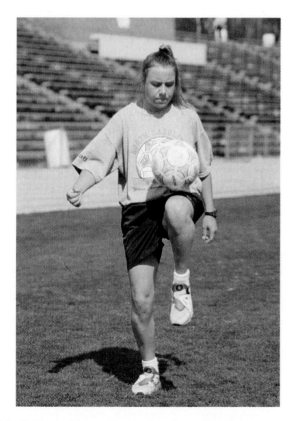

FIGURE 1-9. Neuromuscular Coordination.
The ability to integrate the senses with motor function to produce coordinated movement.

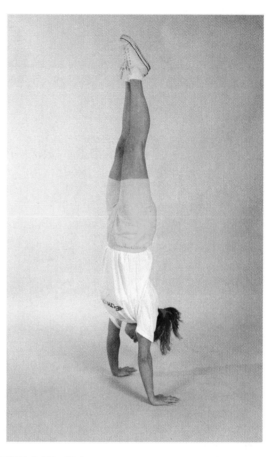

FIGURE 1-10. Balance.
The ability to maintain equilibrium when moving or stationary.

speed ability to perform a particular movement very rapidly
power ability to generate great amounts of force against resistance in a short period of time
agility ability to change or alter, quickly and accurately, the direction of body movement
neuromuscular coordination ability to integrate the senses—visual, auditory, and proprioceptive (knowing the position of your body in space)—with motor function to produce smooth, accurate, and skilled movement
balance ability to maintain a degree of equilibrium while moving or standing still
reaction time time required to produce an appropriate and accurate physiological or mechanical response to a stimulus

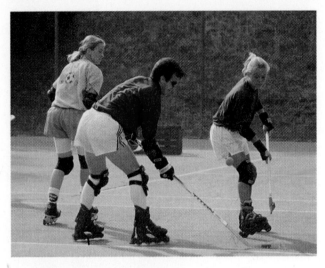

FIGURE 1-11. Reaction Time.
The length of time required to react to a stimulus.

BENEFITS OF BEING PHYSICALLY FIT
Physiological Benefits

Biologically, human beings are designed to be active creatures. Although changes in civilization have resulted in a decrease in the amount of activity needed to accomplish the basic tasks associated with living, the human body has not changed. Therefore it is important to be aware of the requirements for good health and recognize the importance of vigorous physical activity in your life. If you do not, your health, productivity, and effectiveness are likely to suffer. The following is a summary of the physiological effects of physical activity.

Muscular and Skeletal Systems

Regular, vigorous activity increases muscle size, strength, and power and develops endurance for sustaining work. The greatest increase in muscle growth is brought about by those activities that make the muscle work to full capacity. The body's muscular and skeletal systems are responsible for all human locomotion and movement. The condition of these systems depends in large measure on the demands advanced by regular activity. Conversely, your muscular strength, stamina, and efficiency determine the effectiveness of your activity.

Muscles become more efficient as they perform the work of contraction, especially if the work is performed regularly and with gradually increasing loads. The demands of contraction inherent in exercise increase the size and strength of individual muscles and muscle groups. Intense activity involving body movement can increase joint range of motion, improve general coordination, improve general postural tone, increase endurance, and develop specific performance skill.

As a result of exercise, muscles increase in size and strength. They also gain endurance. A chemical change that helps the muscles work more efficiently occurs as a result of exercise. During exercise the rate of muscular fatigue is lower in physically fit persons than in persons with a sedentary lifestyle who exercise only occasionally.

Heart and Circulatory System

Exercise strengthens the heart muscle. Greater demands placed on the heart cause it to increase in size and become stronger. The volume of blood pumped per beat of the heart increases, bringing better nourishment to all parts of the body. Continued and regular exercise develops the heart's network of small vessels, which supply oxygen to the cells and remove waste products. The person who exercises regularly has a lower pulse rate, and this rate returns to normal more quickly after exercise than does the pulse rate of the sedentary person. Moreover, the increase in blood pressure during exercise is smaller in the physically fit person.

Exercise taxes the circulatory system. Muscular activity demands that an increased amount of oxygenated blood be delivered to the working muscle cells. This increase is brought about by more rapid and deeper breathing, by increased heart rate, and by elevated blood pressure. The normal physiological responses become quicker and more efficient when the demands are made with regularity. A severe, infrequent demand such as that made on the circulatory system by a person who participates in athletic activity only occasionally can be extremely fatiguing and can put too much strain on the heart. Vigorous daily activity develops a cardiovascular fitness that produces the quality of physical reserve power and stamina called *endurance*.

Lungs and Respiratory System

Exercise improves the functioning of the lungs by deepening the respiration process. The rate of breathing is slower in the physically fit person, who may take as few as 6 to 8 breaths per minute, than in the sedentary person, who may take 12 to 15. There is deeper diaphragmatic breathing as a result of physical activity, and the blood is exposed to oxygen over a greater area. In the sedentary person a greater portion of the lungs becomes closed off to air that is inhaled. Thus regular exercise results in greater economy in respiration; the physically fit person takes in larger amounts of air and absorbs oxygen from the air in greater amounts than the person who is out of shape.

Digestive and Excretory Systems

Exercise helps to keep the digestive and excretory organs in good condition. The nerves and muscles of the stomach and intestines become well toned and function more efficiently.

Nervous System

Muscles are controlled by nerves. Messages are relayed by nerves to the muscles, which then react in the way the person wishes, whether in running, playing a musical instrument, or hitting a tennis ball. Muscular exercise enhances nerve-muscle coordination. Furthermore, nervous fatigue may be lessened by pleasant physical activity, because the nervous fatigue that has accumulated through anxiety or mental work is offset by muscular activity.

Body Composition

Exercise helps a person to maintain a healthy percentage of body fat by using excess calories. Weight control involves more than merely reducing caloric intake to compensate for sedentary habits and overeating. Regular physical activity takes care of some of our dietary excesses and prevents adding undesired adipose (fat) tissue. Excess body fat results in undue stress on normal body functions, particularly those of the heart. Being overly fat shortens life. Among persons whose body fat percentage exceeds normal by only 15% to 25%, death rates increase by an estimated 30%. Being overly fat can also contribute to the development of orthopedic problems.

Additional Physiological Benefits

Physical exercise contributes to improved posture and appearance through the development of proper muscle tone, greater joint flexibility, and a feeling of well-being. Physical activity generates more energy and thus contributes to greater individual productivity for both physical and mental tasks.

It is often the case that people who become physically active pay more attention to such things as proper nutrition, rest, and relaxation and may also drink less alcohol and stop smoking because they do not want to undo the benefits gained through physical activity. They are likely to be committed to engaging in health promoting rather than health harming behavior.

Besides promoting vigor and fitness, physical activity contributes to improvement in agility, speed, coordination, and skill. A primary objective of collegiate physical education programs is the acquisition of skills that lead to enjoyable recreational sporting performance not only during collegiate years but also throughout life. The benefits of physical fitness are numerous. The person who is physically fit has more strength, energy, and stamina; an improved sense of well-being; better protection from injury (because strong, well-developed muscles safeguard bones, internal organs, and joints and keep moving parts limber); and improved cardiorespiratory function.

Social Rewards

Persons unwilling to acquire or maintain the physical fitness necessary to participate in vigorous activity deny themselves the social outlets, companionship, and feelings inherent in such activities. Participation in physical activity provides an outlet for socializing. Students who maintain ongoing fitness programs may be better able to cope with the intellectual demands of college. Too often students concentrate on developing only their minds and forget to develop as total persons. Physical fitness affects the entire person, and rich dividends accrue to the person who concentrates on the development of the body as well as the mind.

Psychological Benefits

Physical activity is not a panacea for all that ails us, but many people use regular exercise, especially of a recreational nature, as a means of mental relaxation. Many people blame our society for producing stress; stress, however, is an internal physical reaction to the outside environment. Certainly, stress can and does result from all aspects of daily living—work, school, interpersonal relationships, and, occasionally, even leisure activities. Exercise can play a significant role in reducing stress. It diverts attention from stress-producing thoughts to a more relaxing and positive focus. It may also help us to feel better about ourselves and to feel that we are more capable of handling potential stress-producing situations. Chapter 11 describes stress in detail and provides suggestions for stress management.

Benefits of Exercise in the Aging Process

Aging begins immediately at birth and involves a lifelong series of changes in physiological and performance capabilities. These capabilities increase as a function of the growth process throughout adolescence, peak sometime between age 18 and 40, and steadily decline with increasing age. However, this decline may be due as much to the sociological constraints of aging as to biological effects. It is possible to maintain a relatively high level of physiological function if an individual maintains an active lifestyle.

Importance of Staying Active

In most cases, after age 35, qualities such as muscular endurance, coordination, and strength tend to decrease. Furthermore, as we age, recovery from vigorous exercise requires a longer amount of time. Regular physical activity, however, tends to delay and in some cases prevent the appearance of certain degenerative processes. For best results, controlling the effects of the aging process should start early, before its onset (before a person's physical development is completed, which in most cases is between age 14 and 22). If you stay physically fit throughout your life, you will retain greater strength, flexibility, cardiorespiratory health, and a more desirable body composition than if you become sedentary.

Need to Establish Patterns of Exercise

For the average individual, major changes in lifestyle typically coincide with the end of formal education. For many college students, thoughts turn from keeping up with class assignments and arranging weekend parties to going to work every day and trying to pay bills. During the college years, most students are involved in some level of physical activity, whether it is simply walking to and from classes, participating in intramural or recreational activities, or perhaps competing as an intercollegiate athlete. Graduation from a college or university often means that the individual will probably take a job that involves little if any physical activity. The pressure associated with establishing oneself in a new career and profession is intense and time consuming. Thus it is not unusual for a recent graduate to experience a reduction in the physical activity level that he or she enjoyed as a college student. A concerted effort should be made at this point in life to establish patterns of exercise and healthful living that will ultimately become permanent fixtures in the individual's style of living.

Exercising Safely as You Grow Older

Generally, exercise is considered a safe activity for most individuals. In fact, in the long run as you grow older it is safer to exercise than to remain sedentary. The American College of Sports Medicine and the American Heart Association have recommended that individuals under age 40 who are apparently healthy, have no previous history of cardiovascular disease and no known risk factors, and have passed a medical evaluation within the past 2 years can generally begin an exercise program without further evaluation as long as the exercise program progresses gradually and moderately and no unusual signs or symptoms develop.

Males over age 40, females over age 50, and anyone regardless of age who has health problems should have at least some screening before starting an exercise program. Screening may be done by nonmedical personnel in nonmedical settings. Factors such as age, health status, and the type of exercise program to be followed are used to determine the extent of the medical evaluation.

Individuals who are at high risk—those who have two or more major coronary artery disease risk factors or exhibit symptoms of cardiopulmonary or other disease—should have a complete medical examination and undergo an exercise test before beginning an exercise program. Also, if there are any signs of chest pain, shortness of breath, irregular heartbeats, viral infections, or unusual pain in muscles or joints, a physician should be consulted. The physician may decide to prescribe or limit certain activities based on the results.

It seems that consistent participation in vigorous physical activity can result in improvement of many physiological parameters regardless of age. The effects of exercise on the aging process and the long-term health benefits of exercise have been convincingly documented.

IMPORTANCE OF FITNESS FOR COLLEGE STUDENTS

Fitness for college students is similar to fitness for other adults. Maintaining fitness is a lifelong process, and the college years constitute just one portion of the continuum. As mentioned earlier, the period between age 18 and 40 is the formative time for establishing physical fitness. At this time the body reaches the peak of maturity and physiological functioning. These years are a time to learn one's fitness needs and to make lifestyle changes that will enable one to fulfill these individual needs at any time in life.

The college years are an important time for laying the foundations of physical fitness for a lifetime. During these years problems such as excessive weight gain often develop. College students have many demands on their time. Classes, long hours of study, extracurricular activities, work, and other responsibilities take their physical and mental toll. Students become preoccupied with studies, dating, and preparing for careers. As a result they often forget about fitness requirements. Physical ailments, emotional depression, and lack of stamina detract from mental effort and drain the student, potentially resulting in decreased functioning or failure in college. A student may not be able to participate in activities such as swimming, mountain climbing, skiing, backpacking, or scuba diving because of lack of physical fitness. Even if an unfit student does participate in these activities, his or her safety, proficiency, and enjoyment may be considerably less than that of a person with a higher level of physical fitness. However, if the person is in good physical condition, he or she has a better chance of achieving academically and having a more enjoyable college experience than do physically unfit classmates.

Your college years should be the time for incorporating regular physical activity into your lifestyle and for establishing a personal daily regimen that will help to guarantee a productive, healthy, happy, and interesting life.

Help for the Sedentary Student

If you are not fit, you need help and guidance in planning a physical fitness program. Effort must be directed toward eliminating the cause or causes of your poor physical condition. It should be remembered that the causes of poor fitness vary widely. They can involve problems such as being overweight or underweight, having a poor diet, being ill, suffering from emotional disturbances, or leading an unhealthy lifestyle. A fitness program should address the particular cause or causes. If the cause involves infection or illness, then the help of a physician is necessary. If the cause is an emotional disorder or a psychological maladjustment, the college guidance program or health service may provide counseling. If it relates to an unhealthy lifestyle, health and physical education personnel may be of benefit. If the cause is lack of the right kind and amount of physical activity, your school's physical education staff can provide assistance. (See Appendix A for a discussion of college resources that can assist you in planning a fitness program.)

WHERE DO YOU BEGIN?

Just as you are never too sedentary to begin a fitness program, neither are you ever too old. It is wise to start a fitness program early in life, but all of us can benefit from exercise no matter when we begin. Long-term success in sticking with an exercise program undoubtedly has some basis in your underlying motivation for beginning such a program in the first place.

What Is Your Present Level of Physical Fitness?

Before you begin any type of fitness program, it is essential for you to establish some baseline information relative to your existing levels of fitness. Throughout this text, many different Lab Activities will be presented to help you evaluate the various aspects of fitness. They are designed to help you incorporate the information presented to you and include practical application to emphasize important points. By learning to evaluate your fitness, you will be able to maintain an ongoing personal fitness log to help you keep track of your progress.

Many of the Lab Activities in this text are accompanied by a set of norms or standards that allow you to compare your performance with that of the general population. Such standards indicate where special attention should be directed within an individualized fitness program and where fitness counseling and help are needed so that appropriate techniques can be incorporated for improvement. Seeing how you compare with others can serve as a motivational tool to some extent. Remember, however, that what is really important is not your comparison with how everyone else does but rather your improvement from one test to the next. It is important to appraise your daily schedule regularly to determine whether you are devoting the proper amount of time to keeping yourself fit. There is little question that incorporating consistent, regularly scheduled exercise as an essential part of your lifestyle may be difficult, especially in light of the existing demands on your time. **Lab Activity 1-6** at the end of this chapter asks you to keep a daily fitness schedule for 1 week to determine your existing patterns of exercise and leisure-time activities. How good are you about exercising regularly throughout the week?

Fitness is your capacity for a task. The task that concerns you as a student is to be a success in college. A lifetime of ambition and hope lies ahead of you. The degree to which you achieve your goals will be enhanced by how able you are to accomplish the tasks that college and life demand. Many first-year college students do not complete 4 years of college or attain a degree. If a lack of fitness is one of the reasons so many drop out, students can better ensure their success by preparing themselves physically and mentally for the demands of college.

Fitness is not developed in a day or in one easy lesson. It takes time and hard work. If you have overlooked this essential key to success, a good start would be to determine the contribution physical fitness can make to you as a college student.

Why Do You Want to Get Fit?

Before starting your personal fitness program, it may be helpful to examine your attitudes toward physical fitness, your reasons for wanting to be physically fit, and your present level of activity. Identifying your reasons for starting a physical fitness program and what you expect the program to achieve will help you determine the degree to which you are motivated and aspire to a desirable fitness level. **Motivation plays a major role in determining how successful you will be in developing and maintaining a satisfactory degree of fitness.** Certainly, individuals have different motivations for becoming physically fit. **Lab Activity 1-7** at the end of this chapter will help you identify not only your motivations but also the goals you hope to accomplish through participation in a fitness program.

All of us are concerned about physical fitness, but our concern develops as the result of different motivations. Some people want to be physically fit because of the effect that physical fitness can have on their appearance. Others want to be physically fit because of the benefits that it can offer toward healthful living. Still others desire physical fitness because of the implications it has for leisure-time or recreational pursuits.

Determining Your Medical History

At this point in your life, chances are that your health is very good. Nevertheless, it is always a good idea to assess your medical history by identifying any preexisting medical conditions that should be considered before beginning an exercise program. Therefore, before you start any program, you should complete Lab Activity 1-8, a medical history evaluation form located at the end of this chapter. If you answer *yes* to any of the questions on this form, you should consult your physician before beginning your exercise program. Lab Activity 1-9, the Physical Activity Readiness Questionaire (PAR-Q), will also help you determine whether any medical conditions exist that would preclude you from beginning a physical activity program.

WHAT IS YOUR MOTIVATION FOR BEGINNING A FITNESS PROGRAM?

People have many different reasons and motivations for beginning a fitness program. Are you interested in improving your overall health and well-being? Are you concerned about the way you look to your friends? Are you interested in training for some event or activity involving competition? Are you simply tired of being a couch potato? Whatever your motivation happens to be, engaging in fitness activities can have many positive benefits on your style of living (see the following box).

Choosing the Appropriate Fitness Activity

Regardless of the underlying motivation, you must first consider exactly what it is that you are trying to accomplish. You should select the type of activity that will allow you to do two things: (1) achieve the ultimate goals of physical fitness improvement that you have established for yourself, and (2) maintain your interest and motivation throughout your lifetime. For example, if your goal is to increase stamina or endurance, then you will want to choose an

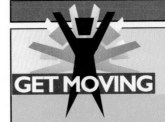

GET MOVING — Motivations for Exercising

1. Exercise can make you healthier
2. Exercise can make you more resistant to illness and disease
3. Exercise can make you feel better
4. Exercise can make you look better
5. Exercise can improve your self-image
6. Exercise can help improve your social life
7. Exercise can make you more resistant to fatigue
8. Exercise can improve your strength
9. Exercise can improve your flexibility
10. Exercise can help you lose fat
11. Exercise can help reduce stress and tension

activity such as jogging, rollerblading, or swimming. If one of your goals is losing weight, you will want to engage in physical activity for a sufficient length of time and on a regular basis to burn calories. If you want to develop strength in your shoulders, you may want to include resistance exercises such as lifting heavy weights.

Sticking With Your Exercise Program

Beginning an exercise program is easy! The hard part comes in making the long-term commitment necessary to make fitness an integral part of your style of living. When you first begin an exercise program you are usually highly motivated and excited. Unfortunately, several things may happen in beginning an exercise program that can be frustrating:

• If you have been relatively inactive, it is likely that you will develop some muscle soreness from performing an activity that you are not used to. Usually this soreness is short-lived and will disappear in a couple of days.

• Initial improvement in strength, cardiorespiratory endurance, and flexibility will be rapid, but after the first 2 to 3 weeks, improvement will be more gradual.

• As the weeks pass, sometimes it becomes difficult to exercise at the same time consistently. Nevertheless, you must look for ways to fit some type of exercise into your routine as often as possible.

• If you go out of town or if friends come to visit you, your normal schedule may be interrupted. You should seek alternative fitness activities such as simply going for a walk if for some reason you can't do what you normally do.

Once you are able to get through these things that may frustrate you initially, there are quite a few things that you can do that will help motivate you to stick with your commitment to exercise. Throughout this text, you will be given many suggestions that will help you get motivated to exercise (see the following box). Use those specific motivational recommendations that are most appropriate and useful to you individually.

How Quickly Can You Expect Results?

"For a change to last, it cannot be obtained fast." You should not expect results in a matter of hours or even days. After a couple of weeks of appropriate activity on a regular basis, some improvement should be noted, depending on what your physical fitness condition was when you started. After an extended period of gradual improvement you may reach a plateau, at which you experience no improvement but instead seem to stay at the same level of fitness. This

is a natural phenomenon. In time, with regular workouts, improvement will occur; after several months, the desired results will be attained. Make a commitment to the fitness program, and keep at it; you will feel better, and this will in turn motivate you to continue. Once you have attained a desirable physical fitness level, you will be strongly motivated to maintain this level through regular workouts.

THERE IS NO SHORTCUT TO FITNESS

Any physical fitness program requires effort to produce results. Steam baths, sauna baths, fitness machines, massages, and gimmicks such as body wraps or fad diets may be relaxing or produce short-term effects, but it is necessary to exert effort to achieve the lasting benefits of physical fitness. The body must do the work. Too often, students look for the easy way to achieve their goals. Physical fitness can be attained, but only after a commitment to an ongoing exercise program and months of work. **There is no shortcut to achieving fitness. You can't sit and be fit.** Although everyone can begin an exercise pro-

GET MOVING

Ways to help you adhere to your fitness commitment on a long-term basis

1. Find a workout partner or perhaps a group of individuals who have a similar commitment to a healthy lifestyle as you. On some days you will find it more difficult to work out than on others, and for one reason or another you simply may not feel like doing it. These individuals can provide social support to you, and you to them, in trying to establish habits of exercise and healthful living.

2. Engage in a variety of activities that can collectively help you to achieve your goals. You don't have to do exactly the same routine every day. In fact, engaging in different activities may help prevent boredom with doing the same thing day-in and day-out and will help you attain a greater degree of generalized fitness.

3. Find positive ways to reward yourself for being faithful to your exercise program. Go out and buy some new clothes, or schedule a trip to the beach or the mountains to take advantage of your improved fitness.

4. Don't get frustrated if you don't meet your short-term goals or if the benefits of exercise are not immediately noticeable. Remember—you are in this for the long term, and the improvement will be gradual.

5. Keep a record or diary of your daily exercise sessions. If you begin to feel frustrated or you don't want to exercise, go to the diary and review how much work you have invested; this may motivate you to continue.

6. Plan your exercise program to fit into your style of living. An exercise program should not seem like a nuisance or interference. It should seem like a welcomed and necessary addition to your life.

7. It is essential to realize that, when necessary, you can skip a day or two of exercise without losing everything you have worked hard to develop. Again, the long-term, consistent practice of regular exercise is the key.

gram, it is especially important to monitor the effects of any program. If you have not exercised for 5 years, you will not achieve fitness in 2 weeks. The program should start with a medical examination, commence at the individual's tolerance level, and be administered progressively.

The purpose of the chapters that follow is to provide you with knowledge about and understanding of the various aspects of fitness. They are designed to show the importance of its essential ingredients. They will explain how you can assess, develop, and maintain your fitness. Finally, they will show you how to plan, develop, and implement a personalized fitness program based on your individual interests.

SUMMARY

- Despite the emphasis on physical fitness, many Americans choose not to engage in physical activity.
- Everyone should try to engage in a total of at least 30 minutes of moderate-intensity physical exercise each day.
- Being physically fit means that the various systems of the body are healthy and function efficiently so as to enable the fit person to engage in activities of daily living, as well as in recreational pursuits and leisure activities, without unreasonable fatigue.
- Anyone can benefit from physical exercise throughout his or her entire lifetime.
- Physical fitness is individualized and varies according to the demands of a specific task.
- Components of health-related physical fitness include muscular strength, muscular endurance, cardiorespiratory endurance, flexibility, and body composition.

- Components of motor skill–related physical fitness include power, balance, agility, neuromuscular coordination, speed, and reaction time.
- There are physiological, psychological, and social benefits associated with physical fitness.
- If you stay physically fit throughout your life, you will retain greater strength, flexibility, cardiorespiratory health, and a more desirable body composition than if you become sedentary.
- The years in college are a time to learn one's fitness needs and to make lifestyle changes that will enable one to fulfill these individual needs at any time in life.
- Before beginning a fitness program it is important to determine your reasons for wanting to get fit, your present level of fitness, and your medical history.
- There is no shortcut to fitness.

REFERENCES

Ainsworth B, Haskell W, Leon, A: Compendium of physical activities, *Med Sci Sports Exerc* 25:71-80, 1993.

American Alliance of Health, Physical Education, Recreation, and Dance: *Lifetime health-related physical fitness*, Reston, Va, 1980, The Alliance.

American Alliance of Health, Physical Education, Recreation, and Dance: *Personal best*, Washington, DC, 1988, The Alliance.

American College of Sports Medicine: *Guidelines for graded exercise testing and exercise prescription*, Baltimore, 1995, Williams & Wilkins.

American College of Sports Medicine: Position stand on recommended quantity and quality of exercise for developing and maintaining cardiorespiratory and muscular fitness in healthy adults, *Med Sci Sports Exerc* 22:265-274, 1990.

American Heart Association: *Exercise standards: a statement for health professionals*, Dallas, 1991, American Heart Association.

American Heart Association: *1996 heart and stroke facts*, Dallas, 1996, American Heart Association.

Bailey CIA, Macphee SJ: Community health-related fitness testing and promoting activity: the North Staffordshire experience, *Br J Phys Educ* 20(2):68, 1989.

Blair S, Kohl N, Gordon R: How much physical activity is good for health? *Ann Rev Public Health* 13:99-126, 1992.

Bockmon DF: Facilitating health pattern change in exercise, *J Holist Nurs* 6(1):21, 1988.

Bouchard C, Shepard R, Stephens T: *Physical activity fitness and health*, Champaign, 1994, Human Kinetics.

Centers for Disease Control and Prevention: Prevalence of sedentary lifestyle: behavioral risk factor surveillance system, *MMWR Morb Mortal Wkly Rep* 42:576-579, 1993.

Debusk R, Stenestrand U, Sheehan M: Training effects of long vs. short bouts of exercise in healthy subjects, *Am J Cardiol* 65:1010-1013, 1990.

Dipietro L, Casperson C: National estimates of physical activity among white and black Americans, *Med Sci Sports Exerc* 23:S105, 1991.

Dishman R: Psychological effects of exercise for disease resistance and health promotion. In Watson R, Eichner M, editors: *Exercise and disease*, Boca Raton, 1992, CRC Press.

Fletcher G, Blair S, Blumenthal J: AHA medical/scientific statement on exercise, *Circulation* 86:340-344, 1992.

Ford HT Jr, Puckett JR, Blessing DL, et al: Effects of selected physical activities on health-related fitness and psychological well-being, *Psychol Rep* 64(1):203, 1989.

Haskell WL, Montoye JH, Orenstein D: Physical activity and exercise to achieve health-related physical fitness components, *Public Health Rep* 100(2):202, 1985.

Hayes D, Ross CE: Body and mind: the effect of exercise, over-weight, and physical health on psychological well-being, *J Health Soc Behav* 27(4):387, 1986.

Katch FI, McArdle WD: *Nutrition, weight control, and exercise,* ed 3, Philadelphia, 1994, Lea & Febiger.

King AC, Taylor C, Haskell W: Effects of differing intensities and formats of 12 months of exercise training on psychological out-comes in older adults, *Health Psychol* 12:292-300, 1993.

King AC, Taylor C, Haskell W, et al: Influence of regular aerobic exercise on psychological health: a randomized, controlled trial of healthy middle-aged adults, *Health Psychol* 8(3):305, 1989.

Leon A: Physical fitness. In Wyinder E, editor: *American health foun-dation: the book of health,* New York, 1981, Franklin Watts.

Long B, Calfas K, Sallis J: Evaluation of patient physical activity after counseling by primary care providers, *Med Sci Sports Exerc* 26:S4, 1994.

McArdle W, Katch F, Katch V: *Exercise physiology, energy, nutrition, and human performance,* Philadelphia, 1994, Lea & Febiger.

McGinnis J: Public health burden of a sedentary lifestyle, *Med Sci Sports Exerc* 24:S196-200, 1992.

Paffenberger R, Hyde R, Wing A: The association of changes in physical-activity level and other lifestyle characteristics with mortality among men, *N Engl J Med* 328:538-545, 1993.

Pate R, Pratt M, Blair S, et al: Physical activity and public health: a recommendation from the Centers for Disease Control and Prevention and the American College of Sports Medicine, *JAMA* 273(5):402-407, 1995.

Sallis J, Hovell M, Hoffstetter C: Predictors of adoption and mainte-nance of vigorous physical activity in males and females, *Prev Med* 21:237-251, 1992.

Sparks A: Health related fitness: an example of innovation without change, *Br J Phys Educ* 20(2):60, 1989.

US Department of Health and Human Services, Public Health Services: *Healthy people 2000: midcourse review and 1995 revisions,* Washington, DC, 1995, USDHHS.

US Department of Health and Human Services, Public Health Services: *Healthy people 2000: national health promotion and disease prevention objectives,* Washington, DC, 1991, USDHHS.

US Department of Health and Human Services, Public Health Service: *Healthy people 2000, national health promotion and disease prevention objectives,* Pub No (PHS) 91-50213, Washington, DC, 1991, US Government Printing Office.

SUGGESTED READINGS

American College of Sports Medicine: *Guidelines for exercise testing and prescription,* Philadelphia, 1995, Lea & Febiger.
Discusses the guidlines and protocols for evaluating different compo-nents of physical fitness in various populations.

Bouchard C, Shepard R, Stephens T: *Physical activity fitness and health,* Champaign, 1994, Human Kinetics.
A complete up-to-date collection of knowledge about the relationships between physical activity, fitness, and health. Well referenced and comprehensive.

Gavin J: *The exercise habit,* Champaign, 1992, Human Kinetics.
Helps answer the question, "How can I stick with my exercise pro-gram?" Helps you pick an exercise program that best suits your per-sonality and lifestyle and develop commitments that will lead to life-long habits of fitness and exercise. Presents the principles underlying the development of aerobic and muscular fitness. Weight control, obe-sity, and the role of fitness in one's life are discussed.

Nieman D: *Fitness and your health,* Palo Alto, 1993, Bull Publishing.
Discusses the impact of incorporating fitness into your style of living on your health. Reveals facts about fitness, nutrition, obesity, aging, and stress.

Lab Activity 1-1

6-Second Dash

Name _____   **Section** _____   **Date** _____

PURPOSE   To measure speed of movement.

PROCEDURE
1. Subject starts from a standing position with both feet behind starting line.
2. Starter uses preparatory commands "get ready," "set," "GO" and starts stopwatch simultaneously.
3. Subject runs as fast as possible in a straight line until whistle is blown at end of 6 seconds. Subject does not stop abruptly but gradually slows down.
4. Scoring assistant marks exact spot where subject was when whistle sounded, then measures and records distance from starting line.
5. Consult Table 1-2 for interpretation.

Distance covered in 6 seconds _____ yards

INTERPRETATION

TABLE 1-2.   Norms in Yards for 6-Second Run, High School and College Students*

Performance Level	Score			
	College Men	College Women	High School Boys	High School Girls
Excellent	54 and above	45 and above	51 and above	43 and above
Good	51-53	42-44	48-50	40-42
Average	42-50	35-41	43-47	35-39
Poor	37-41	29-34	40-42	32-34
Very poor	0-36	0-28	0-39	0-31

*Based on the scores of 50 students for each group as reported by Leroy Scott, Northeast Louisiana University, Monroe, La, 1973.

Performance level _____

Lab Activity 1-2

Vertical Power Jump Test

Name _____   **Section** _____   **Date** _____

PURPOSE
To measure power of the legs in jumping vertically (upward).

EQUIPMENT
A measuring scale marked off in half-inch increments, a scale, and chalk dust.

PROCEDURE
1. The subject should be weighed and the pounds recorded on the worksheet.
2. Subject stands facing sideways to the jump board, preferred arm back with the hand on the back of the shorts, the other arm raised overhead against the wall. Subject stands on toes and reaches as high as possible on the measuring scale; this height is recorded on the worksheet.
3. Chalk is placed on the middle finger; the subject goes into a squat position and then jumps as high as possible, touching the measuring scale with the chalked finger (Figure 1-12). The subject is allowed three trials. The best performance is recorded on the worksheet.
4. On the worksheet, subtract the standing height from the best jumping height, multiply that figure by body weight, and divide the total by 12 to give foot-pounds.
5. Consult Table 1-3 for subject's performance level.

WORKSHEET

Maximum jumping height (inches)
Standing height (inches)   −   _____

                                                    Difference   _____

Body weight (pounds)   ×   _____

                                                    Total   _____
                                                            ÷ 12

                                                    Foot-pounds   _____

Performance level   _____

Continued.

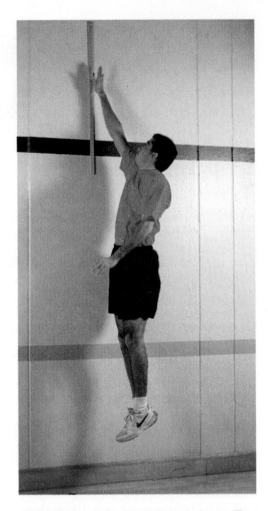

FIGURE 1-12. **Vertical Power Jump Test.**

TABLE 1-3. Norms in Foot-Pounds* for Vertical Power Jump (Work)†

	Score	
Performance Level	**College Men**	**College Women**
Excellent	301 and above	134 and above
Good	240-300	108-133
Average	115-239	55-107
Poor	54-114	30-54
Very poor	0-53	0-29

*(Distance jumped × body weight ÷ 12 = score in foot-pounds.)
† Based on the scores of 125 college men and 100 college women.

SEMO* Agility Test

Name _____   **Section** _____   **Date** _____

PURPOSE   To measure the general agility of the body in moving forward, backward, and sideways.

PROCEDURE

1. Place four rubber cones squarely in the corners of the free-throw lane as indicated in the diagram below (Figure 1-13).
2. Beginning at *A (Start)*, side step to *B*, back pedal to *D*, forward sprint to *A*, back pedal to *C*, forward sprint to *B*, forward sprint to *A (Finish)*.
3. Record time on stopwatch to nearest $1/10$ second. Take the best of two trials.
4. Consult Table 1-4 for interpretation.

Trial # 1   _____ sec

Trial # 2   _____ sec

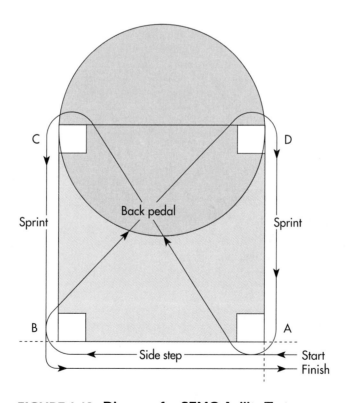

FIGURE 1-13. Diagram for SEMO Agility Test.

Continued.

*Southeast Missouri State University.

INTERPRETATION

Performance Level	Score	
	Men	**Women**
Advanced	10.72 and below	12.19 and below
Advanced intermediate	11.49-10.73	12.99-12.20
Intermediate	13.02-11.50	13.90-13.00
Advanced beginner	13.79-13.03	14.49-13.91
Beginner	13.80 and above	14.50 and above

TABLE 1-4.   Norms in Seconds for SEMO Agility Test, College Students*

*Scores for men were obtained by Dr. Ronald Kirby, Southeast Missouri State University, Cape Girardeau, Mo, 1971. Scores for women were from a small group of subjects from Corpus Christi State University, Corpus Christi, Tex, 1976.

Performance level   _____

Static Balance Test (Stork Test)

Name _____   **Section** _____   **Date** _____

PURPOSE   To measure static balance of the performer supported on the ball of the foot of the dominant leg.

PROCEDURE
1. Subject stands on the foot of the dominant leg and places the other foot on the inside of the supporting knee and hands on the hips (Figure 1-14).
2. On command, subject raises heel of dominant foot and maintains balance as long as possible without moving the ball of the foot from its original position.
3. Record three trials in seconds and take the best of the three.
4. Consult Table 1-5 for interpretation.

Trial # 1 _____ sec

Trial # 2 _____ sec

Trial # 3 _____ sec

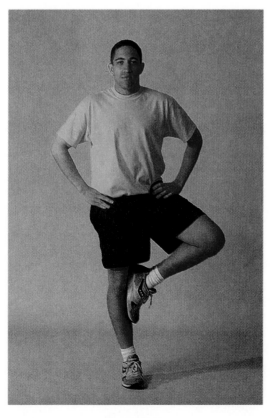

FIGURE 1-14. Stork Stand.   *Continued.*

TABLE 1-5. Norms in Seconds for Stork Stand, College Students*

	Score	
Performance Level	Men	Women
Advanced	51 and above	28 and above
Advanced intermediate	37-50	23-27
Intermediate	15-36	8-22
Advanced beginner	5-14	3-7
Beginner	0-4	0-2

*Based on the scores of 50 men and 50 women, Corpus Christi State University, Corpus Christi, Tex, 1976.

Performance level _____

Lab Activity 1-5

Nelson Choice-Response Movement Test

Name _____   **Section** _____   **Date** _____

PURPOSE   To measure ability to react and move quickly and accurately in accordance with a choice stimulus.

PROCEDURE
1. Two side lines are marked 14 yards apart with a line in the middle (Figure 1-15).
2. Subject assumes a ready stance over the middle line.
3. Tester simultaneously holds a stopwatch in hand and abruptly waves hand in one direction or the other, beginning stopwatch.
4. Subject is timed until over the side line and time is recorded to nearest $1/10$ second.
5. Ten trials are given, five to each side in random order.
6. Rest interval of 20 seconds is used between trials.
7. Calculate average time for the 10 trials.
8. Consult Table 1-6 for interpretation.

Trial # 1 _____ sec
Trial # 2 _____ sec
Trial # 3 _____ sec
Trial # 4 _____ sec
Trial # 5 _____ sec
Trial # 6 _____ sec
Trial # 7 _____ sec
Trial # 8 _____ sec
Trial # 9 _____ sec
Trial #10 _____ sec
TOTAL   _____ sec divided by 10 = _____ sec
                                                          Average

Continued.

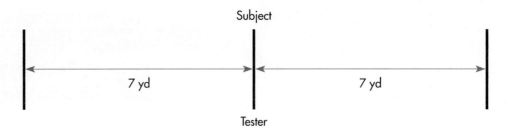

FIGURE 1-15. **Diagram for Nelson Choice-Response Movement Test.**

	Score	
Performance Level	**Men**	**Women**
Advanced	1.30 and below	1.60 and below
Advanced intermediate	1.60-1.35	1.90-1.65
Intermediate	2.40-1.65	2.55-1.95
Advanced beginner	2.70-2.45	2.85-2.60
Beginner	2.75 and above	2.90 and above

TABLE 1-6. **Norms in Seconds for Nelson Choice-Response Movement Test, College Students***

*Data gathered from 200 men, Louisiana State University, Baton Rouge, La, 1968; and 45 women, Corpus Christi State University, Corpus Christi, Tex, 1976.

Performance level _____

Summary Worksheet for Skill-Related Fitness Component Lab Activities

Name _____   **Section** _____   **Date** _____

Lab Activity I-I   **6-Second Dash**

Distance covered in 6 seconds_____ yards

Performance level _____

Lab Activity I-2   **Vertical Power Jump Test**

Maximum jumping power_____ foot-
pounds

Performance level _____

Lab Activity I-3   **SEMO Agility Test**

Best time of two time trials _____ sec

Performance level _____

Lab Activity I-4   **Static Balance Test (Stork Test)**

Best time of three balance trials _____ sec

Performance level _____

Lab Activity I-5   **Nelson Choice-Response Movement Test**

Average time for 10 trials_____ sec

Performance level _____

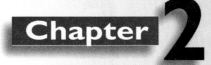

Chapter 2

Choosing a Healthy Lifestyle

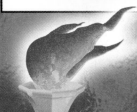

HEALTH 2000 GOALS

- **Increase the Span of Healthy Life.** The active prevention in all communities of premature death, disability, and disease through regular physical activity. *Midpoint Update: no noticeable change reported in this area.*

- **Coronary Heart Disease.** Reduce coronary heart disease deaths to no more than 100 per 100,000 people. In 1987 there were 135 deaths per 100,000 attributable to coronary heart disease. *Midpoint Update: headed in the right direction with current statistic of 114 per 100,000 deaths.*

- **High Blood Pressure.** Increase to at least 50% the proportion of people with high blood pressure whose blood pressure is under control. From 1976 to 1980, 11% of those with high blood pressure had it under control. *Midpoint Update: headed in the right direction with current statistic of 21%.*

- **High Cholesterol.** Reduce the mean serum cholesterol level among adults to no more than 200 mg/dL. From 1976 to 1980 there was an average of 213 mg/dL among people age 20 to 74. *Midpoint Update: headed in the right direction with current average of 205 mg/dL.*

- **Cancer.** Reverse the rise in cancer deaths to achieve a rate of no more than 130 per 100,000 people. In 1987 there were 134 cancer-related deaths per 100,000 people. *Midpoint Update: headed in the right direction with current statistic of 133 per 100,000 deaths.*

OBJECTIVES

After completing this chapter, you will be able to do the following:

- Define the wellness concept and relate the physical, social, emotional, intellectual, and spiritual components.
- Discuss the promotion of the healthy lifestyle in the United States.

- Explain how diseases may be related to an unhealthy lifestyle.
- Discuss the risk factors associated with coronary heart disease.
- Identify cancer warning signs.
- Identify conditions that would seem to indicate a need for some professional medical help.

KEY TERMS

While reading this chapter, you will become familiar with the following terms:

- wellness
- health risk factors
- hypokinetic disease
- coronary artery disease
- cancer

hoosing a healthy lifestyle means that you are concerned about more than simply developing yourself physically. Living healthy also means that you are able to express your emotions effectively; have good relations with others around you; are concerned about your decision-making abilities; and pay some attention to ethics, values, and spirituality. All these aspects of self are interwoven into the fabric of our being. One component affects the others, and we will be only as strong as our weakest link. Stated another way, good health has traditionally been viewed by the public as freedom from disease. Thus if an individual was not sick, he or she was considered to be healthy. This perspective is changing. While it is generally agreed that not being ill is one part of being healthy, at the same time it does not indicate that one is in a state of well-being. Well-being is largely achieved and maintained by the individual who properly manages his or her own lifestyle. Paying attention to aspects of a healthy style of living such as physical fitness, adequate nutrition, stress management, control of alcohol consumption and avoidance of drug abuse, smoking cessation, and weight control management can all contribute to well-being. Regardless of your present state of health, you can still achieve a higher level of wellness by integrating these components into your style of living.

WELLNESS MODEL

Traditional medicine concentrates on curing or alleviating disease, whereas the wellness model encourages people to prevent illness by improving their positive well-being in a variety of ways. The term wellness is a popular word in today's health vocabulary. Wellness workshops are held in hospitals, colleges, and universities. There are community wellness programs in many cities, and the concept of wellness management is being introduced in industry. National wellness associations are being formed that conduct wellness conferences that attract hundreds of participants.

Wellness has a relatively nebulous definition because it emphasizes all aspects of healthful living. Author Don Ardell, who has been instrumental in the wellness movement over the years, has perhaps best defined wellness as "a way of life which you design to enjoy the highest level of health and well-being possible during the years you have in this life." It has also been pointed out that "life is not an illness for which we seek a cure. Instead, life is a journey to be enjoyed—and to enjoy it most, all aspects of self must be in tune and working harmoniously."

Relationship of Fitness to Wellness

Although all the components of wellness exist in concert with one another, each is a single entity. Being physically fit is critical to a healthful style of living but is no more important for total well-being than our social, emotional, mental, or spiritual stability. Arguably, fitness can impact each of these components in either a positive or a negative manner. The bottom line in the wellness approach is a balance between the components, with no more emphasis on any single component than on the others.

This book will emphasize the fitness aspect of the wellness model, in particular the various components of fitness that are considered to be primarily health-related components: muscular strength, muscular endurance, cardiorespiratory endurance, flexibility, and body composition. As indicated in Chapter 1, health-related fitness is concerned with the development of those components of fitness that can potentially facilitate a healthy lifestyle.

Emotional Wellness

Emotions play a major role in healthful living and have a great deal to do with how we feel about ourselves and interact with others. Emotional stability determines how well you are able to deal with stress and how you adjust and adapt to changes in the environment. It is hoped that everyone will at some point in his or her life have a chance to experience all the emotions associated with human beings. If you do not, a significant portion of the life experience will be unfulfilled. However, it is important to maintain your emotional stability at some midrange between the highs and lows. Wide variations in emotional stability may lead to both physical and mental disturbances in health.

Social Wellness

Unless we choose the lifestyle of a hermit, each of us must interact with other people who touch our lives. The development of social skills, communication skills, and interpersonal relationships is critical to psychological development. The ability to show emotion toward another individual is also an extremely important aspect of healthy living.

Intellectual Wellness

One must make wise decisions when faced with the variety of situations that occur throughout life. Individuals develop a set of values and beliefs and consider them when they make choices and solve problems. Personal growth can proceed once a foundation has been established. This permits the individual to act and develop the coping skills needed to adapt to changing conditions.

Spiritual Wellness

Spiritual wellness means different things to people of various religions, cultures, and nationalities. Whether spirituality means believing in some supreme omnipotent entity or simply establishing values, morals, and ethics, the need to establish some basic purpose for our existence is ultimately the glue that holds the wellness model together.

Is spirituality then the most important component of wellness? At different times throughout life each component will take on greater importance than the others. Persistent neglect of any of the components will cause that component to become the most critical, thus destroying the balance of the model. Being *well* means being able to balance all aspects of life in a manner that will promote good health within individual limitations.

NEED FOR WELLNESS

There is an urgent need for wellness in today's world. Health problems exist among a large segment of the population, and often these problems could have been prevented if individuals had paid more attention to their health. Everyone should recognize some of the dividends that can occur with increased attention to personal health needs.

High Health Care Costs

Because of high health care costs today, a large segment of the population cannot afford to be sick. In light of the economics of health care, wellness represents an excellent investment.

Health care spending has grown from 5.3% of the gross domestic product (GDP) in 1960 to 9.2% in 1980 and 13.9% in 1993. In 1993, total health care costs were $884.2 billion or $3299 per person, an increase of 322% since 1980. According to the American Hospital Association the average cost of a hospital stay was $820 per day, with a total-stay average cost of $5794.

Injury alone costs over $120 billion annually, cardiovascular disease costs over $150 billion, and cancer costs over $80 billion. There are nearly 300,000 coronary bypass procedures performed each year, at a cost of approximately $40,000 each. Treatment for a single case of lung cancer is about $38,000. A liver transplant can cost more than $250,000. Lifetime treatment costs for an AIDS patient are $102,000. Yet most of these conditions are preventable. As a result of such health care costs, wellness today represents a market with staggering dollar figures.

Health Risk Factors

There are various human factors that we cannot control, some that we need medical assistance to control, and some that we can control through the lifestyle we adopt. For example, we cannot control age, sex, or heredity. We need medical help in controlling diabetes and hypertension. However, it is possible for humans to control such health risk factors as smoking, obesity, diet, exercise, cardiorespiratory fitness, and stress.

The importance of applying wellness to our lives is especially significant when we examine some of the leading health problems and causes of death in our society. Table 2-1 indicates the number of deaths that occurred from various causes in 1994.

TABLE 2-1. Causes of Death in the U.S. in 1994	
Total deaths (all causes)	2,298,000
Heart disease	733,460
Cancer	540,790
Stroke	153,560
Chronic obstructive pulmonary disease	102,300
Accidents (total)	88,840
Motor vehicle accidents	42,260
Pneumonia	82, 270
Diabetes	55,470
HIV	40,210
Suicide	30,680
Homicide	24,010

Data from US Bureau of the Census: *Statistical abstracts of the United States,* Washington, DC, 1994.

---

wellness emphasizes all aspects of healthful living to help attain the highest level of health and well-being throughout a person's lifespan

health risk factors inherited physical traits or lifestyle conditions that can make one more susceptible to injury or illness, including smoking, obesity, improper diet, insufficient cardiorespiratory fitness, and susceptibility to stress

Statistics concerning deaths among young people age 15 to 24 show the following causes of premature deaths: (1) accidents (motor vehicle), (2) homicide, (3) suicide, (4) cancer, (5) heart disease, and (6) HIV. The incidence of such deaths could be significantly reduced if wellness became a high priority in the lives of young people. These deaths reflect a failure in proper health practices and living with ourselves and each other. In most cases they are related to one's lifestyle. Americans today are expressing an interest in being healthy and fit to enjoy a full life. This interest has been stimulated by the growing realization that one's lifestyle, the way one lives, and the quality of one's environment influence greatly the attainment and maintenance of personal health.

Thus health is affected by every aspect of an individual's life. Physical, psychological, emotional, spiritual, social, and environmental forces all interact to influence one's health. Those who adhere to the wellness doctrine believe that it is the responsibility of the individual to work toward achievement of a healthy lifestyle to realize an optimal sense of well-being. A healthy lifestyle should reflect the integration of such components as proper nutrition, regular and appropriate physical activity, stress management, and elimination of controllable risk factors such as smoking and drug abuse. Unhealthy lifestyles are associated with diseases (particularly stress-related diseases such as hypertension), heart attack, and early mortality for those who do not choose to control their lifestyle. Lab Activity 2-1 will help you assess your lifestyle relative to healthy living.

HEALTH OBJECTIVES FOR THE NATION: HEALTHY PEOPLE 2000

In 1987, the U.S. Department of Health and Human Services of the Public Health Service coordinated a national effort focused on formulating a document titled *Healthy People 2000, National Health Promotion and Disease Prevention Objectives.* Input for this document was received from over 300 national organizations, 8 regional hearings, individual state health departments, and public review and comment from over 10,000 people. This effort was coordinated by the Institute of Medicine of the National Academy of Sciences. *Healthy People 2000* builds on the 1990 objectives and was expanded to 22 priority areas grouped under four broad categories: health promotion, health protection, preventative services, and surveillance and data systems. The three broad goals of *Healthy People 2000* are as follows:

- Increase the span of healthy life for Americans
- Reduce health disparities among Americans
- Achieve access to preventative services for all Americans

Physical activity and fitness are identified as one of the 22 priority areas in which changes in the habits of people would have a positive influence on their health. Figure 2-1 is a summary of the 12 objectives identified to increase physical activity and fitness.

The objectives for the year 2000 encourage people to become better informed and to take more personal

FIGURE 2-1. Twelve Objectives Identified to Increase Physical Activity

- Reduce coronary artery disease deaths to no more than 100 per 100,000 people.
- Reduce overweight to a prevalence of no more than 20% among people age 20 and older and no more than 15% among adolescents age 12 through 19.
- Increase to at least 30% the population of people age 6 and older who engage regularly, preferably daily, in light-to-moderate physical activity for at least 30 minutes per day.
- Increase to at least 20% the proportion of people age 18 and older and to at least 75% the proportion of children and adolescents age 6 through 17 who engage in vigorous physical activity that promotes the development and maintenance of cardiorespiratory fitness 3 or more days per week for 30 or more minutes per occasion.
- Reduce to no more than 15% the proportion of people age 6 and older who engage in no leisure-time physical activity.
- Increase to at least 40% the proportion of people age 6 and older who regularly perform physical activities that enhance and maintain muscular strength, muscular endurance, and flexibility.
- Increase to at least 50% the proportion of overweight people age 12 and older who have adopted sound dietary practices combined with regular physical activity to attain appropriate body weight.
- Increase to at least 50% the proportion of children and adolescents in 1st through 12th grades who participate in daily school physical education.
- Increase to at least 50% the proportion of physical education class time that students spend being physically active, preferably engaged in lifetime physical activities.
- Increase the proportion of worksites offering employer-sponsored physical activity and fitness programs.
- Increase the availability and accessibility of physical activity and fitness facilities including hiking, biking, fitness trails, public swimming pools, and areas of park and recreation open space.
- Increase to at least 50% the proportion of primary care providers who routinely assess and counsel their patients regarding the frequency, duration, type, and intensity of each patient's physical activity practices.

responsibility for their health and fitness. It is also important to reduce health care costs by shifting the focus from treatment to prevention and by extending the benefits of good health to all individuals regardless of socioeconomic status.

HYPOKINETIC DISEASE

Hypokinetic disease is a term referring to those diseases that can be associated in some respects with a sedentary lifestyle. The term implies low activity levels. Many individuals in our society gear their exercise habits to the demands of everyday life. Because the physiological demands of today's society are relatively easy, little activity is experienced. This lack of activity may cause many of the body processes to deteriorate. Thus medical problems such as coronary artery disease, high blood pressure, obesity, osteoporosis, diabetes, stress, insomnia, and low back pain may all be directly or indirectly linked with a lack of physical fitness activity. Frequently, these various types of hypokinetic disease are interrelated, and an increase in activity levels may alter the disease processes to some extent. Activity that builds muscular strength, endurance, and flexibility may protect against injury and disability. The effects of exercise on hypokinetic disease will be addressed in this chapter and in Chapters 10 and 11.

PREVENTION OF CARDIOVASCULAR DISEASE

Coronary artery disease (CAD) is the leading cause of death in the United States. It accounts for nearly one third of all deaths and for more than one half of all cardiovascular deaths. There is no question that the cardiovascular system has not been designed to handle many of the stresses placed on it. American adults form many habits during the college-age years, such as patterns of eating and drinking and levels of physical exercise, that carry over for the rest of their lives. The lifestyle you choose plays a major role in determining whether you develop CAD. Coronary artery disease results from the accumulation of fatty deposits (atherosclerotic plaque) within the coronary arteries (Figure 2-2). The coronary arteries supply blood to the heart muscle, which functions properly only when provided with a steady blood supply. The deposition of fatty plaque often begins early in life, and the continued, gradual deposition of plaque can lead to a significant narrowing of the coronary arteries, or *atherosclerosis.* The partial or complete occlusion of one or more of the major coronary arteries can lead to a condition called *myocardial ischemia,* in which the heart muscle fails to receive an adequate supply of oxygen. This can produce symptoms such as chest pain

(angina pectoris) and if severe can precipitate a heart attack. Each year approximately 1.5 million Americans suffer heart attacks and about one third of these die. A heart attack can occur suddenly and without warning. But the factors that ultimately lead to a cardiac arrest are present early in life and for the most part go undetected until they manifest in a potentially life-threatening heart attack. Signs and symptoms associated with heart attacks are shown in Figure 2-3.

Other Forms of Cardiovascular Disease

Certainly CAD is the most prevalent of the cardiovascular diseases. Other cardiovascular diseases include hypertension, stroke, congenital heart defect, rheumatic heart disease, peripheral artery disease, and congestive heart failure.

Hypertension will be discussed in detail in a later section as a major coronary risk factor. Hypertension refers to a consistently elevated blood pressure. High blood pressure can have a negative effect on virtually all of the physiological systems throughout the body.

A *stroke* results from damage to blood vessels in the brain and is caused either by blockage from a clot or by rupture of an artery resulting in cerebral hemorrhage. Either of these mechanisms will cause disruption of oxygenated blood flow to the brain. The extent of the damage is dependent on the location of the lesion and the specific area of the brain affected.

A *congenital heart defect* is one that is present at birth. The causes of congenital heart defects are not clearly identified. Pregnant women who contract the rubella virus during the first 3 months of pregnancy place the infant at increased risk. Other possible causes include genetics, the use of drugs and alcohol by the pregnant woman, and her exposure to environmental pollutants.

Rheumatic heart disease involves chronic damage to the valves in the heart muscle resulting from a streptococcal bacterial infection. Left untreated, this bacterial infection can result in an inflammatory disease called *rheumatic fever.* Defective heart valves fail to either fully open or close, resulting in a backflow of blood within the heart.

Peripheral artery disease involves restricted blood flow to the extremities, especially to the legs, feet, and hands, which results in damage to the vessels.

Congestive heart failure occurs from an inability of the heart to pump out all of the blood that returns to

---

hypokinetic disease disease associated with a sedentary lifestyle
coronary artery disease disease that results from the accumulation of fatty deposits (atherosclerotic plaque) within the coronary arteries

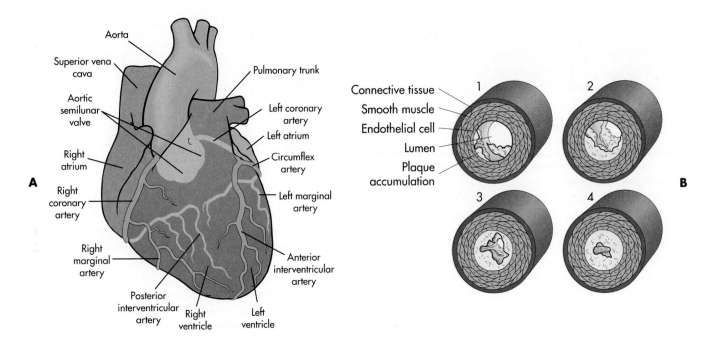

FIGURE 2-2. The Human Heart.
A, The heart muscle showing coronary arteries. **B,** The development of atherosclerosis.
(1) Normal coronary artery. *(2)* Beginning stages of atherosclerosis; fatty plaque is deposited in vessel walls. *(3)* Advanced stage of atherosclerosis leading to diminished blood flow. *(4)* Totally blocked coronary artery. (**A** from Lewis SM, Collier IC, Heitkemper MM: *Medical-surgical nursing: assessment and management of clinical problems,* ed 4, St Louis, 1996, Mosby.)

it. This can lead to dangerous fluid accumulations not only in the heart but also in the veins, lungs, and kidneys.

Risk Factors

Coronary artery disease is related to personal lifestyle, health habits or behaviors, and inherited characteristics known as *risk factors*. These risk factors cannot be labeled as causes but are instead characteristics that increase the probability of developing CAD. The following risk factors have been identified:

- Cigarette smoking
- Hypertension
- Elevated serum cholesterol level
- Elevated triglycerides
- Obesity
- Physical inactivity
- Diabetes
- High-stress lifestyle
- Family history (heredity)
- Age
- Gender

primary risk factors

Each of the risk factors is of great importance in the development of CAD. The risk factors are related to CAD in an additive fashion: the greater the number of risk factors present, the greater the likelihood of developing CAD. Also each of these factors is, at least in part, a function of individual lifestyles and behavior patterns. This observation holds out hope that it may be possible to prevent premature CAD through modification of the risk factors. Of these risk factors, many can be reduced or eliminated by changing your lifestyle or behavior to reduce elevated serum cholesterol levels, stop smoking, reduce hypertension, increase physical activity, reduce body fat, control diabetes, and reduce stress. Family history, age, and gender are risk factors that cannot be altered.

RISKO is an assessment tool designed to give you an estimation of your chances of suffering a heart attack by analyzing the risk factors present in your lifestyle (see Lab Activity 2-2). It must be added that this assessment should be used only to identify personal characteristics and health habits that, if modified, can reduce the likelihood of a heart attack.

Tests That May Indicate the Presence of CAD

ECG Abnormalities During Exercise.   An abnormal electrocardiogram (ECG) recorded during exercise indicates some type of interference with the normal electrical activity that occurs in the heart muscle during periods of stress testings. ECG tracings provide an indication of some impending CAD. Further

---

FIGURE 2-3. Signals of a Heart Attack—and What to Do.

Know the Warning Signals of a Heart Attack

- Uncomfortable pressure, fullness, squeezing or pain in the center of your chest, lasting 2 minutes or more.
- Pain may spread to shoulders, neck, or arms.
- Severe pain, dizziness, fainting, sweating, nausea, or shortness of breath may also occur.
- However, not all these signals are always present.
- Don't wait. Get help immediately.

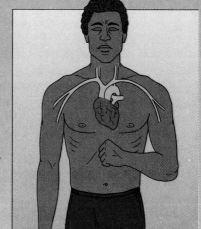

Know What to Do in Case of an Emergency

- If you are having chest discomfort that lasts for 2 minutes or more, call the emergency rescue service.
- If you can get to a hospital faster by car, have someone drive you.
- Find out which hospitals in your area offer 24-hour emergency cardiac care.
- Select in advance the facility nearest your home and office and tell your family and friends so that they will know what to do.
- Keep a list of emergency rescue service numbers next to your telephone and in a prominent place in your pocket, wallet, or purse.

Be a Heart Saver

- If you are with someone who is having the "signals," and if they last for 2 minutes or longer, act at once.
- Expect a "denial." It is normal for someone to deny the possibility of anything as serious as a heart attack, but insist on taking prompt action.
- Call the emergency rescue service, or
- Get to the nearest hospital emergency room that offers 24-hour emergency cardiac care.
- Give mouth-to-mouth breathing and chest compression (CPR) if it is necessary and if you are properly trained.

---

medical testing may be required to determine the reason for the abnormality.

Pulmonary Function Abnormalities. Pulmonary function tests can indicate difficulty in delivering oxygenated blood to the cardiorespiratory system, which makes the heart work harder. For those individuals who have obstructive lung disease, ventilation may require three times the effort necessary for a person without lung disease. Many diseases might result in decreased pulmonary function and lead to asthma, chronic bronchitis, emphysema, cystic fibrosis, or lung cancer. Cigarette smoking is a major cause of lung diseases.

Cigarette Smoking

Cigarette smoking is the most important preventable cause of death in the United States. A 1983 report released by the Surgeon General of the United States stated that "cigarette smoking should be considered the most important of the known risk factors for CAD in the United States." Cigarette smoking is responsible for approximately 21% of all CAD deaths. There has been a great deal of interest in the possible role that smoking plays in heart disease. Some early studies showed a relationship between smoking and coronary death rate. The Framingham, Massachusetts, Heart Epidemiology Study of 2282 middle-age men over a 10-year period and the Albany, New York, study of 1838 middle-age men over an 8-year span found that heart attacks among smokers of 20 or more cigarettes per day were three times more frequent than among nonsmokers, even when such factors as high blood pressure, obesity, and cholesterol level were taken into account.

More recently a study of coronary artery–bypass patients showed that 92% of them were cigarette smokers. A 1988 study indicated that cigarette smoking not only was a leading cause of coronary artery disease but also was responsible for about 80% of the 117,000 deaths resulting from lung cancer. According to 1994 statistics, less than 25% of all adults smoke cigarettes. The number of male adults who smoke has declined steadily from 52.4% in 1965 to 28.1% in 1993. Among females, the number of smokers has declined from 34.1% to 22.4%.

As with the other major CAD risk factors, cigarette smoking is related to CAD risk in a graded fashion: the more you smoke, the greater the risk. Smokers of low-tar, low-nicotine cigarettes are probably at as

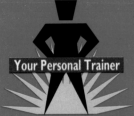

Your Personal Trainer

Lynn Freeman, English major/waitress
Age: 22

Scenario

I've always been quite active, but this year as I am nearing graduation and juggling an increased class load along with my 2 to 3 night a week job, I haven't been able to dedicate myself to exercising as regularly as I used to. I really enjoy roller-blading, and I take advantage of every opportunity I get to strap on my skates. In addition to my regular Saturday morning outings with two of my close friends, I have been roller-blading to work, which is about 2 or 3 miles from campus.

I live in a town of about 200,000 people, and my route only takes me across one congested street, but lately my asthma has been acting up a lot. It gets really bad in the afternoons just before I start waiting tables.

Solution

Exercise-induced asthma (EIA) affects a number of professional and amateur athletes. Onset of an asthma attack due to strenuous exercise can take place anywhere from 5 minutes into the activity up to a half hour after its completion.

The first thing you should do is consult your physician and make sure that you are making proper use of your antiinflammatory inhaler or bronchodilator. It also helps to use your inhaler at least 10 minutes before you start exercising.

You should warm up before you hit the street; if you don't have time, start out at a leisurely pace—give yourself enough time to get to work so you don't feel rushed.

Don't roller-blade to work when the air quality is particularly bad—this information can be found in most daily newspapers, radio, and/or TV news reports. Wearing a scarf over your mouth in cold weather should also help.

Your doctor or the American Lung Association can provide you with more specific information on how to exercise safely and effectively so that your asthma doesn't interfere with your lifestyle.

---

much risk as smokers of cigarettes with higher tar and nicotine content. It should be noted that all cigarette smokers have a much higher risk than nonsmokers. Recently it has been shown that individuals exposed to second-hand smoke (the smoke from a cigarette that enters the environment) are also at higher risk for CAD and lung cancer.

Cessation of smoking is associated with a reduction in the risk of CAD. Within 2 years after smoking cessation, overall mortality risk returns to only slightly higher than that for a nonsmoker. There is no doubt that cigarette smokers are a declining minority. In recent years significant pressure has been exerted by many different governmental and private organizations to curb and restrict the use of tobacco and tobacco products. However, the use of cigarettes and tobacco products, especially among teenage girls, continues to present a major health problem in the United States.

Hypertension

It is estimated that 62 million Americans have hypertension. For unknown reasons, blacks have a higher prevalence of high blood pressure than do whites. Individuals with chronic high blood pressure are three to four times more likely to develop CAD and seven times more likely to have a stroke than those with normal blood pressure. High blood pressure causes the heart to work harder to overcome the arterial resistance to blood flow. Thus it may damage the arterial walls and lead to heart disease and stroke.

Blood pressure is the pressure that the blood exerts against the inner wall of the arteries. Normal blood pressure is considered to be 120/80 mm Hg in adult Americans. The systolic blood pressure (the larger of the two numbers) represents the pressure in the artery at the time the heart beats. Diastolic blood pressure is recorded during the resting phase of the heart. Blood pressure that is continually above 140/90 should be considered hypertension.

Chronic high blood pressure, or *hypertension,* may develop as a condition secondary to another disease. However, the causes of the most common form of hypertension are not fully understood. Fortunately, for many with this condition, weight reduction, cessation of smoking, decreased psychological stress, reduced salt intake, and increased exercise often produce beneficial effects. In more resistant cases, hypertension may be controlled with medication.

Blood pressure varies from minute to minute, going up with excitement or exertion and down with rest and relaxation. Thus a single measurement of blood pressure may differ somewhat from your "normal" blood pressure. Lab Activity 2-3 will help you learn to measure blood pressure.

Elevated Serum Cholesterol Level

Cholesterol is a fatty substance manufactured by the body and is also found in some of the food we eat. Cholesterol is transported in the bloodstream, and if present in excessive amounts, it adheres to the walls of the arteries. This contributes to the deposition of atherosclerotic plaque.

Cholesterol is transmitted through the cardiovascular system in forms called *lipoproteins*, primarily either high-density or low-density varieties. *Low-density lipoprotein* (LDL) is believed to deposit cholesterol on the arterial wall, whereas *high-density lipoprotein* (HDL) seems to be able to remove the cholesterol deposited by LDL from the arterial walls. Thus the more HDL present, the better off you are, because it appears to be an anti–risk factor. Physically active persons have a far more desirable amount of HDL cholesterol in relation to the LDL form (HDL/LDL ratio) than do those who are inactive. An excess of these lipoproteins is referred to as *hyperlipidemia.* This can be detected by blood tests that measure HDL, LDL, and total cholesterol. Many people know their total serum cholesterol level but do not know how much of it is HDL ("good") cholesterol or LDL ("bad") cholesterol. The ratio of total cholesterol (TC) to HDL is important and should be less than 4.0. A ratio greater than 5 indicates an increased risk of CAD.

Serum cholesterol concentration is related to the dietary intake of cholesterol and saturated fats. Cholesterol and saturated fats are found in especially large quantities in egg yolks, organ meats (such as liver and kidney), red meats, and dairy products. Saturated fat is high in tropical plant oils such as palm and coconut oils. Cholesterol is found only in animal products. A reduction of the dietary intake of cholesterol and especially saturated fats usually results in a decrease in the serum cholesterol concentration. The fat found in canola, olive, and peanut oil is a type of unsaturated fat that may help prevent CAD. However, too much fat from all sources has been related to the cause of several different types of cancer, including breast, prostate, and colon cancers.

Americans represent a high-risk population that tends to exhibit rather high serum cholesterol values. Many other societies around the world in which the typical diet is lower in cholesterol and saturated fats show lower average cholesterol levels. Not coincidentally, these societies also tend to show lower rates of death from CAD.

Thus serum cholesterol levels are directly related to the incidence of CAD: the higher the serum cholesterol level, the greater the risk of CAD. It has been recommended that desirable total cholesterol levels for American adults be between 180 and 200 milligrams per deciliter (mg/dl) of blood. The American Dietetics Association has recommended a total cholesterol level under 180 mg/dl for those under age 20. The risk of heart attack with cholesterol levels of 250 mg/dl is twice that with 200 mg/dl, and more than four times greater at 300 mg/dl. The recommended LDL level is less than 130 mg/dl, and the recommended HDL level is greater than 45 mg/dl. The Health Link box on p. 48 provides a quick summary and a few helpful tips.

Elevated Triglycerides

The presence of excess triglycerides (also known as *free fatty acids*) combined with elevated cholesterol levels speeds up the process of atherosclerosis. Individuals who consume a lot of sugar and/or alcohol are likely to have elevated triglyceride levels. A recommended triglyceride level is 125 mg/dl. Reducing the intake of sugar and alcohol and reducing body fat can substantially lower triglyceride levels.

Obesity

Obesity will be discussed in greater detail in Chapter 8. However, obesity is related to CAD only in that people who are obese tend to have not only higher blood pressure but also hyperlipidemia. Also, obese individuals are usually sedentary and are more likely to develop a form of diabetes. All of these are risk factors for CAD. There is little doubt that adopting a style of living that incorporates consistent exercise and decreased caloric intake will have the greatest impact in reducing obesity.

Physical Inactivity

Individuals who lead a relatively sedentary style of living are more likely to suffer from CAD than those who maintain an active lifestyle. The medical literature has clearly determined that physical activity can increase fitness and provide many health benefits. A study published in the *Journal of the American Medical Association* examined the relationship between physical fitness, physical activity, and death rates in men and women. This study measured the fitness levels of 13,344 subjects followed over an average of more than 8 years to determine the contribution of a physically active lifestyle toward decreasing the risk of death

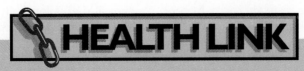

MANAGING YOUR SERUM CHOLESTEROL LEVELS

Categories of Risk for Serum Cholesterol Level

Desirable = <200 mg/dl
Borderline high = 200-239 mg/dl
High = >240 mg/dl

Everyone should know his or her total serum cholesterol value. Ask your doctor if dietary modifications and increased physical activity are all the changes that you need to make. The following strategies can help lower serum cholesterol levels that are between 200 and 250 mg/dl.

Eat Less Fat

Switch to drinking fluid skim milk rather than 2% or whole. (If you are used to drinking whole milk, switch to 2%. Later, you can make the switch to the fluid skim milk found in the dairy case at stores.)
Eat fewer fried foods; breading absorbs fat.
Avoid foods that include sauces, gravies, or oily dressings.
Trim all visible fats from meats before and after cooking.

Don't eat the skin from poultry; it has fat in it.
Choose to eat a meatless dish one or two meals per week.
Choose low-fat snacks such as fresh fruits, raw vegetables, or salt-free pretzels to munch rather than fatty chips, cookies, etc.
Eat fish once a week; baked or broiled, not fried.

Exercise More

Park farther from your destination so you'll have more distance to walk.
Use your bicycle more often (don't forget the helmet).
Take the stairs rather than the elevator.
Turn off the T.V. and take a walk.
For study breaks, take a walk or exercise instead of checking the refrigerator for a snack.

Incorporate More Physical Activity, Even if It's for 20 Minutes a Day, Into Your Routine

---

and illness. The results of this study show an extremely strong, inversely proportional relationship between physical fitness and death from all causes, specifically heart disease and cancer. As physical activity levels increased, deaths declined. These findings are consistent for both men and women. Even moderate levels of physical fitness that are attainable by most adults appear to be protective against early death. Since a significant percentage of adults in the United States are considered to be sedentary, this study strongly suggests that Americans increase their physical activity levels as a deterrent to many disease processes (Figure 2-4).

Exercise reduces the risks associated with hypertension, possibly because exercise maintains the elasticity of the arterial walls and thus retards the arteriosclerotic process (hardening of the arteries). It also increases vessel size, myocardial efficiency, and efficiency of peripheral blood distribution and return.

Exercise also may reduce the occurrence and severity of CAD by decreasing blood cholesterol and triglyceride levels, thus altering the amount of fatty

plaque being deposited on the arterial walls. Exercise increases the amount of HDL, the "good" form of cholesterol. Those who exercise regularly tend to be more able to control their body weight or, more precisely, their percentage of body fat. People with excess body fat often have high LDL ("bad") cholesterol levels.

Exercise can also help to reduce the effects of psychological and emotional stress. The mechanisms of stress reduction are not well understood, and much research is being done to try to explain how exercise reduces stress.

Diabetes

Diabetes mellitus is defined as a condition in which blood sugar levels are not properly controlled by the hormone insulin. In type I diabetes, which usually occurs in young people, the pancreas produces little or no insulin. In type II diabetes, which has an onset in adulthood, the pancreas produces insulin, but the body is unable to use it. Adult-onset diabetes produces abnormalities in lipoproteins, which seems to accelerate atherosclerosis. Increased blood sugar may

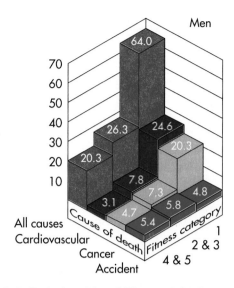

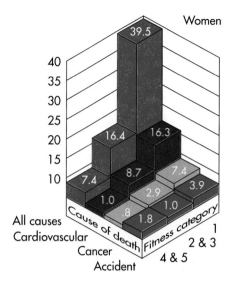

FIGURE 2-4. Relationship of Fitness Levels and Incidence of Death.
There is an inversely proportional relationship between the level of physical activity and the number of deaths resulting from cardiovascular disease and cancer. (Redrawn from Blair S, Kohl H, Paffenberger R, et al: Physical fitness and all-cause mortality; a prospective study of healthy men and women, *JAMA* 262 (17): 2395-2401, 1989.)

also, over time, damage some of the blood vessels not only in the heart but also in the brain, thus potentially predisposing an individual to have a stroke. Other potentially detrimental effects of poorly controlled diabetes include insulin shock and diabetic coma. Many older, overweight individuals develop adult-onset diabetes. With weight loss, blood sugar levels often return to normal.

Stress

Chronic stress is closely associated with CAD. Recent studies have focused mostly on suppressed anger and aggressiveness as causes of increased CAD. Stress reduction techniques have been shown to lower blood pressure and control hypertension. Stress will be discussed in detail in Chapter 11.

Family History

Those individuals who have had some previous history of cardiopulmonary or metabolic disease problems are at "known risk" and have a higher likelihood of CAD than those who are apparently healthy.

A history of CAD in the family is considered to be a predisposing risk factor when parents or siblings experienced evidence of the atherosclerotic disease process before the age of 55 to 60. However, this may be due

more to socioeconomic, cultural, and lifestyle factors within the family unit than to hereditary factors.

Age

As age increases, so do the chances of a person's having some type of CAD. It is well accepted that the onset of CAD occurs early in life. However, it is possible to retard the effects of the aging process by incorporating a healthful style of living that will impact on many of the risk factors already mentioned.

Gender

During their childbearing years, females generally have fewer heart attacks than their male counterparts. This can be attributed in large part to the fact that higher estrogen levels in females tend to increase HDL, which seems to provide a degree of protection against CAD. However, after menopause, a woman's risk of heart disease increases to that of a man. Stereotypical gender roles also may have served to decrease some of the risk factors (such as cigarette smoking and stress) that traditionally have been attributed more to the male in society. However, as the role of the female in society continues to change, the incidence of CAD in the female population will likely increase.

CANCER

Cancer is the second leading cause of death in adults, falling behind CAD. It is estimated that about 30% of all Americans will get cancer during their lifetime, and one of five will eventually die from it. Cancer is a condition in which cellular behavior becomes abnormal. The cells no longer perform their normal functions. In general, cancer cells do not multiply at an increased rate. Instead, whatever causes cancer alters the cell's genetic makeup and changes the way it functions. This abnormal cell then divides, forming additional cancer cells, and over a period of time this tumor or collection of abnormal cells tends to invade and ultimately take over normal tissue.

Tumors may be either *benign* or *malignant*. Benign tumors typically pose only a small threat to a tissue and tend to remain confined in a limited space. Malignant tumors, though, are cancerous and grow out of control and spread within a specific tissue. Unfortunately, malignancies can invade surrounding tissues and spread via the blood and lymphatic systems (metastasize) to the entire body, making it difficult to control the cancer.

Malignancies are classified according to the type of tissues in which they occur and according to the rate at which they affect the tissue. Although different types of cancer cells share similar characteristics, each is separate and distinct. Some types are relatively easy to cure, whereas others are difficult to cure and are even life threatening. Skin cancer is the most common type and, fortunately, one of the easiest to detect and cure. Males and females have a different incidence of other types of cancers. In males, the highest incidence of cancer is in the prostate, followed closely by lung, colon/rectal, urinary, and leukemias/lymphomas. In females the highest incidence is found in the breast, followed by colon/rectal, lung, uterus, and leukemias/lymphomas.

Causes of Cancer

The precise causes of cancer are not easily identified. Researchers have identified more than 100 types of cancer with genetic origins. Certain cancers appear to run along family lines. The onset of most cancer has also been attributed to certain environmental factors, including viruses; exposure to ultraviolet light, radiation, and certain chemicals such as tobacco; and alcohol use. A fatty diet has been linked to cancer. It is likely that a combination of hereditary and environmental factors is responsible for the development of cancer.

Recognizing and Treating Cancer

Unquestionably, early detection and treatment of cancer markedly improves the patient's chances of

---

FIGURE 2-5. American Cancer Society's Cancer Warning Signals.

- Change in bowel or bladder habits
- A sore that does not heal
- Unusual bleeding or discharge
- Thickening or lump in breast or elsewhere
- Indigestion or difficulty in swallowing
- Obvious change in a wart or mole
- Nagging cough or hoarseness

A physician should be consulted if you experience any of these signs.

---

beating the disease. Figure 2-5 identifies the warning signs of cancer described by the American Cancer Society. The presence of any of these signs warrants immediate attention by a physician. Figure 2-6 presents guidelines that can be used for the early detection of cancer before any identifiable symptoms are seen. The most effective forms of treatment involve three traditional techniques: surgery, radiation, and chemotherapy. Lab Activity 2-4 helps you assess whether you are at risk for skin, breast, or cervical cancer by identifying certain risk factors associated with each.

YOU MUST TAKE RESPONSIBILITY FOR YOUR OWN HEALTH

Some people today think of health as the responsibility of doctors, hospitals, clinics, insurance companies, and the government. They feel that health is someone else's responsibility, not their own. If they become sick, they reason that the doctor will prescribe the right medicine or will send them to the hospital or to a specialist who will provide the proper remedy. It is important to realize, however, that health cannot be purchased and that the responsibility cannot be relegated to some other person or agency. Health is an obligation on the part of individuals, and it is erroneous to equate more health service with better health. Instead, individuals must take responsibility for their own health.

The decisions that you make will have an impact on your health. You are the one who decides what to eat and when and if to exercise, drink, engage in drug abuse, smoke, or see a doctor. Thus the decisions you make will leave their imprint on your health and well-being. In many cases if people are sick they have only themselves to blame. See the box on p. 52 for additional reasons to maintain a healthy lifestyle.

FIGURE 2-6. **Cancer-Related Checkups.**

Following are guidelines for the early detection of cancer in people without symptoms. Talk with your doctor—ask how these guidelines relate to you. Remember, these guidelines are not rules and apply only to people without symptoms. If you have any of the seven warning signals of cancer, see your doctor or go to your clinic without delay.

Age 20 to 40: Cancer-Related Checkup Every 3 Years

Should include the procedures listed below, plus health counseling (such as tips on quitting smoking) and examinations for cancers of the thyroid, testes, prostate, mouth, ovaries, skin, and lymph nodes. *Some people are at higher risk for certain cancers and may need to have tests more frequently.*

Breast
- Examination by doctor every 3 years
- Self-exam every month
- One baseline mammogram between ages 35 and 40
  Higher risk for breast cancer: personal or family history of breast cancer, never had children, first child after 30

Uterus
- Pelvic exam every 3 years

Cervix
- Pap test—after three initial negative tests 1 year apart—*at least* every 3 years (includes women under 20 if sexually active)
  Higher risk for cervical cancer: early age at first intercourse, multiple sex partners

Testes
- Self-exam every month
- Consult doctor when an abnormality is present
  Higher risk for testicular cancer: personal or family history of testicular cancer, undescended testicles not corrected during early childhood, more prevalent in Caucasians and in men under age 35

Age 40 and Over: Cancer-Related Checkup Every Year

Should include the procedures listed below, plus health counseling (such as tips on quitting smoking) and examinations for cancers of the thyroid, testes, prostate, mouth, ovaries, skin, and lymph nodes. *Some people are at higher risk for certain cancers and may need to have tests more frequently.*

Breast
- Examinations by doctor every year
- Self-exam every month
- Mammogram every year after age 50 (between age 40 and 50, ask your doctor)
  Higher risk for breast cancer: personal or family history of breast cancer, never had children, first child after 30

Uterus
- Pelvic examination every year

Cervix
- Pap test—after two initial negative tests 1 year apart—*at least* every 3 years
  Higher risk for cervical cancer: early age at first intercourse, multiple sex partners

Endometrium
- Endometrial tissue sample at menopause if at risk
  Higher risk for endometrial cancer: infertility, obesity, failure of ovulation, abnormal uterine bleeding, estrogen therapy

Testes
- Self-exam every month
- Consult doctor when an abnormality is present
  Higher risk for testicular cancer: personal or family history of testicular cancer, undescended testicles not corrected during early childhood, more prevalent in Caucasians, risk declines with increasing age

Colon and Rectum
- Digital rectal examination every year
- Guaiac slide test every year after age 50
- Procto exam—after two initial negative tests 1 year apart—every 3 to 5 years after age 50
  Higher risk for colorectal cancer: personal or family history of colon or rectal cancer, personal or family history of polyps in the colon or rectum, ulcerative colitis

---

Years ago, health factors that humans can control, such as poor nutrition and sanitation, contributed to widespread sickness and poor health. Today, modern medical science has eliminated many health scourges and has provided humans with knowledge about the causes of disease and many preventive measures. However, to be effective this knowledge must be applied. Seat belts are placed in automobiles, for example, because research shows that many deaths and injuries can be prevented if they are worn. Although this knowledge is readily available, some individuals still insist on ignoring the use of this pro-

---

cancer a condition in which cellular behavior becomes abnormal

Reasons for creating a healthy lifestyle

GET MOVING

1. It is critical for you to understand that exercise may be the key to a healthy lifestyle. Significant research indicates that exercising on a consistent basis can have many positive benefits for your health.
2. If you exercise you are more likely to eat a healthier diet, avoiding foods that are high in cholesterol and triglycerides, which helps to reduce body fat.
3. If you exercise you are less likely to be obese, which decreases your chances of having diabetes and hypertension.
4. Exercise can help you reduce stress, which in turn helps to reduce hypertension.
5. If you don't smoke and you eat a healthy diet, you can greatly reduce your chances of cancer.
6. If you are healthy and fit, you generally feel better about yourself, and your social life may be enhanced by the way that others feel about you.
7. If you live a healthy lifestyle you may retard the aging process.

---

tective device. As a result many automobile accidents cause preventable injuries and deaths each year.

Spiraling health care costs and the realization of the benefits to be gained from participation in health and fitness activities have prompted many colleges, corporations, and other organizations to establish programs for their students and clientele. They have found that such programs promote good health and make economic sense, because poor health is costly in terms of illness, absenteeism, decreased productivity, and premature death. Corporations are becoming involved in wellness promotion efforts because fitness is good business; thus executive and other employee fitness programs are being established in thousands of companies. Corporations realize they have a large investment in their employees and want to protect this investment by establishing fitness programs.

The realization that health is a personal responsibility has resulted in many individuals making conscious efforts to adopt sound health practices. Also, it has motivated some to form and participate in self-help groups. People who are motivated to do something about their health problems but need extra support are likely to seek the help of others who have similar difficulties. Groups such as Alcoholics Anonymous, Emphysema Anonymous, weight control groups, and stroke and cancer recovery clubs have been organized and conduct meetings throughout the United States. By openly acknowledging problems and sharing experiences people gain much needed support from other group members.

The challenge of attaining the optimal level of health for ourselves and our loved ones is a lifetime one. No one can do the job for us, nor should they. This is a responsibility each person should assume to the extent he or she is able, with pride and conviction. As Sigerist, the noted medical historian, said, "Health is then something positive; a joyful attitude toward life and the responsibilities which life places upon us. It is both an individual need and a collective one." Lab Activity 2-5 will help you assess how healthy you think you are in relation to others and determine your level of satisfaction with your health status.

WHEN SHOULD YOU SEEK PROFESSIONAL HELP?

One can practice some basic principles of self-treatment, but from time to time professional help is needed to deal with a health problem. Of course competent medical care is needed in case of emergencies, but it is also a part of managing one's state of wellness. It is important to learn about one's body and its needs, to be able to react meaningfully in the event of an emergency, and to know when and how to use medical resources (see the following Safe Tip box).

Having periodic medical and dental checkups is an important part of managing your health. If you do not already have a competent doctor or dentist, you can get the name of one by contacting the college health service office, a local medical school, or the nearest medical or dental society, hospital, or health department.

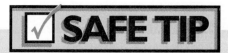

BASIC SELF-TREATMENT GUIDELINES

When trying to determine whether a health problem requires a physician's care, ask yourself the following questions. If you answer *yes* to any of them, consult a doctor.

Generally:

- Is this injury or pain so severe that I can't carry out my usual activities? Does it represent a threat to my health?
- Is this a strange sign or symptom, something that I have not experienced before?
- Is this condition worsening rather than improving?
- Have I had this condition too long?
- Have I had this condition in the past and it keeps recurring?

Specifically:

- Is there blood in my bowel movement or urine?
- Am I unable to control this bleeding?
- Do I have a high fever (102° F or above)?
- Am I becoming dehydrated?
- Do I have a stiff neck and a fever?
- Am I having a crushing sensation in my chest?
- Am I experiencing vomiting or diarrhea that just won't quit?

Choosing a Physician

Before choosing a doctor, consider your most frequent health problems and try to find a physician who is best qualified to help deal with them. When you go to see the doctor, be able to communicate clearly and completely to him or her your reason for the visit. Also, be prepared to provide important background information such as your health history, any medications that you take on a regular basis, and any allergies that you may have, especially to medications. If you do not understand what the doctor says, ask questions. After the visit comply with your doctor's instructions. If a prescription has been given to you, take only the drug that has been prescribed. If you feel that a second professional opinion is in order, do not hesitate to seek such advice.

It is estimated that one third of the people in the United States do not consult a physician for an annual medical checkup. Probably a similar number practice self-diagnosis and self-treatment for many of their health ailments. For them the following is applicable: "He who treats himself has a fool for a patient and an even greater fool for a physician."

Self-Medication

There are varied reasons for self-medication. Some people are afraid to find out about a particular health condition that is bothering them. Some may want to avoid the expense of medical care. Others may be swayed by misleading advertisements for certain health products and services that guarantee quick cures. Many nonprescription medicines can be used with safety if the directions on the label are followed. However, many can be potentially hazardous to your health if misused, used in combination with other medications, or if their use masks a serious condition. If your medicine chest overflows with over-the-counter (nonprescription) high-potency pain relievers, antihistamine and cold remedies, weight-reducing pills, or old prescription drugs, you may be asking for trouble.

Some persons use prescription drugs that have been prepared for someone else. A drug that may be helpful for one person can be harmful to another. The borrower may have an entirely different condition from that of the lender, and the prescription drug may not help his or her condition. Furthermore, it is illegal to use another person's prescription because these medications are ordered by a doctor for one particular individual.

If you self-medicate, your condition may not improve, and you may waste a lot of valuable time and money. If you have a serious medical problem, you should see a doctor. In this way you will feel better physically and emotionally because you will no longer have to worry about what is wrong or what to do about it.

A great many diseases can cause symptoms of pain and discomfort. Their origin may be infectious agents such as bacteria or viruses, exposure to environmental pollutants, lifestyle choices, psychological problems, or unknown factors. Therefore, obtaining expert medical advice early in an illness is important. The layperson cannot, of course, run to the physician with every minor ailment, but if the uncomfortable symptoms do not disappear in a few days or if they worsen, it is wise to seek professional help.

SUMMARY

- The wellness model incorporates aspects of intellectual, physical, social, emotional, and spiritual health in a manner that allows you to enjoy the highest level of health and well-being possible.
- There is a need for wellness in today's society to prevent some of the existing health-related problems.
- *Healthy People 2000, National Health Promotion and Disease Prevention Objectives* has identified three broad goals for health promotion and disease prevention. The need to increase physical activity and fitness was identified as one of 22 priority areas, and specific objectives were proposed.
- Hypokinetic diseases are associated with a sedentary lifestyle.
- Coronary artery disease is the leading cause of death in the United States each year.

- The major risk factors that predispose a person to CAD are cigarette smoking, hypertension, lack of physical activity, family history, elevated serum cholesterol level, elevated triglycerides, diabetes, obesity, age, and gender.
- Cancer is the second leading cause of death in adult Americans. Early detection and treatment is critical for reducing the likelihood of death.
- Health is a personal responsibility, and thus many individuals are incorporating health and wellness practices into their lifestyles.
- Professional medical help is needed periodically, not only in cases of emergency but also as a part of managing one's state of wellness.

REFERENCES

American Cancer Society: *Cancer facts and figures for 1996,* New York, 1996, The Society.

American College of Sports Medicine: Position stand on physical activity, physical fitness, and hypertension, *Med Sci Sports Exerc* 10:i-x, 1993.

American Heart Association: *Coronary risk factor statement for the American public,* Dallas, 1989, The Association.

American Heart Association: *Heart attack,* Dallas, 1989, The Association.

American Heart Association: *1996 heart and stroke facts,* Dallas, 1996, The Association.

American Hospital Association: *Hospital statistics,* Chicago, 1993, The Association.

Bernstien L, Henderson R, Hanish J: Physical exercise and reduced risk of breast cancer in young women, *J Natl Cancer Inst* 86:1403-1408, 1994.

Bijnen F, Caspersen C, Mosterd W: Physical inactivity as a risk factor for coronary heart disease: a WHO and International Society and Federation of Cardiology position statement, *Bull World Health Organ* 72(1):1-4, 1994.

Blair S, Kohl H, Paffenberger R, et al: Physical fitness and all-cause mortality; a prospective study of healthy men and women, *JAMA* 262(17):2395-2401, 1989.

Casperson CJ: Physical activity epidemiology: concepts, methods and application to exercise science. In Pandolf KB, editor: *Exercise and sciences reviews,* vol 17, New York, 1989, Macmillan.

Casperson C, Merritt R: Trends in physical activity patterns in older adults. The behavioral risk factor surveillance system, *Med Sci Sports Exerc* 24:S26, 1992.

Centers for Disease Control and Prevention: Public health focus: physical activity and the prevention of coronary heart disease, *MMWR Morb Mortal Wkly Rep* 42:669-672, 1993.

Haskell W, Alderman E, Fair J: Effects of intensive multiple risk factor reduction on coronary atherosclerosis and clinical cardiac events in men and women with coronary artery disease. The Stanford Coronary Risk Intervention Project (SCRIP), *Circulation* 89:975-990, 1994.

Isreal R, Sullivan M, Marks R: Relationship between cardiorespiratory fitness and lipoprotein in men and women, *Med Sci Sports Exerc* 26:425-431, 1994.

Lee I, Paffenberger R, Hsieh C: Physical activity and the risk of developing colorectal cancer among college alumni, *J Natl Cancer Inst* 83:1324-1329, 1991.

Leon A: Effects of exercise conditioning on physiologic precursors of coronary artery disease, *J Cardiopulm Rehabil* 11:46-57, 1991.

Lewis SM, Collier IC, Heitkemper MM: *Medical-surgical nursing: assessment and management of clinical problems,* ed 4, St Louis, 1996, Mosby.

Moore S: Physical activity, fitness and atherosclerosis. In Bouchard C, Shepard R, Stephens T, editors: *Physical activity fitness and health,* Champaign, 1994, Human Kinetics.

Morris J, Clayton D, Everitt M: Exercise in leisure time: coronary attack and death rates, *Br Heart J* 63:325-334, 1990.

National Center for Health Statistics: *Health, United States, 1989 and prevention profile,* DHHS Pub No (PHS) 91-1232, Hyattsville, Md, 1990, US Department of Health and Human Services.

Nieman D: Physical activity, fitness and infection. In Bouchard C, Shepard R, Stephens T, editors: *Physical activity fitness and health,* Champaign, 1994, Human Kinetics.

Payne WA, Hahn DB: *Understanding your health,* ed 4, St Louis, 1995, Mosby.

Shepard R: Exercise in the prevention and treatment of cancer, *Sports Med* 15:258-280, 1993.

Sternfeld B: Cancer and the protective effect of physical activity: the epidemiological evidence, *Med Sci Sports Exerc* 24:1195-1209, 1992.

Tipton C: Exercise training and hypertension: an update, *Exerc Sport Sci Rev* 19:447-505, 1991.

US Bureau of the Census: *Statistical abstracts of the United States,* Washington, DC, 1994.

US Department of Health and Human Services, Public Health Services: *Healthy people 2000: midcourse review and 1995 revisions,* Washington, DC, 1995, USDHHS.

US Department of Health and Human Services, Public Health Services: *Healthy people 2000: national health promotion and disease prevention objectives,* Washington, DC, 1991, USDHHS.

US Department of Health and Human Services, Public Health Service: *Healthy people 2000, national health promotion and disease prevention objectives,* Washington, DC, 1991, US Government Printing Office.

US Department of Health and Human Services, Public Health Service: *Promoting health/preventing disease, year 2000 objectives for the nation,* Washington, DC, 1989, US Government Printing Office (draft).

SUGGESTED READINGS

Benson H, Stuart E: *The wellness book: a comprehensive guide to maintaining health and treating stress-related injuries,* New York, 1992, Fireside Press.
Gives you the ability to gain control over your body and mind through medical care, which can help you to decrease illness.

Payne WA, Hahn DB: *Understanding your health,* ed 4, St Louis, 1995, Mosby.
An excellent health textbook that discusses in detail the various health-related problems discussed in this chapter. Strongly recommended as a reference.

University of California at Berkeley: *The new wellness encyclopedia,* Boston, 1995, Houghton-Mifflin.
Provides the latest, research-based information on taking care of yourself through diet, exercise, and lifestyle modification.

White T, Editors of the University of California at Berkeley Wellness Letter: *The wellness guide to lifelong fitness,* New York, 1993, Random House.
A total reference guide to wellness addressing all aspects of the wellness lifestyle model. Well illustrated and written in a manner that is easily understood.

Health Style: A Self-Test

Name _____ **Section** _____ **Date** _____

PURPOSE All of us want good health, but many of us do not know how to be as healthy as possible. Health experts now describe lifestyle as one of the most important factors affecting health. In fact, it is estimated that as many as seven of the ten leading causes of death could be reduced through common-sense changes in lifestyle. That's what this brief test, developed by the Public Health Service, is all about. Its purpose is simply to tell you how well you are doing to stay healthy. The behaviors covered in the test are recommended for most Americans. Some of them may not apply to persons with certain chronic diseases or handicaps or to pregnant women. Such persons may require special instructions from their physicians.

PROCEDURE 1. Circle the appropriate response for each question.
2. Add the total number of points for each section.

Behavior	Almost Always	Sometimes	Almost Never
Tobacco Use			
If you *never smoke* or use tobacco products, enter a score of 10 for this section and go to the next section on *Alcohol and Drugs*.			
1. I avoid smoking cigarettes and chewing tobacco.	2	1	0
2. I smoke only low-tar and low-nicotine cigarettes *or* I smoke a pipe or cigars.	2	1	0
Tobacco Use Score: _____			
Alcohol and Drugs			
1. I avoid drinking alcoholic beverages *or* I drink no more than one or two drinks a day.	4	1	0
2. I avoid using alcohol or other drugs (especially illegal drugs) as a way of handling stressful situations or problems in my life.	2	1	0
3. I am careful not to drink alcohol when taking certain medicines (e.g., medicine for sleeping, pain, colds, and allergies) or when pregnant.	2	1	0
4. I read and follow the label directions when using prescribed and over-the-counter drugs.	2	1	0
Alcohol and Drugs Score: _____			

Continued.

Behavior	Almost Always	Sometimes	Almost Never
Eating Habits			
1. I eat a variety of foods each day, such as fruits and vegetables, whole grain breads and cereals, lean meats, dairy products, dry peas and beans, and nuts and seeds.	4	1	0
2. I limit the amount of fat, saturated fat, and cholesterol I eat (including fat in meats, eggs, butter, and other dairy products, shortenings, and organ meats such as liver).	2	1	0
3. I limit the amount of salt I eat by cooking with only small amounts, not adding salt at the table, and avoiding salty snacks.	2	1	0
4. I avoid eating too much sugar (especially frequent snacks of sticky candy or soft drinks).	2	1	0
	Eating Habits Score: _____		
Exercise/Fitness Habits			
1. I maintain a desired weight, avoiding overweight and underweight.	3	1	0
2. I do vigorous exercises for 15-30 minutes at least three times a week (examples include running, swimming, and brisk walking).	3	1	0
3. I do exercises that enhance my muscle tone for 15-30 minutes at least three times a week (examples include yoga and calisthenics).	2	1	0
4. I use part of my leisure time participating in individual, family, or team activities that increase my level of fitness (such as gardening, bowling, golf, and baseball).	2	1	0
	Exercise/Fitness Score: _____		
Stress Control			
1. I have a job or do other work that I enjoy.	2	1	0
2. I find it easy to relax and express my feelings freely.	2	1	0
3. I recognize early and prepare for events or situations likely to be stressful for me.	2	1	0
4. I have close friends, relatives, or others whom I can talk to about personal matters and call on for help when needed.	2	1	0
5. I participate in group activities (such as church and community organizations) or hobbies that I enjoy.	2	1	0
	Stress Control Score: _____		
Safety			
1. I wear a seat belt while riding in a car.	2	1	0
2. I avoid driving while under the influence of alcohol and other drugs.	2	1	0
3. I obey traffic rules and the speed limit when driving.	2	1	0
4. I am careful when using potentially harmful products or substances (such as household cleaners, poisons, and electrical devices).	2	1	0
5. I avoid smoking in bed.	2	1	0
	Safety Score: _____		

What your Scores Mean to You

Scores of 9 and 10: Excellent! Your answers show that you are aware of the importance of this area to your health. More important, you are putting your knowledge to work for you by practicing good health habits. As long as you continue to do so, this area should not pose a serious health risk. It's likely that you are setting an example for your family and friends to follow. Since you got a very high test score on this part of the test, you may want to consider other areas where your scores indicate room for improvement.

Scores of 6 to 8: Good. Your health practices in this area are good, but there is room for improvement. Look again at the items you answered with a "Sometimes" or "Almost Never." What changes can you make to improve your score? Even a small change can often help you achieve better health.

Scores of 3 to 5: Fair. Your health risks are showing! Would you like more information about the risks you are facing and about why it is important for you to change these behaviors? Perhaps you need help in deciding how to successfully make the changes you desire. In either case, help is available.

Scores of 0 to 2: Poor. Obviously, you were concerned enough about your health to take the test, but your answers show that you may be taking serious and unnecessary risks with your health. Perhaps you are not aware of the risks and what to do about them. You can easily get the information and help you need to improve, if you wish. The next step is up to you.

What am I doing to become as healthy as possible?_____

_____

What steps can I take to feel better? _____

_____

_____

What changes do I need to make in my lifestyle?_____

_____

_____

_____

_____

You Can Start Right Now!

The test you just completed gave numerous suggestions to help you reduce your risk of disease and premature death. Here are some of the most significant.

Avoid Cigarettes and Other Tobacco Products. Cigarette smoking is the single most important preventable cause of illness and early death. It is especially risky for pregnant women and their unborn babies. Persons who stop smoking reduce their risk of getting heart disease and cancer. So if you're a cigarette smoker, think twice about lighting that next cigarette. If you choose to continue smoking, try decreasing the number of cigarettes you smoke and switching to a low-tar and low-nicotine brand. If you chew, stop the habit.

Follow Sensible Drinking Habits. Alcohol produces changes in mood and behavior. Most people who drink are able to control their intake of alcohol and to avoid undesired, and often harmful, effects. Heavy, regular use of alcohol can lead to cirrhosis of the liver, a leading cause of death. Also, statistics clearly show that mixing drinking and driving is often the cause of fatal or crippling accidents. So if you drink, do it wisely and in moderation. **Use care in taking drugs.** Today's greater use of drugs—both legal and illegal—is one of our most serious health risks. Even some drugs prescribed by your doctor can be dangerous if taken when drinking alcohol or before driving. Excessive or continued use of tranquilizers (or "pep pills") can cause physical and mental problems. Using or experimenting with illicit drugs such as marijuana, LSD, heroin, cocaine, and PCP may lead to a number of damaging effects or even death.

Eat Sensibly. Overweight individuals are at greater risk for diabetes, gall bladder disease, and high blood pressure. So it makes good sense to maintain proper weight. But good eating habits also mean holding down

Continued.

the amount of fat (especially saturated fat), cholesterol, sugar, and salt in your diet. If you must snack, try nibbling on fresh fruits and vegetables. You'll feel better—and look better, too.

Exercise Regularly. Almost everyone can benefit from exercise—and there's some form of exercise almost everyone can do. (If you have any doubt, check first with your doctor.) Usually, as little as 15-30 minutes of vigorous exercise three times a week will help you have a healthier heart, eliminate excess weight, tone up sagging muscles, and sleep better. Think how much difference all these improvements could make in the way you feel!

Learn to Handle Stress. Stress is a normal part of living: everyone faces it to some degree. The causes of stress can be good or bad, desirable or undesirable (such as a promotion on the job or the loss of a spouse). Properly handled, stress need not be a problem. But unhealthy responses to stress—such as driving too fast or erratically, drinking too much, or prolonged anger or grief—can cause physical and mental problems. Even on a very busy day, find a few minutes to slow down and relax. Talking over a problem with some-one you trust can often help you find a satisfactory solution. Learn to distinguish between things that are "worth fighting about" and things that are less important.

Be Safety Conscious. Think "safety first" at home, at work, at school, at play, and on the highway. Buckle seat belts, and obey traffic rules. Keep poisons and weapons out of the reach of children, and keep emer-gency numbers by your telephone. When the unexpected happens, you'll be prepared.

Where Do You Go From Here?

Start by asking yourself a few frank questions: Am I really doing all I can to be as healthy as possible? What steps can I take to feel better? Am I willing to begin now? If you scored low in one or more sections of the test, decide what changes you want to make for improvement. You might pick an aspect of your lifestyle where you feel you have the best change for success, and tackle that one first. Once you have improved your score there, go on to other areas.

If you already have tried to change your health habits (to stop smoking or to exercise regularly, for exam-ple), don't be discouraged if you haven't yet succeeded. The difficulty you have encountered may be due to influences you've never really thought about—such as advertising—or to a lack of support and encour-agement. Understanding these influences is an important step toward changing the way they affect you.

There's Help Available. In addition to personal actions you can take on your own, there are community programs and groups (such as the YMCA or the local chapter of the American Heart Association) that can assist you and your family to make the changes you want to make. If you want to know more about these groups or about health risks, contact your local health department or the address below. There's a lot you can do to stay healthy or to improve your health—and there are organizations that can help you. Start a new HEALTHSTYLE today!

National Health Information Clearinghouse
PO Box 1133
Washington, DC 20013-1133
1-800-336-4794

Lab Activity 2-2

RISKO

Name _____ **Section** _____ **Date** _____

PURPOSE   To determine your risk of heart disease

PROCEDURE   Complete the appropriate questions for your sex. Find the interpretation for your score at the end of the lab activity. (Categories for women on the following pages.)

MEN   Find the column for your age group. Everyone starts with a score of 10 points. Work down the page *adding* points to your score or *subtracting* points from your score.

			54 or younger	55 or older
1. Weight Locate your weight category in the table on p. 63.	*If you are in …*		**STARTING SCORE** [10]	**STARTING SCORE** [10]
	A	weight category A	SUBTRACT 2	SUBTRACT 2
	B	weight category B	SUBTRACT 1	ADD 0
	C	weight category C	ADD 1	ADD 1
	D	weight category D	ADD 2	ADD 3
			EQUALS	**EQUALS**
2. Systolic Blood Pressure Use the "first" or "higher" number from your most recent blood pressure measurement. If you do not know your blood pressure, estimate it by using the letter for your weight category.	*If your blood pressure is …*			
	A	119 or less	SUBTRACT 1	SUBTRACT 5
	B	between 120 and 139	ADD 0	SUBTRACT 2
	C	between 140 and 159	ADD 0	ADD 1
	D	160 or greater	ADD 1	ADD 4
			EQUALS	**EQUALS**
3. Blood Cholesterol Level Use the number from your most recent blood cholesterol test. If you do not know your blood cholesterol level, estimate it by using the letter for your weight category.	*If your blood cholesterol is …*			
	A	199 or less	SUBTRACT 2	SUBTRACT 1
	B	between 200 and 224	SUBTRACT 1	SUBTRACT 1
	C	between 225 and 249	ADD 0	ADD 0
	D	250 or higher	ADD 1	ADD 0
			EQUALS	**EQUALS**
4. Cigarette Smoking (If you smoke a pipe, but not cigarettes, use the same score adjustment as those cigarette smokers who smoke less than a pack a day.)	*If you …*			
	A	do not smoke	SUBTRACT 1	SUBTRACT 1
	B	smoke less than a pack a day	ADD 0	SUBTRACT 1
	C	smoke a pack a day	ADD 1	ADD 0
	D	smoke more than a pack a day	ADD 2	ADD 3
			FINAL SCORE	**FINAL SCORE**

Modified from American Heart Association: © *RISKO*, 1985.

Continued.

RISKO—cont'd

Name ___Debbie Davenport___   Section _____   Date ___9/16/96___

PURPOSE   To determine your risk of heart disease

PROCEDURE   Complete the appropriate questions for your sex. Find the interpretation for your score at the end of the lab activity.

WOMEN   Find the column for your age group. Everyone starts with a score of 10 points. Work down the page *adding* points to your score or *subtracting* points from your score.

		54 or younger	55 or older
1. Weight Locate your weight category in the table on p. 63.	*If you are in ...* A weight category A B weight category B C weight category C D weight category D	**STARTING SCORE** 10 SUBTRACT 2 · 8 SUBTRACT 1 ADD 1 ADD 2 **EQUALS** 8	**STARTING SCORE** 10 SUBTRACT 2 ADD 0 ADD 1 ADD 3 **EQUALS**
2. Systolic Blood Pressure Use the "first" or "higher" number from your most recent blood pressure measurement. If you do not know your blood pressure, estimate it by using the letter for your weight category.	*If your blood pressure is ...* A 119 or less B between 120 and 139 C between 140 and 159 D 160 or greater	SUBTRACT 1 · 7 ADD 0 ADD 0 ADD 1 **EQUALS** 7	SUBTRACT 5 SUBTRACT 2 ADD 1 ADD 4 **EQUALS**
3. Blood Cholesterol Level Use the number from your most recent blood cholesterol test. If you do not know your blood cholesterol level, estimate it by using the letter for your weight category.	*If your blood cholesterol is ...* A 199 or less B between 200 and 224 C between 225 and 249 D 250 or higher	SUBTRACT 2 · 5 SUBTRACT 1 ADD 0 ADD 1 **EQUALS** 5	SUBTRACT 1 SUBTRACT 1 ADD 0 ADD 0 **EQUALS**
4. Cigarette Smoking (If you smoke a pipe, but not cigarettes, use the same score adjustment as those cigarette smokers who smoke less than a pack a day.)	*If you...* A do not smoke B smoke less than a pack a day C smoke a pack a day D smoke more than a pack a day	SUBTRACT 1 · 4 ADD 0 ADD 1 ADD 2 **FINAL SCORE** 4	SUBTRACT 1 SUBTRACT 1 ADD 0 ADD 3 **FINAL SCORE**

WEIGHT TABLE FOR MEN

Look for your height (without shoes) in the far left column and then read across to find the category into which your weight (in indoor clothing) would fall.

Because both blood pressure and blood cholesterol are related to weight, an estimate of these risk factors for each weight category is printed at the bottom of the table.

Your Height		Weight Category (lb)			
Ft	In	A	B	C	D
5	1	up to 123	124-148	149-173	174 plus
5	2	up to 126	127-152	153-178	179 plus
5	3	up to 129	130-156	157-182	183 plus
5	4	up to 132	133-160	161-186	187 plus
5	5	up to 135	136-163	164-190	191 plus
5	6	up to 139	140-168	169-196	197 plus
5	7	up to 144	145-174	175-203	204 plus
5	8	up to 148	149-179	180-209	210 plus
5	9	up to 152	153-184	185-214	215 plus
5	10	up to 157	158-190	191-221	222 plus
5	11	up to 161	162-194	195-227	228 plus
6	0	up to 165	166-199	200-232	233 plus
6	1	up to 170	171-205	206-239	240 plus
6	2	up to 175	176-211	212-246	247 plus
6	3	up to 180	181-217	218-253	254 plus
6	4	up to 185	186-223	224-260	261 plus
6	5	up to 190	191-229	230-267	268 plus
6	6	up to 195	196-235	236-274	275 plus
Estimate of Systolic Blood Pressure		119 or less	120 to 139	140 to 159	160 or more
Estimate of Blood Cholesterol		199 or less	200 to 224	225 to 249	250 or more

WEIGHT TABLE FOR WOMEN

Look for your height (without shoes) in the far left column and then read across to find the category into which your weight (in indoor clothing) would fall.

Because both blood pressure and blood cholesterol are related to weight, an estimate of these risk factors for each weight category is printed at the bottom of the table.

Your Height		Weight Category (lb)			
Ft	In	A	B	C	D
4	8	up to 101	102-122	123-143	144 plus
4	9	up to 103	104-125	126-146	147 plus
4	10	up to 106	107-128	129-150	151 plus
4	11	up to 109	110-132	133-154	155 plus
5	0	up to 112	113-136	137-158	159 plus
5	1	up to 115	116-139	140-162	163 plus
5	2	up to 119	120-144	145-168	169 plus
5	3	up to 122	123-148	149-172	173 plus
5	4	up to 127	128-154	155-179	180 plus
5	5	up to 131	132-158	159-185	186 plus
5	6	up to 135	136-163	164-190	191 plus
5	7	up to 139	140-168	169-196	197 plus
5	8	up to 143	144-173	174-202	203 plus
5	9	up to 147	148-178	179-207	208 plus
5	10	up to 151	152-182	183-213	214 plus
5	11	up to 155	156-187	188-218	219 plus
6	0	up to 159	160-191	192-224	225 plus
6	1	up to 163	164-196	197-229	230 plus
Estimate of Systolic Blood Pressure		119 or less	120 to 139	140 to 159	160 or more
Estimate of Blood Cholesterol		199 or less	200 to 224	225 to 249	250 or more

Continued.

WHAT YOUR SCORE MEANS	
0-4	You have one of the lowest risks of heart disease for your age and sex.
5-9	You have a low to moderate risk of heart disease for your age and sex, but there is some room for improvement.
10-14	You have a moderate to high risk of heart disease for your age and sex, with considerable room for improvement on some factors.
15-19	You have a high risk of developing heart disease for your age and sex, with a great deal of room for improvement on all factors.
20 & over	You have a very high risk of developing heart disease for your age and sex and should take immediate action on all risk factors.

Warning

If you have diabetes, gout, or a family history of heart disease, your actual risk will be greater than indicated by this appraisal.

If you do not know your current blood pressure or blood cholesterol level, you should visit your physician or health center to have them measured. Then figure your score again for a more accurate determination of your risk.

If you are overweight, have high blood pressure or high blood cholesterol, or smoke cigarettes, your long-term risk of heart disease is increased even if your risk in the next several years is low.

HOW TO REDUCE YOUR RISK

- Try to quit smoking permanently. There are many programs available.
- Have your blood pressure checked regularly, preferably every 12 months after age 40. If your blood pressure is high, see your physician. Remember, blood pressure medicine is only effective if taken regularly.
- Consider your daily exercise (or lack of it). A half hour of brisk walking, swimming, or other enjoyable activity should not be difficult to fit into your day.
- Give some serious thought to your diet. If you are overweight or eat a lot of foods high in saturated fat or cholesterol (whole milk, cheese, eggs, butter, fatty foods, fried foods) then changes should be made in your diet. Look for the *American Heart Association Cookbook* at your local bookstore.
- Visit or write your local Heart Association for further information and copies of free pamphlets on many related subjects, including the following:
  - Reducing your risk of heart attack
  - Controlling high blood pressure
  - Eating to keep your heart healthy
  - How to stop smoking
  - Exercising for good health

SOME WORDS OF CAUTION

- If you have diabetes, gout, or a family history of heart disease, your real risk of developing heart disease will be greater than indicated by your RISKO score. If your score is high and you have one or more of these additional problems, you should give particular attention to reducing your risk.
- If you are a woman under age 45 or a man under age 35, your RISKO score represents an upper limit on your real risk of developing heart disease. In this case, your real risk is probably lower than indicated by your score.
- Using your weight category to estimate your systolic blood pressure or your blood cholesterol level makes your RISKO score less accurate; your score will tend to overestimate your risk if your actual values on these two important factors are average for someone of your height and weight, and your score will underestimate your risk if your actual blood pressure or cholesterol level is above average for someone of your height or weight.

Lab Activity 2-3

Measuring Blood Pressure

Name _____ **Section** _____ **Date** _____

PURPOSE   To gain practice in measuring blood pressure.*

PROCEDURE
1. Have a partner sit comfortably in a chair with the arm supported on a table (Figure 2-7).
2. Place the blood pressure cuff securely around the arm just above the elbow, with the arrow pointing to the center of the elbow joint.
3. Place the stethoscope over the artery in the center of the elbow crease, and have the subject hold it steady with the hand.
4. Hold the bulb in your hand so that the screw valve can be opened and closed with one hand.
5. Close the valve, and inflate the pressure to approximately 160-180 mm Hg as read on the pressure gauge.
6. Slowly open the screw valve, letting air escape, and watch the needle begin to fall on the pressure gauge.
7. Listen for the presence of a beat or thumping sound and mark the pressure at which the sound was first heard. This will be systolic pressure.
8. Continue to decrease the cuff pressure while listening to the beat sound. When the beat sound disappears, mark the pressure level and record that number as diastolic pressure.
9. Your partner can practice on you; fill in your systolic and diastolic pressures below.
10. Practice using the blood pressure cuff on *yourself.* Change arms or stand up to see any differences in blood pressures.

$$\text{Blood Pressure} = \frac{\text{Systolic Pressure}}{\text{Diastolic Pressure}} = \frac{\text{mm Hg}}{\text{mm Hg}}$$

INTERPRETATION   Normal blood pressure is usually considered to be approximately 120/80 mm Hg. Many factors can influence blood pressure. If your blood pressure reading deviates from normal, it is best to repeat this measurement several different times to determine whether a sustained deviation exists. Blood pressures that are consistently in excess of 140/90 are indicative of hypertension, and pressures below 100/60 are considered hypotension. In either case a physician should be consulted.

*It takes a significant amount of practice to become proficient at accurately measuring blood pressure.

Continued.

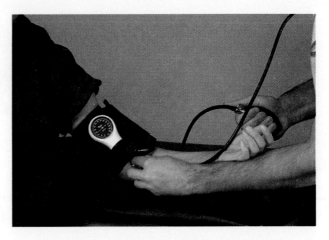

FIGURE 2-7. **Measuring Blood Pressure.**

Lab Activity 2-4

Are You at Risk for Skin, Breast, or Cervical Cancer?

Name _____ **Section** _____ **Date** _____

PURPOSE   Some people may have more than an average risk of developing certain cancers. These people can be identified by certain risk factors. This simple self-testing method is designed by the American Cancer Society to help you assess your risk factors for three common types of cancer. These are the major risk factors but by no means represent the only ones that might be involved.

PROCEDURE   Check your response to each risk factor. Add the number in the parentheses to arrive at a total score for each cancer type. Find out what your score means by reading the information in the right-hand column. You are advised to discuss this information with your physician if you are at higher risk.

Skin Cancer

1. Frequent work or play in the sun.
   a. Yes (10)   b. No (1)

2. Work in mines, around coal tars, or around radioactivity.
   a. Yes (10)   b. No (1)
3. Complexion—fair skin and/or light skin.
   a. Yes (10)   b. No (1)

Your total points _____

Interpretation

Numerical risks for skin cancer are difficult to state. For instance, a person with a dark complexion can work longer in the sun and be less likely to develop cancer than a light complected person. Furthermore, a person wearing a long-sleeved shirt and a wide brimmed hat may work in the sun and be less at risk than a person who wears a bathing suit in the sun for only a short period. The risk goes up greatly with age.

The key here is that if you answered *yes* to any question, you need to realize that you have above-average risk.

Breast Cancer

1. Age groups
   a. 20-34 (10)   c. 50 and over (90)
   b. 35-49 (40)
2. Ethnic group
   a. Oriental (5)   c. White (25)
   b. Black (20)   d. Mexican-American (10)
3. Family history
   a. Mother, sister, aunt, or grandmother with breast cancer (30)
   b. None (10)

Explanation

1. Excessive ultraviolet light causes skin cancer. Protect yourself with a sun screen medication.
2. These materials can cause skin cancer.

3. Light complexions need more protection than others.

Explanation

1. Breast self-exam is recommended for women over age 20.

2. Breast cancer is the second leading cause of death from cancer in white females.

3. Females over age 50, particularly those with family history, are at greatest risk.

Continued.

4. Your history
   a. No breast disease (10)
   b. Previous noncancerous lumps or cysts (25)
   c. Previous breast cancer (100)
5. Maternity
   a. First pregnancy before age 25 (10)
   b. Pregnancy after age 25 (15)
   c. No pregnancies (2)

Your total points _____

Interpretation

Under 100   Low-risk women should practice monthly breast self-examination (BSE) and have their breasts examined by a doctor as part of a cancer-related checkup.

100-199   Moderate-risk women should practice monthly BSE and have their breasts examined by a doctor as part of a cancer-related checkup. Periodic breast x-rays should be included as your doctor may advise.

200 or higher   High-risk women should practice monthly BSE and have the above examinations more often. See your doctor for the recommended frequency of physical and x-ray examinations appropriate for you.

Cervical Cancer*

1. Age group
   a. Under 25 (10)   c. 40-54 (30)
   b. 25-39 (20)   d. 55 and over (30)

2. Ethnic group
   a. Oriental (10)   d. White (10)
   b. Puerto Rican (20)   e. Mexican-American (20)
   c. Black (20)
3. Number of pregnancies
   a. 0 (10)   c. 4 and over (30)
   b. 1 to 3 (20)
4. Viral infections
   a. Herpes and other viral infections or ulcer formations on the vagina (10)
   b. Never (1)
5. Age at first intercourse
   a. Before 15 (40)   c. 20-24 (20)
   b. 15-19 (30)   d. 25 and over (10)
6. Bleeding between periods or after intercourse?
   a. Yes (40)   b. No (1)

Your total points _____

Explanation

1. The highest occurrence is in the 40-year-and-over age group. The numbers represent the relative rates of cancer for different age groups. A 45-year-old woman has a risk three times higher than a 20-year-old.

2. Puerto Ricans, Blacks, and Mexican-Americans have higher rates of cervical cancer.

3. Women who have delivered more children have a higher occurrence.

4. Viral infections of the cervix and vagina are associated with increased risk of cervical cancer.

5. Women with earlier intercourse and with more sexual partners are at a higher risk.

6. Irregular bleeding may be a sign of uterine cancer.

Interpretation

40-69   This is a low-risk group. Ask your doctor for a Pap test. You will be advised how often you should be tested after your first text.

70-99   In this moderate-risk group, more frequent Pap tests and annual pelvic exams may be required.

100 or higher   You are in a high-risk group and should have a Pap test (and pelvic exam) as advised by your doctor.

*The cervix is the lower portion of the uterus. These questions would not apply to a woman who has had a complete hysterectomy.

Lab Activity 2-5

Health Satisfaction Scale

Name _____   **Section** _____   **Date** _____

PURPOSE   This activity will help determine your level of health satisfaction.

PROCEDURE   Indicate how strongly you agree or disagree with the following statements, using the scale provided below.

1 = strongly disagree   2 = disagree   3 = neutral feelings   4 = agree   5 = strongly agree

_____   1. I believe that the amount of regular exercise I obtain is adequate.
_____   2. I think that my weight and amount of body fat are acceptable for someone my age and height.
_____   3. I do not smoke, drink excessively, or use "recreational" drugs such as marijuana because their use is unhealthy.
_____   4. I believe that my emotional health is stable.
_____   5. I think that my concern for personal safety is high. I use safety belts while riding in moving vehicles, wear a helmet while biking, have smoke detectors, etc.
_____   6. I believe that I obtain enough rest.
_____   7. I take the time to engage in various relaxation activities.
_____   8. The quality of the environment in which I live is healthy.
_____   9. My diet is nutritious and varied.
_____ 10. I believe that I am in control of my life and accept the responsibility for my actions.
_____ Total points

INTERPRETATION

Point range	Health satisfaction rating
40-50	Highly satisfied
35-39	Fairly satisfied
<35	Unsatisfied

If your health satisfaction rating is in the fair or low range, what actions can you take to improve it?

Modified from Allen, Hyde: *Investigations in stress control,* Minneapolis, 1981, Macmillan.

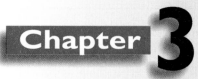

Chapter 3

Overcoming Behaviors That Interfere With Health and Fitness

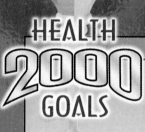

HEALTH 2000 GOALS

- **Drug Abuse.** Reduce drug-abuse–related hospital emergency department visits by at least 20%.
- **Alcohol Abuse.** Reduce the proportion of college students engaging in recent occasions of heavy drinking of alcoholic beverages to no more than 32%. In 1989, 41.7% of college students had, within the past 2 weeks, consumed five or more drinks on one occasion.
- **Tobacco Use.** Tobacco use is the most preventable cause of death and disease. Reduce cigarette smoking to a prevalence of no more than 15% among people age 20 and older. In 1987, 29% of adults smoked. *Midpoint Update: headed in the right direction with current statistic of 25%; however, recent reports indicate that more young people are beginning to smoke.*
- **Sexually Transmitted Diseases (STDs).** By age 21 one out of every five people has required treatment for an STD. Increase to at least 75% the proportion of primary care and mental health care providers who provide age-appropriate counseling on the prevention of HIV and other STDs.
- **HIV Education.** Provide HIV education for students and staff in at least 90% of colleges and universities.

OBJECTIVES

After completing this chapter, you will be able to do the following:

- Discuss the problem of substance abuse and the reasons why an individual may develop a dependency.
- Identify various drugs that are commonly abused and explain the negative effects they can have on a healthy lifestyle.
- Discuss the abuse of alcohol in the college population and explain why so many people develop problems from drinking.
- Discuss how the use of and exposure to tobacco products can affect your health.
- Explain how sexually transmitted diseases are spread, and tell what can be done to minimize this problem.

KEY TERMS

While reading this chapter, you will become familiar with the following terms:

- substance abuse
- psychological dependence
- physical dependence
- addiction
- tolerance
- habituation
- withdrawal syndrome
- anabolic steroids
- alcoholism
- tobacco use
- sexually transmitted diseases (STDs)

To be healthy and physically fit means that a person must develop lifestyle habits that exclude negative practices such as substance abuse, smoking, and unsafe sexual practices. Engaging in these lifestyle behaviors interferes with your efforts to become physically fit, and the long-term effects can potentially pose a major threat to your health and well-being. The following box offers a number of points to consider before making decisions that could have long-term effects on your quality of life.

SUBSTANCE ABUSE

Substance abuse is a crucial problem in American society and on college campuses. In addition, it is a major deterrent to health and fitness.

Substance abuse differs from drug use and drug misuse. *Drug use* refers to the taking of any drug for medical purposes. *Drug misuse* refers to the irresponsibility that many individuals show in their use of drugs. Persons who ignore medical advice about proper use of a prescribed drug or lend prescriptions to others are exhibiting a misuse of drugs. Substance abuse may be defined as the use of various substances for nonmedical reasons; that is, with the intent of getting "high"—altering mood or behavior—or for the purpose of enhancing performance. The terms *addiction* and *dependence* are often associated with substance abuse.

Addiction and Dependence

There are two general aspects of dependence—psychological and physical. Psychological dependence is the desire to repeat the ingestion of a drug to produce pleasure or to avoid discomfort. Physical dependence is the state of drug adaptation that manifests as the development of tolerance and, when the drug is removed, causes a withdrawal syndrome. The term addiction means physical dependence. An addicted individual's body needs a drug to function, builds a tolerance to that drug, and will in most cases suffer from withdrawal symptoms.

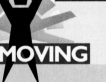

Reasons not to smoke, drink, take drugs, or have unprotected sex

GET MOVING

1. Using drugs or drinking alcohol when you are driving threatens everyone on the road—not just you.
2. Drinking too much the night before makes you feel miserable the next day.
3. The majority of people in this country find smoking, chewing, and spitting tobacco to be a disgusting habit.
4. No one should spend money on something that can cause as many health problems as tobacco does.
5. Getting drunk and abusing drugs makes you more likely to have unprotected sex.
6. Using cocaine or crack just once can lead to an addiction.
7. Excessive drinking or drug abuse can interfere in your relationships with your family, friends, peers, and co-workers.
8. There is no evidence that so-called "performance-enhancing drugs" actually enhance performance.
9. Large doses of anabolic steroids or human growth hormone will make you bigger, stronger, and faster, but they cause a variety of negative, sometimes irreversible, side effects on many organs.
10. Having sex with a number of partners is the best way to contract a sexually transmitted disease.
11. Decisions about having sex should be made before one is influenced by the "heat of the moment" or the effects of alcohol or drugs.
12. In today's world, having unprotected sex can kill you.

The Addictive Personality

There are many possible reasons why certain individuals develop addictions to drugs, alcohol, and tobacco. Certainly, your personality, that complicated set of attitudes and attributes that develop throughout your life as a result of previous experiences, may predispose you to addictive behavior patterns. But personality is not the sole cause of addictive behavior. It has been suggested that addictive behavior is closely related to the family environment and that your behavior is somehow linked to the way your parents and other family members used alcohol, drugs, or tobacco. Some believe that addiction is a disease in itself rather than secondary to some other physical or psychological disorder.

Alcohol and drugs are most commonly abused for their effects on mood and behavior. For example, a drug may produce a feeling of euphoria, often called a "high." These substances are often referred to as *psychoactive* or *psychotropic* drugs. However, certain drugs, when abused, can distort the personality to such a degree that individuals may become dangerous to themselves or society in general. Research has indicated that most individuals who abuse psychoactive substances have the type of personality that is often impressionable, escapist, or fragile. Persons with stronger personalities may experiment with drugs and alcohol but are less likely to become dependent on them because they do not satisfy their needs. The following Health Link box lists signs that may indicate a substance abuse problem.

Tolerance

Tolerance of a drug is the need to increase the dose to create the effect that was obtained previously by smaller amounts. The term *tolerance* refers to the physical reaction of the body to a frequently administered drug. Over time, the body builds tolerance to the usual level of certain drugs. Therefore after abusing one of these drugs for a period of time, a person no longer gets the same "high" unless the dose is increased. This is one reason that chronic drug abusers continually need to increase their number of "fixes" or doses of a drug.

Habituation

Habituation, another term used in connection with drugs, may be defined as psychological dependence as a result of continued use. Individuals may be habituated to the use of alcohol, cigarettes, or drugs. They can become habituated to almost anything if they feel that it is helping them. In other words, drug abuse can become a habit if individuals feel psychologically that it is helping them in some way.

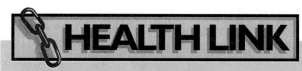

IDENTIFYING THE SUBSTANCE ABUSER

The following are signs of substance abuse:
- Sudden personality changes
- Severe mood swings
- Changing peer groups
- Decreased interest in extracurricular and leisure activities
- Worsening grades
- Disregard for household chores and curfews
- Feeling of depression most of the time
- Breakdown in personal hygiene habits
- Increased sleep and decreased eating
- Clothes and skin smell of alcohol or marijuana
- Sudden weight loss
- Lying, cheating, stealing, etc.
- Arrests for drunk driving or for possessing illegal substances
- Truancies from school
- Loses or changes jobs frequently
- Becomes defensive at the mention of drugs or alcohol
- Increased isolation (spends time in room)
- Family relationship deteriorates
- Drug paraphernalia (needles, empty bottles, etc.) found
- Others make observations about negative behavior
- Shows signs of intoxication
- Constantly misses appointments
- Falls asleep in class or at work
- Has financial problems
- Misses assignments or deadlines
- Diminished productivity

substance abuse the use of various substances for nonmedical reasons with the intent of altering mood or behavior and/or enhancing performance

psychological dependence the desire to repeatedly ingest a drug to produce pleasure or avoid pain/discomfort

physical dependence state of drug adaptation that develops due to the body's tolerance, resulting in physical withdrawal syndrome when the drug is removed

addiction refers to being physically dependent on a drug to function

tolerance physical reaction of the body to a frequently administered drug

habituation psychological dependence as a result of continual drug use

Withdrawal

Withdrawal symptoms are the unpleasant physical problems that occur when the drug is taken away. The withdrawal syndrome consists of an unpleasant physiological reaction when the drug is abruptly stopped. Some drugs that are abused by the athlete overlap with those thought to enhance performance. Examples include amphetamines and cocaine. Tobacco (nicotine), alcohol, cocaine, and marijuana are the most abused recreational drugs.

DRUG ABUSE
Narcotic Drugs

Narcotic drugs are derived directly from opium or are synthetic opiates. Morphine, codeine, heroin, and opium are examples of substances made from the alkaloid of opium. They may be injected, smoked, or taken orally. They produce euphoria, drowsiness, respiratory depression, nausea, and potentially coma or death. They are highly addictive both physically and psychologically.

Narcotic analgesics are used for the management of moderate-to-severe pain. They have a high risk of physical and psychological dependency, and many other problems stem from their use as well. It is believed that slight-to-moderate pain can be effectively dealt with by drugs other than narcotics.

Central Nervous System Stimulants

Central nervous system stimulants may be used to increase alertness, to reduce fatigue, or in some instances to increase competitiveness and even produce hostility. In general, some individuals respond to stimulants with a loss of judgment that may lead to personal injury or injury to others.

Two major categories of stimulants are psychomotor stimulant drugs and adrenergic drugs. Psychomotor stimulants are of two general types, amphetamines (e.g., methamphetamines) and nonamphetamines (e.g., cocaine). The major actions of psychomotor stimulants result from the rapid turnover of catecholamines (e.g., epinephrine and norepinephrine), which have a marked effect on the nervous and cardiovascular systems, metabolic rates, temperature, and smooth muscle. On the other hand, adrenergic drugs act directly on adrenergic receptors, or those that release catecholamines from nerve endings. Ephedrine is an example of this type; in high doses it can cause mental stimulation and increased blood flow. As a result, it may also cause elevated blood pressure, headache, increased and irregular heartbeat, anxiety, and tremors. Cocaine, amphetamines, and caffeine are the most commonly used psychomotor drugs.

Cocaine

Cocaine has become one of the most popular drugs of abuse during recent years. It has been estimated that more than 22 million Americans have tried cocaine at least once, and there has been a 91% increase in cocaine-related deaths since 1982. Cocaine, also known as "coke," "snow," "toot," "happy dust," and "white girl," is a powerful central nervous system stimulant with effects of very short duration. Cocaine use produces immediate feelings of euphoria, excitement, decreased sense of fatigue, and heightened sexual drive. Cocaine may be snorted, taken intravenously, or smoked ("free-based"). The initial effects are extremely intense, and since they are pleasurable, strong psychological dependence is developed rapidly by users regardless of whether they can afford to support this expensive habit.

Habitual use of cocaine will not lead to physical tolerance or dependence. An overdose can lead to overstimulation of the sympathetic nervous system and can cause tachycardia, hypertension, extra heartbeats, coronary vasoconstriction, stroke, pulmonary edema, aortic rupture, or sudden death.

Long-term effects include nasal congestion and damage to the membranes and cartilage of the nose if snorted; bronchitis; loss of appetite leading to nutritional deficiencies; convulsions; impotence; and cocaine psychosis with paranoia, depression, hallucinations, and disorganized mental function.

Crack. *Crack* is a rocklike crystalline form of cocaine that is heated in a small pipe and then inhaled, producing an immediate rush. The effects last for only a matter of minutes and are frequently followed by a state of depression. This sudden, intense stimulation of the nervous system predisposes the user to cardiac failure or respiratory failure and makes this commonly available drug extremely dangerous.

Amphetamines

Amphetamines are also called "uppers," "speed," "bennies," "crystal," "meth," and "crank." Amphetamines are synthetic alkaloids that are extremely powerful and dangerous drugs. They may be injected, inhaled, or taken as tablets. Amphetamines are among the most abused drugs used with the goal of enhancing sports performance. In ordinary doses, amphetamines can produce euphoria, with an increased sense of well-being and heightened mental activity (until fatigue from lack of sleep sets in) accompanied by nervousness, insomnia, and anorexia. In high doses, amphetamines reduce mental activity and impair performance of complicated motor skills. The athlete's behavior may become irrational. The chronic user may be "hung up" or, in other words, get stuck in a repetitious behavioral sequence. This perseveration may last for hours, becoming increasingly more irrational. The long-term, or even short-term, use of amphetamines can lead to "amphetamine psychosis," manifested by auditory and visual hallucinations and paranoid delusions.

Physiologically, high doses of amphetamines can cause mydriasis (abnormal pupillary dilation), increased blood pressure, hyperreflexia (increased reflex action), and hyperthermia.

In terms of sports performance, athletes believe that amphetamines promote quickness and endurance, delay fatigue, and increase confidence, thereby causing increased aggressiveness. Studies indicate that there is no improvement in performance, but there is an increased risk of injury, exhaustion, and circulatory collapse.

Caffeine

Caffeine is found in coffee, tea, cocoa, and cola, and is readily absorbed into the body. It is a central nervous system stimulant and diuretic and also stimulates gastric secretion. One cup of coffee can contain from 100 to 150 mg of caffeine. In moderation, caffeine causes a stimulation of the cerebral cortex and medullary centers in the brain, resulting in wakefulness and mental alertness. In larger amounts and in individuals who ingest caffeine daily, it raises blood pressure, decreases and then increases the heart rate, and increases plasma levels of epinephrine, norepinephrine, and renin. It affects coordination, sleep, mood, behavior, and thinking processes.

Some adverse effects of caffeine ingestion are tremors, nervousness, diuresis, arrhythmias, restlessness, hyperactivity, irritability, dry mouth, tinnitus, insomnia, headaches, and depression. A habitual user of caffeine who suddenly stops may experience withdrawal, including headache, drowsiness, lethargy, rhinorrhea (runny nose), irritability, nervousness, depression, and loss of interest in work. Caffeine also acts as a diuretic when hydration may be important.

Central Nervous System Depressants

Central nervous system depressants are commonly used for medical purposes. Depressants include barbiturates, benzodiazepines (sedatives), inhalants, and alcohol. Common street names for depressants are "downers," "ludes," "barbs," "goofballs," "rainbows," "nemmies," "tooies," and "reds." Depressants may be ingested, injected, or inhaled. They alter consciousness to some extent, promote sleep, relieve pain, relax muscles, relieve anxiety, slow breathing, and impair coordination and judgment.

Inhalants

Inhalants can damage the heart, brain, lungs, and liver. Inhalants are used to produce euphoria, and the initial effects are similar to those of alcohol. Glue, acetone, gasoline, kerosene, fingernail polish, aerosol sprays, lighter fluid, and butane have all been inhaled to create this effect.

Other Drugs

Marijuana

Marijuana is another one of the most abused drugs in Western society. It is more commonly called "grass," "weed," "pot," "dope," or "hemp." The marijuana cigarette is called a "joint," "j," "number," "reefer," or "root." Marijuana is often classified as a hallucinogenic drug. When used in small doses, it produces a "high" feeling and a sense of relaxation lasting for several hours. Larger doses can cause hallucinations.

Marijuana is not a harmless drug. The chemicals in marijuana enter the system either by smoking or ingestion. The components of marijuana smoke are similar to those of tobacco smoke, and the same cellular changes are observed in the user. The immediate effects of use are relaxation and feelings of heightened awareness of visual, auditory, and tactile sensations. It also causes impairment of coordination, performance, perception, attention, and short-term memory. Its effects on attention have linked its use to automobile accidents. Problems associated with long-term use include restlessness, irritability, loss of motivation, sleep disturbances, and possible damage to the lungs. With long-term use, both tolerance and psychological dependence can develop.

Continued use leads to respiratory diseases such as asthma and bronchitis and a decrease in vital capacity of 15% to as much as 40% (certainly detrimental to physical performance). Among other deleterious effects are lowered sperm counts and testosterone levels. Evidence of interference with the functioning of the immune system and cellular metabolism has also been found. The most consistent sign is the increase in pulse rate, which averages close to 20% higher during exercise and is a definite factor in limiting performance. Some decrease in leg, hand, and finger strength has been found at higher doses. Like tobacco, marijuana must be considered carcinogenic.

Psychological effects such as a diminution of self-awareness and judgment, a slowing of thought processes, and a shorter attention span appear early in

> **withdrawal syndrome** unpleasant physiological reaction(s) that can occur when ingestion of a drug is abruptly stopped

the use of the drug. Postmortem examinations of habitual users reveal not only cerebral atrophy but also alterations of anatomical structures, which suggests irreversible brain damage. Marijuana also contains unique substances (cannabinoids) that are stored, in very much the same manner as are fat cells, throughout the body and in the brain tissues for weeks and even months. These stored quantities result in a cumulative deleterious effect on the habitual user.

Hallucinogens

Hallucinogenic drugs have no medical value whatsoever; users take them to create illusions and hallucinations in an attempt to "go on a trip." They cause poor perception of time and distance. Hallucinogenic drugs are also referred to as "mesc," "angel dust," "PCP," "LSD," "hog," "buttons," or "cactus." These drugs have a high degree of psychological dependence.

The so-called "designer drugs" are chemical variations of medically useful drugs whose structure has been altered to produce extremely potent but dangerous street drugs that have somewhat unpredictable effects. Perhaps the most widely used designer drug is currently "ecstacy" (MDMA). Ecstacy causes a euphoric high, along with increased blood pressure, sweating, rapid heartbeat, visual distortion, erratic mood swings, and paranoia.

Anabolic Steroids

Anabolic steroids are synthetically created chemical compounds whose structure closely resembles that of naturally occurring sex hormones—in particular the male hormone testosterone. These drugs are prescribed and used therapeutically in the treatment of diseases in which protein synthesis is an essential component of the healing process. Athletes use these drugs for increasing lean body weight, muscle mass, and strength.

Anabolic steroids have both androgenic and anabolic effects. Androgenic effects include growth development, maintenance of reproductive tissues, and masculinization in males. Anabolic effects promote nitrogen retention, which leads to protein synthesis in skeletal muscles and other tissues and can result in an increase in muscle mass, weight, general growth, and bone maturation. Individuals who choose to take anabolic steroids are seeking to maximize the anabolic effects while minimizing the androgenic side effects. The problem is that no steroids exist that produce only anabolic effects; they also have androgenic effects.

Anabolic steroids do increase muscle size and strength when taken in conjunction with an intense weight-training program over a period of 1 to 2 months. However, it has also been proposed that prolonged use of anabolic steroids may result in harmful side effects such as liver dysfunction, reduced testicular function and loss of sexual interest, headaches, nausea, acne, unpredictable aggressive behavior, increased risk of coronary heart disease, and kidney tumors (Table 3-1).

In 1984, the American College of Sports Medicine (ACSM) reported that anabolic steroids taken with an adequate diet could contribute to an increase in body weight and that with a heavy resistance program could produce a significant gain in strength. However, when used in mass quantities as is typically done by individual athletes, they can have many deleterious and irreversible side effects that constitute a major threat to the health of the athlete. The following Health Link box summarizes the ACSM's worldwide literature review on the effects of anabolic steroids.

Anabolic steroids present an ethical dilemma for the sports world. It is estimated that over a million young male and female athletes are taking or have taken them, with most being purchased through the black market. Approximately 6.5% of male and 1.9% of female athletes are taking anabolic steroids. An estimated 2.5% of intercollegiate athletes take anabolic steroids. The more commonly used anabolic steroids include Anavar, Dianabol, and Anadrol.

TABLE 3-1.   Steroids and Your Body

Tissue/ Body Part	Reported Effects
Brain	Increased hostile or aggressive behavior Psychological dependence
Skin	Excessive growth of facial and body hair in females Female baldness Acne
Breasts	Male development Decreased size and increased risk of cancer in females
Heart	Increased blood pressure, potential for stroke and heart attack
Liver	Cancer and bleeding
Genitals	Male sterility and reduction in testicle size Enlargement of genitals in females
Muscles	Stimulates muscle growth Reduces workout recovery time
Other	Voice deepens or becomes hoarse in females Prostate cancer Kidney damage Menstrual problems

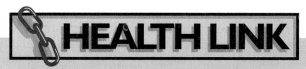

EFFECTS OF ANABOLIC STEROIDS

The following position statement of the American College of Sports Medicine is the result of a worldwide literature review on the effects of anabolic steroids.

- The administration of anabolic-androgenic steroids to healthy humans below age 50 in medically approved therapeutic doses often does not of itself bring about any significant improvements in strength, aerobic endurance, lean body mass, or body weight.
- There is no conclusive scientific evidence that extremely large doses of anabolic-androgenic steroids either aid or hinder athletic performance. The prolonged use of oral anabolic-androgenic steroids has resulted in liver disorders in some persons. Some of these disorders are apparently reversible with the cessation of drug use, but others are not.

- The administration of anabolic-androgenic steroids to male humans may result in a decrease in testicular size and function and a decrease in sperm production. Although these effects appear to be reversible when small doses of steroids are used for short periods of time, the reversibility of the effects of large doses over extended periods of time is unclear.
- Serious and continuing efforts should be made to educate male and female athletes, coaches, physical educators, physicians, trainers, and the general public regarding the inconsistent effects of anabolic-androgenic steroids on improvement of human physical performance and the potential dangers of taking certain forms of these substances, especially in large doses, for prolonged periods.

Human Growth Hormone

Human growth hormone (HGH) is produced by the somatotrophic cells of the anterior region of the pituitary gland, from which it is released into the circulatory system. The amount released varies with age and the developmental periods of a person's life. A lack of HGH can result in dwarfism. In the past, HGH was in limited supply because it was extracted from cadavers. Now, however, it can be made synthetically and is more available.

Experiments indicate that HGH can increase muscle mass, skin thickness, connective tissues in muscle, and organ weight and can produce lax muscles and ligaments during rapid growth phases. It also increases body length and weight and decreases body fat percentage.

The use of HGH by athletes throughout the world is on the increase because it is more difficult to detect in urine than anabolic steroids. There is currently a lack of concrete information about the effects of HGH on the athlete who does not have a growth problem. It is known that an overabundance of HGH in the body can lead to premature closure of long-bone growth sites or, conversely, can cause acromegaly, a condition that produces elongation and enlargement of bones of the extremities and thickening of bones and soft tissues of the face. Also associated with acromegaly are diabetes mellitus,

cardiovascular disease, goiter, menstrual disorders, decreased sexual desire, and impotence. It decreases the life span by up to 20 years. As with anabolic steroids, HGH presents a serious problem for the sports world. At this time there is no proof that an increase of HGH combined with weight training contributes to strength and muscle hypertrophy.

ALCOHOL ABUSE

An estimated three out of every four college students drink, and one out of every five considers himself or herself a heavy drinker. As a result of the high incidence of drinking in colleges and universities, problems have developed such as students missing classes because of hangovers, drinking while driving, engaging in violent behavior, and damaging property while under the influence. In light of these and other problems, some states have raised the minimum drinking age, and colleges and universities are increasingly placing restrictions on the use of alcohol on their campuses.

> **anabolic steroids** organic compounds that primarily contain sterol and sex hormones and are used for increasing lean body weight, muscle mass, and strength

Why Do People Drink?

The reasons that people abstain, drink moderately, or imbibe heavily have never been completely explained. Studies seem to indicate that alcohol serves to meet individual need patterns. It is felt that situations and environmental conditions that produce tension and insecurity may cause some to resort to drinking. People who are uncomfortable and lack poise at social gatherings use drinking as a social lubricant. The alcohol gives them courage and helps them feel at ease. Unfortunately, some people have failed to develop wholesome interpersonal relationships. Alcohol provides a temporary means of escape from those experiences that frustrate and worry them. Drinking does not solve the problem but instead offers a temporary means of escape from reality. Although there are some conflicting views as to its cause, there appears to be agreement that some of the causes are psychological. Some psychologists believe that individuals who are emotionally disturbed, have compulsive personalities, or exhibit obsessive-compulsive behavior are more prone to alcoholism.

What Is Alcoholism?

Alcoholism is called a disease because an alcoholic is sick, totally dependent on the substance and the abuse of it. The National Council on Alcoholism defines an alcoholic as "a person who is powerless to stop drinking, and whose drinking seriously alters his normal living pattern." Many persons may ask, "Why do some people become alcoholics while others in the same situation or environment do not?" Why is it that only 10% to 15% of the more than 100 million drinkers become alcoholics? This is a valid question for which there is no absolute answer. There are many potential alcoholics who do not become alcoholics. Unfortunately, alcoholism is a chronic condition that does not go away. It is progressive and incurable as long as the alcoholic continues drinking. If he or she stops drinking, the disease can be arrested. But most experts believe that the alcoholic cannot drink again. Otherwise that person will be right back where he or she was when the decision was made to stop drinking. Alcoholics are sensitive to alcohol and all other sedatives. The brain of an alcoholic produces a substance called *THIQ*, which is extremely addicting. Years of abstinence will not eliminate the ability to produce THIQ. It is always present and renders the alcoholic powerless to quit once he or she begins drinking.

What Are the Effects of Alcohol?

Alcohol is classified as a drug that depresses the central nervous system. Alcohol is absorbed from the digestive system into the bloodstream very rapidly.

Factors that affect how rapidly absorption takes place include the number of drinks consumed, the rate of consumption, alcohol concentration of the beverage, and the amount of food in the stomach. Some alcohol is absorbed into the blood through the stomach, but the greater part is absorbed through the small intestine. Alcohol is transported through the blood to the liver, where it can be metabolized at a rate of $2/3$ oz per hour. An excess causes an increase in the level of alcohol circulating in the blood. As blood alcohol content (BAC) levels continue to increase, predictable signs of intoxication appear. At 0.1% the person loses motor coordination, and from 0.2% to 0.5% the symptoms become progressively more profound, perhaps even life threatening. Intoxication persists until the remainder of the alcohol can be metabolized by the liver. There is no way to "sober-up" by accelerating the liver's metabolism of alcohol; it just takes time. Figure 3-1 shows how your BAC increases with the rate of alcohol consumption. The following Safe Tip box will clarify the alcohol content of many common drinks.

Alcohol-Related Diseases

Alcohol consumption can directly or indirectly cause numerous physical problems. Gastritis, an inflammation of the stomach, can result from excessive alcohol consumption. Alcoholics suffer from malnutrition because they lose interest in food and are unable to purchase proper foods. Also, alcohol provides considerable calories but lacks important nutrients.

Alcohol is poisonous to cells. The most common cause of liver disorders, cirrhosis (a scarring and hardening of liver tissue), is a result of chronic alcoholism. Over the years there has been some linkage of alcohol to cancer, especially cancer of the liver, larynx, esophagus, and tongue. These represent only a few of the diseases caused when excessive amounts of alcohol are consumed for extended periods of time.

How can you tell whether you currently have or are developing a drinking problem? You must identify the warning signs that let you know that the potential for such a problem exists. Lab Activity 3-1 will give you some indication of how critical your drinking problem is.

TOBACCO USE

The number of deaths caused by tobacco use is alarming. Every year 147,000 tobacco users die from cancer, 240,000 from heart disease, 61,000 from respiratory diseases, and 4000 from injuries such as fires caused by careless smokers. About 4000 infants die annually as a result of their mothers' smoking.

Number of drinks
in 2-hour period
(1½-oz 86-proof liquor
or 12-oz beer)

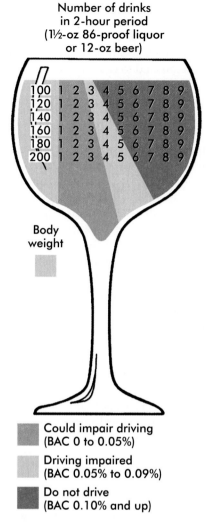

Body
weight

Could impair driving
(BAC 0 to 0.05%)

Driving impaired
(BAC 0.05% to 0.09%)

Do not drive
(BAC 0.10% and up)

FIGURE 3-1. The rate of alcohol consumption influences the blood alcohol content (BAC) level. (Modified from Hahn D, Payne W: *Focus on health,* ed 2, St Louis, 1994, Mosby.)

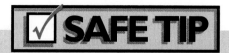

HOW MUCH ALCOHOL IS IN THIS DRINK?

The alcohol in beer is the same form of alcohol as in wine or distilled spirits such as whiskey and rum. However, the *concentration* is different. The following compares the concentration and the amounts you would have to drink to ingest the same amount of alcohol.

- A mixed drink made with 1.5 ounces of distilled spirits (40% alcohol = 80 proof) such as whiskey, rum, or vodka
- A 3-ounce glass of fortified wine (20% alcohol)
- A 5-ounce glass of table wine (12% alcohol)
- A 12-ounce beer (4.5% alcohol)
- A 10-ounce wine cooler (6% alcohol)

What do these figures mean? Each of these contains the same amount of pure alcohol. You can become just as intoxicated by drinking one 12-ounce can of beer as by drinking a 5-ounce glass of table wine. If you choose a mixed drink made with 1.5 ounces of vodka, it is just as intoxicating as a can of beer. However, keep in mind that the more concentrated the alcohol, the faster it can intoxicate. For example, if you drink a straight shot of whiskey (1.5 ounces), you'll feel the effects faster than if you drink a 5-ounce glass of table wine.

Tip: The percentage of alcohol by volume is noted on the label of the beverage container.

Why Do People Smoke?

The pleasure derived from smoking may be due as much to the social ritual that is associated with it as to the physiological effects. Certainly many of the young people who begin to smoke do so because they regard it as symbolic of adulthood. It has been suggested that smokers are not true addicts and that instead the habit-forming nature of tobacco is to a large extent psychologically and socially determined. But as millions of smokers know, smoking is a habit that becomes more difficult to break the more and the longer one smokes. It is known that nicotine is physically addictive. Although a smoker does not suffer the harsh withdrawal symptoms typical of certain addictive drugs, nervousness and irritability are commonly experienced when smoking is stopped.

What Is in Tobacco Smoke?

The major components of tobacco smoke are carbon monoxide, nicotine, and tars, all of which have harmful effects on the body. Tobacco smoke also contains pyridine compounds, ammonia, carbon dioxide, organic acids, aldehydes, and other substances. The more deeply the smoker inhales and the shorter the length to which the cigarette is smoked, the more nicotine is absorbed.

alcoholism a disease in which a person is unable to stop drinking and in which drinking results in a serious alteration of his or her normal living pattern
tobacco use the use of cigarettes, cigars, pipes, or smokeless tobacco

Nicotine

Nicotine, a colorless, oily compound, is extremely poisonous in concentrated form. One drop injected into an average-size man would kill him. Most smokers who inhale will absorb about 10% of the total nicotine content (about 20 to 30 mg in an average filtered cigarette). This small amount has certain physiological effects when absorbed into the bloodstream. However, about 90% of the absorbed nicotine is detoxified in the body before being eliminated by the kidneys.

Nicotine affects the body in a variety of ways. Small doses have a stimulating effect on various brain centers. It constricts the blood vessels of the skin, resulting in a clammy, pallid appearance and a reduction of skin temperature. Nicotine also increases the blood pressure and the heart rate. It has a numbing effect on the taste receptors of the tongue, hence the loss of interest in food by many heavy smokers. Beginning smokers may experience some slight toxic effects such as nausea and vomiting, but as the smoker builds up a tolerance, these generally disappear.

Carbon Monoxide

Approximately 1% of cigarette smoke is composed of carbon monoxide. A highly poisonous gas, carbon monoxide is also a component of automobile exhaust. Many individuals are killed each year by the inhalation of this gas in closed areas such as garages. The carbon monoxide in cigarette smoke reduces the oxygen-carrying capacity of the red blood cells and therefore causes a reduction of oxygen in the body. This is one of the reasons why smokers complain of "shortness of breath" after mild exercise.

Tar

Tobacco tar is a dark, sticky substance that can be condensed from cigarette smoke. It is the substance discussed in advertisements concerning "low tar and nicotine." Tar is extremely toxic and is *carcinogenic* (causing cancerous lesions) on test animals. The chemicals in cigarette tar are believed to contribute to the development of lung cancer.

Passive Smoke

There are dangers associated with the passive ("second hand") inhalation of smoke by nonsmokers. Both smokers and nonsmokers are exposed to smoke containing carbon monoxide, nicotine, ammonia, and cyanide. Obviously smokers inhale the greater quantity of contaminated air. However, it has been estimated that for each pack of cigarettes smoked, the nonsmoker sharing a common air supply will inhale the equivalent of three to five cigarettes. According to a review of passive smoking research, passive smoking may be responsible for as many as 15,000 premature deaths among exposed nonsmokers. It is also true that significant numbers of individuals exposed to passive smoke develop nasal symptoms, eye irritation, headaches, cough, and in some cases allergies to smoke. For these reasons and others, many state, local, and private sector policies have been established to restrict or ban smoking in public areas. There is little doubt that passive smoking poses a significant health threat to the nonsmoker.

Smokeless Tobacco

Unfortunately, the use of smokeless chewing tobacco has seen a tremendous increase in recent years. Once a pinch or pouch of chewing tobacco is placed "between the cheek and gum," nicotine is absorbed through the mucous membranes, and within a short period of time the level of nicotine in the blood is equivalent to that of a cigarette smoker. The user of chewing tobacco experiences the nicotine effects without exposure to the tar and carbon monoxide associated with a burning cigarette. Certainly the use of smokeless tobacco has eliminated many of the risks associated with cigarette smoking. However, inadvertently swallowed saliva contains carcinogens that must be eliminated through the digestive and urinary systems, thus predisposing the user to the risks of cancer. Additionally, the use of chewing tobacco increases the risk of periodontal disease in the gums, destroys the enamel on teeth, and causes the development of white blotches on the mucous membranes of the mouth, which are thought to be associated with development of cancer in the mouth.

Curbing Tobacco Use

Many steps have been taken to caution the nation's 53 million smokers about the dangers of tobacco. A warning from the U.S. Surgeon General is printed on each package of cigarettes. Television commercials for cigarettes have been banned. Group therapy sessions have been organized to help people stop smoking. Patches that deliver nicotine through the skin are often prescribed along with group sessions to help smokers "kick the habit." Special cigarette holders and filter tips have been devised to cut down on tar and nicotine. Many public buildings have been designated as nonsmoking areas. Municipalities are acting to ban smoking altogether in public places. In many states it is illegal to sell tobacco products to individuals under age 18. Yet millions of Americans, including many college students, continue to smoke. Many adults belong to the hard-core group of smokers who will never quit the habit. However, a major focus is educational efforts to prevent young people from choosing to begin to smoke. The following Health Link box lists some facts about smoking and makes suggestions for those who want to quit.

Lab Activity 3-2 will help you assess your knowledge about the use of cigarettes.

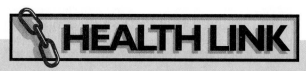

SMOKING: FACTS AND QUITTING TIPS

The Facts

Health Risks

- Smoking is an addiction. Tobacco smoke contains nicotine, a drug that is addictive and can make it very hard to quit.
- Smoking accounts for nearly a third of cancer deaths, including most lung cancer deaths.
- Smoking causes most deaths from lung cancer—a cancer that accounts for more than a quarter of all cancer deaths.
- Smoking is also a major cause of heart disease.

Effects on Others

- Smoking harms not just the smoker but also family members, people you work with, and others who breathe the tobacco smoke.
- Pregnant women who smoke are more likely to deliver babies with weights too low for the babies' good health. If all women quit smoking during pregnancy, about 4000 new babies would not die each year.
- During the first 2 years of life, children whose parents smoke are more likely to need to go to the hospital for bronchitis and pneumonia than children of parents who do not smoke.
- Children whose parents smoke are more likely to have sore throats and ear infections.
- Children whose parents smoke often become smokers themselves.

Who Smokes?

- Black men are more likely to smoke than white men (33% compared with 27%). So black men are more likely to develop cancers that are caused by smoking, especially cancer of the esophagus, lung, and larynx.
- About 23% of black and white American women smoke. Unfortunately, the smoking habits of black American women are not decreasing as quickly as the rate of smoking for American men.

Why Quit?

- Quitting smoking makes a difference right away—you can taste and smell food better. Your breath smells better. Your cough goes away. This happens for men and women of all ages, even those who are older. It happens for healthy people as well as those who already have a disease caused by smoking.
- Quitting smoking cuts the risk of lung cancer, many other cancers, heart disease, stroke, other lung diseases, and other respiratory illnesses.
- People who have stopped smoking have better health than those who smoke, fewer days off sick, fewer complaints about their health, and less bronchitis and pneumonia.
- After 15 years off cigarettes, the risk of death for ex-smokers nearly drops to the level of persons who have never smoked.
- Quitting saves money. The average smoker spends over $1000 per year on cigarettes.
  Questions on quitting? Call the National Cancer Institute's toll-free Cancer Information Service at 1-800-4-CANCER.

Quitting Tips

Getting Ready to Quit...

- Notice when and why you smoke. Try to find the things in your daily life that make you want to smoke (such as during your morning cup of coffee or after a meal).
- Change your smoking routines: Keep your cigarettes in a different place. Smoke with your other hand. Don't do anything else when smoking. Think about how you feel when you smoke.
- Smoke only in certain places, such as outdoors.

Continued.

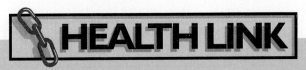

SMOKING: FACTS AND QUITTING TIPS—CONT'D

- When you want a cigarette, wait 1 minute. Try to think of something to do instead of smoking (chew gum, drink a glass of water).
- Buy one pack of cigarettes at a time. Switch to a brand of cigarettes you don't like.
- Set a date for quitting. If possible, have a friend quit smoking with you.

On the Day You Quit...

- Change your morning routine. When you eat breakfast, don't sit in the same place at the kitchen table. Stay busy.
- Get rid of all your cigarettes. Wet them down so you will not be able to get them out of the garbage. Put away your ashtrays.
- When you get the urge to smoke, do something else instead.
- Carry other things to put in your mouth, such as gum, hard candy, or a toothpick.
- Reward yourself at the end of the day for not smoking. See a movie or enjoy your favorite meal.

Staying Quit...

- Don't worry if you are sleepier or more short-tempered than usual; that will pass.
- Try to exercise more (take walks or ride a bike).
- Consider the positive things about quitting, such as how much you like yourself as a nonsmoker, health benefits for you and your family, and the example you set for others around you. A positive attitude will help you through the tough times.
- When you feel tense, try to keep busy, think about ways to solve the problem, tell yourself that smoking won't make it any better, and go do something else.
- Eat regular meals. Feeling hungry is sometimes mistaken for the desire to smoke.
- Start a money jar with the money you save by not buying cigarettes.
- Let others know that you have quit smoking—most people will support you. Many of your smoking friends may want to know how you quit. It's good to talk to others about your quitting.
- If you slip and smoke, don't be discouraged. Many former smokers tried to stop several times before they succeeded. Quit again.

If you need more help, see your doctor. He or she may prescribe nicotine gum or a nicotine patch to help you break your addiction to cigarettes. Or call the National Cancer Institute's toll-free Cancer Information Service at 1-800-4-CANCER for information.

Modified from National Cancer Institute: *Smoking: facts and quitting tips for black Americans,* NIH Pub No 92-3405, March, 1992.

SEXUALLY TRANSMITTED DISEASES

Sexually transmitted diseases (STDs) are infectious diseases that can be contracted through sexual contact. Any of the STDs can potentially be transmitted through sexual contact (including vaginal and anal intercourse and oral-genital contact) with an infected partner who may or may not show any signs or symptoms. STDs may be caused by bacteria or viruses. Bacterial infections such as gonorrhea, syphilis, and chlamydia may be cured with antibiotics in the majority of cases. Serious health problems are prevented if these infections are diagnosed and treated early. Viral infections such as herpes, genital warts, and HIV are much more difficult to treat, and in some cases no cure exists. Table 3-2 discusses the common STDs, their symptoms, treatment, and potential effects.

The current trend is to emphasize prevention through "safer sex" practices and treatment of STDs

TABLE 3-2. Common STDs

Any of these STDs can be transmitted through sexual contact (including vaginal and anal intercourse and oral-genital contact) with an infected partner who may or may not have symptoms.

STD	What Are the Signs?	How Do You Take Care of It?	Possible Problems
Chlamydia	About 75% of infected people have no symptoms. However, there may be a mild mucuslike discharge from the genitals or stinging when urinating. Also, there may be pain in the testicles (men) or abdomen (women).	Infected persons and their sexual partners must be tested and treated with antibiotics.	Painful infections of the reproductive organs, which may lead to infertility in both men and women.
Genital herpes	Sores around genitals or anus, often with small, painful blisters. Some people have no symptoms but are still infected and contagious.	Infected persons should avoid intimate sexual contact while sores persist. Acyclovir capsules or ointment may be helpful but will not cure herpes.	May contribute to cervical cancer and be transmitted to infants during childbirth.
Crab lice	Visible, blood-sucking lice in pubic hair. Causes itching. Eggs (nits) attached to hair shafts.	Treatments to kill lice. Recent sexual partners, clothing, and bed linen should be treated.	None.
Genital warts	Usually painless growths around the genitals or anus occur about 1-3 months after contact. In rare cases, growths may itch, burn, or bleed, or may not appear for years.	Chemical treatment, liquid nitrogen, laser beam, or surgery. May return after treatment.	May obstruct the urethra or complicate vaginal delivery in childbirth; may be connected to cervical cancer.
Trichomoniasis	Among women, symptoms may include a vaginal discharge, discomfort during sexual intercourse, abdominal pain, pain when urinating, and itching in the genital area. Most men have no symptoms, but some men may experience a penile discharge, painful urination, or a "tingly" feeling in the penis.	Infected persons and their partners are treated with antibiotics.	If untreated, may lead to bladder and urethral infections in men and women.

Continued.

rather than focus on the ethics of sexual behavior. Most important, some of these diseases have the potential to cause serious, long-term health problems, even death.

The American College Health Association emphasizes that "you do not have to feel guilty, ashamed or embarrassed if you think you have a sexually transmitted disease. But if you do have these feelings, do not let them prevent you from getting treatment. STDs do not go away by themselves, and in many cases, relatively quick, painless treatments are available. No one is immune to STDs. Everyone who is sexually active can get or transmit an STD. It does not matter if you are rich or poor, gay, or straight. It is not who you are that makes you vulnerable to a sexually transmitted disease—it is what you do. Reduce your risk by protecting yourself." Practicing safer sex may help

sexually transmitted diseases (STDs) infectious diseases that can be contracted through sexual contact

TABLE 3-2. Common STDs—cont'd

STD	What Are the Signs?	How Do You Take Care of It?	Possible Problems
Gonorrhea	Men may have a creamy puslike penile discharge and pain when urinating, or they may have no symptoms. Women may have vaginal discharge and pain when urinating, but often have no symptoms.	Infected persons and their sexual partners must be tested and treated with antibiotics.	If untreated, can cause arthritis, dermatitis, heart problems, and reproductive problems in both men and women. Can be transmitted to infants at birth, causing blindness.
Syphilis	Painless ulcer (chancre) at point of contact, usually penile shaft, around vaginal opening, or anus. Secondary stage may include rash or swollen lymph nodes.	Infected persons and their sexual partners must be tested and treated with antibiotics.	If untreated, may affect brain or heart, or even be fatal. Pregnant women can transmit to unborn infant.
Aids (Acquired Immunodeficiency Syndrome)	Increased susceptibility to common infections and unusual cancers. Most people infected with the virus may show no symptoms for many years but are still contagious.	No current proven treatment. Avoid sexual contact or practice "safer sex."	Full-blown AIDS almost always is fatal. Outlook for carriers of the virus is uncertain.

Modified from American College Health Association: *Making sex safer*, Baltimore, 1990, American College Health Association.

you to avoid contracting an STD. Your risk can be substantially decreased by following the guidelines in Figure 3-2.

Lab Activity 3-3 enables you to assess your safer sex practices and determine whether you are at risk for contracting a sexually transmitted disease.

HIV

Some special consideration must be given to the human immunodeficiency virus (HIV). *HIV* is a virus that may be transmitted from person to person through contact with different body fluids (e.g., blood, semen, and vaginal fluid). Within approxi-

---

FIGURE 3-2. Safer Sex Guidelines.

- **Form a monogamous relationship in which you and your partner make an agreement to be faithful sexually, and stick to it.** Avoid sexual intimacy until you and your partner have been tested for preexisting STDs.
- **Use condoms.** Although condoms do not provide 100% protection, they do provide the best protection now available. (For tips on the proper use of condoms, see the ACHA brochures "Making Sex Safer" and "Safer Sex.") If possible, also use a spermicide to create an additional barrier against some STDs. Women who feel hesitant about providing condoms and insisting on their use need to remember that

many STDs are more dangerous for them—females have fewer obvious symptoms and a higher risk of serious health consequences.
- **Include STD testing as part of your regular medical checkup, especially if you have changed partners or have more than one partner.** Do not wait for symptoms to appear.
- **Learn the common symptoms of STDs.** Seek medical help immediately if any suspicious symptoms develop, even mild ones.
- **Do not use drugs, including alcohol, in potentially intimate situations.** Drugs lower your ability to make sensible, self-protecting decisions.

mately 6 weeks after exposure to the virus, antibodies to HIV can be detected through a blood test. Unfortunately, in some cases symptoms do not become evident for up to 10 years after exposure. AIDS is a disease caused by HIV. AIDS is an acronym for acquired immunodeficiency syndrome. A *syndrome* is a collection of signs and symptoms that are recognized as the effects of an infection. HIV destroys a person's immune system so it does not battle other infections. Someone who has AIDS has no protection against even the simplest infections and thus is extremely vulnerable to developing a variety of illnesses, even cancers that cannot be stopped. Tests that detect the presence of HIV cannot predict when or if the individual will show the symptoms of AIDS. About 50% of people who are HIV positive develop AIDS within 10 years of becoming HIV infected. Those individuals who develop AIDS generally die within 2 years after the symptoms appear.

AIDS is the disease of the 1990s. Since it was first identified in 1981, more than 450,000 Americans have been reported as having AIDS. Approximately 250,000 have died from this disease through 1994. It is believed that over 1.5 million Americans are now infected with HIV (1 in 250), although most may not display signs or symptoms of HIV. One out of 100 adult males between age 20 and 49 is HIV positive. It is now the leading cause of death in people age 25 to 44 in the United States. There are 40,000 to 50,000 new cases each year. The World Health Organization estimates that worldwide there are 10 to 12 million adult

carriers of the virus, with 40 million estimated by the year 2000.

Even though some drug therapy may extend the lives of AIDS patients, there is currently no available treatment to cure those with this disease. Much work is being done to find a preventive vaccine and an effective treatment. Presently, antiviral drugs such as AZT have slowed replication of the virus and improved survival prospects.

Initially, symptoms of AIDS are similar to those of the flu: night sweats, fever, chills, excessive tiredness, sore throat, and persistent cough. The person may become free of symptoms for a while, but many proceed to develop full-blown AIDS. With AIDS, the individual develops a variety of life-threatening infections; the vast majority die within a few years.

HIV is transmitted by intimate sexual contact or by exposure to infected blood or other body fluids. You cannot get the virus simply by being around someone or touching someone who is infected with HIV. The virus enters the body through damaged skin or membranes. You can dramatically reduce your chances of contracting HIV by making careful choices about sexual activity, such as by knowing your sexual partner, using condoms during any type of sexual contact, avoiding injury to body tissues that results in bleeding during sex, and not mixing alcohol or drugs with sex. Drugs tend to cloud your judgment about sexual behavior. Also, avoid contact with the blood of others, and do not abuse intravenous (IV) drugs. A major way this virus is spread is through the sharing of IV drug needles by addicts.

SUMMARY

- Substance abuse is a crucial problem in American society and on college campuses. It is also a major deterrent to health and fitness.
- There are many possible reasons why certain individuals develop addictions to drugs, alcohol, and tobacco.
- Among the most common drugs of abuse are narcotics, stimulants (cocaine, amphetamines, caffeine), depressants (inhalants), hallucinogens, marijuana, anabolic steroids, and human growth hormone.
- An estimated three out of every four college students drink, and one out of every five considers

himself or herself a heavy drinker. The reasons that some people abstain, drink moderately, or imbibe heavily have never been completely explained.
- The number of deaths caused by tobacco use is alarming. There are dangers associated with the passive inhalation of smoke by nonsmokers. The use of smokeless chewing tobacco has seen a tremendous increase in recent years.
- Sexually transmitted diseases are extremely common and certainly have a negative impact on health. AIDS and other STDs are life-threatening diseases.

REFERENCES

Alcoholics Anonymous World Service: *Is AA for you?* New York, 1988, Alcoholics Anonymous.

American College Health Association: *Alcohol and other drugs: risky business,* Rockville, Md, 1991, The Association (pamphlet).

American College Health Association: *Making sex safer,* Baltimore, 1990, The Association (pamphlet).

American College of Sports Medicine: Position statement on the use and abuse of anabolic-androgenic steroids in sports, *Med Sci Sports Exerc* 16:13-18, 1984.

American Medical Association Department of HIV, Division of Health Science: *Digest of HIV/AIDS policy,* Chicago, 1993, American Medical Association Department of HIV.

American Red Cross: *First aid: responding to emergencies,* St Louis, 1991, Mosby.

American School Health Association: *Sex talk,* Research Triangle Park, NC, 1994, ASHA (pamphlet).

Burroughs-Wellcome: *There's something you should know: important information about sexually transmitted diseases,* Research Triangle Park, NC, 1995, Burroughs-Wellcome (pamphlet).

Byrd JC, Shapiro RS: Passive smoking: a review of medical and legal issues, *Am J Public Health,* 79(2):209, 1989.

Carroll CR: *Drugs in modern society,* ed 2, Dubuque, Iowa, 1989, William C Brown.

Centers for Disease Control and Prevention: *HIV/AIDS surveillance report,* Atlanta, 1991, CDC.

Fiore M, Novotny T, Pierce J: Methods used to quit smoking in the United States. Do cessation programs help? *JAMA* 263:2760, 1990.

Ray O, Ksir C: *Drugs, society, and human behavior,* ed 5, St Louis, 1996, Mosby.

Sachs D: Advances in smoking cessation treatment, *Curr Pulmonol* 12:139, 1991.

US Department of Health and Human Services: *The health benefits of smoking cessation,* DHHS Pub No (CDC) 90-8416, 1990.

US Department of Health and Human Services, Public Health Services: *Healthy people 2000: midcourse review and 1995 revisions,* Washington, DC, 1995, USDHHS.

US Department of Health and Human Services, Public Health Services: *Healthy people 2000: national health promotion and disease prevention objectives,* Washington, DC, 1991, USDHHS.

Wagner J: Enhancement of athletic performance with drugs: an overview, *Sports Med* 12:250-265, 1991.

SUGGESTED READINGS

Payne W, Hahn D: *Understanding your health,* ed 4, St Louis, 1995, Mosby.
Health text with separate chapters on drugs, alcohol, smoking, and sexually transmitted diseases.

Ray O, Ksir C: *Drugs, society, and human behavior,* ed 5, St Louis, 1996, Mosby.
A comprehensive and up-to-date text that looks at the problem of substance abuse and its effects on our society and individual behaviors.

Lab Activity 3-1

How Do You Use Alcoholic Beverages?

Name _____   **Section** _____   **Date** _____

PURPOSE   To determine your pattern of alcohol use.

PROCEDURE Answer these questions in terms of your own alcohol use. Record your number of *yes* and
no responses at the bottom of the questionnaire.

Do you:	Yes	No
1. Drink more frequently than you did a year ago?	_____	_____
2. Drink more heavily than you did a year ago?	_____	_____
3. Plan to drink, sometimes days in advance?	_____	_____
4. Gulp or "chug" your drinks, perhaps in a contest?	_____	_____
5. Set personal limits on the amount you plan to drink but then consistently disregard these limits?	_____	_____
6. Drink at a rate greater than two drinks per hour?	_____	_____
7. Encourage or even pressure others to drink with you?	_____	_____
8. Frequently want a nonalcoholic beverage but then end up drinking an alcoholic drink?	_____	_____
9. Drive your car while under the influence of alcohol or ride with another person who has been drinking?	_____	_____
10. Use alcoholic beverages while taking prescription or OTC medications?	_____	_____
11. Forget what happened while you were drinking?	_____	_____
12. Have a tendency to disregard information about the effects of drinking?	_____	_____
13. Find your reputation fading because of alcohol use?	_____	_____
Total	_____	_____

Continued.

INTERPRETATION

If you indicate *yes* on any of these questions, you may be demonstrating aspects of irresponsible alcohol use. Two or more *yes* responses indicate an unacceptable pattern of alcohol use and may reflect problem drinking behavior.

Test Your Knowledge About Cigarette Smoking

Name _____   **Section** _____   **Date** _____

PURPOSE   To determine your understanding of the factors involved in cigarette smoking.

PROCEDURE Answer *true* (T) or *false* (F) to each question; then consult the discussion section to determine the correct answer.

T or F		T or F	
____	1. There are now safe cigarettes on the market.	____	11. The "smoker's cough" reflects underlying damage to the tissue of the airways.
____	2. A small number of cigarettes can be smoked without risk.	____	12. Cigarette smoking does not appear to be associated with damage to the heart and blood vessels.
____	3. Most early changes in the body resulting from cigarette smoking are temporary.	____	13. Because of the design of the placenta, smoking does not present a major risk to the developing fetus.
____	4. Filters provide a measure of safety to cigarette smokers.	____	14. Women who smoke cigarettes and use an oral contraceptive should decide which they wish to continue, because there is a risk in using both.
____	5. Low-tar, low-nicotine cigarettes are safer than high-tar, high-nicotine brands.	____	15. Air pollution is a greater risk to our respiratory health than is cigarette smoking.
____	6. Mentholated cigarettes are better for the smoker than are nonmetholated brands.	____	16. Addiction, in the sense of physical addiction, is found in conjunction with cigarette smoking.
____	7. It has been scientifically proven that cigarette smoking causes cancer.	____	17. The best "teachers" a young smoker has are his or her parents.
____	8. No specific agent capable of causing cancer has ever been identified in the tobacco used in smokeless tobacco.	____	18. Nonsmoking and higher levels of education are directly related.
____	9. The cure rate of lung cancer is so good that no one should fear developing this form of cancer.	____	19. About as many women smoke cigarettes as do men.
____	10. Smoking is not harmful as long as the smoke is not inhaled.	____	20. Fortunately, for those who now smoke, stopping is relatively easy.

Continued.

Discussion	Discussion
1. F Depending on the brand, some cigarettes contain less tar and nicotine; none are safe, however.	12. F Cigarette smoking is, in fact, the single most important risk factor in the development of cardiovascular disease.
2. F. Even a low level of smoking exposes the body to harmful substances in tobacco smoke.	13. F Children born to women who smoke during pregnancy show a variety of health impairments, including smaller birth size, premature birth, and more illnesses during the first year of life. Smoking women also have more stillbirths.
3. T Some, however, cannot be reversed—particularly changes associated with emphysema.	
4. T However, the protection is far from adequate.	14. T Women over age 35 are particularly at risk for experiencing serious heart disease if they continue using both cigarettes and an oral contraceptive.
5. T Many persons, however, smoke low-tar, low-nicotine cigarettes in a manner that makes them just as dangerous as stronger cigarettes.	15. F Although air pollution does expose the body to potentially serious problems, the risk is considerably less than that associated with smoking.
6. F Menthol simply makes cigarette smoke feel cooler. The smoke contains all of the harmful agents found in the smoke from regular cigarettes.	16. T Dependency, including true physical addiction, is widely recognized in cigarette smoking.
7. T Particularly for lung cancer and cancers of the larynx, esophagus, oral cavity, and urinary bladder.	17. T There is strong correlation between cigarette smoking of parents and the subsequent smoking of their children. Parents who do not want their children to smoke should not smoke.
8. F Unfortunately, smokeless tobacco is no safer than the tobacco that is burned. The user of smokeless tobacco swallows much of what the smoker inhales.	18. T The higher one's level of education, the less likely one is to smoke.
9. F Approximately 10% of those persons having lung cancer will live the 5 years required to meet the medical definition of "cured."	19. T Although in the past more men smoked than did women, the trend is changing. Cigarette smoking is becoming a women's pastime.
10. F Because of the toxic material in smoke, even its contact with the tissue of the oral cavity introduces a measure of risk from this form of cigarette use.	20. F Unfortunately, smoking cessation is difficult, but many people have been successful in quitting. The best advice is never to begin smoking.
11. T The "cough" occurs in response to an inability to clear the airway of mucus as a result of changes in the cells that normally keep the air passages clear.	

What Is Your Risk of Contracting a Sexually Transmitted Disease?

Name _____   **Section** _____   **Date** _____

PURPOSE   A variety of factors interact to determine your risk of contracting a sexually transmitted disease (STD). This inventory is intended to provide you with an estimate of your level of risk.

PROCEDURE   Circle the number in each row that best characterizes you. Enter the number on the line at the end of the row (score line). After assigning yourself a number in each row, total the number appearing in the score column. Your total score will allow you to interpret your risk of contracting an STD.

							Score
Points **Age**	1 0-9	3 10-14	4 15-19	5 20-29	3 30-34	2 35+	_____
Points **Sexual practices**	0 Never engage in sex	1 One sex partner	2 More than one sex partner, but never more than one at a time	4 Two to five sex partners	6 Five to ten sex partners	8 Ten or more sex partners	_____
Points **Sexual attitudes**	0 Will not engage in premarital sex	1 Premarital sex is okay if it is with future spouse	8 Any kind of premarital sex is okay	1 Extramarital sex is not for me	7 Extramarital sex is okay	8 Believe in complete sexual freedom	_____
Points **Attitudes toward contraception**	1 Would use condom to prevent pregnancy	1 Would use condom to prevent STDs	6 Would never use a condom	5 Would use the birth control pill	4 Would use other contraceptive measure	8 Would not use anything	_____
Points **Attitudes toward STD**	3 Am not sexually active so I do not worry	3 Would be able to talk about STDs with my partner	4 Would check an infection to be sure	6 Would be afraid to check out an infection	6 Can't even talk about an infection	6 STDs are no problem—easily cured	_____

Your total score _____

Continued.

INTERPRETATION

5-8   Your risk is well below average

9-13   Your risk is below average

14-17 Your risk is at or near average

18-21 Your risk is moderately high

22+   Your risk is high

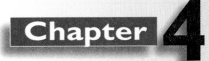

Chapter 4 — Getting Your Fitness Program Started

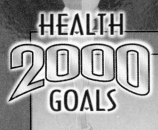

HEALTH 2000 GOALS

■ **Physical Activity and Fitness.** Participation in regular activity depends in part on the availability and proximity of community facilities and conducive environments.

• Fifty-one percent of adults agreed that greater availability of exercise facilities would help them become more involved in regular exercise.

• Leisure-time sedentariness increases with advancing age—33% of people age 45 to 64 and 43% of those age 65 and older engage in no leisure-time physical activity.

OBJECTIVES

After completing this chapter, you will be able to do the following:

■ Discuss the various principles of training and conditioning.
■ Identify the importance and the roles of warm-up, workout, and cool-down in a training program.

■ Discuss the precautions that should be exercised when working out in either a hot or a cold environment.
■ Discuss the impact of fitness activities on the menstrual cycle.
■ Describe the role of exercise during pregnancy.

KEY TERMS

While reading this chapter, you will become familiar with the following terms:

- overload
- SAID principle
- progression
- consistency

- specificity
- individuality
- exercise tolerance
- warm-up

- workout/activity
- cool-down
- heat stress

- hypothermia
- menstruation
- dysmenorrhea

Being healthy and physically fit is your own personal responsibility. To achieve an optimal state of fitness you must be willing and committed to making the effort. No one else can do it for you. If you make that effort you will see results that can change the the way you feel about yourself—and the way that others see you (Figure 4-1).

This chapter sets forth basic principles for a fitness program to help those who want to become physically fit. Much information has been generated regarding principles that should be observed to design the right kind of fitness program. The principles of fitness identified in this chapter will be followed and developed in subsequent chapters that focus on improving the components of health-related fitness.

BASIC PRINCIPLES OF A FITNESS PROGRAM

Regardless of the type of fitness activity in which you choose to participate, there are certain principles that should be incorporated into each and every program. These principles and guidelines apply to both those individuals who participate recreationally and those who are competitive athletes; the only difference is the level of intensity required. Incorporation of the seven principles we will discuss will help you to create an effective yet safe environment for fitness activities.

The Program Must Be Fun and Enjoyable

Enjoying yourself may be one of the most critical factors in a successful training program in the long run. The activity you select must be one that you enjoy and that provides motivation to continue with for a lifetime (Figure 4-2). For example, a quick look at the streets on a sunny day will show that running is a popular form of physical activity. There is no question that a running program will result in significant improvement in cardiorespiratory endurance over a period of time. However, some people simply hate to run and would prefer to do any other activity. If these people select running as their activity because it is "in" and not because they enjoy doing it, then chances are that they will not stick with it for very long. You

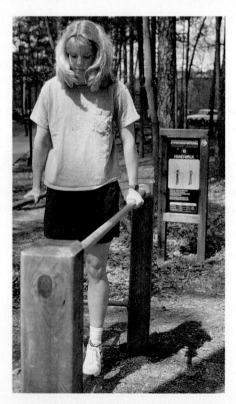

FIGURE 4-1. **Personal Fitness.**
Each person has his or her own reasons for engaging in a fitness program.

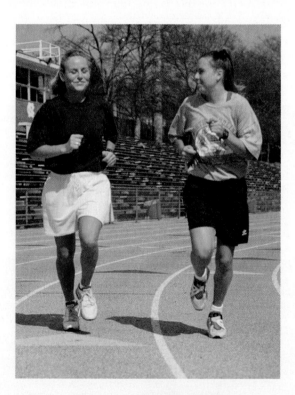

FIGURE 4-2. **Fitness is Fun.**

should enjoy getting into good physical condition, and a successful training program will be considered fun rather than work. The following Fit List box provides some suggestions to make physical activity more attractive.

Overload

To achieve the greatest benefits from the exercise program, you should recognize the principle of overload. For a physiological component of fitness to improve, the system must work harder than it is used to working. The system must experience stress so that over a period of time it will improve to the point at which it can easily accommodate additional stress (Figure 4-3).

The SAID Principle

The SAID principle (an acronym for Specific Adaptation to Imposed Demands) states that when the body is subjected to stresses and overloads of varying intensities, it will gradually adapt, over time, to overcome whatever demands are placed on it. Even though overload is a critical factor in training and conditioning, the stress must not be great enough to produce damage or injury. The body needs to have a chance to adjust to the imposed demands. Therefore overload is a gradual increase in the frequency, duration, or intensity of the physical activity that is a part of the training program. This is one of the most critical factors in any activity program.

For example, if you are on a running program to improve cardiorespiratory endurance and you go out and run 1 mile in 10 minutes, the cardiorespiratory

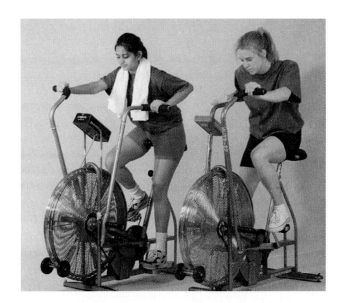

FIGURE 4-3. **Overload.**

system will be able to accommodate this distance and intensity very easily. However, if the long-range goal of your training program is to run the Boston Marathon, it is foolish to believe that you could finish a race of this distance and intensity by running only one 10-minute mile a day. If you gradually overload the system by running farther at a faster pace, you will force the cardiorespiratory system to work more efficiently to keep up with increased physiological demands. In weight training, adding more weight and decreasing the number of sets and repetitions will help in the development of muscular strength. Also, flexibility may be increased by stretching a muscle to a greater length than normal. Therefore by overloading the system over a long period of time, one should expect to produce significant improvement in that system's ability to handle a stressful exercise bout.

Progression

A little today and a little more tomorrow is a good principle to follow in any training program. You should start gradually and add a little each day in terms of repetitions of an exercise, speed, or endurance required. The rate of progression should be within your capabilities to adapt physiologically. In other words, the workout should gradually become a

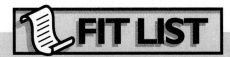

SUGGESTIONS FOR MAKING PHYSICAL ACTIVITY MORE ATTRACTIVE

Some students find physical activity dull. Here are some ways to make it more inviting:
- Exercise to music.
- Exercise with classmates.
- Keep your program simple.
- Instill variety into activity: for example, dancing, hiking, tennis, and swimming.
- Reward yourself when fitness goals are met.
- Don't become upset when goals are not met and benefits are not immediate.
- Keep a record of things such as your weight and the distance you jog.
- Plan the program to fit into your daily life.

---

overload   for a physiological component of fitness to improve, the system must work harder than it is used to working

SAID principle   acronym for Specific Adaptation to Imposed Demands: states that when the body is subjected to stresses and overloads of varying intensities, it will gradually adapt, over time, to overcome whatever demands are placed on it

little longer or more intense until you reach the desired level of physical fitness.

Progression is closely related to overload. Without overloading the system, progression does not occur. For example, in weight training, exercises are commonly referred to as a progressive resistive exercise (PRE). In a PRE program, a particular muscle is exercised through a full range of motion against resistance. Improvement in strength occurs only when the muscle is overloaded; progression in weight should occur only when the muscle has adapted to the increased overload.

Progression is also important for motivation. Interest level in an activity remains high as long as you continue to see improvement in your physical ability. Even though weight increases may be minimal in strength training, a progression of even 1 pound is often enough to maintain interest and motivation.

There comes a time in many fitness programs when *improving* fitness levels becomes less critical than maintaining fitness levels. When you reach this point, consistency becomes extremely important.

Consistency

One of the biggest problems with beginning a fitness program is finding time during the day to fit in an hour or so of activity. For the competitive varsity athlete, consistency is not a problem because a specific hour is assigned for practice, and everyone is required to be there at that time. The recreational athlete frequently has a problem finding a specific time unless he or she is involved in a class that meets on a scheduled basis. It is important to select a specific period of time for exercising each day and stick to it.

The best time of day to exercise is whenever you have the time and are motivated to do so. The important thing is to set aside some time for a fitness program and make it part of your daily routine. The least desirable times are probably after a meal, when activity may make you uncomfortable, and just before bedtime, when the activity may be so invigorating that it is difficult to fall asleep. The number of days per week you are involved with a specific activity will vary depending on a number of personal factors. Remember—even though you may be able to go walking or lift weights only three times a week, it is recommended that you try to engage in a minimum total of 30 minutes of accumulated activity each day. For the competitive athlete, three times per week is usually insufficient; he or she should attempt to work out five or six times per week.

"If you don't use it you will lose it." If you are not consistent in your exercise program, the many positive gains you have made may begin to reverse themselves.

Specificity

The type of physiological changes that occur are directly related to the type of training used. To realize the maximal gains in a physiological system, activities and programs should be selected and designed with specificity to achieve this aim. Once again according to the SAID principle, a particular physiological system will respond and adapt over time to whatever specific demands are placed on it. For example, to develop flexibility in a specific joint, stretching exercises must be incorporated that progressively lengthen the musculotendinous structures that surround that joint. To develop muscular strength in the upper arms, resistive exercises must be designed that overload the biceps and triceps muscles.

Individuality

When you become involved in an activity program, it is important to remember that no two persons are exactly the same; therefore training regimens should meet the criterion of individuality. People differ in things such as fitness goals, makeup of their physical resources, motivation, body build, and state of physical fitness. A training program for one person will not necessarily satisfy the needs of another person. Furthermore, not all persons involved in similar activities will progress at the same rate, nor will they be able to overload their systems to the same degree. Exercise is good, but it must be adapted to individuals' needs and abilities. Just as a medical prescription must be related to a person's health needs, so should a physical fitness prescription. A person's exercise prescription should be based on the individual's objectives, needs, functional capacity, and interests.

Stress levels also vary among individuals. It is important to consider the degree to which stress affects you and how it may interfere with your fitness program. Actually, some people tend to view physical activity as an outlet to release the stress that builds up during a day. However, for competitive athletes, the stress of competition may become detrimental to their well-being. Therefore, whether it is stress or any other individual characteristic, you should establish goals for your program before getting started.

Safety

Another factor to consider when planning a training program is safety. The purpose of the activity program should be to improve selected components of fitness through physical exercise. Unfortunately, injuries often occur as the result of poorly planned activity programs. Too often people who have been sedentary for long periods of time overestimate their physical abilities and "overdo" it. This overdoing may result in musculoskeletal injuries or other health problems. Therefore start out gradually with your exercise program to avoid injuries.

Other rules to observe to avoid injury or tragedy are to seek a safe route to walk or jog, especially when it is dark; engage in activities appropriate for your age; use safe exercise equipment; "listen" to your body for potential problems; and observe necessary precautions on cold or extremely hot days. Finally, participate at the appropriate intensity for your level of fitness.

Exercise tolerance means the manner in which the body responds to exercise. Physical activity should not produce prolonged fatigue and pain. Instead, the body should respond favorably to exercise. Afterward, you should feel invigorated and relaxed. In other words, exercise should be adapted to your tolerance level. The response of the body to physical activity will indicate what the tolerance level is. All things being equal, if there is a positive reaction to the physical activity, then it is suitable for your training program.

The rule of thumb to follow is to start out slowly and progress according to your own capabilities. Adherence to the rule "train don't strain" can certainly reduce the likelihood of injury. If you are unsure of how to get started or perhaps how quickly to progress in a personal fitness program, seek professional advice from persons with some background in exercise science, such as certified athletic trainers, physical educators, or physicians (see Appendix A for other sources of help).

THREE BASIC ELEMENTS OF EVERY TRAINING PROGRAM

You should be aware of the three basic elements of any physical fitness program: warm-up, workout/activity, and cool-down (Figures 4-4 and 4-5).

Warm-Up

A period of warm-up exercises should take place before the workout. The warm-up increases body temperature, stretches ligaments and muscles, and increases flexibility. Related warm-ups, those similar to the activity engaged in, are preferable to unrelated ones because of the rehearsal or practice effect that results.

Warm-ups have been found to be important in preventing injury and muscle soreness. It appears that muscle injury can result when vigorous exercises are not preceded by a related warm-up. An effective, quick warm-up can also be an effective motivator. If you get satisfaction from a warm-up, you probably will have a stronger desire to participate in the activ-

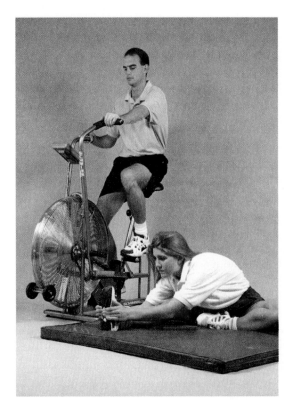

FIGURE 4-4. Warm-Up.
Warm-up should begin with an activity to elevate core temperature, followed by stretching.

progression starting gradually and adding a little each day in terms of repetitions of an exercise, speed, or endurance to increase performance

consistency selecting a specific period of time for exercising each day helps make exercise a part of one's regular routine

specificity to realize maximum gains in the physiological system, activities and programs should be selected with the end goal in mind

individuality exercise programs should be specifically designed for the *individual* because no two people have the same fitness goals, physical abilities, motivation, body composition, or preliminary level of physical fitness

exercise tolerance exercising at one's tolerance level should not result in prolonged fatigue, physical pain, or discomfort but should instead create feelings of invigoration and relaxation

warm-up prepares the body physiologically for exercise by increasing body temperature, stretching ligaments and muscles, and increasing flexibility

workout/activity period of physical activity consisting of a warm-up, stretching, cardiorespiratory exercise, and a cool-down

cool-down prevents pooling of the blood and enables the body to cool and return to a resting state

---

FIGURE 4-5. The Three Basic Elements of Training Programs.

The Warm-Up

- Take from 10 to 15 minutes to warm up.
- Engage in exercises that stretch muscles and put body joints through a full range of motion. Walking, slow jogging, and other activities can also be used to warm up.
- Exercise all body segments and muscle groups, including neck, shoulder girdle and joints, trunk, thigh joints, thighs, knees, and legs.
- Engage in exercises that cause a gradual increase in heart and circulatory system action.

The Workout

- Take from 30 minutes to 1 hour to work out.
- Engage in exercises and activities that will develop muscular strength and endurance, cardiorespiratory endurance, and flexibility.
- Adapt to individual needs.
- Alternate work and rest periods.
- As a beginner, increase duration of exercise intervals and keep exercise intensity constant.
- Monitor heart rate (see Chapter 5).

The Cool-Down

- Take from 5 to 10 minutes to cool down after working out.
- Engage in relaxing forms of exercise.
- Activities can include slow jogging, walking, and stretching exercises.
- Check heart rate, which should show recovery from acceleration during the workout.

---

ity. By contrast, a poor warm-up can lead to fatigue and boredom, limiting your attention and ultimately resulting in a poor program. There is some evidence that a good warm-up may also improve certain aspects of performance.

The function of the warm-up is to prepare the body physiologically for some upcoming physical work bout. Most professionals view the warm-up period as a precaution against unnecessary musculoskeletal injury and possible muscle soreness. The purpose is to very gradually stimulate the cardiorespiratory system to a moderate degree. This produces an increased blood flow to working skeletal muscles and results in an increase in muscle temperature.

Moderate activity speeds up the metabolic processes, producing an increase in core body temperature. Furthermore, an increase in the temperature of skeletal muscle causes an increased speed of contraction and relaxation, probably because the

speed of nerve impulse conduction is increased. The elastic properties (the length of stretch) of the muscle are increased, whereas the viscous properties (the rate at which the muscle can change shape) are decreased.

Before any workout/activities there should be a two part warm-up. This warm-up should include a general warm-up that precedes a specific warm-up. The general warm-up involves elevating the core temperature by static stretching exercises. The specific warm-up involves activities related to the workout/activity to be performed. These activities are sport-specific and should gradually increase in intensity. Also, the type of warm-up should be related to the muscles used in the activity. For example, a soccer player uses the upper extremity considerably less than the lower extremity. His or her specific warm-up should be directed more toward the lower extremity, perhaps by adding some stretching exercises for the lower extremity. The specific warm-up should also be sport-specific. For example, a basketball player should warm up by shooting lay-ups and jump shots and dribbling; a tennis player should hit forehand and backhand shots and serves.

The warm-up should last approximately 10 to 15 minutes. You should not wait longer than 15 minutes to start the activity after the warm-up, although the effects generally last for about 45 minutes. Thus the third-string football player who warms up before the game and then does nothing more than stand around until he enters the game during the fourth quarter runs a much higher risk of injury. This player should be encouraged to stay warmed up and ready to play throughout the course of a game. In general, sweating is a good indication that the body has been sufficiently warmed up and is ready for more strenuous activity.

A good warm-up should begin with 2 or 3 minutes of light jogging to increase metabolic rate and core temperature. This should be followed by a period of flexibility exercises in which the muscles are stretched to take advantage of the increase in muscle elasticity. Finally, the intensity of the warm-up should be increased gradually by performing body movements and skills associated with the specific activity in which you are going to participate.

Workout/Activity

Before beginning any activity, you should dress appropriately for the workout/activity, wearing clothes that will enable you to move freely and safely. Some exercise physiologists have suggested that a workout, or conditioning period, might consist of the following:

1. 10 to 15 minutes of warm-up
2. 10 minutes of strength exercises

3. 20 minutes of cardiorespiratory exercises at target heart rate (see Chapter 5)
4. 5 minutes of cool-down

Specific exercises for the workout are discussed in Chapters 5, 6, 7, and 12.

Cool-Down

After a vigorous workout, a cool-down period is essential. This part of the training program helps in returning blood to the heart for reoxygenation. After vigorous activity, enough blood may not circulate back to the brain, heart, and intestines. This causes a pooling of the blood in the muscles of the arms and legs. Pooling of blood in the extremities places additional stress and strain on the heart. Symptoms such as dizziness or faintness may occur without a cool-down period. The cool-down period prevents pooling of blood by relying on continued muscle contraction to help pump blood back through the venous system toward the heart.

The cool-down period should last about 5 to 10 minutes. During the cool-down, you should engage in stretching activities as done during the warm-up. Some feel that stretching during cool-down is more effective for preventing injury than stretching during warm-up. Although the value of warm-up and workout periods is well accepted, the importance of a cool-down period is often ignored. Again, experience and observation seem to indicate that persons who stretch during the cool-down period tend to have fewer problems with muscle soreness after strenuous activity.

PRECAUTIONS FOR BEGINNING A FITNESS PROGRAM

For the normal healthy college student, there is virtually no reason to expect that participation in any type of fitness activity will pose a threat to health or well-being. However, if your medical history as indicated in Lab Activity 1-8 identifies any health-related problem, it is advisable to consult appropriate medical personnel before engaging in any type of activity.

Paying attention to the principles and guidelines of training and conditioning as detailed earlier in this chapter can markedly reduce your chances of suffering injuries associated with exercise. Many of the injuries that occur with exercise can be eliminated by an awareness of the way you exercise, by "listening" to what your body is telling you through aches and pains, and by understanding the potential dangers associated with exercise in extreme environmental conditions (Figure 4-6). Common musculoskeletal injuries that can occur with exercise are discussed in Chapter 10. The following section discusses exercise in both hot and cold weather.

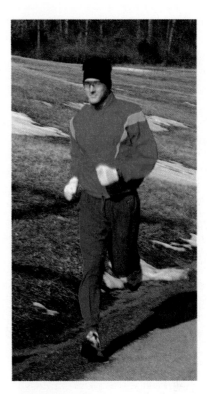

FIGURE 4-6. Environmental Conditions Are an Important Consideration.

SPECIAL CONSIDERATIONS FOR BEGINNING AN EXERCISE PROGRAM
Heat Stress

Regardless of your level of physical conditioning, extreme caution must be taken when exercising in hot, humid weather. Prolonged exposure to extreme heat can result in heat cramps, heat exhaustion, or heatstroke. Heat stress is certainly preventable, but each year many people will suffer illness or perhaps death from some heat-related cause. People who exercise in the heat are particularly vulnerable to heat stress. The physiological processes in the body will continue to function when body temperature is maintained within a normal range. Maintenance of normal temperature in a hot environment depends on the ability of the body to eliminate heat. Body temperature can be affected by five factors.

> **heat stress** prolonged exposure to extreme heat resulting in heat cramps, heat exhaustion, or heat-stroke

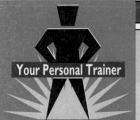

Jeffery Lakins, Journalism major
Age: 20

Scenario

I will be returning to school this August in the south, and I am not looking forward to the hot and humid conditions. I have been active all summer in a range of outdoor activities, including my two favorites: cross-country running and mountain biking. There are a number of good trails around campus, and I look forward to the new environment.

Last year getting off the plane was like running into a wall, but I continued to work out after getting to campus. I thought I was in pretty good shape, and then one day it all snuck up on me. On the way to an afternoon class I collapsed and had to be treated for heat illness.

Solution

It is a good thing you are thinking ahead. For the most part heat-related illnesses are totally preventable. Give your body time to become acclimatized to working out in a hot, humid environment. Start off slow and gradually increase intensity as you become more accustomed to the new conditions.

If the heat, humidity, or combined heat index is too high, you should reschedule your workout to avoid the most intense times of the day; if it is air-conditioned, use your campus fitness center as an alternative.

Wear loose, cotton clothing to maximize evaporation and minimize your body's heat absorption. Sunscreen should be worn as appropriate. Drink plenty of water before, during, and after your workout. Keeping an accurate record of your weight will help you monitor for dehydration.

Metabolic Heat Production. Normal metabolic function in the body results in the production of heat. Consequently, metabolism will always cause a heat gain dependent on the intensity of the physical activity. The higher the metabolic rate, the more heat is produced.

Conductive Heat Exchange. Body heat can be either gained or lost when the body comes into contact with other objects. If you are in contact with a surface that has a temperature lower than your body temperature, heat will be lost. Direct contact with any object or surface that has a temperature greater than your skin temperature will result in a heat gain.

Convective Heat Exchange. Body heat can be either lost or gained, depending on the temperature of the circulating medium. A cool breeze will always tend to cool the body by removing heat from the body surface. Conversely, if the temperature of the circulating air is higher than the temperature of the skin, there will be a gain in body heat.

Radiant Heat Exchange. Radiant heat from sunshine will definitely cause an increase in body temperature. However, on a cloudy day your body is also emitting radiant heat energy, and thus radiation may also result in either heat loss or heat gain. Obviously the effects of the sun's radiation are much greater in the sunshine than in the shade.

Evaporative Heat Loss. Sweat glands in the skin allow water to be transported to the surface, where it evaporates, taking large quantities of heat with it. When the temperature and radiant heat of the environment become higher than body temperature, loss of body heat becomes highly dependent on the process of sweat evaporation.

A person can sweat off about 1 quart of water per hour for about 2 hours, but the air must be relatively free of water for evaporation to occur. Heat loss through evaporation is severely impaired when the relative humidity reaches 65% and virtually stops when the humidity reaches 75%.

It should be obvious that heat-related problems have the greatest chance of occurrence on those days when the sun is bright and the temperature and relative humidity are high. But it is certainly true that heat cramps, heat exhaustion, and heatstroke can occur whenever the body's ability to dissipate heat is impaired.

Heat Cramps

Heat cramps are extremely painful muscle spasms that most commonly occur in the calf and abdomen, although any muscle can be involved. The person most likely to get heat cramps is one who is in fairly good condition but who simply overexerts in the heat. Heat cramps are related to an imbalance between water and several *electrolytes* (sodium, chloride, potassium, magnesium, and calcium ions), which are essential for muscle contraction. Profuse sweating causes losses of large amounts of water and minimal quantities of the electrolytes. This may destroy the balance of water and the concentration of these elements in skeletal muscle and result in painful muscle contraction.

Heat cramps may be prevented by adequate replacement of water and the electrolytes. Ingestion of salt tablets is not recommended. Fluid replacement drinks are effective in replacing both water and electrolytes. The electrolytes may also be replaced by normal ingestion of foods; most fruits are high in potassium, and calcium can be obtained through milk and cheese products. The immediate treatment for heat cramps is ingestion of large quantities of water and mild stretching, with ice massage of the muscle in spasm.

Heat Exhaustion

Heat exhaustion results from inadequate replacement of fluids lost through sweating. Clinically, the victim of heat exhaustion will collapse and manifest profuse sweating, pale skin, mildly elevated temperature, dizziness, hyperventilation, and rapid pulse.

It is sometimes possible to spot a person who is having problems with heat exhaustion. The individual may begin to develop heat cramps and may become disoriented and light-headed. The person's physical performance may not be up to usual standards when fluid replacement has been inadequate. In general, persons in poor physical condition who attempt to exercise in the heat are most likely to get heat exhaustion.

Immediate treatment of heat exhaustion requires ingestion of large quantities of cool water. If possible, the person should be placed in a cool environment, although it is more essential to replace fluids.

Heatstroke

Unlike heat cramps and heat exhaustion, *heatstroke* is a serious, life-threatening emergency. The specific cause of heatstroke is unknown; however, it is clinically characterized by sudden collapse with loss of consciousness; flushed, relatively dry skin; and most important, a core temperature of 106° F or higher. Basically there is a breakdown of the sweating mechanism, and the body loses the ability to dissipate heat by sweating.

Heatstroke can occur suddenly and without warning. With heat-related illnesses there is not a progression from heat cramps to heat exhaustion to heatstroke. To have heatstroke it is not necessary to first have heat cramps and/or heat exhaustion. The possibility of death from heatstroke can be significantly reduced if body temperature is lowered to normal within 45 minutes.

Every first-aid effort should be directed to lowering body temperature. Strip *all* clothing from the victim, douse him or her with cool water, and fan him or her with a towel. It is imperative that the victim be transported to a hospital as quickly as possible, preferably by paramedics. However, if they are delayed, transport the victim in whatever vehicle happens to be available. The replacement of fluid is not critical in initial first aid.

Prevention of Heat-Related Illness

Acclimatization. Of all the factors listed, it is most important to acclimatize yourself to the existing heat and humidity conditions. This is the process of gradually preparing the body to be able to work in heat by slowly exposing the system to the stresses of a hot, humid environment. Heat dramatically reduces performance capabilities, and abrupt exposure to these conditions can predispose a person to heat-related illness. Acclimatization to heat generally occurs rapidly, usually within 5 to 7 days of gradually increasing periods of exercise in the heat. It is enhanced by being in good physical condition and by adequate fluid replacement.

Water and Electrolyte Replacement. During hot weather it is essential to continually replace fluids lost through evaporation by drinking large quantities of fluid, regardless of whether you are thirsty. There is little question that adequate replacement of fluids is the best defense against heat stress.

Rapid absorption of fluids from the gastrointestinal tract is of key importance. Colder fluids are emptied more rapidly from the stomach. If the stomach is partially filled with fluid, the rate of emptying is greater. Gastric emptying seems to be impaired when the fluid ingested contains concentrated simple sugars, although recent studies have indicated that gastric emptying may be actually improved using lower concentrations of simple sugars and sodium.

A number of commercial drinks containing simple sugars and electrolytes are available, including Gatorade, Powerade, All-Sport, Exceed, 10-K, Squencher, and Thirst Quencher. These drinks are good for replenishing fluids and electrolytes before and after activity in the heat. They also may be useful in activities lasting longer than an hour, in which replacement of simple sugars needed for energy becomes important. Nevertheless, water is still considered to be the best form of fluid replacement during exercise. Fluids should be replenished as often and in as great a quantity as necessary during exercise.

Clothing. When exercising in the heat, wear as little clothing as possible to allow maximal evaporation. Light-colored, 100% cotton material allows maximal evaporation. Caution should be used when wearing a hat because about 40% of all heat lost from the body is lost through the head. Thus a hat tends to interfere with keeping cool. Wearing a rubberized suit for the purpose of losing weight during hot weather is ineffective and dangerous. The only weight lost will be water weight, which must be replaced immediately after activity. Rubberized suits severely limit the body's ability to dissipate heat and may predispose you to heat exhaustion or possibly heatstroke.

The use of sunscreens and sunglasses is also recommended to reduce the long-term effects of exposure to the sun.

Exercise Your Common Sense When Exercising. If possible, do not exercise during the hottest parts of the day—between 11:00 AM. and 4:00 PM. The temperature is usually highest at about 4:00 PM. Try to avoid exercising on surfaces such as asphalt, concrete, or Astroturf, which tend to absorb and hold heat.

If you experience any of the heat-related problems, stop the activity immediately, get into a cool environment, and drink large quantities of cool water. Common sense is the best prevention of heat stress.

Exercising in the Cold

Although being able to dissipate heat is a problem in hot, humid weather, conserving heat becomes a major concern when exercising in cold weather. It is essential to consider the factors that may combine to significantly lower body temperature or produce hypothermia. These major factors are temperature, dampness, wind, and fatigue.

Each of these factors when considered independently will probably not result in hypothermia. However, collectively they can be a real problem. Most cases of hypothermia occur when the temperature is in the 50° to 60° F range and when it is also damp and windy. Hypothermia results when the body's temperature drops below 35° C (95° F). Essentially it is a breakdown in the body's ability to produce heat. Initially there is shivering, followed by loss of coordination and difficulty speaking. As the body's temperature continues to drop, shivering stops, the

muscles stiffen, and the person becomes unconscious. People who have hypothermia should be taken to the hospital for treatment, and all efforts should be directed toward elevating core temperature. The following Fit List box provides recommendations to help reduce the chances of hypothermia.

Women and Exercise

Exercising During the Menstrual Period

The approach that has been taken toward participation in physical activities during menstruation has changed drastically during recent years. Twenty years ago it was not uncommon for a female to be excused from a physical education class or from a team practice during her menstrual period, regardless of how she was feeling. As female participation in physical activity and competitive sports continues to grow, many myths about the impact of the menstrual cycle on performance are being discarded. Today it is generally accepted that there is no reason to restrict physical activity during a woman's period. However, individual responses to the menstrual cycle may cause problems for some women.

The menstrual cycle averages about 28 days in length. The cycle can be divided into three phases: the first is the menstrual period or menstruation, the second is the time period in which the woman is most likely to become pregnant, and the third is the pre-

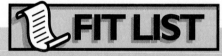

REDUCING THE CHANCES OF HYPOTHERMIA

- Use common sense, and be aware of the environmental conditions that predispose to hypothermia.
- Wear a hat to reduce loss of body heat through the head.
- Dress in layers of thin clothing, which can be removed layer by layer to prevent sweating. Remember that dampness is one of the more critical factors. If possible, wear materials such as Goretex that allow moisture to escape from the body while keeping out moisture from the environment.
- Wear sufficiently protective clothing on the feet, hands, ears, and neck to prevent frostbite.
- Gradually acclimatize yourself to exercising in the cold. Acclimatization to exercising in the cold is just as important as when exercising in a hot, humid environment.

menstrual phase that ends with the onset of menstruation. Menstruation is a normal biological event that does not pose any threat to the active female. Usually the first menstrual period (menarche) occurs between the ages of 10 and 17. At first, most young women experience irregular menstrual cycles. Within a few years, the body adjusts, and cycles become more regular. The cycle repeats monthly unless a pregnancy has occurred. At some time in middle age, generally between ages 44 and 55, the menstrual cycle ceases (menopause).

During the phase of the cycle when the female is most likely to become pregnant, many report feeling "upbeat." However, during the premenstrual period it is not unusual for women to experience a variety of physical and emotional problems. They may experience headaches, bloating, weight gain, and tender breasts. Reports of feeling irritable and depressed are common. The symptoms disappear with the start of the menstrual period. This has been widely reported in the popular press as "premenstrual syndrome" or PMS. Indeed, the normal changes in the female's hormonal cycle explain these symptoms. A variety of treatments have been proposed, from vitamins to psychotherapy. Some women find relief for a few months, but for many, no long-term treatment has been found effective. If symptoms are severe and interfere with normal functioning, the woman should seek professional help. The disorder may be managed with hormonal treatment. However, for most females whose experience with PMS is not severe, learning to expect these feelings and symptoms and how to cope is helpful. Physical activity provides an excellent method to deal with the physical and emotional stresses created by these hormonal changes.

Menstruation creates varying degrees of discomfort. The pain or cramping results from the contractions of the muscular uterus. These mid- to lower abdominal cramps begin a few hours before the onset of menstrual bleeding and generally last 12 to 24 hours after the flow has begun. Cramps may be accompanied by pain in the lower back, buttocks, or upper thighs. For some the cramps are mild and controlled by pain relievers such as ibuprofen. For others, the cramps are severe enough to be incapacitating for hours or a couple of days. Painful menstrual periods are called dysmenorrhea. The headaches and tender breasts experienced before menstruation usually resolve within the first couple of days of the period. These symptoms may be so severe that they interfere with a woman's ability to perform physical activities. Medical evaluation is advised in cases of severe symptoms in either the premenstrual or the menstrual period.

Recent medical knowledge of the relationship between exercise and the menstrual cycle concludes that there are no harmful effects of one on the other. Published studies indicate the following:

- Menarche does not occur earlier in physically active girls. In fact, it may be delayed.
- Disruption of the normal menstrual cycle occurs when percentage of body fat drops to less than about 12%. Low percentages of body fat are characteristic of endurance and highly fit athletes.
- In general, physical performance seems best in the immediate postmenstrual phase. However, there have been reports of record-breaking achievements occurring during menstruation.
- Changes in a female's hormone levels may affect her desire and motivation to engage in physical activity or compete. Reduced motivation may be noticed just before menstruation, particularly if the female experiences depression, irritability, and mood changes.

All females should chart and keep records of their menstrual cycle to determine if the hormonal changes are influencing their feelings. Disruptions in the normal pattern may be caused by physical or psychological problems such as fatigue, severe illness, extreme weight reduction efforts, or anxiety. Pregnancy will disrupt the cycle too. If a regular cycle pattern changes to a more irregular one, the cause should be investigated.

Moderate exercise does not disturb the menstrual cycle. In fact, it may have some beneficial effects. Exercise during the premenstrual and menstrual phases may reduce the severity of symptoms often experienced during these times. Females also report a heightened sense of well-being after exercising.

Dysmenorrhea is neither cured nor aggravated by physical activity. However, it does appear to be less of a complaint in active female atheletes.

It is not unusual for the physically active female to experience changes in the usual pattern of her menstrual cycle. *Oligomenorrhea* refers to irregular menstrual periods that involve diminished bleeding. *Amenorrhea* is a condition in which menstruation disappears altogether. Amenorrhea is not necessarily caused by weight loss but may be related to a low calorie intake. Those with body fat less than 17% may

---

hypothermia breakdown of the body's ability to produce heat, which can result in shivering, loss of coordination, and difficulty speaking

menstruation a normal biological event that should not restrict physical activity

dysmenorrhea painful menstrual periods that may interfere with a woman's ability to participate in physical activities; medical consultation is recommended for severe and repeated cases

exhibit amenorrhea. Some females involved in endurance activities such as long-distance running, swimming, and cycling tend to report such changes in their menstrual cycle. Menstruation often returns to normal after the intense participation in the activity ends.

Physical Activity During Pregnancy

Traditionally, women have been asked to avoid strenuous exercise during pregnancy because it might endanger the health of the woman and unborn baby. The woman's condition was described as delicate. More recently, the recognition that exercise is beneficial for everyone's health has led concerned women to ask their doctors if it is safe to go cycling or continue aerobics classes. Will it harm the baby or cause a miscarriage?

In the past, pregnancy was considered to be an abnormal condition. Today it is recognized as an altered physical state in which the woman's body undergoes a variety of changes to support the development of an unborn baby. The internal environment is very protective of the unborn baby. The developing baby is surrounded by the amniotic fluid, which acts as a shock absorber, dispersing the force of a direct blow to the mother's abdomen.

It is recommended that the pregnant female not begin a new exercise program during the first and third trimesters. She should not increase the intensity or duration of the exercise before the fifteenth week or after the twenty-eighth week. However, mild-to-moderate physical activities are recommended during the second trimester of pregnancy when the discomfort and possible risks to the fetus are low. The woman should be encouraged to perform activities that are comfortable and within her capabilities (Figure 4-7). The mother-to-be should exercise at an intensity at which she can continue to carry on a conversation during exercise. By continuing her prepregnancy exercise habits, the woman can prevent muscle weakness that would occur from disuse, help to prevent excessive weight gain, and reduce emotional stress. Extreme exercise and highly competitive sports should be avoided. Certain conditions such as hypertension and kidney and heart disease place the health of the pregnant woman at risk. These pregnancies are called *high-risk* and may require extreme limitation of physical activity.

The type of exercise recommended will depend on the condition of the woman when her pregnancy begins and the health of the pregnancy. The pregnant

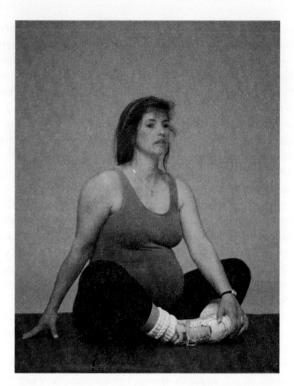

FIGURE 4-7. Exercise Is Generally Safe Throughout Pregnancy.

woman should avoid becoming overheated. When a woman's body temperature rises, the unborn baby's environment also heats up. This temperature increase has been linked to birth defects, especially if it occurs during the first 3 months of pregnancy.

The key to being able to exercise during pregnancy is to become fit before getting pregnant. It is advisable to curtail contact sports and sports with severe exertion, especially in highly competitive situations.

The following are suggested activities that can be done during pregnancy:

- Swimming seems to be suitable throughout the pregnancy. It is self-limiting, and the individual may perform at her own speed. Water is good for relaxation of muscles and provides a soothing effect. Changes in body composition make the female more buoyant, and swimming remains easy as pregnancy advances. Swimming may be started during pregnancy even though the woman had not been swimming before.
- Bicycling is another non–weight-bearing activity. A stationary bike may be preferable to standard cycling because of weight and balance changes dur-

ing pregnancy. Also, it is possible to control climate indoors so that the expectant mother does not become overheated.

- Walking is an excellent activity during pregnancy, even though it is weight bearing. Walking keeps the muscles of the trunk, pelvis, and legs in good tone during pregnancy. Like swimming and cycling, it offers aerobic benefits as well.
- Running is an activity of questionable value for the pregnant female. It is likely that few problems would develop during the first two trimesters of pregnancy. However, during the last trimester, running should be done with extra caution because of expected increases in body weight.
- Aerobic exercise, like running, should be avoided during the third trimester, especially because it involves a considerable amount of bouncing.

The American College of Obstetrics and Gynecology has developed guidelines for pregnant women to follow when exercising. The following Safe Tip box summarizes guidelines designed to ensure the safety, health, and fitness of the pregnant woman and her developing baby.

ARE YOU READY TO BEGIN?

At this point you have been given the basic guidelines and considerations for beginning a fitness program (see the box on p. 106 for a quick review). **Lab Activity 4-1** is a checklist that will help you in designing a program that will be effective, fun, enjoyable, and safe. Remember—you can't sit and be fit—so let's get started.

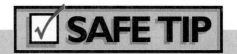

GUIDELINES FOR EXERCISE DURING PREGNANCY

- Consult your physician before starting an exercise program.
- It is better to modify your prepregnancy exercise program than to start a new one.
- Do not exercise to exhaustion.
- Avoid any activities that involve bouncing, jarring, or twisting motions.
- Avoid any activities that require rapid stops and starts.
- Do not perform any activity that puts the abdomen in jeopardy.
- Be aware that your body's center of gravity changes during pregnancy; it may be harder to keep your balance during some exercises.
- Do not exercise while lying on your back, particularly after the fourth month.
- Do not exercise during hot, humid weather.
- Drink plenty of fluids before, after, and sometimes during the workout.
- During your workout, make sure your temperature stays below 100° F and your heart rate does not exceed 140 beats per minute.

Modified from Alexander LL, LaRosa JH: *New dimensions in women's health,* Boston, 1994, Jones & Bartlett; and Agostini R: *Medical and orthopedic issues of active and athletic women,* Philadelphia, 1994, Hanley & Belfus.

GET MOVING

Things to consider when you're ready to start exercising

1. Choose to participate in any fitness activity that you truly enjoy. If you hate running, swimming, cycling, aerobic dance, and rollerblading but you absolutely love to play golf—choose golf.
2. No matter what kind of exercise program you choose to participate in, if you consistently exercise at a higher level than you are used to, and progress within your own limitations, you will see improvement.
3. Exercising promotes good health as long as you pay attention to creating an environment that is conducive to safety and injury prevention.
4. Going through a thorough warm-up and following the workout with a cool-down can help minimize muscle soreness and muscle strain.
5. Nothing tastes better than an ice-cold glass of water on a hot day. The more you drink, the better.
6. If you are going to exercise outdoors during the summer months, remember that there are some beautiful sunrises and sunsets. Why not exercise when they are happening to avoid the hottest part of the day?
7. If you want to continue to exercise outdoors when the weather turns cold, realize that sporting goods stores have some great looking warm-up suits, jackets, and exercise clothes. Buy them and dress appropriately.
8. For some women exercise decreases the discomfort associated with menstruation.
9. If mom stays fit and healthy during pregnancy, baby is more likely to be healthy.

SUMMARY

- Fitness is a personal responsibility.
- Much scientific knowledge has been generated regarding principles that should be observed when designing the right kind of training program needed to be physically fit.
- Before starting a personal training program, it is helpful to examine your attitude toward physical fitness, reasons for wanting to be physically fit, and present level of activity.
- Most college students, after careful analysis, are not satisfied with their physical condition.
- Your fitness goals should be considered when planning a training program.
- Physical activities should be enjoyable.
- To achieve the greatest benefits from the exercise program, you should recognize and use the principle of overload.
- The training program should be progressive and within your capabilities to adapt physiologically.
- Consistency in exercising is important.
- Training programs should be individualized.
- Safety should be a consideration in the training program.
- Three basic elements of every training program are warm-up, workout/activity, and cool-down.
- Individuals should know whether they meet desirable physical fitness standards as determined by scientific methods of measurement and evaluation.
- A general assessment of the training program you are following may be obtained by monitoring your reaction to exercise.
- Results will not be seen overnight. It will take some time, but the results are worth the wait.
- It is important to understand the dangers involved in exercising in extreme environmental conditions.
- There are few reasons that a female cannot continue to exercise during menstruation.
- Exercise during pregnancy is generally safe; in fact, it is usually recommended.

REFERENCES

Agostini R: *Medical and orthopedic issues of active and athletic women,* Philadelphia, 1994, Hanley & Belfus.

Alexander LL, LaRosa JH: *New dimensions in women's health,* Boston, 1994, Jones & Bartlett.

American College of Obstetrics and Gynecology: *Exercise during pregnancy and postnatal period home exercise programs,* Washington, DC, 1985, ACOG.

American College of Sports Medicine: Position stand on recommended quantity and quality of exercise for developing and maintaining cardiorespiratory and muscular fitness in healthy adults, *Med Sci Sports Exerc* 22:265-274, 1990.

Chwalbinska MJ, Hanninen O: Effect of active warming-up on thermoregulatory, circulatory and metabolic responses to incremental exercise in endurance trained athletes, *Int J Sports Med* 10(1):25, 1989.

Clapp J: A clinical approach to exercise in pregnancy, *Clin Sports Med* 13:443-458, 1994.

Coleman E: Sports drink update, *Sports Sci Exchange* 1(5):1, 1988.

Constantini N: Clinical consequences of athletic amenorrhea, *Sports Med* 17:213-223, 1994.

Dishman RK: Determinants of participation in physical activity. In Bouchard C, editor: *Exercise, fitness, and health: a consensus of current knowledge,* Champaign, 1990, Human Kinetics.

Fishbein EG, Phillips M: How safe is exercise during pregnancy? *J Obstet Gynecol Neonatal Nurs* 19:45, 1990.

Fletcher G, Froelicher L, Hartley L: Exercise standards: a statement for professionals from the American Heart Association, *Circulation* 82:2286-2322, 1990.

Gisolfi C: Exercise, intestinal absorption, and rehydration, *Sports Sci Exchange* 4(32):1, 1991.

Hubbard R: An introduction: the role of exercise in the etiology of exertional heatstroke, *Med Sci Sports Exerc* 22:2-5, 1990.

Lecroart J, Deklunder G: Thermoregulation. In Fahey T, editor: *Encyclopedia of sports medicine and exercise physiology,* New York, 1995, Garland.

Marshall L: Clinical evaluation of amenorrhea in active and athletic women, *Clin Sports Med* 13:371-387, 1994.

Murray R: The effects of consuming carbohydrate-electrolyte beverages on gastric emptying and fluid absorption during and following exercise, *Sports Med* 4:322, 1987.

Nielsen B: Heat stress and acclimatization, *Ergonomics* 37:49-58, 1994.

Neilsen B, Hales J, Strange S: Human circulatory and thermoregulatory adaptations with heat acclimatization and exercise in a hot dry environment, *J Physiol* 460:467-485, 1993.

Okazaki Y, Kodama K, Sato H: Attenuation of increased myocardial oxygen consumption during exercise as a major cause of warm-up phenomenon, *J Am Coll Cardiol* 21:1597-1604, 1993.

Paglone A, Worthington S: Cautions and advice on exercise during pregnancy, *Contemp Obstet Gynecol* 25:160, 1985.

Pandolf K: Avoiding heat illness during exercise. In Torg J, Shepard R, editors: *Current therapy in sports medicine,* St Louis, 1995, Mosby.

Pate RR: Principles of training. In Kulund D, editor: *The injured athlete,* Philadelphia, 1986, JB Lippincott.

Payne WA, Hahn DB: *Understanding your health,* St Louis, 1995, Mosby.

Safran MR: The role of warm-up in muscular injury prevention, *Am J Sports Med* 16:123, 1988.

Shellock F, Prentice W: Warming-up and stretching for improved physical performance and prevention of sport-related injuries, *Sports Med* 2:267-278, 1985.

Sonstroem R: Improving compliance with exercise programs. In Torg J, Shepard R, editors: *Current therapy in sports medicine,* St Louis, 1995, Mosby.

US Department of Health and Human Services, Public Health Services: *Healthy people 2000: national health promotion and disease prevention objectives,* Washington, DC, 1991, USDHHS.

Webb P: Heat storage and body temperature during cooling and rewarming, *Eur J Appl Physiol* 66:18-24, 1993.

Wells C: *Women, sport and performance,* Champaign, 1985, Human Kinetics.

Wolf L, Amey M, McGrath M: Exercise and pregnancy. In Torg J, Shepard R, editors: *Current therapy in sports medicine,* St Louis, 1995, Mosby.

SUGGESTED READINGS

American College of Sports Medicine: *ACSM fitness book,* Champaign, 1992, Human Kinetics.
A beginner's guide to starting an exercise program. Shows the reader how to update the fitness program when improvement occurs.

Pearl A: *The athletic female,* Champaign, 1993, Human Kinetics.
Provides an in-depth look at medical, physiological, and behavioral issues for athletic females from pubescence through maturity.

Rejeski W, Kenney E: *Fitness motivation,* Champaign, 1988, Human Kinetics.
Brings research in exercise psychology and in-depth case studies together to look at what motivates exercise participants to want to keep fit. Ideas and techniques are recommended to reduce drop-out rate in fitness programs.

Shangold M, Merkin G: *Women and exercise: physiology and sports medicine,* Philadelphia, 1994, FA Davis.
Written by one of the leading researchers in the field of women in sports; provides guidelines and recommendations for females engaged in exercise.

Thein L: Environmental conditions affecting the athlete, *J Orthop Sports Phys Ther* 21(3):158-171, 1995.
Very comprehensive paper that looks at managing problems that may occur when exercising in extreme environmental conditions.

Lab Activity 4-1

Planning for a Physical Activity Program

Name _____ **Section** _____ **Date** _____

PURPOSE To determine whether you have addressed the necessary considerations for beginning a physical activity program.

PROCEDURE In the space provided, indicate your best response.

1. Based on your responses in **Lab Activity 1-7**, list the goals you wish to accomplish by engaging in a physical activity program._____

    _____

    _____

    _____

    _____

    _____

    _____

2. What are the components of fitness that you want to concentrate on to accomplish these goals (e.g., muscular strength, flexibility, cardiorespiratory endurance)? _____

    _____

    _____

    _____

3. What are the physical activities that you most enjoy participating in that you think will be the most effective in accomplishing these goals? _____

    _____

    _____

4. When do you think will be the best time during the day for you to work out? _____

    _____

5. How many days a week do you plan to engage in physical activity? _____

    _____

6. Do you plan to work out on your own, or will you choose a workout partner? List the people with whom you might like to work out. _____

    _____

Continued.

7. How long do you think your warm-up, workout/activity, cool-down will take?_____

_____

8. What will your warm-up activity consist of?_____

_____

_____

9. Briefly describe what you plan to do during your workout. (Specific exercises and instructions relative to the various health-related components of fitness will be covered in subsequent chapters.) _____

_____

_____

_____

10. What will your cool-down activity consist of?_____

_____

_____

_____

_____

_____

11. What things can you do to make your physical activity program safe and reduce the possibility of injury?

_____

_____

_____

_____

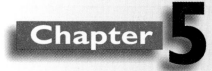

Chapter 5

Developing Cardiorespiratory Fitness

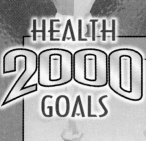

HEALTH 2000 GOALS

■ **Development and Maintenance of Cardiorespiratory Fitness.** To have at least 20% of people age 18 and older and at least 75% of children and adolescents age 6 to 17 engage in vigorous physical activity 3 or more days per week, for 20 minutes or more per session. In 1985, 12% of people age 18 and older met these criteria; in 1984, 66% of youth age 10 to 17 exercised at this level.

• Higher levels of cardiorespiratory fitness enable people to carry out their daily occupation tasks and leisure pursuits more easily.
• Activities such as stair climbing, strenuous housework, yardwork, certain occupational tasks, and some childhood pursuits may qualify as vigorous activity if they are sustained and elevate the heart rate to at least 60% of the maximum recommended level for a person's age.

OBJECTIVES

After completing this chapter, you will be able to do the following:

■ Explain the relationships of heart rate, stroke volume, cardiac output, and rate of oxygen use.
■ Describe the function of the heart, blood vessels, and lungs in oxygen transport.
■ Describe the oxygen transport system and the concept of maximal rate of oxygen use.
■ Describe the differences between aerobic and anaerobic activity.

■ Describe the principles of continuous, interval, fartlek, and par cours training and the potential of each technique for improving cardiorespiratory endurance.
■ Identify methods for assessment of cardiorespiratory endurance.
■ Demonstrate a method to assess your level of cardiorespiratory endurance.

KEY TERMS

While reading this chapter, you will become familiar with the following terms:

• cardiorespiratory endurance
• stroke volume
• training effect

• maximal oxygen consumption ($\dot{V}O_2$max)
• slow-twitch muscle fibers
• fast-twitch muscle fibers
• metabolism

• anaerobic metabolism
• aerobic metabolism
• aerobic activity
• anaerobic activity
• continuous training

• target heart rate (THR)
• rating of perceived exertion (RPE)
• interval training
• fartlek
• par cours

Of all the components of physical fitness listed in Chapter 1, none is more important than *cardiorespiratory endurance*, sometimes referred to as *cardiovascular endurance*. By definition, cardiorespiratory endurance is the ability to perform whole-body activities and continue movement for extended periods of time without undue fatigue. The cardiorespiratory system provides a means by which oxygen is supplied to the various tissues of the body. Without oxygen the cells within the human body cannot possibly function, and ultimately death will occur. Thus the cardiorespiratory system is the basic life-support system of the body.

TRAINING EFFECTS ON THE CARDIORESPIRATORY SYSTEM

Basically, transport of oxygen throughout the body involves the coordinated function of four components: (1) the heart, (2) the blood vessels, (3) the blood, and (4) the lungs. The improvement of cardiorespiratory endurance through training occurs because of increased capability of each of these four elements in providing necessary oxygen to the working tissues. A basic discussion of the training effects and response to exercise that occur in the heart, blood vessels, blood, and lungs should make it easier to understand why the training techniques to be discussed later are so effective in improving cardiorespiratory endurance.

Adaptation of the Heart to Exercise

The heart is the main pumping mechanism and circulates oxygenated blood throughout the body to the working tissues. The heart receives deoxygenated blood from the venous system and then pumps the blood through the pulmonary vessels to the lungs, where carbon dioxide is exchanged for oxygen. The oxygenated blood then returns to the heart, from which it exits through the aorta to the arterial system and is circulated throughout the body, supplying oxygen to the tissues (Figure 5-1).

Heart Rate

As the body begins to exercise, the muscles use the oxygen at a much higher rate, and the heart must pump more oxygenated blood to meet this increased demand. The heart is capable of adapting to this increased demand through several mechanisms. *Heart*

rate shows a gradual adaptation to an increased workload by increasing proportionally to the intensity of the exercise and will plateau at a given level after about 2 to 3 minutes (Figure 5-2).

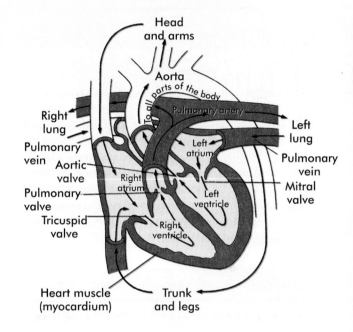

FIGURE 5-1. **Anatomy of the Heart and Blood Flow.**

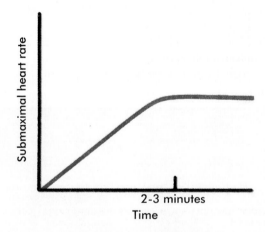

FIGURE 5-2. **Heart Rate and Workload.**
Two to three minutes are required for heart rate to plateau at a given workload.

Monitoring heart rate is an indirect method of estimating oxygen consumption. In general, heart rate and oxygen consumption have a linear relationship, although at very low intensities and at high intensities this linear relationship breaks down (Figure 5-3). During higher-intensity activities maximum heart rate may be achieved before maximal oxygen consumption, which will continue to rise. The greater the intensity of the exercise, the higher the heart rate. Because of these existing relationships it should become apparent that the rate of oxygen consumption can be estimated by taking the heart rate.

Stroke Volume

A second mechanism by which the heart is able to adapt to increased demands during exercise is to increase the stroke volume, the volume of blood being pumped out with each beat. The heart pumps out approximately 70 ml of blood per beat. Stroke volume can continue to increase only to the point at which there is simply not enough time between beats for the heart to fill up. This occurs at about 40% to 50% of maximal oxygen consumption or at a heart rate of 110 to 120 beats per minute, and above this level increases in the volume of blood being pumped out per unit of time must be caused entirely by increases in heart rate (Figure 5-4).

Cardiac Output

Stroke volume and heart rate together determine the volume of blood being pumped through the heart in a given unit of time. Approximately 5 L of blood is pumped through the heart during each minute at rest. This is referred to as the *cardiac output*, which indicates how much blood the heart is capable of pumping in exactly 1 minute. Thus cardiac output is the primary determinant of the maximal rate of oxygen consumption possible (Figure 5-5). During exercise, cardiac output increases to approximately four times that experienced during rest in the normal individual (about 20 L) and may increase as much as six times in the elite endurance athlete (about 30 L).

Cardiac output = Stroke volume × Heart rate

A training effect that occurs with regard to cardiac output of the heart is that the stroke volume increases while exercise heart rate is reduced at a given standard exercise load. The heart becomes more efficient because it is capable of pumping more blood with each stroke. Because the heart is a muscle, it will hypertrophy, or increase in size and strength to some extent, but this is in no way a negative effect of training.

Training Effect

Increased stroke volume × Decreased heart rate = Cardiac output

During exercise females tend to have a 5% to 10% higher cardiac output than males do at all intensities. This is likely due to a lower concentration of hemo-

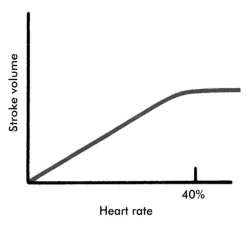

FIGURE 5-4. Stroke Volume.
Stroke volume plateaus at about 40% of maximum heart rate.

---

cardiorespiratory endurance the ability to perform whole-body activities and continue movement for extended periods of time without undue fatigue
stroke volume volume of blood being pumped out of the heart with each beat
training effect improvement of cardiorespiratory endurance as a result of athletic training

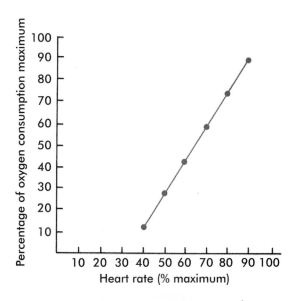

FIGURE 5-3. Maximum Heart Rate and V̇o₂max.
Maximum heart rate is achieved at about the same time as V̇o₂max.

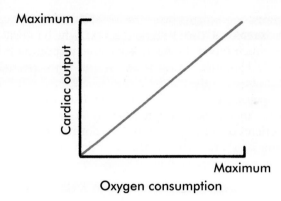

FIGURE 5-5. Cardiac Output.
Cardiac output limits $\dot{V}O_2$ max.

globin in the female, which is compensated for during exercise by an increased cardiac output.

Adaptation in Blood Flow

The amount of blood flowing to the various organs increases during exercise. However, there is a change in overall distribution of cardiac output; the percentage of total cardiac output to the nonessential organs is decreased, whereas it is increased to active skeletal muscle. Volume of blood flow to the heart muscle or *myocardium* increases substantially during exercise, even though the percentage of total cardiac output supplying the heart muscle remains unchanged. In skeletal muscle there is increased formation of blood vessels or capillaries, although it is not clear whether new ones form or dormant ones simply open up and fill with blood.

The total peripheral resistance is the sum of all forces that resist blood flow within the vascular system. Total peripheral resistance decreases during exercise primarily because of vessel vasodilation in the active skeletal muscles.

Blood Pressure. Blood pressure in the arterial system is determined by the cardiac output in relation to total peripheral resistance to blood flow. Blood pressure is created by contraction of the heart muscle. Contraction of the ventricles of the heart creates systolic pressure, and relaxation of the heart creates diastolic pressure. During exercise, there is a decrease in total peripheral resistance and an increase in cardiac output. Systolic pressure increases in proportion to oxygen consumption and cardiac output; diastolic pressure shows little or no increase. Blood pressure falls below preexercise levels after exercise and may stay low for several hours. There is general agreement that engaging in consis-

tent aerobic exercise will produce modest reductions in both systolic and diastolic blood pressure at rest and during submaximal exercise.

Adaptations in the Blood

Oxygen is transported throughout the system bound to *hemoglobin*. Found in red blood cells, hemoglobin is an iron-containing protein that has the capability of easily accepting or giving up molecules of oxygen as needed. Training for improvement of cardiorespiratory endurance produces an increase in total blood volume, with a corresponding increase in the amount of hemoglobin. The concentration of hemoglobin in circulating blood does not change with training; it may actually decrease slightly.

Adaptation of the Lungs

As a result of training, pulmonary function is improved in the trained individual relative to the untrained individual. The volume of air that can be inspired in a single maximal ventilation is increased. The diffusing capacity of the lungs is also increased, facilitating the exchange of oxygen and carbon dioxide. Pulmonary resistance to air flow is also decreased. Figure 5-6 summarizes the effects of training on the cardiorespiratory system.

MAXIMAL OXYGEN CONSUMPTION

The maximal amount of oxygen that can be used during exercise is referred to as maximal oxygen consumption ($\dot{V}O_2$max). It is considered to be the best indicator of the level of cardiorespiratory endurance. $\dot{V}O_2$max is most often presented in terms of the volume of oxygen used relative to body weight per unit of time (ml/kg/min). A normal $\dot{V}O_2$max for most college-age men and women would fall in the range of 38 to 46 ml/kg/min. A world-class male marathon runner may have a $\dot{V}O_2$max in the 70 to 80 ml/kg/min range, and a female marathoner will have a 60 to 70 ml/kg/min range.

Rate of Oxygen Consumption

The performance of any activity requires a certain rate of oxygen consumption that is relatively the same for all persons, depending on each person's present level of fitness. Generally the greater the rate or intensity of the performance of an activity, the greater the oxygen consumption. Each person has his or her own maximal rate of oxygen consumption. A person's ability to perform an activity is closely related to the amount of oxygen required by that activity. This ability is limited by the maximal rate of oxygen consumption of which the person is capable of delivering into

FIGURE 5-6. The Effects of Continuous Training on the Cardiorespiratory System.

- Decreased resting heart rate
- Decreased heart rate at specific workloads
- Increased stroke volume
- Increased cardiac output
- Decreased recovery time
- Increased capillarization in muscle
- Increased functional capacity in the lungs
- Increased oxygen utilization
- Decreased muscle glycogen utilization.

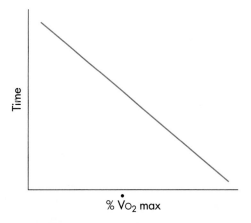

FIGURE 5-7. $\dot{V}O_2$max and Activity Duration. The greater the percentage of $\dot{V}O_2$max required during an activity, the less time for the duration of the activity.

the lungs. Fatigue occurs when insufficient oxygen is supplied to the muscles. It should be apparent that the greater percentage of maximal oxygen consumption required during an activity, the less time the activity may be performed (Figure 5-7).

Three factors determine the maximal rate at which oxygen can be used: (1) external respiration, involving the ventilatory process, or pulmonary function; (2) gas transport, which is accomplished by the cardiovascular system (i.e., the heart, blood vessels, and blood); and (3) internal respiration, which involves the use of oxygen by the cells to produce energy. Of these three factors the most limiting is generally the ability to transport oxygen through the system; thus the cardiovascular system limits the overall rate of oxygen consumption. A high $\dot{V}O_2$ max within a person's range indicates that all three systems are working well.

$\dot{V}O_2$max: An Inherited Characteristic

The maximal rate at which oxygen can be used is a genetically determined characteristic; we inherit a certain range of $\dot{V}O_2$ max, and the more active we are, the higher the existing $\dot{V}O_2$ max will be within that range. Therefore a training program is capable of increasing $\dot{V}O_2$ max to its highest limit within our range.

Fast-Twitch Versus Slow-Twitch Muscle Fibers

The range of maximal oxygen consumption that we inherit is in a large part determined by the metabolic and functional properties of skeletal muscle fibers. Basically there are two distinct types of muscle fibers: slow-twitch and fast-twitch fibers, each of which has distinctive metabolic and contractile capabilities. Because they are relatively fatigue resistant, slow-twitch fibers are associated primarily with long-duration, aerobic-type activities. Fast-twitch fibers are useful in short-term, high-intensity activities, which mainly involve the anaerobic system. Chapter 6 will

further examine the relation of muscle fiber type to athletic ability.

Cardiorespiratory Endurance and Work Ability

Cardiorespiratory endurance plays a critical role in our ability to carry out normal daily activities. Fatigue is closely related to the percentage of $\dot{V}O_2$max that a particular workload demands. For example, Figure 5-8 presents two persons, A and B. A has a $\dot{V}O_2$max of 50 ml/kg/min, whereas B has a $\dot{V}O_2$max of only 40 ml/kg/min. If both A and B are exercising at the same intensity, then A will be working at a much lower percentage of $\dot{V}O_2$max than B is. Consequently, A should be able to sustain his or her activity over a much longer period of time. Everyday activities may be adversely affected if your ability to use oxygen efficiently is impaired. Thus improvement of cardiorespiratory endurance should be an essential component of any training program.

Regardless of the training technique used for the improvement of cardiorespiratory endurance, one principal goal remains the same. **You are trying to increase the ability of the cardiorespiratory system**

maximal oxygen consumption ($\dot{V}O_2$max) measured in a laboratory to determine how much oxygen can be used during 1 minute of maximal exercise

slow-twitch muscle fibers relatively fatigue resistant, these muscle fibers are utilized in long-duration, aerobic-type activities

fast-twitch muscle fibers type of muscle fibers used in short-term, high-intensity (anaerobic) activities for speed or power and in activities such as sprinting or weight lifting

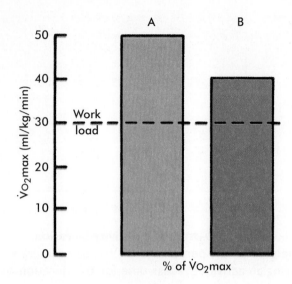

FIGURE 5-8.   Fitness and $\dot{V}O_2$max.
Student A should be able to work longer than student B as a result of lower use of $\dot{V}O_2$max.

to supply a sufficient amount of oxygen to working muscles. Without oxygen, the body is incapable of producing energy for an extended period of time.

PRODUCING ENERGY FOR EXERCISE

All living systems need to perform a variety of activities such as growing, generating energy, repairing damaged tissues, and eliminating waste. All of these activities are referred to as metabolic or cellular metabolism.

Muscles are metabolically active and must generate energy to move. Energy is produced from the breakdown of certain nutrients from foodstuffs. This energy is stored in a compound called *adenosine triphosphate (ATP)*, which is the ultimate usable form of energy for muscular activity. ATP is produced in the muscle tissue from blood glucose or glycogen. Fats and proteins can also be metabolized to generate ATP. Glucose not needed immediately is stored as *glycogen* in the resting muscle and liver. Stored glycogen in the liver can later be converted back to glucose and transferred to the blood to meet the body's energy needs.

If the duration or intensity of the exercise increases, the body relies more heavily on fats stored in *adipose* tissue to meet its energy needs. The longer the duration of an activity, the greater the amount of fat used, especially during the later stages of endurance events. During rest and submaximal exertion, both fat and carbohydrates are used to provide energy in approximately a 60% to 40% ratio. Carbohydrates must be

available to use fat. If glycogen is totally depleted, fat cannot be completely metabolized. Regardless of the nutrient source that produces ATP, it is always available in the cell as an immediate energy source. When all available sources of ATP are used, more must be regenerated for muscular contraction to continue.

Various sports activities involve specific demands for energy. For example, sprinting and jumping are high-energy output activities, requiring a relatively large production of energy for a short time. Long-distance running and swimming, on the other hand, are mostly low-energy output activities per unit of time, requiring energy production for a prolonged time. Other physical activities demand a blend of both high- and low-energy output. These various energy demands can be met by the different processes in which energy can be supplied to the skeletal muscles.

Anaerobic Versus Aerobic Metabolism

Two major energy-generating systems function in muscle tissue: anaerobic and aerobic metabolism. Each of these systems produces ATP. During sudden outbursts of activity in intensive, short-term exercise, ATP can be rapidly metabolized to meet energy needs. After a few seconds of intensive exercise, however, the small stores of ATP are used up. The body then turns to stored glycogen as an energy source. Glycogen can be broken down to supply glucose, which is then metabolized within the muscle cells to generate ATP for muscle contractions.

Glucose can be metabolized to generate small amounts of ATP energy without the need for oxygen. This energy system is referred to as anaerobic metabolism (occurring in the absence of oxygen). As exercise continues, the body has to rely on a more complex form of carbohydrate and fat metabolism to generate ATP. This second energy system requires oxygen and is therefore referred to as aerobic metabolism (occurring in the presence of oxygen). The aerobic system of producing energy generates considerably more ATP than the anaerobic one.

In most activities both aerobic and anaerobic systems function simultaneously. The degree to which the two major energy systems are involved is determined by the intensity and duration of the activity (Table 5-1). If the intensity of the activity is such that sufficient oxygen can be supplied to meet the demands of working tissues, the activity is considered to be aerobic. Conversely, if the activity is of high enough intensity or the duration is such that there is insufficient oxygen available to meet energy demands, the activity becomes anaerobic.

Table 5-2 provides a comparison summary between aerobic and anaerobic activities.

TABLE 5-1. Energy Systems Used According to Length of Time and Type of Activity

Energy System	Length of Time	Type of Activity
Anaerobic	6-60 sec	Any type of sprint (running, swimming, cycling) Short-duration, explosive activities
Combined systems	1-3 min	Medium-distance activities (400 and 800 meters) Intermittent sports activities
Aerobic	>3 min	Long-distance events Long-duration intermittent activities

TABLE 5-2. Comparison of Aerobic Versus Anaerobic Activities

	Mode	Relative Intensity	Intensity	Frequency	Duration	Miscellaneous
Aerobic activities	Continuous, long-duration, sustained activities	Less intense	50%-85% of HRR 60%-90% of MHR	At least three but not more than six times per week	20 to 60 min	Less risk to sedentary or older individuals
Anaerobic activities	Explosive, short-duration, burst-type activities	More intense	85%-100% of HRR 90%-100% of MHR	Three to four days per week	10 sec to 2 min	Used in sport and team activities

HRR, heart rate reserve; *MHR,* maximum heart rate.

Excess Postexercise Oxygen Consumption (Oxygen Deficit)

As the intensity of the exercise increases and insufficient amounts of oxygen are available to the tissues, an oxygen deficit is incurred. Oxygen deficit occurs in the beginning of exercise (within the first 2 to 3 minutes) when the oxygen demand is greater than the oxygen supplied. It has been hypothesized that this oxygen debt is caused by lactic acid produced during anaerobic activity and that this "debt" must be "paid back" during the postexercise period. However, there is now a different rationale for this oxygen deficit, which is currently being referred to as "excess postexercise oxygen consumption." It is theoretically caused by disturbances in mitochondrial funtion from an increase in temperature.

SPECIFIC TRAINING TECHNIQUES TO IMPROVE CARDIORESPIRATORY ENDURANCE

As emphasized in Chapter 1, cardiorespiratory endurance may be improved by engaging in a total of 30 minutes of cumulative exercise that may involve a number of different activities each day. This new guideline certainly makes it easier for many people to meet at least the minimum criteria for consistent exercise. However, there are many people who are interested in a more structured activity for improving cardiorespiratory endurance. The box on p. 118 offers a number of tips for including activities that utilize and strengthen your cardiorespiratory endurance in your regular routine.

There are a number of specific training methods through which cardiorespiratory endurance may be improved, including (1) continuous or sustained

metabolism term used to describe metabolic or cellular activities common to all living systems, which include growing, generating energy, repairing damaged tissues, and eliminating waste

anaerobic metabolism metabolizing small amount of glucose without the need for oxygen

aerobic metabolism process that generates more ATP than anaerobic metabolism, requires oxygen, and breaks down more complex forms of carbohydrate and fats

aerobic activity an activity in which the intensity of the activity is low enough that the cardiovascular system can supply enough oxygen to continue the activity for long periods

anaerobic activity an activity in which the intensity is so great that the demand for oxygen is greater than the body's ability to deliver oxygen

training, (2) interval training, (3) fartlek, and (4) par cours. To a large extent the amount of improvement possible will be determined by initial levels of cardiorespiratory endurance.

Continuous Training

Continuous training involves the FITT principles:
Frequency of the activity
Intensity of the activity
Type of activity
Time (duration) of the activity

Frequency

To see at least minimal improvement in cardiorespiratory endurance, it is necessary for the average person to engage in no less than three sessions per week. If possible, you should aim for five sessions per week. A competitive athlete should be prepared to train as often as six times per week. Everyone should take off at least 1 day per week to give damaged tissues a chance to repair themselves.

Intensity

The intensity of the exercise is also a critical factor even though recommendations regarding training intensities vary. This is particularly true in the early stages of training, when the body is forced to make a lot of adjustments to increased workload demands.

Because heart rate is linearly related to the intensity of the exercise and to the rate of oxygen consumption, it becomes a relatively simple process to identify a specific workload (pace) that will make the heart rate plateau at the desired level. By monitoring heart rate we can determine whether the pace is too fast or too slow to get the heart rate into a target range.

Monitoring Heart Rate. Lab Activity 5-1 will help you learn to assess your pulse rate. There are several points at which heart rate is easily measured. The most reliable is the radial artery, located on the thumb side of the wrist joint. By placing your index and middle fingers on the thumb side of the flexor tendon, you should be able to locate a strong pulse (Figure 5-9, *A*). Do not use your thumb to monitor pulse rate. Each pulse represents one heartbeat. By counting the number of beats that occur in 1 minute, you will get an accurate heart rate. Because the heart rate will slow down during a 1-minute period, you should monitor your heart rate for 10 seconds and then multiply by 6 to give you the number of beats per minute. An alternative method is to count for 6 seconds and then add a zero.

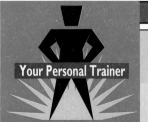

Your Personal Trainer

Marie Anastasia, Information systems manager
Age: 31

Scenario

I am taking an extended bike tour of western Oregon this summer and will be cycling 25 to 75 miles a day, both on- and off-road. I've started training after work and have been frustrated by a sharp cramp in my side on the final downhill sprint before I get back to my apartment. If I slow down the cramp goes away, but once I get back up to speed the pain returns.

Solution

Your cramps may be due to your current level of conditioning, weak abdominal muscles, or improper breathing techniques that may be causing a lack of oxygen in the diaphragm.

Try using a strong, consistent pace throughout your ride and gradually increase either your mileage or the intensity of your training.

The problem may also be as simple as what you have been eating for lunch. Modify your eating habits to avoid foods that might produce constipation or gas. If you are training right after work, start taking an earlier lunch; in addition, avoid spicy snacks, fatty or fried foods, sugars, fruit juices, and drinks with caffeine before working out.

If your abdominal pain persists, seek evaluation by your physician.

A second area in which the pulse is easily located is the carotid artery in the neck. Again using your index and middle fingers, locate the Adam's apple and then slide your fingers into the groove on either side (Figure 5-9, *B*). The carotid artery is simple to find, especially during exercise. However, there are pressure receptors located in the carotid artery that if subjected to hard pressure from the two fingers will slow down the heart rate, giving a false indication of what the heart rate really is. Thus the pulse at the radial artery provides the most accurate measure of heart rate. Regardless of where the heart rate is taken, it should be monitored within 15 seconds after stopping exercise.

The objective of aerobic exercise is to elevate your heart rate to a specified target rate and maintain it at that level during your entire workout. Heart rate can be increased or decreased by speeding up or slowing down your pace. It has already been indicated that heart rate increases proportionately with the intensity of the workload and will plateau after 2 to 3 minutes of activity. Thus you should be actively engaged in the workout for 2 to 3 minutes before measuring your pulse.

Calculating Maximum Heart Rate. Exact determination of maximum heart rate (MHR) involves exercising an individual at a maximal level and monitoring the heart rate using an electrocardiogram. This is a difficult process outside of a laboratory. However, an approximate estimate of maximum heart rate for both males and females is about 220 beats per minute. Maximum heart rate is related to age. As you get older, your maximum heart rate decreases. Thus a relatively simple estimate of your maximum heart rate would be: MHR = 220 − Age.

Thus for a 20-year-old college student, maximum heart rate would be about 200 beats per minute (220 − 20 = 200) (Figure 5-10).

Calculating Heart Rate Reserve. Heart rate reserve (HRR) or heart rate range indicates the range in heart rate between resting heart rate (RHR) and maximum heart rate (MHR). It is calculated by the following equation: HRR = MHR − RHR. It has been shown that 60% to 80% of the HRR corresponds to 60% to 80% of $\dot{V}O_2$max. Thus a percentage of HRR can be used to calculate a target heart rate.

Target Heart Rate. There are several formulas that will easily allow you to identify a target heart rate (THR).

If you are interested in working at 70% of your maximum rate, the target heart rate can be calculated by multiplying 0.7 × (220 − Age). Again using a 20-year-old student as an example, target heart rate would be 140 beats per minute (0.7 × [220 − 20] = 140).

---

continuous training a technique that uses exercises performed at the same level of intensity for long periods

target heart rate (THR) a specific heart rate to be achieved and maintained during exercise

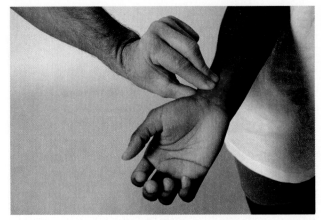
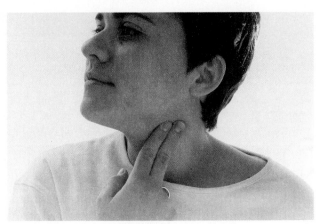

A   B

FIGURE 5-9. Measuring Pulse.
Measuring pulse rate at **A,** radial artery and **B,** carotid artery.

FIGURE 5-10. Sample Worksheet for Calculating Training Heart Rate.

Estimation of Maximum

Heart Rate		Example
220		220
−	Age	− 20
	Predicted maximum heart rate	200
×%	Intensity	× 0.7
	Training heart rate	140 beats/min

Karvonen Equation   **Example**

	Maximum heart rate	200
−	Resting heart rate	− 70
		130
×%	Intensity	× 0.6
		78
+	Resting heart rate	+ 70
	Training heart rate	148 beats/min

Another commonly used formula that takes into account your current level of fitness is the Karvonen equation:

$$THR = RHR* + (0.6\,[MHR - RHR]).$$

Resting heart rate generally falls between 60 and 80 beats per minute. A 20-year-old person with a resting pulse of 70 beats per minute, according to the Karvonen equation, would have a target training heart rate of 148 beats per minute (70 + 0.6 [200 − 70] = 148).

---

*True resting heart rate should be monitored with the subject lying down.

Regardless of the formula you use, it should be clear that to see minimal improvement in cardiorespiratory endurance, you must train with the heart rate elevated to at least 60% of its maximum rate. The American College of Sports Medicine recommends that for the healthy college-age student it is more desirable to train at 50% to 85% of heart rate reserve ($\dot{V}O_2max$), or 60% to 90% of maximum heart rate when training continuously. Exercising at a 70% level is considered a moderate level since activity can be continued for a long period of time with little discomfort and still produce a training effect. In a trained individual it is not difficult to sustain a heart rate at the 85% level. ACSM has also indicated that individuals with a low fitness level may respond to a low exercise intensity of 40% to 50% of heart rate reserve or $\dot{V}O_2$ max.

Rating of Perceived Exertion. Rating of perceived exertion (RPE) can be used in addition to monitoring heart rate to indicate exercise intensity. During exercise, individuals are asked to rate subjectively on a numerical scale from 6 to 20 exactly how they feel relative to their level of exertion (Table 5-3). More intense exercise that requires a higher level of oxygen consumption and energy expenditure is directly related to higher subjective ratings of perceived exertion. Over a period of time, individuals can be taught to exercise at a specific RPE that relates directly to more objective measures of exercise intensity.

Type

The type of activity used in continuous training must be aerobic. Aerobic activities are activities that generally involve repetitive, whole-body, large-muscle movements that are rhythmical in nature and that use large amounts of oxygen, elevate the heart rate, and maintain it at that level for an extended period of time. Examples of aerobic activities are walking, running, jogging, cycling, swimming, rope skipping, stepping, aerobic dance exercise, roller blading, and cross-country skiing.

The advantage of these aerobic activities as opposed to more intermittent activities, such as racquetball, squash, basketball, or tennis, is that with aerobic activities it is easy to regulate intensity by either speeding up or slowing down the pace. Because we already know that the given intensity of the workload elicits a given heart rate, these aerobic activities allow us to maintain heart rate at a specified or target level. Intermittent activities involve variable speeds and intensities that cause the heart rate to fluctuate considerably. Although these intermittent activities will improve cardiorespiratory endurance, they are much more difficult to monitor in terms of intensity. It is important to point out that any type of activity, from gardening to aerobic exercise, can improve fitness and reduce the risks for several chronic diseases discussed in Chapter 2. Again, the fact that you enjoy a specific type of activity should be an important factor in the selection of a particular aerobic activity.

Time (Duration)

For minimal improvement to occur, you must participate in at least 20 minutes of continuous activity with the heart rate elevated to its working level. ACSM recommends 20 to 60 minutes of workout/activity with the heart rate elevated to training levels. Generally, the greater the duration of the workout, the greater the improvement in cardiorespiratory endurance. The competitive athlete should train for at least 45 minutes.

Guidelines for Continuous Training

In summary, when using the continuous training method, the activity selected must be aerobic and should be enjoyable. To see minimal improvement in cardiorespiratory endurance, training must be done for a period of 20 to 60 minutes, three to five times per week with the heart rate elevated to an intensity of no less than 60% of its maximum rate. As mentioned in Chapter 4, each training program should be designed to meet individual needs and abilities. The principle of overload states that you must stress the system if you are to see improvement and progress from one level to another. Everyone should begin slowly with the idea that he or she will progress as quickly as possible at his or her own rate. If you are able to perform an activity at a given level without undue stress and it seems that you are not being "challenged" at that particular level, you may progress to the next level. Remember, however, that beginning at a level that is too high will probably produce various musculoskeletal injuries that will often result in setbacks in a training program.

All training programs are based on monitoring heart rate during some type of aerobic activity. Heart rate can be increased or decreased by altering the pace. The following rough guidelines can be applied to beginning, intermediate, and advanced levels (Table 5-4).

TABLE 5-3. Rating of Perceived Exertion

Scale	Verbal Rating
6	
7	Very, very light
8	
9	Very light
10	
11	Fairly light
12	
13	Somewhat hard
14	
15	Hard
16	
17	Very hard
18	
19	Very, very hard
20	

From Borg GA: Psychophysical basis of perceived exertion, *Med Sci Sports Exerc* 14:377, 1982.

TABLE 5-4. Guidelines for Continuous Training

Training Level*	Frequency (Sessions per Week)	Duration (Minutes)†	Intensity of Exercise (% of $\dot{V}O_2$max or HRR)
Beginner	3	20	40%-50%
Intermediate	4-5	30-45	50%-75%
Advanced	5-6	45-60	75%-85%

*Determine your training level by completing the Lab Activities at the end of this chapter.
† The heart rate should be elevated to training levels during this entire period.

---

rating of perceived exertion (RPE) a technique used to subjectively rate exercise intensity on a numerical scale

ADVANCED TRAINING METHODS
Interval Training

Unlike continuous training, interval training involves activities that are more intermittent. Interval training consists of alternating periods of relatively intense work and active recovery. It allows for performance of much more work at a more intense workload over a longer period of time than if working continuously. We have stated that it is most desirable in continuous training to work at an intensity of about 60% to 80% of maximum heart rate. Obviously, sustaining activity at a relatively high intensity over a 20-minute period would be extremely difficult. The advantage of interval training is that it allows work at this 80% or higher level for a short period of time followed by an active period of recovery during which you may be working at only 30% to 45% of maximum heart rate. Thus the intensity of the workout and its duration can be greater than with continuous training.

Most sports are anaerobic, involving short bursts of intense activity followed by a sort of active recovery period (e.g., football, basketball, soccer, and tennis). Training with the interval technique allows you to be more sport-specific during the workout. With interval training you can apply the overload principle by making the training period much more intense. There are several important considerations in interval training. The *training period* is the amount of time that continuous activity is actually being performed, and the *recovery period* is the time between training periods. A *set* is a group of combined training and recovery periods, and a *repetition* is the number of training/recovery periods per set. *Training time* or *distance* refers to the rate or distance of the training period. The *training/recovery ratio* indicates a time ratio for training versus recovery.

Table 5-5 indicates recommended training intervals in terms of both time and distance. This information may be used as a guide for establishing an interval workout.

An example of interval training would be a soccer player running sprints. An interval workout would involve running two sets of four 400 meter dashes in under 70 seconds, with a 2-minute 20-second walking recovery period between each dash. During this training session the soccer player's heart rate would probably increase to 85% to 95% of maximum level during the dash and should probably fall to the 35% to 45% level during the recovery period.

Older adults should exercise some caution when using interval training as a method for improving cardiorespiratory endurance. The intensity levels attained during the active periods may be too high for the older adult.

Fartlek Training

Fartlek is a training technique that is a type of cross-country running originated in Sweden. Fartlek literally means "speed play." It is similar to interval training in that you must run for a specified period of time; however, specific pace and speed are not identified. It is recommended that the course for a fartlek workout be some type of varied terrain with some level running, some uphill and downhill running, and some running through obstacles such as trees or rocks. The object is to put surges into a running workout, varying the length of the surges according to individual purposes.

One big advantage of fartlek training is that because the pace and terrain are always changing, the training session is less regimented and allows for an effective alternative in the training routine.

Again, if fartlek training is going to improve cardiorespiratory endurance, it must elevate the heart rate to at least minimum training levels. Fartlek may best be used as an off-season conditioning activity or as a change of pace activity to counteract the boredom of a training program that uses the same activity day after day.

Par Cours

Par cours is a technique for improving cardiorespiratory endurance that basically combines continuous training and circuit training. This technique involves jogging a short distance from station to station and performing a designated exercise at each station according to guidelines and directions provided on an instruction board located at that station. Par cours circuits provide an excellent means for gaining some aerobic benefits while incorporating some of the benefits of calisthenics. Typically, par cours circuits are found in parks or recreational areas within metropolitan areas.

TABLE 5-5. Recommended Interval Training Workouts

Level	Intensity During Training Period	Intensity During Recovery Period
Beginner	70%-75% of MHR	30%-35% of MHR
Intermediate	75%-85% of MHR	35%-40% of MHR
Advanced	85%-95% of MHR	40%-45% of MHR

indicated by the maximal capacity of the working tissues to use oxygen ($\dot{V}O_2$max). We know from an earlier discussion that $\dot{V}O_2$max can be predicted or estimated by measuring heart rates at varying workloads. You can use Lab Activities 5-2 through 5-6 as tests to determine your specific levels of cardiorespiratory endurance. It must be remembered that each of these activities is based to a large extent on one or both of the following factors: (1) the motivation of the person and (2) the minimal level of cardiovascular endurance.

EVALUATION OF CARDIORESPIRATORY ENDURANCE

How fit is your cardiorespiratory system? Numerous tests have been developed to evaluate fitness levels. Most of these tests are based on the idea that cardiorespiratory endurance capacity is best

interval training alternating periods of relatively intense work with periods of active recovery
fartlek a type of workout that involves jogging at varying speeds over varying terrain
par cours a technique for improving cardiorespiratory endurance that combines continuous training and circuit training

SUMMARY

- Cardiorespiratory endurance involves the coordinated function of the heart, lungs, blood, and blood vessels to supply sufficient amounts of oxygen to the working tissues.
- The best indicator of how efficiently the cardiorespiratory system functions is the maximal rate at which oxygen can be used by the tissues.
- Heart rate is directly related to the rate of oxygen consumption. It is therefore possible to estimate the intensity of the workout in terms of rate of oxygen use by monitoring heart rate.
- Aerobic exercise involves an activity in which the level of intensity and duration is low enough to provide a sufficient amount of oxygen to supply the demands of the working tissues. In anaerobic exercise the intensity of the activity is so high that oxygen is being used more quickly than it can be supplied.

- Continuous or sustained training for improvement of cardiorespiratory endurance involves selecting an activity that is aerobic in nature and training at least three times per week for a time period of no less than 20 minutes with the heart rate elevated to at least 60% of maximum rate.
- Interval training involves alternating periods of relatively intense work followed by active recovery periods. Interval training allows performance of more work at a relatively higher workload than continuous training does.
- Fartlek makes use of jogging or running over varying types of terrain at changing speeds.
- Par cours is a training technique that combines continuous training with exercises done at stations along the course.

REFERENCES

American College of Sports Medicine: *Guidelines for exercise testing and prescription,* Philadelphia, 1995, Lea & Febiger.

Åstrand PO: *Ergometry test of physical fitness,* Varberg, Sweden, 1989, Monark-Crescent AB.

Åstrand PO: Åstrand-Rhyming nomogram for calculation of aerobic capacity from pulse rate during submaximal work, *J Appl Physiol* 7:218, 1954.

Borg GA: Psychophysical basis of perceived exertion, *Med Sci Sports Exerc* 14:377, 1982.

Brooks G, Mercier J: The balance of carbohydrate and lipid utilization during exercise: the crossover concept, *J App Physiol* 76:2253-2261, 1994.

Cerretelli P: Energy sources for muscle contraction, *Sports Med* 13:S106-S110, 1992.

Cox M: Exercise training programs and cardiorespiratory adaptation, *Clin Sports Med* 10(1):19-32, 1991.

Dicarlo L, Sparling P, Millard-Stafford M: Peak heart rates during maximal running and swimming: implications for exercise prescription, *Int J Sports Med* 12:309-312, 1991.

Durstein L, Pate R, Branch D: Cardiorespiratory responses to acute exercise. In American College of Sports Medicine: *Resource manual for guidelines for exercise testing and prescription,* Philadelphia, 1993, Lea & Febiger.

Gaesser GA, Wilson LA: Effects of continuous and interval training on the parameters of the power-endurance time relationship for high-intensity exercise, *Int J Sports Med* 9(6):417, 1988.

Glass S, Whaley M, Wegner M: A comparison between ratings of perceived exertion among standard protocols and steady state running, *Int J Sports Med* 12:77-82, 1991.

Green J, Patla A: Maximal aerobic power: neuromuscular and metabolic considerations, *Med Sci Sports Exerc* 24:38-46, 1992.

Hawley J, Myburgh K, Noakes T: Maximal oxygen consumption: a contemporary perspective. In Fahey T, editor: *Encyclopedia of sports medicine and exercise physiology,* New York, 1995, Garland.

Honig C, Connett R, Gayeski T: O_2 transport and its interaction with metabolism, *Med Sci Sports Exerc* 24:47-53, 1992.

Karvonen MJ, Kentala E, Mustala O: The effects of training on heart rate: a longitudinal study, *Ann Med Exp Biol* 35:305, 1957.

Koyanagi A, Yamamoto K, Nishijima K: Recommendation for an exercise prescription to prevent coronary heart disease, *Med Syst* 17:213-217, 1993.

Levine G, Balady G: The benefits and risks of exercise testing: the exercise prescription, *Adv Intern Med* 38:57-79, 1993.

Londeree B, Moeschberger M: Effect of age and other factors on maximal heart rate, *Res Q Exerc Sport* 53:297, 1982.

McArdle W, Katch F, Katch V: *Exercise physiology, energy, nutrition, and human performance,* Philadelphia, 1994, Lea & Febiger.

Monahan T: Perceived exertion: an old exercise tool finds new applications, *Phys Sports Med* 16:174, 1988.

Pate R, Pratt M, Blair S: Physical activity and public health: a recommendation from the CDC and ACSM, *JAMA* 273(5):402-407, 1995.

Powers S: Fundamentals of exercise metabolism. In American College of Sports Medicine: *Resource manual for guidelines for exercise testing and prescription,* Philadelphia, 1993, Lea & Febiger.

Saltin B, Strange S: Maximal oxygen uptake: old and new arguments for a cardiovascular limitation, *Med Sci Sports Exerc* 24:30-37, 1992.

Smith M, Mitchell J: Cardiorespiratory adaptations to exercise training. In American College of Sports Medicine: *Resource manual for guidelines for exercise testing and prescription,* Philadelphia, 1993, Lea & Febiger.

Stachenfeld N, Eskenazi M, Gleim G: Predictive accuracy of criteria used to assess maximal oxygen consumption, *Am Heart J* 123:922-925, 1992.

Swain D, Abernathy K, Smith C: Target heart rates for the development of cardiorespiratory fitness, *Med Sci Sports Exerc* 26:112-116, 1994.

US Department of Health and Human Services, Public Health Services: *Healthy people 2000: national health promotion and disease prevention objectives,* Washington, DC, 1991, USDHHS

Wagner P: Central and peripheral aspects of oxygen transport and adaptations with exercise, *Sports Med* 11:133-142, 1991.

Weltman A, Weltman J, Rutt R, et al: Percentage of maximal heart rate reserve, and $\dot{V}O_2$ peak for determining endurance training intensity in sedentary women, *Int J Sports Med* 10(3):212, 1989 (review).

Williford H, Scharff-Olson M, Blessing D: Exercise prescription for women: special considerations, *Sports Med* 15:299-311, 1993.

Zhang Y, Johnson M, Chow N: Effect of exercise testing protocol on parameters of aerobic function, *Med Sci Sports Exerc* 23:625-630, 1991.

SUGGESTED READINGS

Brooks G, Fahey T, White T: *Exercise physiology: human bioenergetics and its applications,* Mountain View, Calif, 1996, Mayfield.
An up-to-date advanced text in exercise physiology that contains a comprehensive listing of the most current journal articles relative to exercise physiology.

Fahey T: *Encyclopedia of sports medicine and exercise physiology,* New York, 1995, Garland.
A text that includes a wide range of topics relative to fitness and that does a particularly good job of discussing cardiorespiratory endurance.

Wilmore J, Costill D: Physiology of sport and exercise, Champaign, 1994, Human Kinetics.
An excellent introductory text for undergraduate students. It is well illustrated with color photographs and explains difficult material in a clear and understandable manner.

Calculating Resting Heart Rate, Maximum Heart Rate, and Training Target Heart Rate

Name _____ Section _____ Date _____

PURPOSE   The purpose of this Lab Activity is to practice counting resting heart rate (RHR) at the radial and carotid arteries, calculating maximum heart rate (MHR), and determining training target heart rate (TTHR).

PROCEDURE   **Calculating Resting Heart Rate**

1. Practice counting the number of pulses felt for a given peiod of time at both the carotid and radial locations. Use a clock or watch to count for 10, 15, 30, and 60 seconds. To establish your resting heart rate in beats per minute, multiply the 10-second count by 6, multiply the 15-second count by 4, and multiply the 30-second count by 2.
2. Practice locating your carotid and radial pulses quickly. This is important when trying to count your pulse after exercise. Counting pulse after exercise will be necessary in labs.
3. Practice counting the pulse of another person using both the wrist and carotid locations (do not use your thumb).

Results

Record the various pulse counts you have taken in the spaces provided here:

Carotid Pulse Count (Self)		Heart Rate per Minute	Carotid Pulse Count (Partner)		Heart Rate per Minute
_____	10 seconds × 6	_____	_____	10 seconds × 6	_____
_____	15 seconds × 4	_____	_____	15 seconds × 4	_____
_____	30 seconds × 2	_____	_____	30 seconds × 2	_____
_____	60 seconds × 1	_____	_____	60 seconds × 1	_____

Carotid Pulse Count (Self)		Heart Rate per Minute	Carotid Pulse Count (Partner)		Heart Rate per Minute
_____	10 seconds × 6	_____	_____	10 seconds × 6	_____
_____	15 seconds × 4	_____	_____	15 seconds × 4	_____
_____	30 seconds × 2	_____	_____	30 seconds × 2	_____
_____	60 seconds × 1	_____	_____	60 seconds × 1	_____

Continued.

Calculating Maximum Heart Rate

Maximum Heart Rate = 220 beats/min −   _20_   = _200_   beats/min
                                     (your age in years)

Calculating Training Target Heart Rate

To calculate a training target heart rate, use the Karvonen equation.

$$TTHR = RHR + (0.6 [MHR-RHR])$$

TTHR = _____ + (0.6 X [_____ − _____]) = _____ beats/min
        (your resting   (your maximum   (your resting
        heart rate)   heart rate)   heart rate)

What is your resting heart rate?   _____

What is your maximum heart rate?   _____

What is your training target heart rate?   _____

Target
THR range = MHR x (.70) = _140 bpm_
              200
140-170 bpm   MHR x (.85) = _170 bpm_

Recovery Heart Rate = ≤ 100 bpm after 10 min.

Lab Activity 5-2

1.5-Mile Test*

Name _____ **Section** _____ **Date** _____

PURPOSE To determine the level of cardiorespiratory endurance by recording the time required to complete a 1.5-mile measured distance course.

EQUIPMENT
1. Measured course of 1.5 miles, preferably on flat surface
2. Stopwatch

PROCEDURE Subjects are instructed to cover the 1.5-mile distance as quickly as possible by either running, jogging, or walking.

TREATMENT OF DATA
1. Time required to cover the distance should be recorded to the nearest second.
2. Consult Table 5-6 (p. 128) to determine appropriate fitness category.

SAMPLE WORKSHEET FOR 1.5-MILE TEST

		Example
1. Record the time required to complete the 1.5-mile distance.	_____	1. 11:00
2. Record your age.	_____	2. 20
3. Record your sex.	_____	3. Male
4. Record your fitness category as indicated in Table 5-6 (p. 128).	_____	4. Moderate

---

*This test may be too difficult for beginners because of the distance.

Fitness Category		Time (Age 17-25)	Time (Age 26-35)
TABLE 5-6. 1.5 Mile Run Standards for Moderately Fit* College Students†			
Superior	(females)	<10:30	<11:30
	(males)	<8:30	<9:30
Excellent	(females)	10:30-11:49	11:30-12:49
	(males)	8:30-9:29	9:30-10:29
Good	(females)	11:50-13:09	12:50-14:09
	(males)	9:30-10:29	10:30-11:29
Moderate	(females)	13:10-14:29	14:10-15:29
	(males)	10:30-11:29	11:30-12:29
Fair	(females)	14:30-15:49	15:30-16:49
	(males)	11:30-12:29	12:30-13:29
Poor	(females)	>15:49	>16:49
	(males)	>12:29	>13:29

* Moderately fit college students are not athletes but laypersons who engage in continuous aerobic activity lasting a minimum of 20 minutes, three times a week.
† Based on data collected n = 427 females, 511 males.

Åstrand-Rhyming Nomogram for Estimation of Physical Fitness

Name _____ **Section** _____ **Date** _____

PURPOSE
To determine the physical fitness of a subject based on cardiac and oxygen transport changes that occur during a 6-minute bicycle ergometer test (Figure 5-11).

EQUIPMENT
1. Monarch bicycle ergometer
2. Metronome
3. Stopwatch
4. Towel

PRETEST PROCEDURE
1. Record the resting heart rate of the subject after a 5-minute rest period.
2. Adjust the saddle height of the ergometer for the subject.
   a. With the front part of the foot on the pedal there should be a slight bend in the knee joint.
   b. The pedal should be at its lowest point.

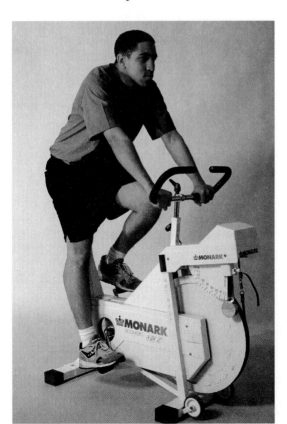

FIGURE 5-11. Bicycle Ergometer.
Equipment used in Åstrand-Rhyming nomogram test.

Continued.

3. Set the metronome to produce 100 beats per minute.
    a. The setting is equal to 50 complete pedal turns per minute. Each time the metronome clicks, one foot should reach the bottom of a pedal revolution.
    b. Both the light and sound stimuli are switched to the "on" position.
4. Work is started with a slack brake belt.
    a. The subject should begin pedaling 15 seconds before the timed work period begins.
    b. Tighten the brake belt with the handwheel until the red pointer is on 1,2, or 3 kp (kilopounds).
    c. A suitable beginning workload for women is 2 kp (600 kilopound meters [kpm] per minute).
    d. A suitable beginning workload for men is 3 kp (900 kpm/min).

SAMPLE WORKSHEET FOR ÅSTRAND-RHYMING NOMOGRAM TEST

			Example
1. Count heartbeat at end of			
minute 5	_____	HR	168
minute 6 +	_____	HR	+164
	_____	Total	332
÷ 2			÷ 2
= _____		Mean HR	166

2. Note workload setting on ergometer _____   1200 kpm/min
3. Find points on nomogram (Figure 5-12) under "Pulse rate" and "Workload" columns, and connect them with a straight line.
4. Predicted $\dot{V}O_2$max _____   3.6 L/min

TEST PROCEDURE

1. Begin timing the work period, which is 6 minutes long.
2. Count the heart rate at the end of the fifth and sixth minutes during the last 30 seconds of each minute.
3. Using the average heart rate of the last 2 minutes of exercise, cross-reference it with the workload level (kpm/min) for men or women.
4. The mean value of the heart rate at the end of the fifth and sixth minutes is designated as the "working pulse" for the load being used. If the difference between the last two readings is five beats or more, the test should be continued another minute or more until a steady-state heart rate occurs.
5. Consult the Åstrand-Rhyming nomogram, and follow the directions to calculate maximal oxygen uptake (Figure 5-12, p. 132). Record on the worksheet on p. 132. (The heart rate during minutes 5 and 6 should range between 150 and 170.)

OR

6. Calculate mean heart as indicated above.
7. Note the workload setting on the ergometer, and record it on the worksheet above and on p. 132.
8. Consult Table 5-7, which predicts maximal oxygen uptake from heart rate and workload on a bicycle ergometer. Locate the appropriate mean heart rate in the left column and the appropriate workload at the top, and determine maximal oxygen uptake in L/min.
9. Multiply by the appropriate age correction factor in Table 5-8, and record it on the worksheet.
10. Consult Table 5-9 to calculate maximal oxygen uptake in ml/kg × min.

TABLE 5-7. Prediction of Maximal Oxygen Uptake From Heart Rate and Workload on a Bicycle Ergometer*

Heart rate	Part A—Men Maximal oxygen uptake (L/min⁻¹)					Heart rate	Part B—Women Maximal oxygen uptake (L/min⁻¹)				
	300 kpm/min 50W	600 kpm/min 100W	900 kpm/min 150W	1200 kpm/min 200W	1500 kpm/min 250W		300 kpm/min 50W	450 kpm/min 75W	600 kpm/min 100W	750 kpm/min 125W	900 kpm/min 150W
120	2.2	3.5	4.8			120	2.6	3.4	4.1	4.8	
121	2.2	3.4	4.7			121	2.5	3.3	4.0	4.8	
122	2.2	3.4	4.6			123	2.4	3.1	3.9	4.7	
123	2.1	3.4	4.6			123	2.4	3.1	3.9	4.6	
124	2.1	3.3	4.5	6.0		124	2.4	3.1	3.8	4.5	
125	2.0	3.2	4.4	5.9		125	2.3	3.0	3.7	4.4	
126	2.0	3.2	4.4	5.8		126	2.3	3.0	3.6	4.3	
127	2.0	3.1	4.3	5.7		127	2.2	2.9	3.5	4.2	
128	2.0	3.1	4.2	5.6		128	2.2	2.8	3.5	4.2	4.8
129	1.9	3.0	4.2	5.6		129	2.2	2.8	3.4	4.1	4.8
130	1.9	3.0	4.1	5.5		130	2.1	2.7	3.4	4.0	4.7
131	1.9	2.9	4.0	5.4		131	2.1	2.7	3.4	4.0	4.6
132	1.8	2.9	4.0	5.3		132	2.0	2.7	3.3	3.9	4.5
133	1.8	2.8	3.9	5.3		133	2.0	2.6	3.2	3.8	4.4
134	1.8	2.8	3.9	5.2		134	2.0	2.6	3.2	3.8	4.4
135	1.7	2.8	3.8	5.1		135	2.0	2.6	3.1	3.7	4.3
136	1.7	2.7	3.8	5.0		136	1.9	2.5	3.1	3.6	4.2
137	1.7	2.7	3.7	5.0		137	1.9	2.5	3.0	3.6	4.2
138	1.6	2.7	3.7	4.9		138	1.8	2.4	3.0	3.5	4.1
139	1.6	2.6	3.6	4.8		139	1.8	2.4	2.9	3.5	4.0
140	1.6	2.6	3.6	4.8	6.0	140	1.8	2.4	2.8	3.4	4.0
141		2.6	3.5	4.7	5.9	141	1.8	2.3	2.8	3.4	3.9
142		2.5	3.5	4.6	5.8	142	1.7	2.3	2.8	3.3	3.9
143		2.5	3.4	4.6	5.7	143	1.7	2.2	2.7	3.3	3.8
144		2.5	3.4	4.5	5.7	144	1.7	2.2	2.7	3.2	3.8
145		2.4	3.4	4.5	5.6	145	1.6	2.2	2.7	3.2	3.7
146		2.4	3.3	4.4	5.6	146	1.6	2.2	2.6	3.2	3.7
147		2.4	3.3	4.4	5.5	147	1.6	2.1	2.6	3.1	3.6
148		2.4	3.2	4.3	5.4	148	1.6	2.1	2.6	3.1	3.6
149		2.3	3.2	4.3	5.4	149		2.1	2.6	3.0	3.5
150		2.3	3.2	4.2	5.3	150		2.0	2.5	3.0	3.5
151		2.3	3.1	4.2	5.2	151		2.0	2.5	3.0	3.4
152		2.3	3.1	4.1	5.2	152		2.0	2.5	2.9	3.4
153		2.2	3.0	4.1	5.1	153		2.0	2.4	2.9	3.3
154		2.2	3.0	4.0	5.1	154		2.0	2.4	2.8	3.3
155		2.2	3.0	4.0	5.0	155		1.9	2.4	2.8	3.2
156		2.2	2.9	4.0	5.0	156		1.9	2.3	2.8	3.2
157		2.1	2.9	3.9	4.9	157		1.9	2.3	2.7	3.2
158		2.1	2.9	3.9	4.9	158		1.8	2.3	2.7	3.1
159		2.1	2.8	3.8	4.8	159		1.8	2.2	2.7	3.1
160		2.1	2.8	3.8	4.8	160		1.8	2.2	2.6	3.0
161		2.0	2.8	3.7	4.7	161		1.8	2.2	2.6	3.0
162		2.0	2.8	3.7	4.6	162		1.8	2.2	2.6	3.0
163		2.0	2.8	3.7	4.6	163		1.7	2.2	2.6	2.9
164		2.0	2.7	3.6	4.5	164		1.7	2.1	2.5	2.9
165		2.0	2.7	3.6	4.5	165		1.7	2.1	2.5	2.9
166		1.9	2.7	3.6	4.5	166		1.7	2.1	2.5	2.8
167		1.9	2.6	3.5	4.4	167		1.6	2.1	2.4	2.8
168		1.9	2.6	3.5	4.4	168		1.6	2.0	2.4	2.8
169		1.9	2.6	3.5	4.3	169		1.6	2.0	2.4	2.8
170		1.8	2.6	3.4	4.3	170		1.6	2.0	2.4	2.7

From Åstrand PO: *Ergometry test of physical fitness*, Varberg, Sweden, 1989, Monark-Crescent AB.
*The value should be corrected for age according to Table 5-8.

Continued.

TABLE 5-8. Age Correction Factors for Estimating Maximal Oxygen Uptake

Age	Factor
15	1.10
25	1.00
35	0.87
40	0.83
45	0.78
50	0.75
55	0.71
60	0.68
65	0.65

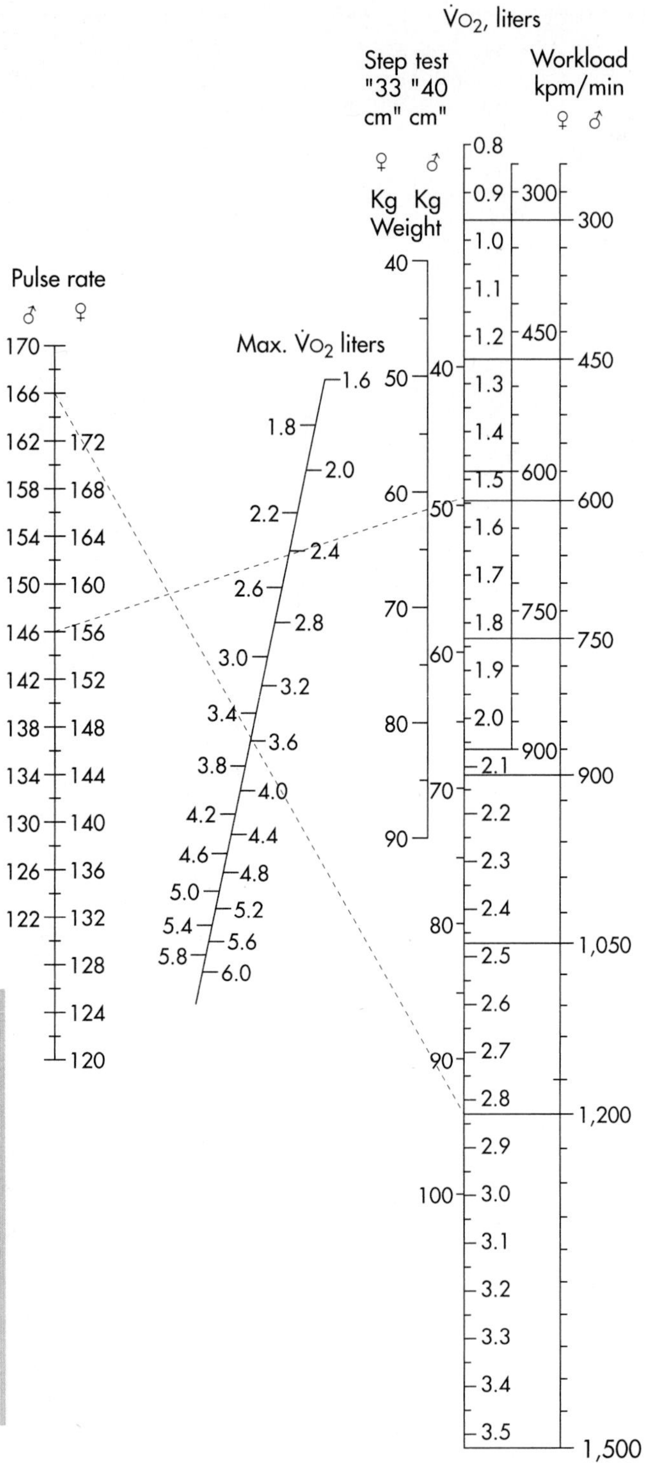

WORKSHEET FOR FIGURE 5-12

Ergometer workload _____

Maximal oxygen uptake _____ L/min

Age correction factor _____

_____ L/min_____ = _____

$\dot{V}_{O_2}$max × Age correction factor   Adjusted $\dot{V}_{O_2}$max

To convert L/min to ml/kg/min:

$$\frac{L/min \times 1000}{Body\ weight\ (kg)} = ml/kg/min$$

FIGURE 5-12. The Adjusted Nomogram.
This nomogram is used for calculating maximal oxygen uptake from submaximal pulse rate and O_2 uptake values during cycling. In tests without direct oxygen uptake measurement, it can be estimated by reading horizontally from the "workload" scale (cycle test) to the O_2 uptake scale. The point on the "O_2 uptake" scale ($\dot{V}_{O_2}$, liters) shall be connected with the corresponding point on the pulse rate scale. The predicted maximal O_2 uptake is read on the middle scale. For example, a male subject reaches a heart rate of 166 at cycling test on a workload of 1200 kpm/min; predicted $\dot{V}_{O_2}$max = 3.6 liters/min (exemplified by dotted lines).

TABLE 5-9. Calculation of Maximal Oxygen Uptake (ml/kg × min)

Body Weight — Maximal Oxygen Uptake (L/min)

Pound	Kg	1.5	1.6	1.7	1.8	1.9	2.0	2.1	2.2	2.3	2.4	2.5	2.6	2.7	2.8	2.9	3.0	3.1	3.2	3.3	3.4	3.5	3.6	3.7
96		33	35	37	39	41	43	45	47	49	51	53	55	57	59	61	63	65	67	69	71	73	75	77
99		32	34	36	38	40	42	44	46	48	50	52	54	56	58	60	62	64	66	68	70	72	74	64
101		32	34	36	38	40	42	44	46	48	50	52	54	56	58	60	62	64	66	68	70	72	74	76
103		31	33	35	37	39	41	43	45	47	49	51	53	55	57	59	61	63	65	67	69	71	73	75
106		31	33	35	37	39	41	43	45	47	49	51	53	55	57	59	61	63	65	67	69	71	73	75
108		30	32	34	36	38	40	42	44	46	48	50	52	54	56	58	60	62	64	66	68	70	72	74
110	50	30	32	34	36	38	40	42	44	46	48	50	52	54	56	58	60	62	64	66	68	70	72	74
112	51	29	31	33	35	37	39	41	43	45	47	49	51	53	55	57	59	61	63	65	67	69	71	73
115	52	29	31	33	35	37	38	40	42	44	46	48	50	52	54	56	58	60	62	63	65	67	69	71
117	53	28	30	32	34	36	38	40	42	43	45	47	49	51	53	55	57	58	60	62	64	66	68	70
119	54	28	30	31	33	35	37	39	41	43	44	46	48	50	52	54	56	57	59	61	63	65	67	69
121	55	27	29	31	33	35	36	38	40	42	44	45	47	49	51	53	55	56	58	60	62	64	65	67
123	56	27	29	30	32	34	36	38	39	41	43	45	46	48	50	52	54	55	57	59	61	63	64	66
126	57	26	28	30	32	33	35	37	39	40	42	44	46	47	49	51	53	54	56	58	60	61	63	65
128	58	26	28	29	31	33	34	36	38	40	41	43	45	47	48	50	52	53	55	57	59	60	62	64
130	59	25	27	29	31	32	34	36	37	39	41	42	44	46	47	49	51	53	54	56	58	59	61	63
132	60	25	27	28	30	32	33	35	37	38	40	42	43	45	47	48	50	52	53	55	57	58	60	62
134	61	25	26	28	30	31	33	34	36	38	39	41	43	44	46	48	49	51	52	54	56	57	59	61
137	62	24	26	27	29	31	32	34	35	37	39	40	42	44	45	47	48	50	52	53	55	56	58	60
139	63	24	25	27	29	30	32	33	35	37	38	40	41	43	44	46	48	49	51	52	54	56	57	59
141	64	23	25	27	28	30	31	33	34	36	38	39	41	42	44	45	47	48	50	52	53	55	56	58
143	65	23	25	26	28	29	31	32	34	35	37	38	40	42	43	45	46	48	49	51	52	54	55	57
146	66	23	24	26	27	29	30	32	33	35	36	38	39	41	42	44	45	47	48	50	52	53	55	56
148	67	22	24	25	27	28	30	31	33	34	36	37	39	40	42	43	45	46	48	49	51	52	54	55
150	68	22	24	25	26	28	29	31	32	34	35	37	38	40	41	43	44	46	47	49	50	51	53	54
152	69	22	23	25	26	28	29	30	32	33	35	36	38	39	41	42	43	45	46	48	49	51	52	54
154	70	21	23	24	26	27	29	30	31	33	34	36	37	39	40	41	43	44	46	47	49	50	51	53
157	71	21	23	24	25	27	28	30	31	32	34	35	37	38	39	41	42	44	45	46	48	49	51	52
159	72	21	22	24	25	26	28	29	31	32	33	35	36	38	39	40	42	43	44	46	47	49	50	51
161	73	21	22	23	25	26	27	29	30	32	33	34	36	37	38	40	41	42	44	45	47	48	49	51
163	74	20	22	23	24	26	27	28	30	31	32	34	35	36	38	39	41	42	43	45	46	47	49	50
165	75	20	21	23	24	25	27	28	29	31	32	33	35	36	37	39	40	41	43	44	45	47	48	49
168	76	20	21	22	24	25	26	28	29	30	32	33	34	36	37	38	39	41	42	43	45	46	47	49
170	77	19	21	22	23	25	26	27	29	30	31	32	34	35	36	38	39	40	42	43	44	45	47	48
172	78	19	21	22	23	24	26	27	28	29	31	32	33	35	36	37	38	40	41	42	44	45	46	47
174	79	19	20	22	23	24	25	27	28	29	30	32	33	34	35	37	38	39	41	42	43	44	46	47
176	80	19	20	21	23	24	25	26	28	29	30	31	33	34	35	36	38	39	40	41	43	44	45	46
179	81	19	20	21	22	23	25	26	27	28	30	31	32	33	35	36	37	38	40	41	42	43	44	46
181	82	18	20	21	22	23	24	26	27	28	29	30	32	33	34	35	37	38	39	40	41	43	44	45
183	83	18	19	20	22	23	24	25	27	28	29	30	31	33	34	35	36	37	39	40	41	42	43	45
185	84	18	19	20	21	23	24	25	26	27	29	30	31	32	33	35	36	37	38	39	40	42	43	44
187	85	18	19	20	21	22	24	25	26	27	28	29	31	32	33	34	35	36	38	39	40	41	42	44
190	86	17	19	20	21	22	23	24	26	27	28	29	30	31	33	34	35	36	37	38	40	41	42	43
192	87	17	18	20	21	22	23	24	25	26	28	29	30	31	32	33	34	36	37	38	39	40	41	43
194	88	17	18	19	20	22	23	24	25	26	27	28	30	31	32	33	34	35	36	38	39	40	41	42
196	89	17	18	19	20	21	22	24	25	26	27	28	29	30	31	33	34	35	36	37	38	39	40	42
198	90	17	18	19	20	21	22	23	24	26	27	28	29	30	31	32	33	34	36	37	38	39	30	41
201	91	16	18	19	20	21	22	23	24	25	26	27	29	30	31	32	33	34	35	36	37	38	40	41
203	92	16	17	18	20	21	22	23	24	25	26	27	28	29	30	32	33	34	35	36	37	38	39	40
205	93	16	17	18	19	20	22	23	24	25	26	27	28	29	30	31	32	33	34	35	37	38	39	40
207	94	16	17	18	19	20	21	22	23	24	26	27	28	29	30	31	32	33	34	35	36	37	38	39
209	95	16	17	18	19	20	21	22	23	24	25	26	27	28	29	31	32	33	34	35	36	37	38	39
212	96	16	17	18	19	20	21	22	23	24	25	26	27	28	29	30	31	32	33	34	35	36	38	39
214	97	15	16	18	19	20	21	22	23	24	25	26	27	28	29	30	31	32	33	34	35	36	37	38
216	98	15	16	17	18	19	20	21	22	23	24	26	27	28	29	30	31	32	33	34	35	36	37	38
218	99	15	16	17	18	19	20	21	22	23	24	25	26	27	28	29	30	31	32	33	34	35	36	37
220	100	15	16	17	18	19	20	21	22	23	24	25	26	27	28	29	30	31	32	33	34	35	36	37

Continued.

TABLE 5-9. Calculation of Maximal Oxygen Uptake (ml/kg × min)—cont'd

Body Weight Pound	Kg	__Maximal Oxygen Uptake (L/min)__																						
		3.8	3.9	4.0	4.1	4.2	4.3	4.4	4.5	4.6	4.7	4.8	4.9	5.0	5.1	5.2	5.3	5.4	5.5	5.6	5.7	5.8	5.9	6.0
96		79	81	83	85	87	89	91	93	95	97	99	101	103	105	107	109	111	113	115	117	119	121	123
99		78	80	82	84	86	88	90	92	94	96	98	100	102	104	106	108	110	112	114	116	118	120	122
101		78	80	82	84	86	88	90	92	94	96	98	100	102	104	106	108	110	112	114	116	118	120	122
103		77	79	81	83	85	87	89	91	93	95	97	99	101	103	105	107	109	111	113	115	117	119	121
106		77	79	81	83	85	87	89	91	93	95	97	99	101	103	105	107	109	111	113	115	117	119	121
108		76	78	80	82	84	86	88	90	92	94	96	98	100	102	104	106	108	110	112	114	116	118	120
110	50	76	78	80	82	84	86	88	90	92	94	96	98	100	102	104	106	108	110	112	114	116	118	120
112	51	75	76	78	80	82	84	86	88	90	92	94	96	98	100	102	104	106	108	110	112	114	116	118
115	52	73	75	77	79	81	83	85	87	88	90	92	94	96	98	100	102	104	106	108	110	112	113	115
117	53	72	74	75	77	79	81	83	85	87	89	91	92	94	96	98	100	102	104	106	108	109	111	113
119	54	70	72	74	76	78	80	81	83	85	87	89	91	93	94	96	98	100	102	104	106	107	109	111
121	55	69	71	73	75	76	78	80	82	84	85	87	89	91	93	95	96	98	100	102	104	105	107	109
123	56	68	70	71	73	75	77	79	80	82	84	86	88	89	91	93	95	96	98	100	102	104	105	107
126	57	67	68	70	72	74	75	77	79	81	82	84	86	88	89	91	93	95	96	98	100	102	104	105
128	58	66	67	69	71	72	74	76	78	79	81	83	84	86	88	90	91	93	95	97	98	100	102	103
130	59	64	66	68	69	71	73	75	76	78	80	81	83	85	86	88	90	92	93	95	97	98	100	102
132	60	63	65	67	68	70	72	73	75	77	78	80	82	83	85	87	88	90	92	93	95	97	98	100
134	61	62	64	66	67	69	70	72	74	75	77	79	80	82	84	85	87	89	90	92	93	95	97	98
137	62	61	63	65	66	68	69	71	73	74	76	77	79	81	82	84	85	87	89	90	92	94	95	97
139	63	60	62	63	65	67	68	70	71	73	75	76	78	79	81	83	84	86	87	89	90	92	94	95
141	64	59	61	63	64	66	67	69	70	72	73	75	77	78	80	81	83	84	86	88	89	91	92	94
143	65	58	60	62	63	65	66	68	69	71	72	74	75	77	78	80	82	83	85	86	88	89	91	92
146	66	58	59	61	62	64	65	67	68	70	71	73	74	76	77	79	80	82	83	85	86	88	89	91
148	67	57	58	60	61	63	64	66	67	69	70	72	73	75	76	78	79	81	82	84	85	87	88	90
150	68	56	57	59	60	62	63	65	66	68	69	71	72	74	75	76	78	79	81	82	84	85	87	88
152	69	55	57	58	59	61	62	64	65	67	68	70	71	72	74	75	77	78	80	81	83	84	86	87
154	70	54	56	57	59	60	61	63	64	66	67	69	70	71	73	74	76	77	79	80	81	83	84	86
157	71	54	55	56	58	59	61	62	63	65	66	68	69	70	72	73	75	76	77	79	80	82	83	85
159	72	53	54	56	57	58	60	61	63	64	65	67	68	69	71	72	74	75	76	78	79	81	82	83
161	73	52	53	55	56	58	59	60	62	63	64	66	67	68	70	71	73	74	75	77	78	79	81	82
163	74	51	53	54	55	57	58	59	61	62	64	65	66	68	69	70	72	73	74	76	77	78	80	81
165	75	51	52	53	55	56	57	59	60	61	63	64	65	67	68	69	71	72	73	75	76	77	79	80
168	76	50	51	53	54	55	57	58	59	61	62	63	64	66	67	68	70	71	72	74	75	76	78	79
170	77	49	51	52	53	55	56	57	58	60	61	62	64	65	66	68	69	70	71	73	74	75	77	78
172	78	49	50	51	53	54	55	56	58	59	60	62	63	64	65	67	68	69	71	72	73	74	76	77
174	79	48	49	51	52	53	54	56	57	58	59	61	62	63	65	66	67	68	70	71	72	73	75	76
176	80	48	49	50	51	53	54	55	56	58	59	60	61	63	64	65	66	68	69	70	71	72	74	75
179	81	47	48	49	51	52	53	54	56	57	58	59	60	62	63	64	65	67	68	69	70	72	73	74
181	82	46	48	49	50	51	52	54	55	56	57	59	60	61	62	63	65	66	67	68	70	71	72	73
183	83	46	47	48	49	51	52	53	54	55	57	58	59	60	61	63	64	65	66	67	69	70	71	72
185	84	45	46	48	49	50	51	52	54	55	56	57	58	60	61	62	63	64	65	67	68	69	70	71
187	85	45	46	47	48	49	51	52	53	54	55	56	58	59	60	61	62	64	65	66	67	68	69	71
190	86	44	45	47	48	49	50	51	52	53	55	56	57	58	59	60	62	63	64	65	66	67	69	70
192	87	44	45	46	47	48	49	51	52	53	54	55	56	57	59	60	61	62	63	64	66	67	68	69
194	88	43	44	45	47	48	49	50	51	52	53	55	56	57	58	59	60	61	63	64	65	66	67	68
196	89	43	44	45	46	47	48	49	51	52	53	54	55	56	57	58	60	61	62	63	64	65	66	67
198	90	42	43	44	46	47	48	49	50	51	52	53	54	56	57	58	59	60	61	62	63	64	66	67
201	91	42	43	44	45	46	47	48	49	51	52	53	54	55	56	57	58	59	60	62	63	64	65	66
203	92	41	42	43	45	46	47	48	49	50	51	52	53	54	55	57	58	59	60	61	62	63	64	65
205	93	41	42	43	44	45	46	47	48	49	51	52	53	54	55	56	57	58	59	60	61	62	63	65
207	94	40	41	43	44	45	46	47	48	49	50	51	52	53	54	55	56	57	59	60	61	62	63	64
209	95	40	41	42	43	44	45	46	47	48	49	50	51	52	53	54	55	56	57	58	59	60	61	63
212	96	40	41	42	43	44	45	46	47	48	49	50	51	52	53	54	55	56	57	58	59	60	61	63
214	97	39	40	41	42	43	44	45	46	47	48	49	51	52	53	54	55	56	57	58	59	60	61	62
216	98	39	40	41	42	43	44	45	46	47	48	49	50	51	52	53	54	55	56	57	58	59	60	61
218	99	38	39	40	41	42	43	44	45	46	47	48	49	51	52	53	54	55	56	57	58	59	60	61
220	100	38	39	40	41	42	43	44	45	46	47	48	49	50	51	52	53	54	55	56	57	58	59	60

Lab Activity 5-4

Cooper's 12-Minute Walking/Running Test

Name _____ Section _____ Date _____

PURPOSE To determine the level of cardiorespiratory endurance of college students during a 12-minute running or walking activity.

EQUIPMENT
1. Measured running course, preferably a track
2. Stopwatch

PROCEDURE
1. During a 12-minute period the subject attempts to cover as much distance as possible by either running or walking.

TREATMENT OF DATA
1. Distance covered should be rounded off to the nearest $1/8$ mile.
2. Consult Table 5-10 (p. 136). Locate the distance covered for either men or women under the appropriate age classification, and determine the level of fitness.

SAMPLE WORKSHEET FOR COOPER'S 12-MINUTE WALKING/RUNNING TEST

	Example
1. Measure distance covered, and round off to nearest $1/8$ mile.	_____ 1. 1.50
2. Record your age.	_____ 2. Age 20
3. Determine fitness level.	_____ 3. Good

TABLE 5-10.	12-Minute Walking/Running Test: Distance (Miles) Covered in 12 Minutes						
Fitness Category		**Distance by Age (Years)**					
		13-19	20-29	30-39	40-49	50-59	60+
Superior	(males)	>1.87	>1.77	>1.70	>1.66	>1.59	>1.56
	(females)	>1.52	>1.46	>1.40	>1.35	>1.31	>1.19
Excellent	(males)	1.73-1.86	1.65-1.76	1.57-1.69	1.54-1.65	1.45-1.58	1.33-1.55
	(females)	1.44-1.51	1.35-1.45	1.30-1.39	1.25-1.34	1.19-1.30	1.10-1.18
Good	(males)	1.57-1.72	1.50-1.64	1.46-1.56	1.40-1.53	1.31-1.44	1.21-1.32
	(females)	1.30-1.43	1.23-1.34	1.19-1.29	1.12-1.24	1.06-1.18	.99-1.09
Fair	(males)	1.38-1.56	1.32-1.49	1.31-1.45	1.25-1.39	1.17-1.30	1.03-1.20
	(females)	1.19-1.29	1.12-1.22	1.06-1.18	.99-1.11	.94-1.05	.87-.98
Poor	(males)	1.30-1.37	1.22-1.31	1.18-1.30	1.14-1.24	1.03-1.16	.87-1.02
	(females)	1.00-1.18	.96-1.11	.95-1.05	.88-.98	.84-.93	.78-.86
Very Poor	(males)	<1.30	<1.22	<1.18	<1.14	<1.03	<.87
	(females)	<1.0	<.96	<.94	<.88	<.84	<.78

The Rockport Fitness Walking Test

Name _____ **Section** _____ **Date** _____

PURPOSE To determine relative fitness.

PROCEDURE
1. Walk 1 mile as fast as you can. Stretch for 5 to 10 minutes before and after. Wear good walking shoes and loose-fitting clothes. Maintain a steady pace.
2. Record your time. Do this to the nearest second. Most people walk between 3.0 and 6.0 miles per hour, so it should take 10 to 20 minutes to walk the mile.
3. Record your heart rate immediately at the end of the mile. (It begins to slow almost immediately after you stop walking.) Count your pulse for 15 seconds and multiply by 4, then record this number. This gives you your heart rate per minute after your test walk.

FIND YOUR FITNESS LEVEL

The information in the following charts pertains to both the non–treadmill walker and the treadmill walker.

Turn to the appropriate Rockport Fitness Walking Test™ charts according to your age and sex. These show the established fitness norms from the American Heart Association.

Using your Relative Fitness Level chart, find your time in minutes and your heart rate per minute. Follow these lines until they meet, and mark this point on the chart. This point is designed to tell you how fit you are compared to other individuals of your same age and sex. For example, if your mark places in the "above average" section of the chart, you are in better shape than the average person in your category.

The charts are based on weights of 170 lb for men and 125 lb for women. If you weigh substantially less, your relative cardiovascular fitness level will be slightly underestimated. Conversely, if you weigh substantially more, your relative cardiovascular fitness level will be slightly overestimated.

HOW TO DETERMINE YOUR 20-WEEK WALKING PROGRAM

EXERCISE PROGRAM CHARTS

Using the exercise program chart, find your time in minutes and your heart rate per minute. Follow these lines until they meet, and mark this point on your chart. Note the color area you fall into and turn to the exercise program, starting on p. 140, corresponding to that color.

You can improve your aerobic capacity and promote lifelong health with the walking program outlined here. Your designated program is designed specifically for your current fitness level.

At the end of the 20-week period, retake the Rockport Fitness Walking Test™ to determine your new fitness level and exercise program.

On each program there are columns labeled "pace" and "heart rate." Pace is only an approximation. Your walking speed should be determined by the pace that keeps your heart rate at the percentage of maximum listed. For your percentage of maximum heart rate, use the chart provided.

From The Rockport Company, 1993.

Continued.

THE WALKING TEST

1. Find a measured track or measure out a mile, using your car's odometer, on a flat uninterrupted road.
2. Walk 1 mile as fast as you can, maintaining a steady pace.
3. Upon completion, record your time to the nearest second.
4. Continue walking, but slow down the pace. Count your pulse beginning with zero for 15 seconds and multiply the number of beats by four; record this number in the space provided. This gives you your heart rate per minute after your test walk. NOTE: Your heart rate begins to slow almost immediately after you stop walking, so continue moving while you take your pulse.
5. Cool down. Remember to repeat the stretching exercises once you've cooled down.

Resting heart rate _____

_____

Heart rate at the end of the mile _____

_____

Time to walk the mile _____

_____

Helpful items needed for test: loose-fitting clothes, comfortable walking shoes (we recommend Rockports!), and a watch with a second hand.

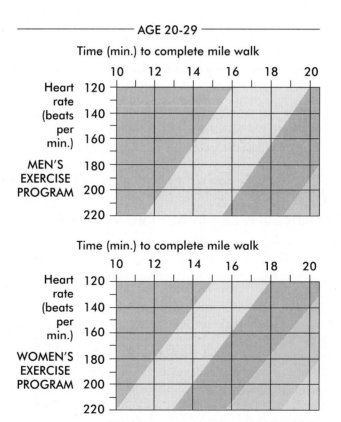

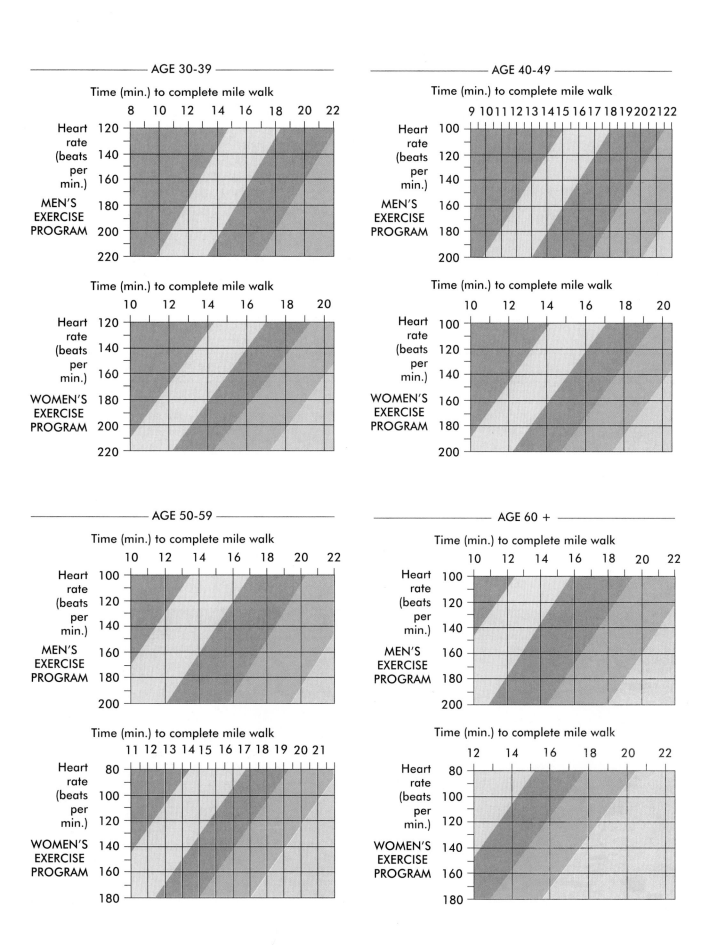

% of Maximum Heart Rate Chart (10-Second Count)			
Age	60%	70%	80%
20-29	19-20	22-23	25-27
30-39	18-19	21-22	24-25
40-49	17-18	20-21	23-24
50-59	16-17	19-20	21-23
60+	14-16	16-18	19-21

Week	1-2	3-4	5	6	7-8	9	10	11	12-13	14	15-16	17-18	19-20
WARM-UP/COOL-DOWN (stretches before and after walk in min.)	5-7	5-7	5-7	5-7	5-7	5-7	5-7	5-7	5-7	5-7	5-7	5-7	5-7
MILEAGE	1.0	1.25	1.5	1.5	1.75	2.0	2.0	2.0	2.25	2.5	2.5	2.75	3.0
PACE (mph)	3.0	3.0	3.0	3.5	3.5	3.5	3.75	3.75	3.75	3.75	4.0	4.0	4.0
HEART RATE (% of max)	60	60	60	60-70	60-70	60-70	60-70	70	70	70	70	70-80	70-80
FREQUENCY (times per week)	5	5	5	5	5	5	5	5	5	5	5	5	5

Week	1-2	3-4	5-6	7	8-9	10-12	13	14	15-16	17-18	19-20
WARM-UP/COOL-DOWN (stretches before and after walk in min.)	5-7	5-7	5-7	5-7	5-7	5-7	5-7	5-7	5-7	5-7	5-7
MILEAGE	1.5	1.75	2.0	2.0	2.25	2.5	2.75	2.75	3.0	3.25	3.5
PACE (mph)	3.0	3.0	3.0	3.5	3.5	3.5	3.5	4.0	4.0	4.0	4.0
HEART RATE (% of max)	60-70	60-70	60-70	70	70	70	70	70-80	70-80	70-80	70-80
FREQUENCY (times per week)	5	5	5	5	5	5	5	5	5	5	5

Week	1	2	3-4	5	6-8	9-10	11-12	13-14	15	16-17	18-20	Maintenance
WARM-UP/COOL-DOWN (stretches before and after walk in min.)	5-7	5-7	5-7	5-7	5-7	5-7	5-7	5-7	5-7	5-7	5-7	5-7
MILEAGE	2.0	2.25	2.5	2.75	2.75	3.0	3.0	3.25	3.5	3.5	4.0	4.0
PACE (mph)	3.0	3.0	3.0	3.0	3.5	3.5	4.0	4.0	4.0	4.5	4.5	4.5
HEART RATE (% of max)	70	70	70	70	70	70	70-80	70-80	70-80	70-80	70-80	70-80
FREQUENCY (times per week)	5	5	5	5	5	5	5	5	5	5	5	3-5

Week	1	2	3-4	5	6	7	8	9-10	11-14	15-20	Maintenance
WARM-UP/COOL-DOWN (stretches before and after walk in min.)	5-7	5-7	5-7	5-7	5-7	5-7	5-7	5-7	5-7	5-7	5-7
MILEAGE	2.5	2.75	3.0	3.25	3.25	3.5	3.75	4.0	4.0	4.0	4.0
PACE (mph)	3.5	3.5	3.5	3.5	4.0	4.0	4.0	4.0	4.5	4.5	4.5
HEART RATE (% of max)	70	70	70	70	70-80	70-80	70-80	70-80	70-80	70-80	70-80
FREQUENCY (times per week)	5	5	5	5	5	5	5	5	5	5	3-5

Week	1	2	3	4	5	6	7-20	Maintenance
WARM-UP/COOL-DOWN (stretches before and after walk in min.)	5-7	5-7	5-7	5-7	5-7	5-7	5-7	5-7
MILEAGE	3.0	3.25	3.5	3.5	3.75	4.0	4.0	4.0
PACE (mph)	4.0	4.0	4.0	4.5	4.5	4.5	4.5	4.5
HEART RATE (% of max)	70	70	70	70-80	70-80	70-80	70-80	70-80
FREQUENCY (times per week)	5	5	5	5	5	5	5	3-5

Measuring Vital Capacity

Name _____   **Section** _____   **Date** _____

PURPOSE   To measure vital capacity of the lungs. This is a measure of the maximum volume of air that can be exhaled after a maximum inhalation (or inhaled after maximum exhalation).

PROCEDURE
1. Have the subject sit in a chair facing the spirometer (Figure 5-13).
2. Check the spirometer to make certain that it has been calibrated according to manufacturer's specifications. The recording pen should be at baseline.
3. Place a new mouthpiece on the tube, insert into the subject's mouth, and apply a nose clip.
4. Allow the subject three to five practice trials to become comfortable with the equipment and breathing procedure.
5. After a brief 1 minute rest period during which the subject breathes normally, have the subject maximally inhale, then immediately exhale as much air as possible at a slow, steady pace. This should be repeated two or three times until maximal and equal volumes have been obtained.
6. Record the maximum volume of air expired by measuring the deflection of the recording pen from baseline in cubic centimeters. _____ cc
7. Consult Table 5-11 to compare the subject's vital capacity measurement with normal vital capacities. Find the appropriate height in inches and the nearest age correction factors.

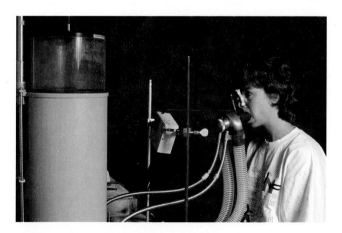

FIGURE 5-13. Spirometry.
Spirometer for measuring vital capacity.

INTERPRETATION In individuals with obstructive airway disease the vital capacity is frequently less than normal. Many factors can decrease your lungs' ability to fill up with air. Cigarette smoking and inhalation of other air pollutants can actually destroy lung tissue. Poor posture or a weak diaphragm muscle can limit your capacity to inhale. Strengthening exercises may be implemented to correct existing strength deficits.

TABLE 5-11. Vital Capacity (cc)

Men: Height in Inches	Age in Years					
	20	30	40	50	60	70
60	3885	3665	3445	3225	3005	2785
62	4154	3925	3705	3485	3265	3045
64	4410	4190	3970	3750	3530	3310
66	4675	4455	4235	4015	3795	3575
68	4940	4720	4500	4280	4060	3540
70	5206	4986	4766	4546	4326	4106
72	5571	5251	5031	4811	4591	4371
74	5736	5516	5296	5076	4856	4636

Women: Height in Inches	Age in Years					
	20	30	40	50	60	70
58	2989	2809	2629	2449	2269	2089
60	3198	3018	2838	2658	2478	2298
62	3403	3223	3043	2863	2683	2503
64	3612	3632	3252	3072	2892	2710
66	3822	3642	3462	3282	3102	2922
68	4031	3851	3671	3491	3311	3131
70	4270	4090	3910	3730	3550	3370
72	4449	4269	4089	3909	3729	3549

Summary Worksheet for Cardiorespiratory Endurance Lab Activities

Name _____   **Section** _____   **Date** _____

Lab Activity 5-1   **Calculating Resting Heart Rate, Maximum Heart Rate, and Training Target Heart Rate**

Counted resting heart rate _____ beats/min

Calculated maximum heart rate _____ beats/min

Calculated training target heart rate_____ beats/min

Lab Activity 5-2   **1.5 Mile Test**

Total time required to complete 1.5-mile distance_____ min

Fitness rating _____

Lab Activity 5-3   **Åstrand-Rhyming Nomogram for Estimation of Physical Fitness**

Predicted $\dot{V}O_2$max _____

Lab Activity 5-4   **Cooper's 12-Minute Walking/Running Test**

Total distance covered _____ mi

Fitness rating _____

Lab Activity 5-5   **The Rockport Fitness Walking Test**

Total time required to walk 1 mile _____ min

Heart rate at the end of the mile _____ beats/min

Fitness rating _____

Lab Activity 5-6   **Measuring Vital Capacity**

Maximum volume of air expired _____ cc

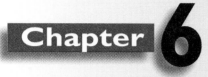

Chapter 6

Improving Muscular Strength and Endurance

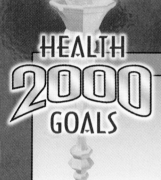

HEALTH 2000 GOALS

- **Muscular Strength and Endurance.** Increase to at least 40% the proportion of people age 6 and older who regularly perform physical activities that enhance and maintain muscular strength and endurance.

- Muscular strength and endurance greatly affect the ability to perform the tasks of daily living without undue physical stress and fatigue.
- A combination of activities that vary type, frequency, duration, and intensity may be needed to increase muscular strength and endurance.

OBJECTIVES

After completing this chapter, you will be able to do the following:

- Define strength and indicate its significance to health and skill of performance.
- Discuss the anatomy and physiology of skeletal muscle.
- Discuss the physiology of strength development and factors that determine strength.
- Describe specific methods for improving muscular strength.

- Differentiate between muscular strength and muscular endurance.
- Discuss differences between males and females in terms of strength development.
- Identify strength-training exercises for developing specific muscle groups.
- Demonstrate proper techniques for using weights to develop strength and muscular endurance.
- Demonstrate various calisthenic exercises that can be used for increasing muscular strength and endurance.

KEY TERMS

While reading this chapter, you will become familiar with the following terms:

- muscular strength
- power
- muscular endurance
- isometric contraction
- concentric contraction
- eccentric contraction
- hypertrophy
- atrophy
- isometric exercise
- progressive resistive exercise
- isotonic training
- isokinetic exercise
- circuit training
- plyometric exercise
- calisthenic exercise

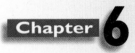

IMPORTANCE OF MUSCULAR STRENGTH

The development of muscular strength is an essential component of fitness for anyone involved in a physical activity program. By definition, muscular strength is the ability or capacity of a muscle or muscle group to exert a maximal force against resistance, one time through a full range of motion. The development of muscular strength may be considered a health-related component of physical fitness. Maintenance of at least a normal level of strength in a given muscle or muscle group is important for normal healthy living. Muscle weakness or imbalance can result in abnormal movement or gait and can impair normal functional movement. Muscle weakness can also produce poor posture, which can affect your appearance. Strength training may play a critical role not only in training programs but also in injury prevention and rehabilitation.

Most movements in sports are explosive and must include elements of both strength and speed if they are to be effective. If a large amount of force is generated quickly, the movement can be referred to as a power movement. Without the ability to generate power, an athlete will be limited in his or her performance capabilities.

IMPORTANCE OF MUSCULAR ENDURANCE

Muscular strength is closely associated with muscular endurance. Muscular endurance is the ability of a muscle or muscle group to perform a series of dynamic contractions or to sustain a static submaximal muscle contraction repeatedly over a period of time. As we will see later, as muscular strength increases, there tends to be a corresponding increase in endurance. For example, a person can lift a weight 25 times. If muscular strength is increased by 10% through weight training, it is very likely that the maximum number of repetitions will also be increased because it is easier for the person to lift the weight. For most people, developing muscular endurance is more important than developing muscular strength, since muscular endurance is probably more critical in carrying out the everyday activities of living. This becomes increasingly true with age. However, a tremendous amount of strength is necessary for anyone involved in certain types of competition.

ANATOMY AND PHYSIOLOGY OF SKELETAL MUSCLE CONTRACTION
Muscle and Tendons

Skeletal muscle consists of two portions: (1) the muscle belly and (2) its tendons, which are collectively referred to as a *musculotendinous unit* (Figure 6-1). The muscle belly is composed of separate, parallel elastic fibers called *myofibrils*. Myofibrils are composed of thousands of small *sarcomeres*, which are the functional units of the muscle. Sarcomeres contain the contractile elements of the muscle and a substantial amount of connective tissue that holds the fibers together (Figure 6-2).

Myofilaments are small contractile elements of protein within the sarcomere. There are two distinct types of myofilaments referred to as *actin* and *myosin*. Fingerlike projections or *crossbridges* connect the actin

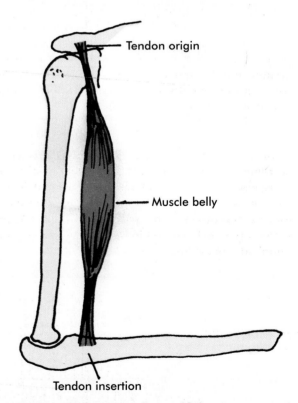

FIGURE 6-1. Musculotendinous Unit.
This unit consists of the muscle belly and its tendon that attaches the contractile portion of the muscle to the bone.

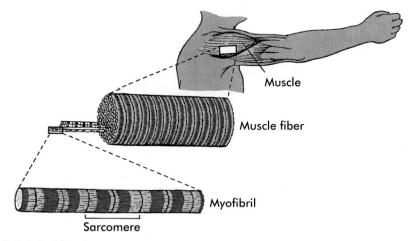

FIGURE 6-2. Muscle.
The muscle is composed of myofibrils, which contain sarcomeres.

and myosin myofilaments. When a muscle is stimulated to contract, the crossbridges pull the myofilaments closer together, thus shortening the muscle and producing movement at the joint that the muscle crosses (Figure 6-3).

The muscle tendon attaches muscle directly to bone. The muscle tendon is composed primarily of connective tissue and is relatively inelastic when compared with muscle fibers. Muscles may be connected to bone by a single tendon or by two or three separate tendons at each end. Those muscles that have two separate muscle and tendon attachments are called *biceps,* and those with three separate muscle and tendon attachments are called *triceps.*

Characteristics of Skeletal Muscle

All skeletal muscles exhibit four characteristics: (1) the ability to change in length, or stretch, *elasticity;* (2) the ability to shorten and return to normal length, *extensibility;* (3) the ability to respond to stimulation from the nervous system, *excitability;* and (4) the ability to shorten and contract in response to some neural command, *contractility.*

Muscle Shape and Size

Skeletal muscles show considerable variation in size and shape. Large muscles generally produce gross motor movements at large joints, such as knee flexion produced by contraction of the large, bulky hamstring muscles. Smaller skeletal muscles, such as the long flexors of the fingers, produce fine motor movements. Muscles producing movements that are powerful in nature are usually thicker and long, whereas those producing finer movements requiring coordination are thin and relatively shorter. Other muscles may be flat, round, or fan shaped.

Motor Unit

Muscles contract in response to stimulation by the central nervous system. A single motor nerve controls a group of muscle fibers that is collectively referred to as a *motor unit.* To contract, an electrical impulse is transmitted from the central nervous system to the specific motor unit. This causes depolarization to occur. Depolarization is a series of complex chemical events that transmit messages by nerves. The end result is that the muscle contracts. Furthermore, the electrical impulse from the central nervous system that travels to the motor unit causes *all* of the muscle fibers in that unit to contract. This is referred to as the *all-or-none response;* it applies to all muscles in the body.

Skeletal Muscle Contraction

Skeletal muscle is capable of three different types of contraction: (1) an isometric contraction, (2) a concentric, or positive, contraction, and (3) an eccentric, or negative, contraction. An isometric contraction

muscular strength the ability of a muscle to generate force against resistance
power generating a large amount of force quickly
muscular endurance the ability to perform repetitive muscular contractions against resistance for an extended period of time
isometric contraction contraction of a muscle to produce tension without a change in the length of the muscle
concentric contraction a contraction in which the muscle shortens in length while developing tension to overcome resistance
eccentric contraction a contraction in which the resistance is greater than the muscular force being produced, causing the muscle to lengthen while producing tension

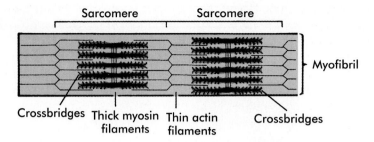

FIGURE 6-3. Muscle Contraction.
Muscles contract when an electrical impulse from the central nervous system causes the myofilaments in a muscle fiber to move closer together.

occurs when the muscle contracts to produce tension but there is no change in length of the muscle. Considerable force can be generated against some immovable resistance, even though no movement occurs. In a concentric contraction, the muscle shortens in length while tension is developed to overcome or move some resistance. In an eccentric contraction, the resistance is greater than the muscular force being produced, and the muscle lengthens while producing tension. Concentric and eccentric contractions must occur to allow most movements.

Fast-Twitch Versus Slow-Twitch Fibers

As mentioned in Chapter 5, all fibers in a particular muscle unit are either *slow-twitch* or *fast-twitch* fibers.

Slow-Twitch Fibers

Slow-twitch fibers are also referred to as type I or *slow-oxidative (SO) fibers.* They are more resistant to fatigue than are fast-twitch fibers. However, the time required to generate force is much greater in slow-twitch fibers.

Fast-Twitch Fibers

Fast-twitch fibers are capable of producing quick, forceful contractions but have a tendency to fatigue more rapidly than do slow-twitch fibers. Fast-twitch fibers are capable of producing powerful contractions, whereas slow-twitch fibers produce a long-endurance type of force. There are two subdivisions of fast-twitch fibers. Both types of fast-twitch fibers are capable of rapid contraction. However, type IIa or *fast-oxidative-glycolytic (FOG) fibers* are moderately resistant to fatigue, and type IIb or *fast-glycolytic (FG) fibers* fatigue rapidly and are considered the "true" fast-twitch

fibers. Recently, a third group of fast-twitch fibers, type IIx, has been identified in animal models. Type IIx fibers are fatigue resistant and are thought to be greater than type IIb but less than type IIa fibers in terms of their maximum power capacity.

Ratio in Muscle

Within a particular muscle are both types of fibers, and the ratio in an individual muscle varies for each person. Those muscles whose primary function is to maintain posture against gravity require more endurance and have a higher percentage of slow-twitch fibers. Muscles that produce powerful, rapid, explosive strength movements tend to have a much greater percentage of fast-twitch fibers. Because this ratio is genetically determined, it may play a large role in determining ability for a given sport activity. Sprinters and weight lifters, for example, have a large percentage of fast-twitch fibers in relation to slow-twitch fibers. Conversely, marathon runners generally have a higher percentage of slow-twitch fibers.

The metabolic capabilities of both fast-twitch and slow-twitch fibers may be improved through specific strength and endurance training. It now appears that there can be an almost complete change from slow- to fast- or from fast- to slow-twitch fiber types in response to training.

FACTORS THAT DETERMINE LEVELS OF MUSCULAR STRENGTH AND ENDURANCE
Size of the Muscle

Muscular strength is proportional to the cross-sectional diameter of the muscle fibers in both males and females. The greater the cross-sectional diameter or the bigger a particular muscle, the stronger it is, and thus the more force it is capable of generating. The size of a muscle tends to increase in cross-sectional diameter with weight training. This increase in muscle size is referred to as hypertrophy. Conversely, a decrease in the size of a muscle is referred to as atrophy.

Number of Muscle Fibers

Strength is a function of the number and diameter of muscle fibers composing a given muscle. The number of fibers is an inherited characteristic. A person with a large number of muscle fibers to begin with has the potential to hypertrophy to a much greater degree than does someone with relatively few fibers.

Neuromuscular Efficiency

Strength is also directly related to the efficiency of the neuromuscular system and the function of the motor unit in producing muscular force. As will be indicated later in this chapter, initial increases in strength during a weight-training program can be attributed primarily to increased neuromuscular efficiency.

Biomechanical Factors

Strength in a given muscle is determined not only by the physical properties of the muscle but also by biomechanical factors that dictate how much force can be generated through a system of levers to an external object.

Position of Tendon Attachment

If we think of the elbow joint as one of these lever systems, we would have the biceps muscle producing flexion of this joint (Figure 6-4). The position of attachment of the biceps muscle on the forearm will largely determine how much force this muscle is capable of generating. If there are two persons, A and B, and A has a biceps attachment that is closer to the fulcrum (the elbow joint) than B, then A must produce a greater effort with the biceps muscle to hold the weight at a right angle because the length of the effort arm will be greater than with B.

Length-Tension Relationship

The length of a muscle determines the tension that can be generated. By varying the length of a muscle, different tensions may be produced. This length-tension relationship is illustrated in Figure 6-5. At position B in the curve, the interaction of the crossbridges between the actin and myosin myofilaments within the sarcomere is at a maximum. Setting a muscle at this particular length will produce the greatest amount of tension. At position A, the muscle is shortened, and at position C the muscle is lengthened. In either case the interaction between the actin and myosin myofilaments through the crossbridges is greatly reduced, and the muscle is not capable of generating significant tension.

Age

The ability to generate muscular force is also related to age. Both men and women seem to be able to increase strength throughout puberty and adolescence, reaching a peak around 20 to 25 years of age, at which time this ability begins to level off and in some cases decline. After about age 25 a person generally loses an average of 1% of his or her maximal remaining strength each year. Thus at age 65 a person would have only about 60% of the strength he or she had at age 25.

The loss in muscle strength and endurance is definitely related to individual levels of physical activity. Those people who are more active, or perhaps those who continue to strength train, considerably reduce the tendency toward declining muscle strength and endurance. In addition, exercise may have an effect in slowing the decrease in cardiorespiratory endurance and flexibility and in slowing increases in body fat that tend to occur with aging. Therefore strength maintenance is important for all individuals regardless of age or the level of competition if total wellness and health is an ultimate goal.

Overtraining

Overtraining can have a negative effect on the development of muscular strength and endurance. The statement "if you abuse it you will lose it" is very applicable. Overtraining can result in psychological breakdown ("staleness") or physiological breakdown, which may involve musculoskeletal injury, fatigue, or sickness. Engaging in proper and efficient resistance training, eating a proper diet, and getting appropriate rest can all minimize the potential negative effects of overtraining.

Gains in muscular strength resulting from resistance training are reversible. Individuals who interrupt or stop resistance training altogether will see rapid decreases in strength gains. "If you don't use it, you'll lose it."

---

hypertrophy an increase in muscle size in response to training
atrophy a decrease in muscle size caused by inactivity

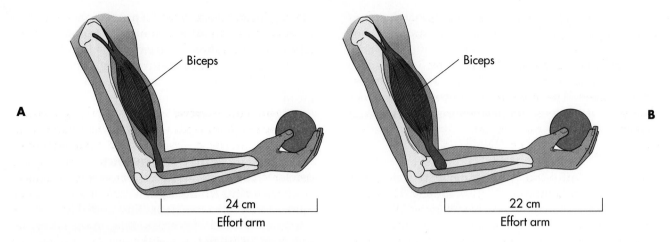

FIGURE 6-4. Muscle Tendon Attachments.
The position of attachment of the muscle tendon on the arm can affect the ability of that muscle to generate force. Person **B** should be able to generate greater force than person **A** because the tendon attachment is closer to the resistance.

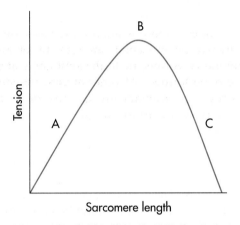

FIGURE 6-5. Length-Tension Relation of Muscle.
The greatest tension is developed at point *B*, with less tension developed at points *A* and *C*.

PHYSIOLOGY OF STRENGTH DEVELOPMENT
Muscle Hypertrophy

There is no question that weight training to improve muscular strength results in an increased size, or hypertrophy, of a muscle. What causes a muscle to hypertrophy? A number of theories have been proposed to explain this increase in muscle size.

It is generally accepted that the number of fibers is genetically determined and does not seem to increase with training. Some evidence exists that there is an *increase in the number of muscle fibers (hyperplasia)* due to the splitting of fibers in response to training. However, this research has been conducted in animals and should not be generalized to humans.

Secondly, it has been hypothesized that because the muscle is working harder in weight training, more blood is required to supply that muscle with oxygen and other nutrients. As a result, it is thought that the *number of capillaries increases,* which in turn increases muscle size. Research indicates that no *new* capillaries are formed during strength training; however, a number of dormant capillaries may become filled with blood to meet this increased demand for blood supply.

A third theory to explain the increase in muscle size seems the most credible. It was mentioned earlier that muscle fibers are composed primarily of small contractile protein filaments called *myofilaments*. These *myofilaments increase in both size and number* as a result of strength training, causing the individual muscle fibers to increase in cross-sectional diameter. This increase is particularly true in men, although women will also see some increase in muscle size. It is certainly true that more research is needed to further clarify and determine the specific causes of muscle hypertrophy.

Reversibility

If strength training is discontinued or interrupted, the muscle will atrophy, decreasing in both strength and mass. Adaptations in skeletal muscle that occur in response to resistance training may begin to reverse in as little as 48 hours. It does appear that consistent exercise of a muscle is essential to prevent reversal of the hypertrophy that occurs due to strength training.

Other Physiological Adaptations to Resistance Exercise

In addition to muscle hypertrophy, there are a number of other physiological adaptations to resistance training. The strength of noncontractile structures such as tendons and ligaments is increased. The mineral content of bone is increased, making the bone stronger and more resistant to fracture.

Maximal oxygen uptake is improved when resistance training is of sufficient intensity to elicit heart rates at or above training levels. However, it must be emphasized that these increases are minimal and if increasing VO_2max is the goal, aerobic exercise rather than weight training is recommended. There are also increases in the levels of several enzymes important in aerobic and anaerobic metabolism. All of these adaptations contribute to strength and endurance.

TECHNIQUES OF RESISTANCE TRAINING

There are a number of different techniques of resistance training for improving strength and endurance, including isometric exercise, progressive resistive exercise, isokinetic training, circuit training, and plyometric exercise.

Understanding and execution of proper techniques alone aren't enough to ensure that one will commit to a specific exercise program. The tips in the box on p. 154 offer a number of motivational strategies that can help one work through common problems or setbacks that people have encountered in working to increase muscular strength and endurance.

Importance of Overload

Regardless of specific techniques used, to improve strength and endurance the muscle must be overloaded in a progressive manner. The amount of weight used and the number of repetitions performed must be sufficient to make the muscle work at a higher intensity than it is used to. Without overloading the muscle, strength and endurance will not improve. However, the muscle should be able to maintain existing levels of strength and endurance as long as training is continued at a level of resistance to which the muscle is accustomed.

It is certainly true that many individuals can benefit more in terms of overall health by concentrating on improving muscular endurance. However, to most effectively build muscular strength, weight training requires a consistent, increasing effort against progressively increasing resistance.

The principle of overload applies to isometric, progressive resistive, and plyometric exercise. All three training techniques produce improvement of muscular strength and endurance over a period of time. Table 6-1 summarizes the five different techniques for improving muscular strength and endurance.

Isometric Exercise

An isometric exercise involves a muscle contraction in which the length of the muscle remains constant while tension develops toward a maximal force against an immovable resistance (Figure 6-6). To develop strength, the muscle should generate a maximal force for 10 seconds at a time, and this contraction should be repeated five to ten times per day.

Isometric exercises were popular in the late 1960s and early 1970s. Several books were published that discussed a series of isometric exercises that could be done while sitting at a desk. The exercises included techniques such as putting your arms underneath the middle desk drawer and pushing up as hard as you could or pushing out on the inside of the chair space with your knees. It was claimed that these brief maximal isometric contractions were capable of producing some rather dramatic increases in muscular strength. Indeed, these isometric exercises are capable of increasing muscular strength; unfortunately, strength gains are specific to the joint angle at which training is performed. At other angles, the strength curve drops off dramatically because of a lack of motor activity at those angles. Therefore arm strength is increased at the specific angle pressed against the desk drawer, but there is no corresponding increase in strength at other positions in the range of motion.

Another major disadvantage of these isometric, "sit at your desk" exercises is that they tend to produce a spike in blood pressure that can result in potentially life-threatening cardiovascular accidents. This sharp increase in blood pressure results from holding your breath and increasing pressure within the chest cavity. Consequently, the heart experiences a significant increase in blood pressure. This has been referred to as the *Valsalva effect*. To avoid or minimize this effect, it is recommended that breathing be done during the maximal contraction.

This does not mean to imply that isometric exercises have no place in a fitness program. There are certain instances in which an isometric contraction can greatly enhance a particular movement. For example,

> **isometric exercise** an exercise in which the muscle contracts against resistance but does not change in length

Ways to help you build muscular strength and endurance

GET MOVING

1. Get a camera or a video recorder and take pictures of yourself from all angles. Tape those pictures up right next to a mirror and after about a month of consistent weight training see how your body has changed.
2. Get a tape measure and take measurements of your chest, waist, hips, arms, and thighs. Record these numbers and remeasure in about a month.
3. If you are trying to lose body fat at the same time, don't get frustrated. Make sure that you measure losses of body fat with a skin-fold caliper rather than by stepping on a scale to see how much you weigh. Muscle weighs more than fat; thus even though you may be losing body fat, your weight may stay the same or perhaps even increase because your muscles are getting bigger.
4. You should vary the type of lifting exercise that you do to strengthen each body part. For example, to strengthen your biceps, on one day you can do biceps curls with dumbells, on the next day do chin-ups on a bar, and on the next use a biceps curl exercise machine. Varying the exercise will result in better overall development.
5. Don't try to lift heavy weights every day. At least once each week you should back off and go with lighter weights, with either a higher number of repetitions or a longer wait between sets.
6. It is really helpful to find a lifting partner who has about your same level of strength and endurance to work out with. The two of you can help to encourage and motivate each other.
7. If you like to lift by yourself, you can either buy some weight equipment and work out at home or choose a time to go to the weight room when it is not very crowded. If you are more motivated when there are a lot of people around to watch you exercise, go to the weight room when it is most crowded and show everyone what you can do.
8. Choose a type of weight-training facility where people of similar interest are working out. If you are lifting to simply tone your muscles and perhaps get a little stronger or develop more endurance, a health club or spa is likely most appropriate. If you are becoming a serious body builder or if you are an athlete, a no-frills, hard-core, gym-type atmosphere may be more appropriate.
9. Realize that when you first begin lifting weights, it is likely that you will develop some degree of muscle soreness. You can avoid this by starting with light weights and gradually progressing the amount of weight on each exercise. Remember—you have to overload the muscle to increase strength and endurance.
10. Most people find that music can help motivate them to lift. Different people have different ideas about the type of music they want to work out to. If you don't like what is being played in the weight room, use your own cassette or CD player.

one of the exercises in power weight lifting is a squat. A squat is an exercise in which the weight is supported on the shoulders in a standing position. The knees are then flexed and the weight is lowered to a three-quarter squat position, from which the lifter must stand completely straight once again. It is not uncommon for there to be one particular angle in the range of motion at which smooth movement through that specific angle is difficult because of insufficient strength. This joint angle is referred to as a *sticking point.* A power lifter will typically use an isometric contraction against some immovable resistance to increase strength at this sticking point. If strength can be improved at this joint angle, then a smooth, coordinated power lift can be performed through a full range of movement.

A more common use for isometric exercises would be for injury rehabilitation or reconditioning. There are a number of conditions or ailments resulting from either trauma or overuse that must be treated with strengthening exercises. Unfortunately, these problems may be exacerbated with full range-of-motion strengthening exercises. It may be more desirable to make use of isometric exercises until the injury has healed to the point that full-range activities can be performed.

TABLE 6-1. Techniques for Improving Muscular Strength		
Technique	**Action**	**Equipment/Activity**
Isometric exercise	Force develops while muscle length remains constant	Any immovable resistance
Progressive resistive exercise	Force develops while the muscle shortens or lengthens	Free weights, Universal, Nautilus, Eagle, Body Master
Isokinetic training	Force develops while muscle is contracting at a constant velocity	Cybex, Orthotron, Mini-gym, Kincom, Brodex, Lido, Merac
Circuit training	Used as a combination of isometric, PRE or isokinetic exercises organized into a series of stations	May use any of the equipment listed above. Calisthenics
Plyometric exercise	Uses a rapid eccentric stretch of the muscle to facilitate an explosive concentric contraction	Hops, bounds, and depth jumping

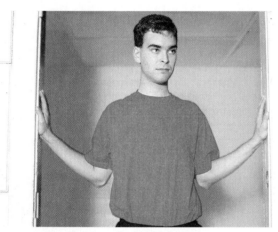

FIGURE 6-6. Isometric Exercise.

Progressive Resistive Exercise

A second technique of resistance training is perhaps the most commonly used and most popular technique for improving muscular strength. Progressive resistive exercise training uses exercises that strengthen muscles through a contraction that overcomes some fixed resistance such as with dumbells, barbells, or various exercise machines. Progressive resistive exercise uses isotonic contractions in which force is generated while the muscle is changing in length.

Eccentric Versus Concentric Contractions

Isotonic contractions may be either concentric or eccentric. Suppose you are going to perform a biceps curl (see Figure 6-21). To lift the weight from the starting position, the biceps muscle must contract and shorten in length (*concentric* or *positive contraction*). If

the biceps muscle does not remain contracted when the weight is being lowered, gravity will cause this weight to simply fall back to the starting position. Thus to control the weight as it is being lowered, the biceps muscle must continue to contract while at the same time gradually lengthening (*eccentric* or *negative contraction*).

It is possible to generate greater amounts of force against resistance with an eccentric contraction than with a concentric contraction. Eccentric contractions require a much lower level of motor unit activity to achieve a certain force than do concentric contractions. Since fewer motor units are firing to produce a specific force, additional motor units may be recruited to generate increased force. In addition, oxygen use is much lower during eccentric exercise than in comparable concentric exercise. Thus eccentric contractions are less resistant to fatigue than are concentric contractions. The mechanical efficiency of eccentric exercise may be several times higher than that of concentric exercise.

In progressive resistive exercise it is essential to incorporate both concentric and eccentric contractions. Research has clearly demonstrated that the muscle should be overloaded and totally fatigued both concentrically and eccentrically for the greatest strength improvement to occur.

When training specifically for the development of muscular strength, the concentric or positive portion of the exercise should require 1 to 2 seconds, and the eccentric or negative portion of the lift should require

> **progressive resistive exercise**   a technique that gradually strengthens muscles through a muscle contraction that overcomes fixed resistance

2 to 4 seconds. The ratio of negative to positive should be approximately 1:2. Physiologically the muscle will fatigue much more rapidly concentrically than eccentrically. Arthur Jones, the inventor of Nautilus equipment, stresses the use of these positive and negative contractions in his training program, although this principle should be applied regardless of which brand of equipment is being used.

Free Weights Versus Exercise Machines

There are various types of exercise equipment that can be used with progressive resistive exercise, including free weights (barbells and dumbells) or exercise machines such as Universal, Cybex, Nautilus, Eagle, and Body Master, to name a few (Figure 6-7, *A*). Dumbells and barbells require the use of iron plates of varying weights that can be easily changed by adding or subtracting equal amounts of weight to both sides of the bar. The exercise machines have a stack of weights that is lifted through a series of levers or pulleys. The stack of weights slides up and down on a pair of bars that restrict the movement to only one plane (Figure 6-7, *B*). Weight can be increased or decreased simply by changing the position of a weight key.

There are advantages and disadvantages to both the free weights and machines. The machines are relatively safe to use in comparison with free weights. If you are doing a bench press with free weights, it is essential to have someone "spot" you (help you lift the weights back onto the support racks if you don't have enough strength to complete the lift); otherwise you may end up dropping the weight on your chest. With the machines you can easily and safely drop the weight without fear of injury. It is also a simple process to increase or decrease the weight with the exercise machines by moving a single weight key, although changes can generally be made only in increments of 10 or 15 pounds. With free weights, iron plates must be added or removed from each side of the barbell. Regardless of which type of equipment is used, the same principles of *isotonic training* may be applied.

Persons who have strength trained using both free weights and exercise machines realize the difference in the amount of weight that can be lifted. Unlike the machines, free weights have no restricted motion and can thus move in many different directions depending on the forces applied. Also, with free weights an element of muscular control on the part of the lifter is required to prevent the weight from moving in any direction other than vertical. This control will usually decrease the amount of weight that can be lifted.

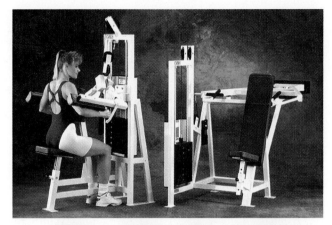

A

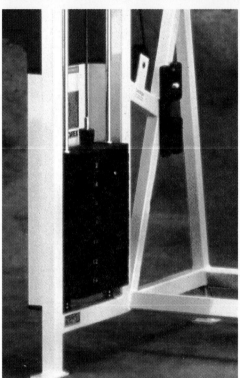

B

FIGURE 6-7. Cybex Equipment.
A, This Cybex equipment is isotonic. **B,** Resistance may be easily altered by changing the key in the stack of weights. (Courtesy CYBEX, Division of LUMEX Inc, New York.)

Variable Resistance

One problem often mentioned in relation to isotonic training is that the amount of force necessary to move a weight through a range of motion changes according to the angle of pull of the contracting muscle. It is greatest when the angle of pull is approximately 90 degrees (see Figure 6-5). In addition, once the inertia of the weight has been overcome and momentum has been established, the force required to move the resistance varies according to the force that muscle can produce through the range of motion. Thus it has been argued that a disadvantage of any type of isotonic exercise is that the force required to move the resistance is constantly changing throughout the range of movement.

Nautilus (Figure 6-8, *A*), has attempted to alleviate this problem of changing force capabilities by using a cam in its pulley system (Figure 6-8, *B*). The cam has been individually designed for each piece of equipment so that the resistance is variable throughout the movement. It attempts to alter resistance so that the muscle can handle a greater load. At the points where the joint angle or muscle length is mechanically disadvantageous, it reduces the resistance to muscle movement. This change in resistance at different points in the range has been labeled *variable resistance* or *accommodating resistance*. Whether this design does what it claims to do is debatable. It must be remembered that in real-life situations it does not matter whether the resistance is changing. What is important is that you develop enough strength to move objects from one place to another. The amount of strength necessary for each person is largely dependent on his or her lifestyle and occupation.

Progressive Resistive Exercise Techniques

There is no such thing as an optimal strength-training program. Even though there are many fallacies and misconceptions associated with resistance training, a considerable amount of research has been done in the area of resistance training to determine optimal techniques in terms of (1) the intensity or the amount of weight to be used, (2) the number of repetitions, (3) the number of sets, (4) the length of the recovery period, and (5) the frequency of training (Table 6-2). It seems that everyone has his or her own ideas about the best techniques for increasing muscular strength and endurance. Achieving total agreement among researchers and/or other experts in resistance training on a resistance training program is impossible.

It is important to realize that there are many effective techniques and training regimens that weight lifters and body builders can use. One may decide from looking at the size of a muscle or seeing the amount of weight these people are able to lift that they are doing something right even though their training regimens may not always follow the recommendations of researchers.

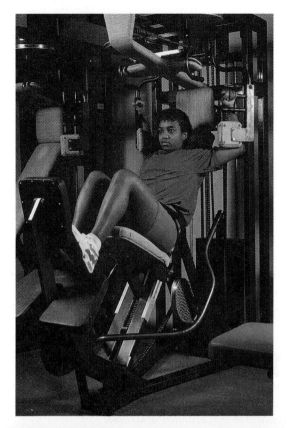

A

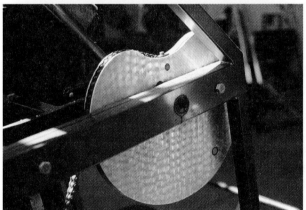

B

FIGURE 6-8. Nautilus.
A, Nautilus bench press machine. **B,** The cam on Nautilus is designed to equalize resistance throughout the full range of motion.

---

isotonic training   exercise that involves a muscle contraction in which force is being generated while the muscle is changing in length

TABLE 6-2.	**PRE Terminology**

Perhaps the most confusing aspect of progressive resistive exercise is the terminology used to describe specific programs. The following list of terms with their operational definitions may provide some clarification.

Terms	Definitions
Repetitions	Number of times you repeat a specific movement.
Repetition maximum (RM)	Maximum number of repetitions at a given weight.
Set	A particular number of repetitions.
Intensity	The amount of weight or resistance lifted.
Recovery period	The rest interval between sets.
Frequency	The number of times an exercise is done in a week's period.

Muscular Strength Versus Muscular Endurance

Muscular endurance was defined as the ability to perform submaximal repeated muscle contractions against resistance for an extended period of time. Most weight-training experts believe that muscular strength and muscular endurance are closely related. As one improves, there is a tendency for the other to improve also. People who possess great levels of strength tend to also exhibit greater muscular endurance when asked to perform repeated submaximal contractions against resistance.

Sets and Reps. Although there is not agreement as to the specific number of sets and reps, it is generally accepted that to develop muscular strength you should use heavier weights with a lower number of repetitions. Conversely, to improve muscular endurance you should use relatively lighter weights with a higher number of repetitions.

When trying to increase muscular strength, for any given exercise the amount of weight selected should be sufficient to allow six to eight repetitions maximum (RM) in each of the three sets with a recovery period of 1 to 2 minutes between sets. Initial selection of a starting weight may require some trial and error to achieve this six to eight RM range. If at least three sets of six repetitions cannot be completed, the weight is too heavy and should be reduced. If it is possible to do more than three sets of eight repetitions, the weight is too light and should be increased. Progression to heavier weights is then determined by the ability to perform at least eight repetitions maximum in each of three sets. When progressing weight, an increase of about 10% of the current weight being lifted should still allow at least six RM in each of three sets.

To concentrate more on muscular endurance you should use three sets of 10 to 12 repetitions. The amount of weight used should be selected and progressed according to the same procedure described above. Thus suggested training regimens for both muscular strength and endurance are similar in terms of sets and number of repetitions.

Frequency of Exercise. There are various recommendations as to how often you should strength train, yet there is once again no consensus among the "experts." ACSM has recommended lifting twice per week. It has also been suggested that one maximal workout per week can maintain muscular strength for months.

To most effectively improve muscular strength and endurance, a particular muscle or muscle group should be exercised consistently every other day. Thus the frequency of weight training should be at least three times per week but no more than four times per week. It is common for serious weight trainers to lift every day; however, they exercise different muscle groups on successive days. For example, Monday, Wednesday, and Friday may be used for upper body muscles, whereas Tuesday, Wednesday, and Saturday are used for lower body muscles (Figure 6-9).

Periodization. The concept of periodization is an approach to conditioning that attempts to bring about peak performance while reducing injuries and overtraining by developing a resistance training program that varies throughout the year. The idea of periodization takes into account that an individual cannot lift at his or her maximum all the time. There should be periods of time when weight training is performed at submaximal levels. Periodization modifies the program according to individual needs that may occur at different times.

Isokinetic Exercise

An isokinetic exercise involves a muscle contraction in which the length of the muscle is changing while the contraction is performed at a constant velocity. In theory, maximal resistance is provided throughout the range of motion by the machine. The resis-

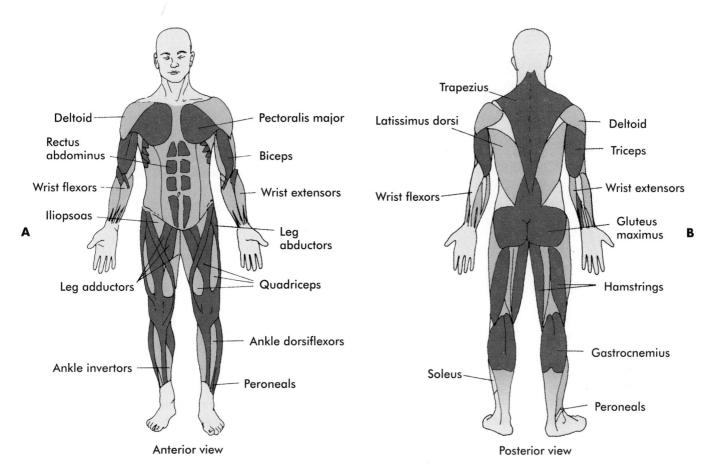

FIGURE 6-9. **Major Muscles of the Body.**

tance provided by the machine will move only at some preset speed, regardless of the force applied to it by the individual. Thus the key to isokinetic exercise is not the resistance but the speed at which resistance can be moved.

Several isokinetic devices are available commercially: Cybex, Orthotron, Biodex, KinCom, and Mini-gym are among the more common isokinetic devices (Figure 6-10). In general, they rely on hydraulic, pneumatic, and mechanical pressure systems to produce this constant velocity of motion. The majority of the isokinetic devices are capable of resisting both concentric and eccentric contractions at a fixed speed to exercise a muscle.

A major disadvantage of these units is their cost. Many of them come with a computer and printing device and are used primarily as diagnostic and rehabilitative tools in the treatment of various injuries.

Isokinetic devices are designed so that regardless of the amount of force applied against a resistance, it can only be moved at a certain speed. That speed will be the same whether maximal force or only half the maximal force is applied. Consequently, when training isokinetically it is absolutely necessary to exert as much force against the resistance as possible (maximal

effort) for maximal strength gains to occur. This is another one of the major problems with an isokinetic strength-training program. Anyone who has been involved in a weight-training program knows that on some days it is difficult to find the motivation to work out. Because isokinetic training requires a maximal effort, it is very easy to "cheat" and not go through the workout at a high level of intensity. In a progressive resistive exercise program, you know how much weight has to be lifted with how many repetitions. Therefore isokinetic training is often more effective if a partner system is used primarily as a means of motivation toward a maximal effort.

When done properly with a maximal effort, it is theoretically possible that maximal strength gains are best achieved through the isokinetic training method, in which the velocity is equal throughout the range of motion. However, there is no conclusive research to support this theory.

> **isokinetic exercise**   an exercise in which the length of the muscle changes, although the contraction is performed at a constant velocity against resistance

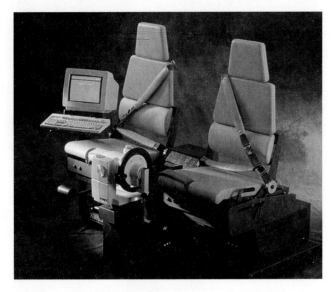

FIGURE 6-10. **Cybex-6000.**
The Cybex-6000 is an isokinetic device that provides resistance at a constant velocity. (Courtesy CYBEX, Division of LUMEX Inc, New York.)

FIGURE 6-11. **Example of Circuit Training Setup.**

- Station 1 Push-ups (30 repetitions)
- Station 2 Hamstring: low back stretching
- Station 3 Bent-knee sit-ups (25 repetitions)
- Station 4 Bench press (10 repetitions at 75% maximum weight)
- Station 5 Rope skipping (100 repetitions)
- Station 6 Knee extensions (15 repetitions at 80% maximum weight)
- Station 7 Shoulder adduction (15 repetitions)
- Station 8 Knee flexions (15 repetitions at 80% maximum weight)

There would be 60 seconds to complete each station, and the entire circuit would be repeated three times in succession.

Circuit Training

Circuit training uses a series of exercise stations that consist of various combinations of weight training, flexibility, calisthenics, and brief aerobic exercises. Circuits may be designed to accomplish many different training goals. With circuit training, you move rapidly from one station to the next and perform whatever exercise is to be done at that station within a specified time period. A typical circuit would consist of eight to twelve stations, and the entire circuit would be repeated three times.

Circuit training is definitely an effective technique for improving strength and flexibility. Certainly, if the pace or the time interval between stations is rapid and if workload is maintained at a high level of intensity with heart rates at or above target training levels for a minimum of 20 minutes, the cardiorespiratory system may benefit from this circuit. However, there is little research evidence that shows that circuit training is very effective in improving cardiorespiratory endurance. It should be and is most often used as a technique for developing and improving muscular strength and endurance. Figure 6-11 provides an example of a simple circuit training setup that can be easily completed by healthy college students.

Plyometric Exercise

Plyometric exercise is a technique that uses specific exercises that encompass a rapid stretch of a muscle eccentrically followed immediately by a rapid concentric contraction of that muscle for the purpose of facilitating and developing a forceful explosive movement over a short period of time. The greater the stretch put on the muscle from its resting length immediately before the concentric contraction, the greater the resistance the muscle can overcome.

Plyometrics emphasize the speed of the eccentric phase. The rate of stretch is more critical than the magnitude of the stretch. An advantage to using plyometric exercise is that it can help develop eccentric control in dynamic movements. Plyometric exercises involve hops, bounds, and depth jumping for the lower extremity and the use of medicine balls and other types of weighted equipment for the upper extremity. Depth jumping is an example of a plyometric exercise in which an individual jumps to the ground from a specified height and then quickly jumps again as soon as ground contact is made.

Plyometrics tend to place a great deal of stress on the musculoskeletal system. The learning and perfection of specific jumping skills and other plyometric exercises must be technically correct and specific to one's age, activity, and physical and skill development.

GENDER AND STRENGTH TRAINING

Strength and endurance are just as important to women as to men. Unfortunately, some women remain reluctant to engage in a weight-training program because of the fear of developing bulky muscles. This fear is unfounded; the average woman is incapable of building significant muscle bulk through weight training. Significant muscle hypertrophy is dependent on the presence of an anabolic steroidal hormone known as *testosterone.* Testosterone is considered a male hormone, although all women possess some testosterone in their systems. Women with higher testosterone levels tend to have more masculine characteristics such as increased facial and body hair, a deeper voice, and the potential to develop a little more muscle bulk.

For the average college-age woman, there is no need to worry about developing large bulky muscles with strength building. What does happen is that muscle tone is improved. Muscle tone basically refers to the firmness, or tension, of the muscle during a resting state. For example, doing sit-ups increases the firmness of the abdominal muscles and makes them more resistant to fatigue. All of us would agree that a person who has a firm, well-toned body is physically attractive.

A woman in weight training will probably see some remarkable gains in strength initially, even though her muscle bulk does not increase. How is this possible? For a muscle to contract, an impulse must be transmitted from the nervous system to the muscle. Each muscle fiber is innervated by a specific motor unit. By overloading a particular muscle, as in weight training, the muscle is forced to work efficiently. Efficiency is achieved by getting more motor units to fire, causing a stronger contraction of the muscle. Consequently, it is not uncommon for a woman to see extremely rapid gains in strength when a weight-training program is first begun. These tremendous initial strength gains, which can be attributed to improved neuromuscular system efficiency, tend to plateau, and minimal improvement in muscular strength will be realized during a continuing strength-training program. These initial neuromuscular strength gains will also be seen in men, although their strength will continue to increase with appropriate training. It must be reiterated that women who do possess higher testosterone levels have the potential to further increase their strength because of the development of greater muscle bulk.

Perhaps the most critical difference between men and women regarding physical performance is the ratio of strength to body weight. The reduced strength/body weight ratio in women is the result of their higher percentage of body fat. The strength/body weight ratio may be significantly improved through weight training by decreasing the body fat percentage while increasing lean weight. Strength training programs for women should follow the same guidelines as those for men.

USE OF ANABOLIC STEROIDS IN WEIGHT TRAINING

Unfortunately, the use of anabolic steroids by persons attempting to develop high levels of strength is becoming commonplace. Athletes use the drug for increasing lean body weight, muscle mass, and strength. Often these drugs are obtained by body builders through mail order advertisements in magazines or through illegal channels. As discussed in Chapter 3, anabolic steroids have many harmful side effects. For this reason, the use of anabolic steroids for the purpose of strength improvement cannot be recommended and is in fact now illegal in most states. Despite the uncertainty about the long-range effects of these drugs, anabolic steroid use is a continuing problem for many persons involved with heavy weight training at all levels.

RESISTANCE TRAINING EXERCISES

To say that a person is strong is probably incorrect. We should instead refer to a specific muscle, muscle group, or movement as being strong because increases in strength occur only in muscles that are regularly subjected to overload. Because muscle contractions result in joint movement, the goal of weight training should be to increase strength in every movement possible about a given joint. Exercises must be designed to place stress on those groups of muscles collectively to produce a specific joint movement.

For this reason this approach to specific strength-training exercises deviates from the traditional approach. The following illustrations (pp. 163 to 173) are organized to show exercises for all motions about a particular joint rather than for each specific muscle. These exercises are demonstrated using free weights (barbells, dumbells, weights, and some machine weights). Any of the exercises described may be applied to various commercial weight machines such as Universal or Nautilus. Positions may differ slightly when different pieces of equipment are used. However, the joint motions that affect the various muscles indicated are still the same.

> **circuit training** a series of exercise stations for strength training, flexibility, and calisthenics
> **plyometric exercise** strength training exercises (hops, bounds and depth jumping) that involve a rapid eccentric (lengthening) stretch of a muscle, followed immediately by a rapid concentric contraction of that muscle to produce a forceful, explosive movement

Figure 6-12 provides guidelines and precautions to follow during strength training. Figures 6-13 to 6-36 describe exercises for strength improvement of shoulder, hip, knee, and ankle joint movements. Complete the worksheets on p. 191 to assess your progress in strength increases while doing the following exercises.

FIGURE 6-12. Guidelines and Precautions in Resistance Training

The following guidelines can improve both your effectiveness and safety during strength training.

- Do appropriate warm-up activities before beginning workout.
- Use proper lifting techniques as recommended on the following pages. Improper lifting techniques can result in injury.
- To ensure balanced development, exercise all muscle groups.
- Avoid doing one-repetition maximum lifts. This can result in muscle strains, especially if you are not properly warmed up.
- Always have a spotter if you are lifting free weights.

- Before using a machine (e.g., Nautilus or Universal), make sure you understand how to use it properly.
- Progress gradually and within your individual limits.
- Always train throughout a full range of motion.
- Use both concentric and eccentric contractions.
- Try to exercise the larger muscle groups first, and alternate exercises to allow previously exercised muscle groups a chance to recover.
- Do not hold your breath during a lift.
- Do not overtrain. Overtraining may result in injury.
- If you have questions about weight training, seek out an expert who can give you specific, correct advice.
- Do not try to show off; always work within your own limits.

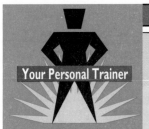

Your Personal Trainer

Cynthia Williamson, Graduate student
Age: 41

Scenario

I've been consistently running a 2.5 mile course three to four times a week for the past 2 years. A few weeks ago I ran a 10K race with one of my friends who is more of a distance runner. I really enjoyed the race and have increased the distance of my weekly runs.

Endurance isn't a problem, but since the race my left knee has been getting sore when I run more than 4 miles. Lately the pain has become more persistent. My knee bothers me going down stairs and when I stand or sit for long periods of time.

Solution

Knee injuries usually present a complex problem. Any number of factors could be involved, ranging from your strength, flexibility, physical conditioning, and agility to your speed, balance, gait, and shoe type.

Repeated minor injuries can make your knees more susceptible to major injury, and it would probably be best to cut back on your running until the pain goes away.

Focus on increasing the strength and flexibility of the muscles around your knee. You can strengthen the muscles around your knees by adding a series of straight leg raises, hip flexion, hip abduction, hip extension, and hip adduction exercises to your exercise routine. Before your workout remember to stretch your hamstring, groin, Achilles tendon, and hip flexor.

When your knee pain subsides, gradually increase the distance you run. Running increased distances may require new shoes, and it may be worthwhile to have your gait analyzed.

After you get back up the speed, add a half mile to your course every week. And, as always, if you experience persistent or recurring pain, be sure to follow up with an athletic trainer, physical therapist, or your physician.

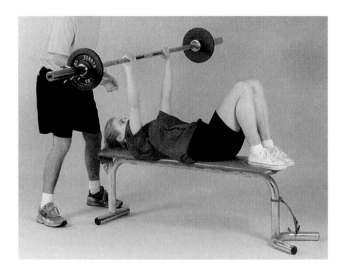

FIGURE 6-13. Bench Press: Free Weights.
Joints affected: Shoulder, elbow.
Movement: Pushing away.
Position: Supine, feet flat on bench, back flat on bench.
Primary muscles: Pectoralis major, triceps.

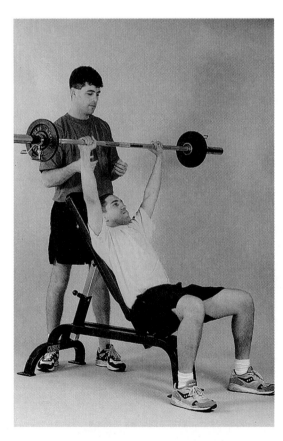

FIGURE 6-14. Incline Press.
Joints affected: Shoulder, elbow.
Movement: Pushing upward and away.
Position: Supine at an inclined angle, feet flat on floor, back flat against bench.
Primary muscles: Pectoralis major, triceps.

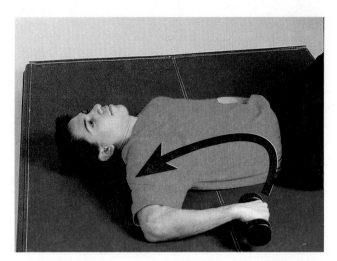
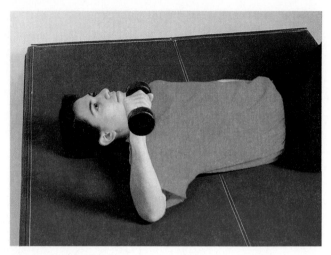

FIGURE 6-15. **Shoulder Rotation.**
Joint affected: Shoulder.
Movement: External rotation.
Position: Supine, shoulder at 90-degree angle and
elbow flexed at 90-degree angle.

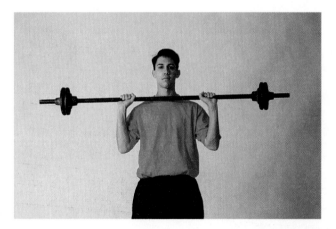
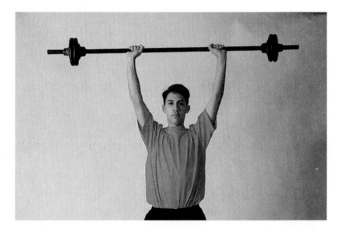

FIGURE 6-16. **Military Press.**
Joints affected: Shoulder, elbow.
Movement: Pressing the weight overhead.
Position: Standing, back straight.
Primary muscles: Deltoid, trapezius, triceps.

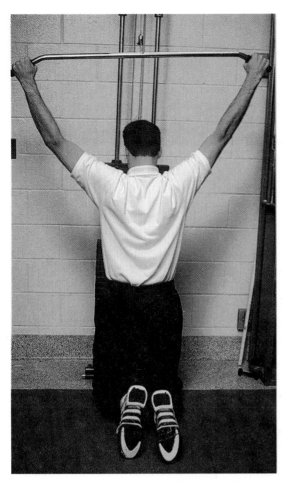
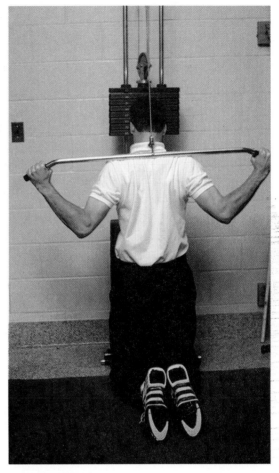

FIGURE 6-17. **Lateral Pull Downs.**
Joints affected: Shoulder, elbow.
Movement: Pulling the bar down behind the neck.
Position: Kneeling, back straight, head up.
Primary muscles: Latissimus dorsi, biceps.

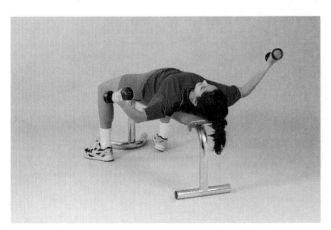
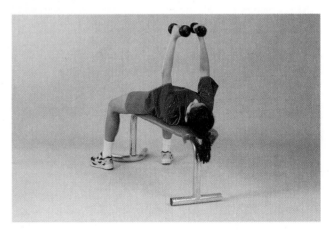

FIGURE 6-18. **Flys.**
Joint affected: Shoulder.
Movement: Horizontal flexion. Bring arms together over head.
Position: Lying on back, feet flat on floor, back flat on bench.
Primary muscles: Deltoid, pectoralis major.

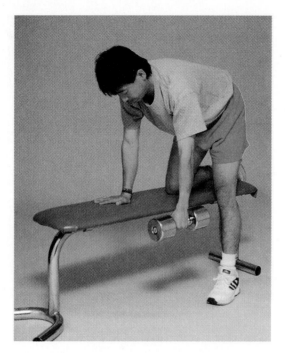
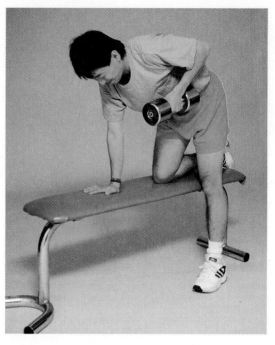

FIGURE 6-19. **Bent Over Rows.**
Joint Affected: Shoulder.
Movement: Adduction of the scapula.
Position: Standing bent over at waist, knee on bench.
Primary muscles: Trapezius, rhomboids.

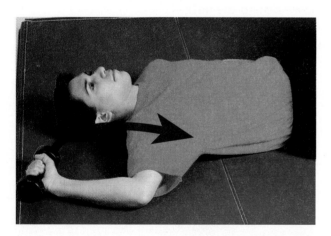
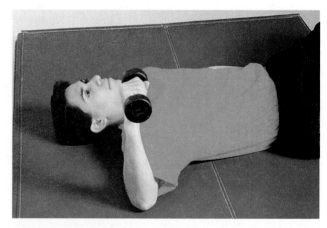

FIGURE 6-20. **Shoulder Medial Rotation.**
Joint affected: Shoulder.
Movement: Internal rotation. Lifting weight off the floor.
Position: Supine, shoulder abducted and elbow flexed.
Primary muscles: Subscapularis.

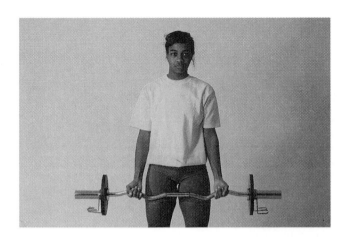
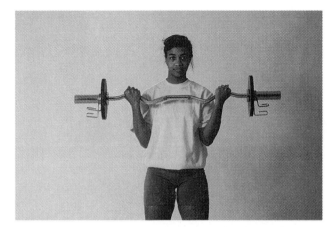

FIGURE 6-21. **Biceps Curls.**
Joint affected: Elbow.
Movement: Elbow flexion. Curling the weight up to the shoulder.
Position: Standing feet front and back rather than side to side, back straight, arms extended.
Primary muscles: Biceps.

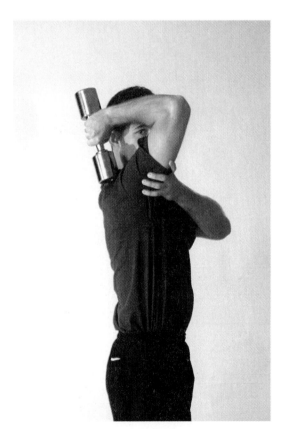
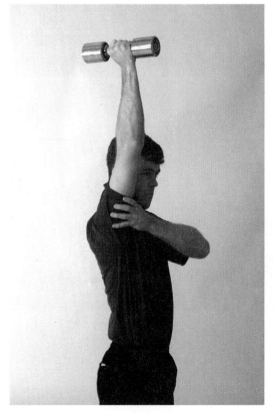

FIGURE 6-22. **Triceps Extensions.**
Joint affected: Elbow.
Movement: Elbow extension. Pressing weight toward ceiling.
Position: Standing, elbow pointing directly toward ceiling beside ear.
Primary muscles: Triceps.

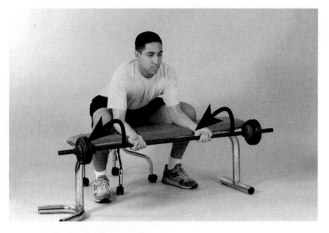

FIGURE 6-23. Wrist Curls.
Joint affected: Wrist.
Movement: Wrist flexion. Curling weight upward.
Position: Seated, forearms on table, palms up.
Primary muscles: Long flexors of forearm.

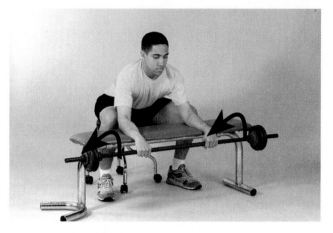

FIGURE 6-24. Wrist Extensions.
Joint affected: Wrist.
Movement: Extension. Curling weight upward.
Position: Seated, forearms on table, palms down.
Primary muscles: Long extensors of forearm.

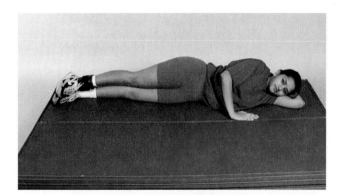

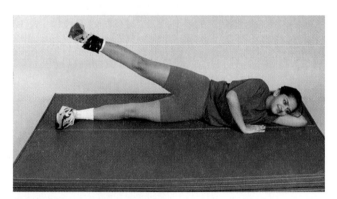

FIGURE 6-25. **Leg Raises.**
Joint affected: Hip.
Movement: Hip abduction. Lifting leg up.
Position: Sidelying. Weight band strapped around ankle.
Primary muscles: Hip abductors.

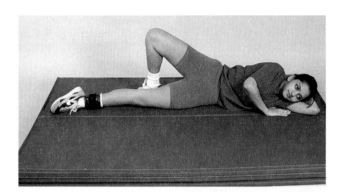
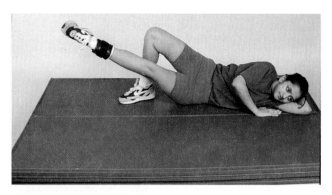

FIGURE 6-26. **Leg Lifts.**
Joint affected: Hip.
Movement: Hip adduction. Lifting bottom leg up.
Position: Sidelying, one leg lifted upward, weight band around ankle.
Primary muscles: Hip adductors.

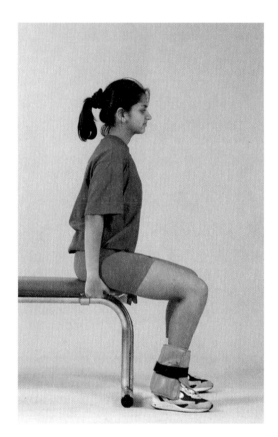
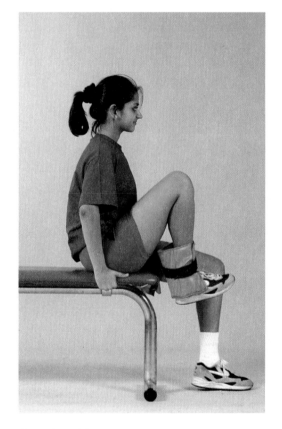

FIGURE 6-27. **Bent-Knee Leg Lifts.**
Joint affected: Hip.
Movement: Hip flexion. Lifting knee up.
Position: Sitting, knee flexed, weight around ankle.
Primary muscles: Iliopsoas.

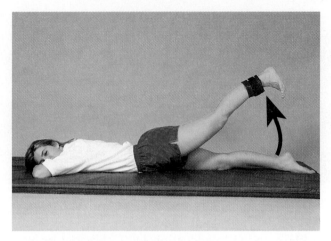

FIGURE 6-28. **Reverse Leg Lifts.**
Joint affected: Hip.
Movement: Hip Extension. Lifting leg toward ceiling.
Position: Prone, knee extended, weight band around ankle.
Primary muscles: Gluteus maximus, hamstrings.

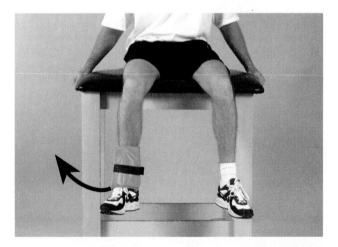 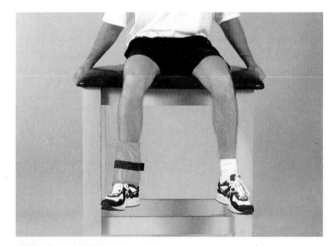

FIGURE 6-29. **Hip Medial Rotation.**
Joint affected: Hip.
Movement: Internal rotation. Rotating lower leg outward.
Position: Sitting, knee flexed, weight on ankle.
Primary muscles: Medial rotators.

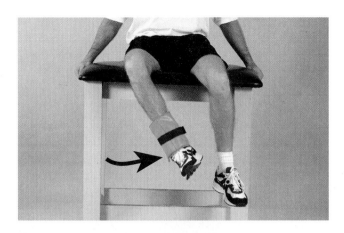

FIGURE 6-30. **Hip Lateral Rotation.**
Joint affected: Hip.
Movement: Lateral rotation. Rotating lower leg inward.
Position: Sitting, knee flexed, weight on ankle.
Primary muscles: Lateral rotators.

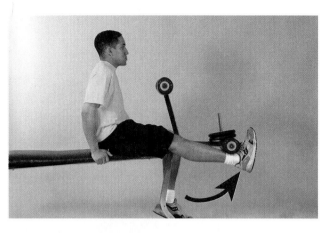

FIGURE 6-31. **Quadriceps Extensions.**
Joint affected: Knee.
Movement: Extension. Straightening knee.
Position: Sitting, on knee machine.
Primary muscles: Quadriceps group.

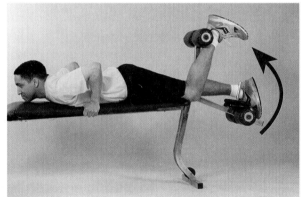

FIGURE 6-32. **Hamstring Curls.**
Joint affected: Knee.
Movement: Flexion. Bending knee and lifting the weight up.
Position: Prone, on knee machine.
Primary muscles: Hamstring group.

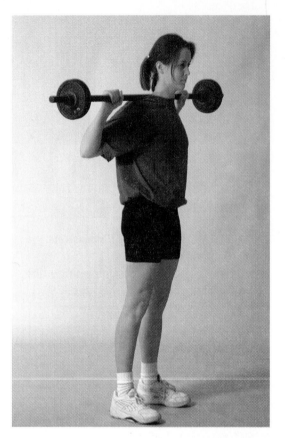
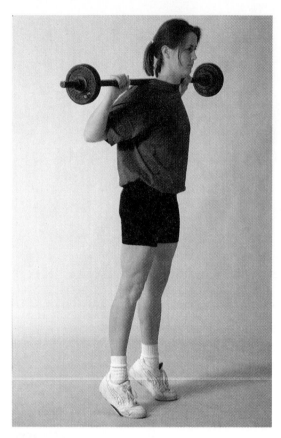

FIGURE 6-33. Toe Raises.
Joint affected: Ankle.
Movement: Plantar flexion. Pressing up on toes.
Position: Standing on one leg and lifting body weight.
Primary muscles: Gastrocnemius and soleus.

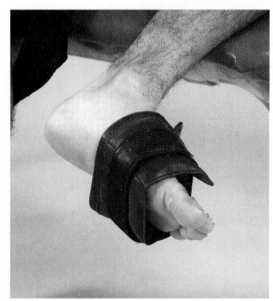
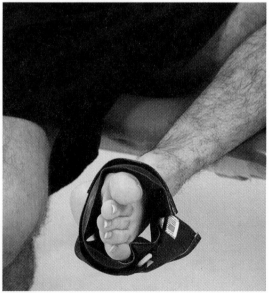

FIGURE 6-34. Ankle Inversion.
Joint affected: Ankle.
Movement: Inversion. Lifting the sole of the foot up and in.
Position: Sitting, knee flexed, instep up, weight on foot.
Primary muscles: Anterior tibialis.

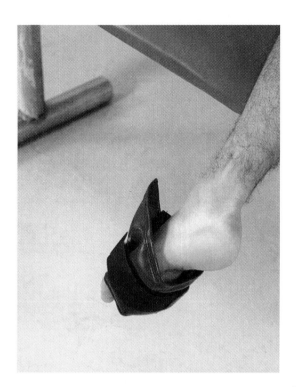
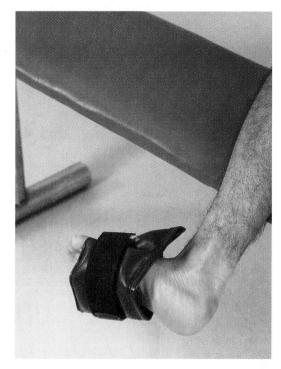

FIGURE 6-35. **Ankle Eversion.**
Joint affected: Ankle.
Movement: Eversion. Lifting the sole of the foot up and out.
Position: Sitting, knee flexed, instep down, weight on foot.
Primary muscles: Peroneals.

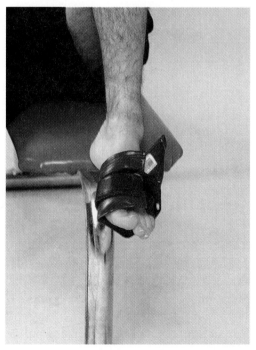
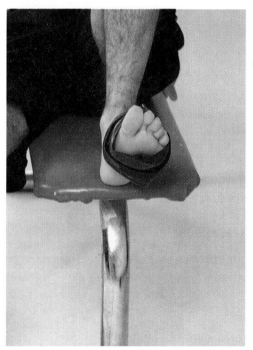

FIGURE 6-36. **Ankle Dorsiflexion.**
Joint affected: Ankle.
Movement: Dorsiflexion. Lifting the toes upward.
Position: Sitting, knee flexed, heel on edge of table, weight on foot.
Primary muscles: Dorsiflexors in shin.

CALISTHENIC STRENGTHENING EXERCISES

Until recently the thought of doing calisthenic exercise probably conjured up the image of a hard-nosed Marine drill instructor leading a group of recruits through a boring, regimented exercise session. But add music and bright-colored exercise clothing and change the name to aerobic exercise, aerobic dance, or jazzercise, and you have a multimillion dollar industry that has swept a large segment of the American population into exercise fanaticism. This new fascination with aerobic exercise has shown that calisthenic exercise can be enjoyable without being excessively regimented.

Calisthenic exercises, if done properly, can improve muscular strength and endurance, flexibility, and cardiorespiratory endurance. However, they are best suited as a supplemental activity to other previously discussed techniques rather than as a substitute for resistance training exercises.

Muscle Strength and Endurance

Calisthenics can help to increase muscular strength, tone, and endurance by using the weight of the body and its extremities as resistance. For example, chinning exercises (see Figure 6-44) use the weight of the body to resist the biceps and brachialis muscles in elbow flexion. The primary advantage of calisthenics over training with weights is that you do not need any expensive equipment or machines to provide resistance for you. Most of these exercises can be accomplished without the use of any equipment.

Flexibility

Calisthenic exercises can also help to improve flexibility as long as each exercise is done through a full range of motion. The weight of a body part can assist in passively stretching a muscle to its greatest length. However, caution must be used when doing calisthenic exercise to improve flexibility. The repetitive, bouncing nature of many of these exercises causes a muscle to be stretched ballistically, which can predispose a muscle to injury, particularly in an untrained person. Through calisthenic exercises the muscle should be progressively stretched during the set of exercises. Do not neglect the importance of a warm-up that includes flexibility exercises before engaging in calisthenics.

Cardiorespiratory Endurance

There is some question as to whether calisthenic exercises can increase resting heart rate significantly, but as stated in Chapter 5, if exercise is of sufficient intensity, frequency, and duration, cardiorespiratory endurance can be improved. Anyone who has gone through a 20- to 30-minute aerobics class will agree that heart rate is elevated to training levels. Calisthenic exercises should be done at a quick pace and without much rest between sets for optimal improvement of cardiorespiratory endurance.

Specific Exercises

The exercises illustrated in Figures 6-37 to 6-45 are recommended because they work on specific muscle

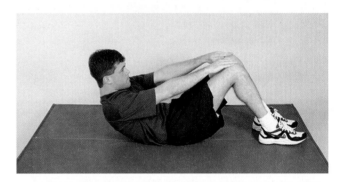

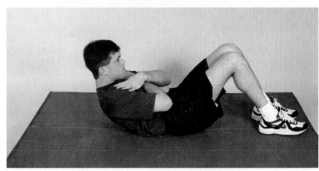

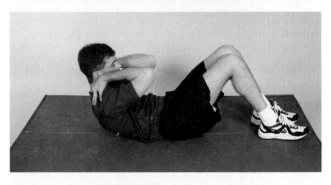

FIGURE 6-37. **Exercise: Curl-ups. A, Beginning. B, Intermediate. C, Advanced.**
Joints affected: Spinal vertebral joints.
Movement: Trunk flexion.
Instructions: Lying on back, hands either on chest or behind back, knees flexed to 90-degree angle, feet on floor, curl trunk and head to approximately 45-degree angle.
Primary muscles: Rectus abdominis.

groups and with a specific purpose. If all exercises are done, most of the major muscle groups in the body will be both stretched and contracted against resistance with the objective of improving strength, flexibility, and endurance. Each exercise can be done at your own pace, although the greater the pace, the greater the stress placed on the cardiorespiratory system. Thus it is recommended that you work quickly and move from one exercise to the next without delay.

These exercises can be done to music if you so desire. Most people find it easier to exercise to fast-paced music with a hard, rhythmic beat. However, you should select the type of music most enjoyable to you.

ASSESSING MUSCULAR STRENGTH AND ENDURANCE

Lab Activities 6-1 through 6-3 will help you assess your levels of muscular strength, endurance, and power. In Lab Activity 6-4, a worksheet is provided on which you can monitor and record your progress on each of the exercises as described in this chapter.

> **calisthenic exercise** exercises using body weight as resistance to improve strength, endurance, flexibility, and body composition

A 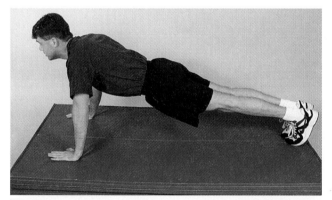 B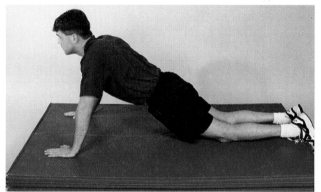

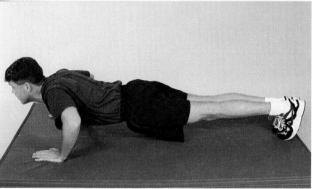 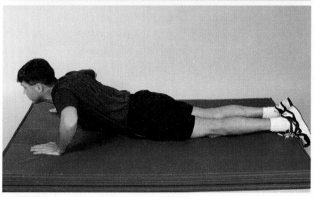

FIGURE 6-38. A, Push-Ups. B, Modified Push-Ups.
Purpose: Strengthening.
Muscles: Triceps and pectoralis major.
Repetitions: Beginner 10; Intermediate 20; Advanced 30.
Instructions: Keep the upper trunk and legs extended in a straight line. Touch floor with chest.
Caution: Avoid hyperextending the back, especially in modified push-ups.

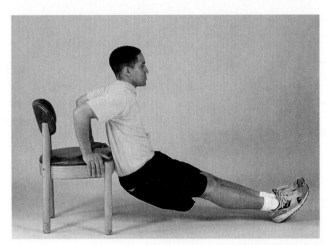 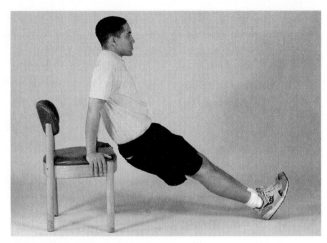

FIGURE 6-39. Triceps Extensions.
Purpose: Strengthening and range of motion at shoulder joint.
Muscles: Triceps and trapezius.
Repetitions: Beginner 7; intermediate 12; advanced 18.
Instructions: Begin with arms extended and body straight. Lower buttocks until they touch the ground, then press back up.

A 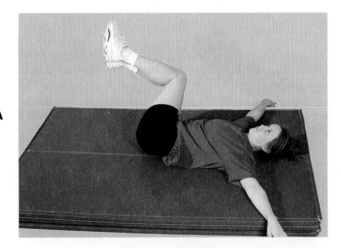 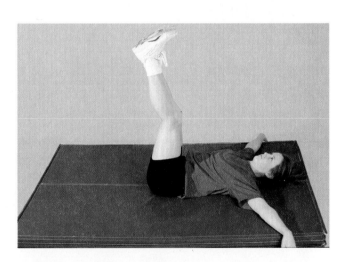 B

FIGURE 6-40. Trunk Rotation. A, Beginner. B, Advanced.
Muscles: Internal and external obliques.
Repetitions: Beginner 10 each direction; intermediate 15 each direction; advanced 20 each direction
Instructions: Rotate trunk from side to side until knees touch the floor, keeping knees slightly bent.
Caution: This exercise should be done only by those who already have strong abdominals.

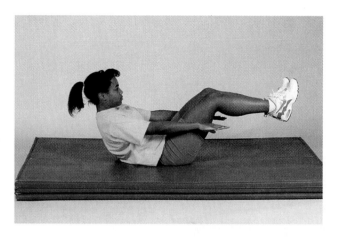

FIGURE 6-41. Sitting Tucks.
Purpose: Strengthen abdominals and stretch low back.
Muscles: Rectus abdominis and erector muscles in low back.
Repetitions: Beginner 10; intermediate 20; advanced 30.
Instructions: Keep legs and upper back off the ground and pull knees to chest.
Caution: This exercise should be done only by those who already have strong abdominals.

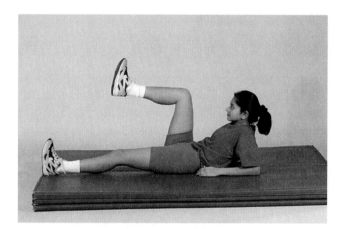

FIGURE 6-42. Bicycle.
Purpose: Strengthen hip flexors and stretch lower back.
Muscles: Iliopsoas.
Repetitions: Beginner 10 each side; intermediate 20 each side; advanced 30 each side.
Instructions: Alternately flex and extend legs as if you were pedaling a bicycle.

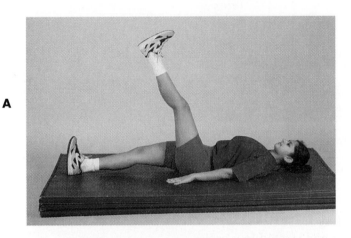 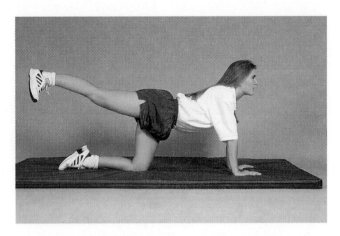

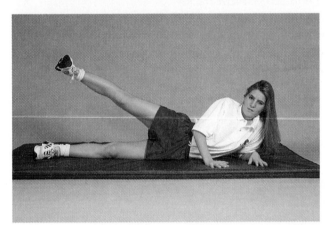 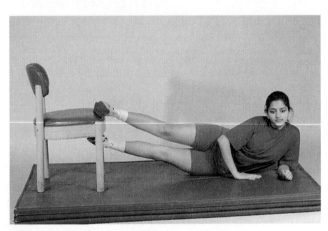

FIGURE 6-43. Leg Lifts. A, Front. B, Back. C, Side (leg up). D, Side (leg down).
Purpose: Strengthen *A*, hip flexors; *B*, hip extensors; *C*, hip abductors; and D, hip adductors.
Muscles: *A*, Iliopsoas; *B*, gluteus maximus; *C*, gluteus medius; and *D*, adductor group.
Repetitions: Beginner 10 each leg: intermediate 15 each leg; advanced 20 each leg.
Instructions: Raise the exercising leg up as far as possible in each position. To prevent injury, avoid ballistic movements or overextension.

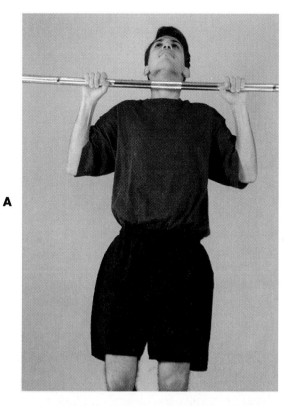

A

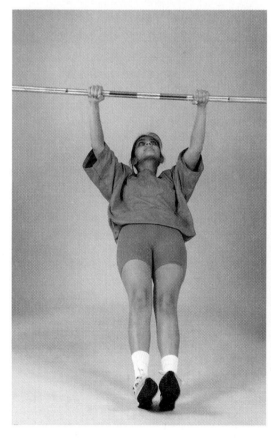

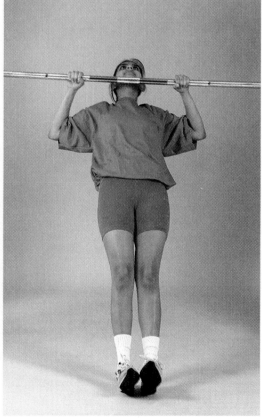

B

FIGURE 6-44. A, Chin-Ups. B, Modified Chin-Ups.
Purpose: Strengthening and stretch of shoulder joint.
Muscles: Biceps, brachialis, and latissimus dorsi.
Repetitions: Beginner 7; intermediate 10; advanced 15.
Instructions: Pull up until chin touches top of bar.

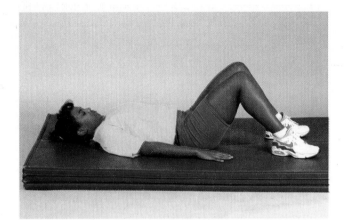 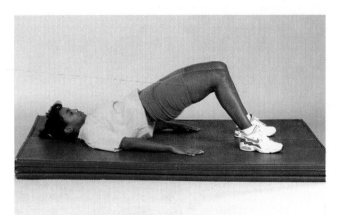

FIGURE 6-45. Buttock Tucks.
Purpose: Strengthen muscles of buttocks.
Muscles: Gluteus maximus and hamstrings.
Repetitions: Beginner 10; intermediate 15; advanced 20.
Instructions: Lying flat on back with knees bent, arch back and thrust the pelvis upward.

SUMMARY

- Strength is an essential component of physical fitness for anyone involved in a physical activity program. Strength may be defined as the maximal force that can be generated against resistance by a muscle during a single maximal contraction.
- Muscular strength and endurance are important health-related components of fitness. Power is a skill-related component of fitness.
- The ability to generate force is dependent both on the physical properties of the muscle and on the mechanical factors that dictate how much force can be generated through the lever system to an external object.
- Muscular power involves the speed with which a forceful muscle contraction is performed.
- Hypertrophy of a muscle is caused by increases in the size of the protein myofilaments, which results in an increased cross-sectional diameter of the muscle.
- The key to improving strength through resistance training is using the principle of overload.
- Five resistance training techniques can improve muscular strength: isometric exercise, progressive resistive exercise, isokinetic training, circuit training, and plyometric training.
- Improvements in strength with isometric training occur at specific joint angles.
- Perhaps the best progressive resistive exercise technique for improving strength involves three

sets of six to eight repetitions done every other day.
- Circuit training involves a series of exercise stations consisting of weight training, flexibility, and calisthenic exercises in which you move rapidly from one station to the next.
- Isokinetic training provides resistance to a muscle at a fixed speed.
- Plyometric exercise uses a quick eccentric stretch to facilitate a concentric contraction.
- Muscular endurance is the ability to perform repeated isotonic or isokinetic muscle contractions or to sustain an isometric contraction without undue fatigue.
- Muscular endurance tends to improve with muscular strength; thus training techniques for these two components are similar.
- The use of anabolic steroids has many negative physiological side effects and cannot be recommended for the purpose of increasing muscular size and strength.
- Women can significantly increase strength levels but generally will not build large muscle bulk as a result of strength training because of a relative lack of the hormone testosterone.
- If done properly, calisthenic exercises can improve muscular strength and endurance, flexibility, and cardiorespiratory endurance.

REFERENCES

Alway SE, MacDougal D, Sale G, et al: Functional and structural adaptations in skeletal muscle of trained athletes, *J Appl Physiol* 64:1114, 1988.

American Medical Association Council on Scientific Affairs: Medical and non-medical uses on anabolic-androgenic steroids, *JAMA* 264:2923-2927, 1990.

Arnheim D, Prentice WE: *Principles of athletic training*, St Louis, 1996, Mosby.

Baker D, Wilson G, Carlyon B: Generality vs. specificity: a comparison of dynamic and isometric measures of strength and speed-strength, *Eur J Appl Physiol* 68:350-355, 1994.

Berger R: Effect of varied weight training programs on strength, *Res Q Exerc Sport* 33:168, 1962.

Booth F, Thomason D: Molecular and cellular adaptation of muscle in response to exercise; perspectives of various models, *Physiol Rev* 71:541-585, 1991.

DeLorme T, Wilkins A: *Progressive resistance exercise*, New York, 1951, Appleton-Century-Crofts.

Duda M: Plyometrics: a legitimate form of power training, *Phys Sports Med* 16:213, 1988.

Dudley GA, Fleck SJ: Strength and endurance training: are they mutually exclusive? *Sports Med* 4(2):79, 1987 (review).

Faulkner J, Green H, White T: Response and adaptation of skeletal muscle to changes in physical activity. In Bouchard C, Shepard R, Stephens J, editors: *Physical activity, fitness, and health*, Champaign, 1994, Human Kinetics.

Fleck SJ, Kramer WJ: Resistance training: physiological responses and adaptations, *Phys Sports Med* 16:108, 1988.

Graves JE, Pollack M, Jones A, et al: Specificity of limited range of motion variable resistance training, *Med Sci Sports Exerc* 21:84, 1989.

Hickson R, Hidaka C, Foster C: Skeletal muscle fiber type, resistance training and strength-related performance, *Med Sci Sports Exerc* 26:593-598, 1994.

Hortobagyi T, Katch FI: Role of concentric force in limiting improvement in muscular strength, *J Appl Physiol* 68:650, 1990.

Huie M: An acute myocardial infarction occuring in an anabolic steroid user, *Med Sci Sports Exerc* 26:408-413, 1994.

Komi P: *Strength and power in sport*, London, 1992, Blackwell Scientific.

Kramer J, Morrow A, Leger A: Changes in rowing ergometer, weight lifting, vertical jump and isokinetic performance in response to standard and standard plus plyometric training programs, *Int J Sports Med* 14(8):440-454, 1993.

Mastropaolo J: A test of maximum power theory for strength, *Eur J Appl Physiol* 65:415-420, 1992.

McComas A: Human neuromuscular adaptations that accompany changes in activity, *Med Sci Sports Exerc* 26(12):1498-1509, 1994.

McArdle W, Katch F, Katch V: *Exercise physiology, energy, nutrition, and human performance*, Philadelphia, 1994, Lea & Febiger.

Meredith CN, Frontera W, Fisher E: Peripheral effects of endurance training in young and old subjects, *J Appl Physiol* 66(6):2844, 1989.

Nicholas JJ: Isokinetic testing in young nonathletic able-bodied subjects, *Arch Phys Med Rehabil* 70(3):210, 1989 (review).

Ozmun J, Mikesky A, Surburg P: Neuromuscular adaptations following prepubescent strength training, *Med Sci Sports Exerc* 26:514, 1994.

Pope H, Katz D: Psychiatric and medical effects of anabolic-androgenic steroid use. A controlled study of 160 athletes, *Arch Gen Psychiatry* 51:375-382, 1994.

Rehfeldt H, Caffiber G, Kramer H, et al: Force, endurance time, and cardiovascular responses in voluntary isometric contractions of different muscle groups, *Biomed Biochem Acta* 48(5-6):S509, 1989.

Sale D, MacDougall D: Specificity in strength training: a review for the coach and athlete, *Can J Appl Sports Sci* 6:87, 1981.

Sanders B: *Sports physical therapy*, Norwalk, Conn, 1990, Appleton & Lange.

Soest A, Bobbert M: The role of muscle properties in control of explosive movements, *Biol Cybern* 69:195-204, 1993.

Strauss RH, editor: *Sports medicine*, Philadelphia, 1991, WB Saunders.

Ulmer H, Knierieman W, Warlo T, et al: Interindividual variability of isometric endurance with regard to the endurance performance limit for static work, *Biomed Biochem Acta* 48(5-6):S504, 1989.

US Department of Health and Human Services, Public Health Services: *Healthy people 2000: national health promotion and disease prevention objectives*, Washington, DC, 1991, USDHHS.

Van Etten L, Verstappen F, Westerterp K: Effect of body building on weight training induced adaptations in body composition and muscular strength, *Med Sci Sports Exerc* 26:515-521, 1994.

SUGGESTED READINGS

Andes K: *A woman's book of strength*, New York, 1995, Perigee.
Written from a woman's perspective on how to eat, exercise, relax, and deal with emotions through strength training.

Baechle T, Groves B: *Weight training: steps to success*, Champaign, 1992, Leisure Press.
Explains the various concepts of exercise, identifies correct lifting techniques, corrects common weight training errors, and lists personal goals for weight training.

Chu D: *Jumping into plyometrics*, Champaign, 1992, Human Kinetics.
Well-illustrated text that helps you develop a safe plyometric training program with exercises designed to improve your quickness, speed, upper body strength, jumping ability, balance, and coordination.

Fahey T: *Basic weight training for men and women*, Mountain View, Calif, 1994, Mayfield.
Details specific weight training principles and techniques for both males and females; well illustrated.

Garhamner J: *Sports Illustrated strength training*, New York, 1987, Harper & Row.
A comprehensive look at weight training, including recommendations on a high-quality strength and conditioning program, various types of equipment, places to train, nutrition, and individualized training programs.

Whitehead N: *Learn weight training in a weekend*, New York, 1992, Alfred A Knopf.
An extremely well-illustrated text that provides a handbook of weight-training exercises on all types of equipment for all muscle groups.

Lab Activity 6-1

Push-Ups

Name _____   **Section** _____   **Date** 9/23/96

PURPOSE   To test muscular strength.

PROCEDURE   1. *Men:* Begin in the standard push-up position with the weight supported on the hands and toes, with trunk and back straight (Figure 6-46).
Women: Begin in the push-up position with the weight on the hands and knees (Figure 6-47).
2. Have a partner place his or her fist on the floor directly under the chest.
3. Lower yourself until your chest touches your partner's fist.
4. Count the number of consecutive correctly done push-ups.
5. Consult Table 6-3 to determine your score.

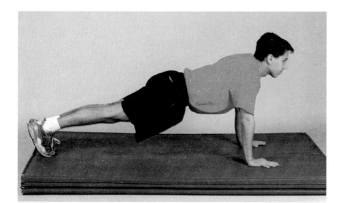
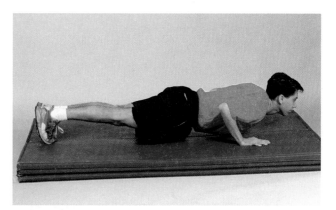

FIGURE 6-46. **Push-Ups.**

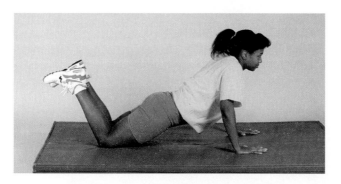

FIGURE 6-47. **Modified Push-Ups.**

Continued.

TABLE 6-3. Push-Up Muscular Endurance Test Standards								
				Fitness Level				
	Age (Years)	Superior	Excellent	Very Good	Good	Average	Poor	Very Poor
Males: Push-Up	15-29	55+	51-54	45-50	35-44	25-34	20-24	15-19
	30-39	45+	41-44	35-40	25-34	20-24	15-19	8-14
	40-49	40+	35-39	30-34	20-29	14-19	12-13	5-11
	50-59	30+	26-29	20-25	10-19	8-9	5-7	0-4
Females: Modified Push-Up	15-29	49+	46-48	34-45	17-33	10-16	6-9	0-5
	30-39	38+	34-37	25-33	12-24	8-11	4-7	0-3
	40-49	33+	29-32	20-28	8-19	6-7	3-5	0-2
	50-59	26+	22-25	15-21	6-14	4-5	2-3	0-1
	60-69	20+	16-19	5-15	3-4	2-3	1-2	0

Lab Activity 6-2

Bent-Knee Curl-Ups

Name _____ **Section** _____ **Date** 9/23/96

PURPOSE   To measure abdominal muscle strength.

PROCEDURE 1. Lie flat on your back and cross your arms across your chest, resting your hands on your shoulders. Knees should be bent to 90 degrees with the feet flat and 18 inches from the buttocks (Figure 6-48).
2. Count the number of curl-ups you are able to complete in 1 minute.
3. Consult Table 6-4 to determine your fitness level.

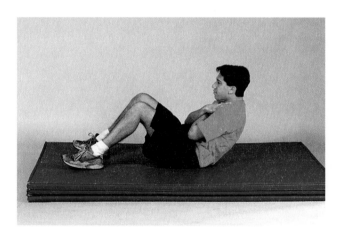

29

FIGURE 6-48. Bent-Knee Curl-Ups.

Continued.

TABLE 6-4.   Bent-Knee Curl-Ups Score

	Age (Years)	Fitness Level						
		Superior	Excellent	Very Good	Good	Average	Poor	Very Poor
Males	17-29	55+	51-55	48-50	42-47	36-41	17-35	0-17
	30-39*	48+	44-48	39-43	33-38	27-32	13-26	0-13
	40-49	43+	39-43	34-38	28-33	23-27	11-22	0-11
	50-59	38+	34-38	29-33	22-28	17-21	8-16	0-8
	60-69	35+	31-35	25-30	18-24	13-17	6-12	0-6
Females	17-29	47+	43-47	36-42	33-35	29-32	14-28	0-14
	30-39*	45+	41-45	35-40	29-34	23-28	11-22	0-11
	40-49	40+	35-40	31-34	24-30	19-23	9-18	0-9
	50-59	35+	31-35	25-30	18-24	13-17	6-12	0-6
	60-69	30+	26-30	21-25	15-20	11-14	5-10	0-5

*The number of curl-ups for ages over 30 is estimated.

Muscular Endurance Test

Name _____ **Section** _____ **Date** _____

PURPOSE To test general levels of muscular endurance.

EQUIPMENT NEEDED Chinning bar and a 16-inch bench.

PROCEDURE 1. Perform the following exercises as indicated:

Men: Bent-leg sit-ups, push-ups, static push-ups, pull-ups, bench jumps.

Women: Bent-leg sit-ups, static push-ups, flexed arm hang, modified pull-ups, bench jumps.

Bent-leg sit-ups. Hands on shoulders, knees flexed to 90 degrees. One elbow must touch knee. Fingers must touch the floor between repetitions. Record total number in 1 minute (Figure 6-49).

Push-ups. Standard push-up position. Chest must touch floor during each repetition. Record total number performed consecutively (see Figure 6-38).

Static push-up. From a standard push-up potition, lower the body until the elbow is flexed at 90 degrees or less. Record the number of seconds this position can be maintained without the body touching the floor or losing the proper form (Figure 6-50).

Pull-ups. Subject grasps bar over overhand grip. The body is raised until the chin is above the bar and lowered until the arms are fully extended. Record the number of repetitions to failure (Figure 6-51).

Flexed-arm hang. Using an overhand grip, raise the body until the chin is above the bar. Record the number of seconds the chin can be held above the level of the bar (Figure 6-52).

Modified pull-ups. Chinning bar is lowered to the height of the chest. Heels remain in contact with the floor underneath the bar. Arms are fully extended. Then pull up until chin touches bar. Record maximum number of repetitions (Figure 6-53).

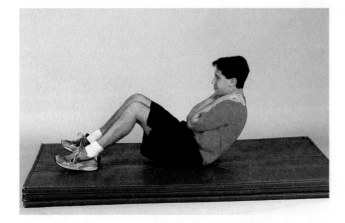

FIGURE 6-49. Bent-Leg Curl-Ups.

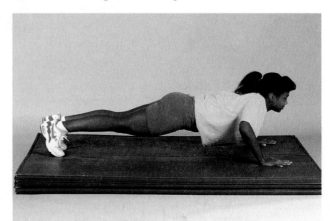

FIGURE 6-50. Static Push-Ups.

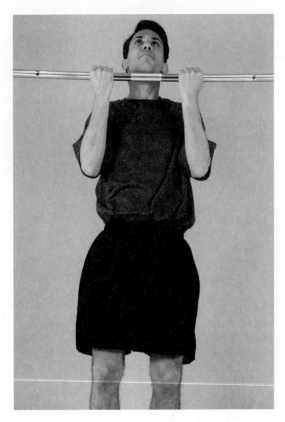

FIGURE 6-51. **Pull-Ups.**

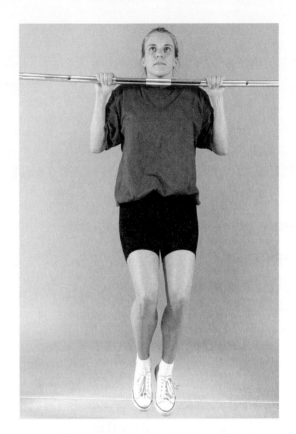

FIGURE 6-52. **Flexed-Arm Hang.**

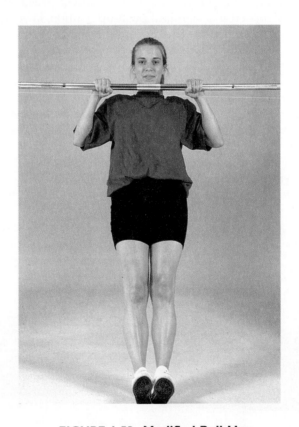

FIGURE 6-53. **Modified Pull-Ups.**

Bench Jumps. Using a 16-inch bench, record the number of times the subject can either jump or step up onto the bench in a 1-minute period (Figure 6-54).

2. Record the information as indicated on the worksheet.
3. Determine the percentile rank for each exercise by consulting Table 6-5.
4. Determine the overall percentile rank as indicated in the worksheet.

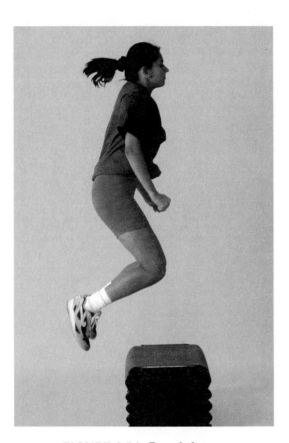

FIGURE 6-54. Bench Jumps.

WORKSHEET

Women			Men		
Exercise	*Score*	*Percentile*	*Exercise*	*Score*	*Percentile*
Bent-leg sit-ups	_____	_____	Bent-leg sit-ups	_____	_____
Static push-ups	_____	_____	Push-ups	_____	_____
Flexed-arm hang	_____	_____	Static push-ups	_____	_____
Modified pull-ups	_____	_____	Pull-ups	_____	_____
Bench jumps	_____	_____	Bench jumps	_____	_____

Total of all five percentiles _____   Total of all five percentiles _____

Overall percentile rank _____ (divide by 5)   Overall percentile rank _____ (divide by 5)

TABLE 6-5.   Muscular Endurance Scoring Table

	Percentile Rank	Bent-Leg Sit-Ups (1 Minute Maximum)	Push-Ups (Men) Static Push-Ups (Women)	Static Push-Ups (Men) Flexed Arm Hang (Women)	Pull-Ups (Men) Modified Pull-Ups (Women)	Bench Jumps
Men	95	50	53	97	14	38
	90	47	49	72	12	36
	80	44	44	67	10	34
	70	41	41	63	9	33
	60	39	38	60	8	31
	50	37	35	57	7	30
	40	35	32	54	6	29
	30	33	29	51	5	27
	20	30	26	47	4	26
	10	27	21	42	2	24
	5	24	17	37	0	22
Women	95	36	38	34	43	28
	90	33	35	28	40	26
	80	30	32	19	36	24
	70	28	30	14	33	22
	60	26	28	10	30	21
	50	24	26	8	28	20
	40	22	24	6	26	19
	30	20	22	4	23	18
	20	18	20	2	20	16
	10	15	17	1	16	14
	5	12	14	0	13	12

Strength Training Log

Name _____ **Section** _____ **Date** _____

PURPOSE To record your progress in building strength in the upper and lower body.

PROCEDURE Fill in the appropriate date and weight used during each exercise session.

Strength Training Worksheet I: Upper Body Exercises

Exercise	Reps	Sets	Date and Weight		
			Date		
Shoulder rotation	6-8	3	Weight		
Bench press	6-8	3	Weight		
Incline press	6-8	3	Weight		
Military press	6-8	3	Weight		
Lateral pull downs	6-8	3	Weight		
Flys	6-8	3	Weight		
Bent Over Rows	6-8	3	Weight		
Shoulder medial rotation	6-8	3	Weight		
Biceps curls	6-8	3	Weight		
Triceps extensions	6-8	3	Weight		
Wrist curls	6-8	3	Weight		
Wrist extensions	6-8	3	Weight		

Strength Training Worksheet II: Lower Body Exercises

Exercise	Reps	Sets	Date and Weight		
			Date		
Leg raises (sidelying)	6-8	3	Weight		
Leg lifts	6-8	3	Weight		
Bent-knee leg lifts	6-8	3	Weight		
Reverse leg lifts	6-8	3	Weight		
Hip medial rotation	6-8	3	Weight		
Hip lateral rotation	6-8	3	Weight		
Quadriceps extensions	6-8	3	Weight		
Hamstring curls	6-8	3	Weight		
Toe raises	6-8	3	Weight		
Ankle inversion	6-8	3	Weight		
Ankle eversion	6-8	3	Weight		
Ankle dorsiflexion	6-8	3	Weight		
Curl-ups	6-8	3	Weight		

Summary Worksheet for Muscular Strength and Muscular Endurance Lab Activities

Name _____ **Section** _____ **Date** _____

Lab Activity 6-1   **Push-Ups**

Total number of push-ups performed _____

Fitness level_____

Lab Activity 6-2   **Bent-Knee Curl-Ups**

Total number of curl-ups performed in 1 minute_____

Fitness level_____

Lab Activity 6-3   **Muscular Endurance Test**

Overall percentile rank for all five tests_____

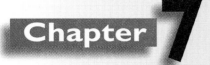

Chapter 7 Stretching to Improve Flexibility

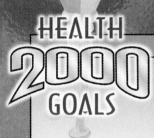

HEALTH 2000 GOALS

- **Flexibility.** Increase to at least 40% the proportion of people age 6 and older who regularly perform physical activities that enhance and maintain flexibility.
  - Stretching exercises and engaging regularly in a variety of physical activities can help maintain and enhance one's flexibility.
  - Individuals with greater flexibility may be at lower risk of future back injury.

OBJECTIVES

After completing this chapter, you will be able to do the following:

- Define flexibility and describe its importance as a health-related component of fitness.
- Identify factors that limit flexibility.
- Differentiate between active and passive range of motion.
- Explain the difference between ballistic, static, and PNF stretching.
- Discuss the neurophysiological principles of stretching.
- Describe stretching exercises that may be used to improve flexibility at specific joints throughout the body.
- Develop a program of flexibility exercises to meet the needs of a healthy, active lifestyle.

KEY TERMS

While reading this chapter, you will become familiar with the following terms:

- flexibility
- active range of motion (dynamic flexibility)
- passive range of motion (static flexibility)
- ballistic stretching
- static stretching
- synergistic muscles
- proprioceptive neuromuscular facilitation (PNF)
- agonist muscle
- antagonist muscle

Flexibility may best be defined as the range of motion possible about a given joint or series of joints. Flexibility can be discussed in relation to movement involving only one joint, such as in the knees, or movement involving a whole series of joints, such as the spinal vertebral joints, which must all move together to allow smooth bending, or rotation, of the trunk.

You may often hear someone say that "Joe has good flexibility." It is incorrect to talk about the entire person as being flexible; flexibility is specific to a given joint or movement. A person may have good range of motion in the ankles, knees, hips, back, and one shoulder joint. However, if the other shoulder joint lacks normal movement, then a problem exists that needs to be corrected before that person can function normally.

WHY IS GOOD FLEXIBILITY IMPORTANT?

Flexibility was discussed earlier as a health-related as opposed to skill-related component of fitness, although for most of us it may be considered important for both. The ability to move smoothly and easily throughout a full range of motion is certainly essential to healthy living. The arthritic person who suffers from degeneration in one or more joints loses the capacity of painless, nonrestricted motion and is hampered in the performance of daily acts of healthful living. Likewise, an individual who has a restricted range of motion will probably realize a decrease in performance capabilities. For example, a sprinter with tight, inelastic hamstring muscles probably loses some speed because the hamstring muscles restrict the ability to flex the hip joint, thus shortening stride length.

Lack of flexibility may result in uncoordinated or awkward movements and probably predisposes a person to muscle strain. Low back pain is sometimes associated with tightness of the musculature in the lower spine and of the hamstring muscles.

Most activities we engage in require relatively "normal" amounts of flexibility. However, some activities such as gymnastics, ballet, diving, karate, and yoga require increased flexibility for superior performance (Figure 7-1). Increased flexibility may increase one's performance through improved balance and reaction time.

Experts in the field of training and the development of physical fitness would all agree that good flexibility is essential to successful physical performance, although their ideas are based primarily on observa-

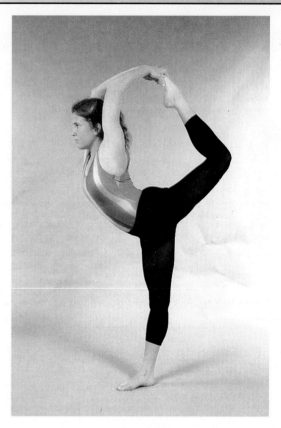

FIGURE 7-1. Extreme Flexibility.
Certain athletic activities require extreme flexibility for successful performance.

tion rather than scientific research. Most people feel that maintaining good flexibility is important in prevention of injury to the musculotendinous unit, and they will generally insist that stretching exercises be included as part of the warm-up before engaging in strenuous activity, although little or no research evidence is available to support this contention.

FACTORS THAT LIMIT FLEXIBILITY

A number of factors may limit the ability of a joint to move through a full, unrestricted range of motion.

The *bony structure* may restrict the endpoint in the range. An elbow that has been fractured through the joint may form excess calcium in the joint space, causing the joint to lose its ability to fully extend. However, in many instances we rely on bony prominences to stop movements at normal endpoints in the range.

Fat may also limit the ability to move through a full range of motion. A person who has a large amount of fat on the abdomen may have severely restricted trunk flexion when asked to bend forward and touch the toes. The fat may act as a wedge between two lever arms, restricting movement wherever it is found.

Skin might also be responsible for limiting movement. For example, a person who has had some type of injury or surgery involving a tearing incision or laceration of the skin, particularly over a joint, will have inelastic scar tissue formed at that site. This scar tissue is incapable of stretching with joint movement.

Muscles and their *tendons*, along with their surrounding fascial sheaths, are most often responsible for limiting range of motion. When performing stretching exercises for the purpose of improving a particular joint's flexibility, you are attempting to take advantage of the highly elastic properties of a muscle. Over time it is possible to increase the elasticity, or the length that a given muscle can be stretched. Persons who have a good deal of movement at a particular joint tend to have highly elastic and flexible muscles.

Connective tissue surrounding the joint, such as ligaments on the joint capsule, may be subject to *contractures.* Ligaments and joint capsules do have some elasticity; however, if a joint is immobilized for a period of time, these structures tend to lose some elasticity and actually shorten. This condition is most commonly seen after surgical repair of an unstable joint, but it can also result from long periods of inactivity.

It is also possible for a person to have relatively slack ligaments and joint capsules. These people are generally referred to as being "double-jointed" or "loose-jointed." Examples of this would be an elbow or knee that hyperextends beyond 180 degrees (Figure 7-2). Frequently there is instability associated with loose-jointedness that may present as great a problem in movement as ligamentous or capsular contractures.

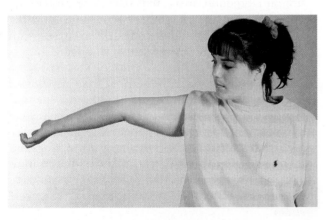

FIGURE 7-2 . Excessive Joint Movement.
A joint can be predisposed to injury, such as in a hyperextended elbow.

FIGURE 7-3. Other Factors Affecting Flexibility.	
Age	For the average person, flexibility tends to decrease through early childhood until age 10 to 12, after which it steadily improves through the college-age years. From about age 20, flexibility gradually declines with age.
Sex	It appears that women generally tend to be more flexible than men. However, this factor may be related to the fact that women tend to spend more time on activities such as dance and gymnastics in which flexibility is essential to performance.
Activity	Those persons who are physically active and remain so throughout life seem to exhibit better flexibility than sedentary persons.

Contractures caused by scarring, ligaments, joint capsules, and musculotendinous units are each capable of improved elasticity to varying degrees through stretching over time.

With the exception of bony structure, age, and gender, all the other factors that limit flexibility may be altered to increase range of joint motion. Figure 7-3 identifies other factors that affect flexibility.

ACTIVE AND PASSIVE RANGE OF MOTION

Active range of motion, also called *dynamic flexibility*, refers to the degree to which a joint can be moved by a muscle contraction, usually through the midrange of movement. Dynamic flexibility is not necessarily a good indicator of the stiffness or looseness of a joint because it applies to the ability to move a joint efficiently, with little resistance to motion.

Passive range of motion, sometimes called *static flexibility*, refers to the degree to which a joint may be passively moved to the endpoints in the range of

flexibility the range of movement possible about a given joint or series of joints
active range of motion (dynamic flexibility) that portion of the total range of motion through which a joint may be moved by an active muscle contraction
passive range of motion (static flexibility) that portion of the total range of motion through which a joint may be moved passively with no muscle contraction

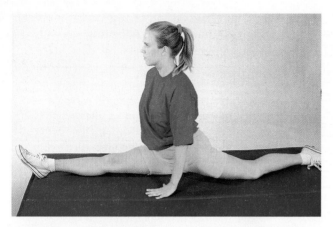

FIGURE 7-4.   Flexibility.
Good flexibility is essential to successful performance in many sport activities.

motion. No muscle contraction is involved to move a joint through a passive range of motion. When a muscle actively contracts, it produces a joint movement through a specific range of motion. However, if passive pressure is applied to an extremity, it is capable of moving farther in the range of motion.

It is essential in sport activities that an extremity be capable of moving through a nonrestricted range of motion. For example, a hurdler who cannot fully extend the knee joint in a normal stride is at considerable disadvantage because stride length and thus speed will be reduced significantly (Figure 7-4).

Passive range of motion is important for injury prevention. There are many situations in sport in which a muscle is forced to stretch beyond its normal active limits. If the muscle does not have enough elasticity to compensate for this additional stretch, it is likely that the musculotendinous unit will be injured.

STRETCHING TECHNIQUES

The goal of any effective flexibility program should be to improve the range of motion at a given articulation by altering the extensibility of the musculotendinous units that produce movement at that joint. It is well documented that exercises that stretch these musculotendinous units over a period of time will increase the range of movement possible about a given joint.

Stretching techniques for improving flexibility have evolved over the years. The oldest technique for stretching is called ballistic stretching, which makes use of repetitive bouncing motions. A second technique, known as static stretching, involves stretching a muscle to the point of discomfort and then holding it at that point for an extended time. This technique

has been used for many years. Recently another group of stretching techniques known collectively as proprioceptive neuromuscular facilitation (PNF), involving alternating contractions and stretches, has also been recommended. Researchers have had considerable discussion about which of these techniques is most effective for improving range of motion.

Agonist Versus Antagonist Muscles

Before discussing the three different stretching techniques, it is essential to define the terms *agonist* and *antagonist*. Most joints in the body are capable of more than one movement. The knee joint, for example, is capable of flexion and extension. Contraction of the quadriceps group of muscles on the front of the thigh causes knee extension, whereas contraction of the hamstring muscles on the back of the thigh produces knee flexion.

To achieve knee extension, the quadriceps group contracts while the hamstring muscles relax and stretch. Muscles that work in concert with one another in this manner are called synergistic muscle groups. The muscle that contracts to produce a movement, in this case the quadriceps, is referred to as the agonist muscle. Conversely, the muscle being stretched in response to contraction of the agonist muscle is called the antagonist muscle. In this example of knee extension, the antagonist muscle would be the hamstring group.

Some degree of balance in strength must exist between agonist and antagonist muscle groups. This is necessary for normal, smooth, coordinated movement and for reducing the likelihood of muscle strain due to the muscular imbalance.

Comprehension of this synergistic muscle action is essential to understanding the three techniques of stretching.

Ballistic Stretching

If you were to walk out to the track on any spring or fall afternoon and watch people who are warming up to run by doing their stretching exercises, you would probably see them using bouncing movements to stretch a particular muscle. This bouncing technique is more appropriately known as *ballistic stretching*, in which repetitive contractions of the agonist muscle are used to produce quick stretches of the antagonist muscle. Ballistic stretching takes advantage of both momentum created by an active contraction and gravity to stretch a muscle. The ballistic stretching technique, although apparently effective in improving range of motion, is seldom recommended.

Increased range of motion is achieved through a series of jerks or pulls on the resistant muscle tissue. It has been suggested that if the forces generated by the jerks are greater than the tissues' extensibility, muscle injury may result.

Successive forceful contractions of the agonist that result in stretching of the antagonist may cause muscle soreness. For example, forcefully kicking a soccer ball 50 times may result in muscular soreness of the hamstrings (antagonist muscle) as a result of eccentric contraction of the hamstrings to control the dynamic movement of the quadriceps (agonist muscle). Ballistic stretching that is controlled usually does not cause muscle soreness.

Static Stretching

The *static stretching* technique is still an extremely effective and popular technique of stretching. This technique involves passively stretching a given antagonist muscle by placing it in a maximal position of stretch and holding it there for an extended time. Recommendations for the optimal time for holding this stretched position vary, ranging from as short as 3 seconds to as long as 60 seconds. Data are inconclusive at present; however, it appears that 30 seconds may be a good time. The static stretch of each muscle should be repeated three or four times. Much research has been done comparing ballistic and static stretching techniques for the improvement of flexibility. Both static and ballistic stretching are effective in increasing flexibility, and there are no significant differences between the two. However, with static stretching there is less danger of exceeding the extensibility limits of the involved joints because the stretch is more controlled. Ballistic stretching is apt to cause muscular soreness, whereas static stretching generally does not and is commonly used in injury rehabilitation of sore or strained muscles.

Static stretching is certainly a much safer stretching technique, especially for sedentary or untrained individuals. However, many physical activities involve dynamic movement. Thus stretching as a warm-up for these types of activities should begin with static stretching followed by ballistic stretching, which more closely resembles the dynamic activity.

Proprioceptive Neuromuscular Facilitation (PNF) Techniques

PNF techniques were first used by physical therapists for treating patients who had various types of neuromuscular paralysis. Only recently have PNF stretching exercises been used as a stretching technique for increasing flexibility. There are a number of different PNF techniques currently being used for stretching, including slow-reversal-hold-relax, con-

tract-relax, and hold-relax techniques. All involve some combination of alternating contraction and relaxation of both agonist and antagonist muscles (a 10-second pushing phase followed by a 10-second relaxing phase).

Using a hamstring stretching technique as an example (Figure 7-5), the slow-reversal-hold-relax technique would be done as follows. Lying on your back with the knee extended and the ankle flexed to 90 degrees, a partner passively flexes your leg at the hip joint to the point at which you feel slight discomfort in the muscle. At this point you begin pushing against your partner's resistance by contracting the hamstring muscle. After pushing for 10 seconds, the hamstring muscles are relaxed and the agonist quadriceps muscle is contracted while your partner applies passive pressure to further stretch the antagonist hamstrings. This should move the leg so that there is increased hip joint flexion. The relaxing phase lasts for 10 seconds, at which time you again push against your partner's resistance, beginning at this new joint angle. The push-relax sequence is repeated at least three times.

The contract-relax and hold-relax techniques are variations on the slow-reversal-hold-relax method. In the contract-relax method, the hamstrings are isotonically contracted so that the leg actually moves toward the floor during the push phase. The hold-relax method involves an isometric hamstring contraction against immovable resistance during the push phase. During the relax phase, both techniques involve relaxation of hamstrings and quadriceps while the hamstrings are passively stretched. This same basic PNF technique can be used to stretch any

---

ballastic stretching technique involving repetitive contractions (bouncing) of the agonist muscle that are used to produce quick stretches of the antagonist muscle

static stretching technique involving passively stretching a given antagonist muscle by placing it in a maximal position of stretch and holding it there for an extended time

proprioceptive neuromuscular facilitation (PNF) a group of stretching techniques including slow-reversal-hold-relax, contract-relax, and hold-relax techniques, all of which involve a combination of alternating contraction and relaxation of both agonist and antagonist muscles

synergistic muscle groups a group of muscles that work together to produce smooth, coordinated movement

agonist muscle the muscle that contracts to produce a movement

antagonist muscle the muscle being stretched in response to contraction of the agonist muscle

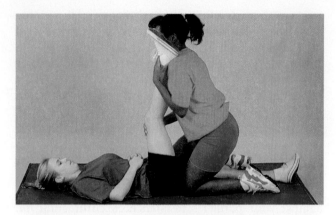

FIGURE 7-5. **Slow-Reversal-Hold-Relax Technique.** Technique stretches hamstring muscles.

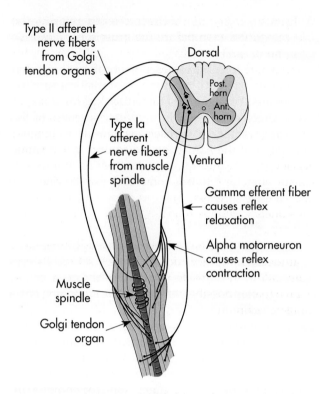

FIGURE 7-6. **Stretch Reflex.** The muscle spindle produces a reflex resistance to stretch, while the Golgi tendon organ causes a reflex relaxation of the muscle in response to stretch.

muscle in the body. PNF stretching techniques are perhaps best performed with a partner, although they may also be done using a wall as resistance.

NEUROPHYSIOLOGICAL BASIS OF STRETCHING

All three stretching techniques are based on a neurophysiological phenomenon involving the *stretch reflex* (Figure 7-6). Every muscle in the body contains various types of receptors that when stimulated inform the central nervous system of what is happening with that muscle. Two of these receptors are important in the stretch reflex: the *muscle spindle* and the *Golgi tendon organ.* Both types of receptors are sensitive to changes in muscle length. The Golgi tendon organs are also affected by changes in muscle tension. When a muscle is stretched, the muscle spindles are also stretched, sending a volley of sensory impulses to the spinal cord that inform the central nervous system that the muscle is being stretched. Impulses return to the muscle from the spinal cord, which causes the muscle to reflexively contract, thus resisting the stretch.

If the stretch of the muscle continues for an extended period of time (at least 6 seconds), the Golgi tendon organs respond to the change in length and the increase in tension by firing off sensory impulses of their own to the spinal cord. The impulses from the Golgi tendon organs, unlike the signals from the muscle spindle, cause a reflex relaxation of the antagonist muscle. This reflex relaxation serves as a protective mechanism that will allow the muscle to stretch through relaxation before the extensibility limits are exceeded, preventing damage to the muscle fibers.

With the jerking, bouncing motion of ballistic stretching the muscle spindles are being repetitively

stretched; thus there is continuous resistance by the muscle to further stretch. The ballistic stretch is not continued long enough to allow the Golgi tendon organs to have any relaxing effect.

The static stretch involves a continuous sustained stretch lasting anywhere from 6 to 60 seconds, which is sufficient time for the Golgi tendon organs to begin responding to the increase in tension. The impulses from the Golgi tendon organs have the ability to override the impulses coming from the muscle spindles, allowing the muscle to reflexively relax after the initial reflex resistance to the change in length. Thus lengthening the muscle and allowing it to remain in a stretched position for an extended period of time is unlikely to produce any injury to the muscle.

The effectiveness of the PNF techniques may be attributed in part to these same neurophysiological principles. The slow-reversal-hold-relax technique discussed previously takes advantage of two additional neurophysiological phenomena. The maximal isometric contraction of the muscle that will be stretched during the 10-second "push" phase again causes an increase in tension, which stimulates the

Golgi tendon organs to effect a reflex relaxation of the antagonist even before the muscle is placed in a position of stretch. This relaxation of the antagonist muscle during contractions is referred to as *autogenic inhibition.*

During the relaxing phase the antagonist is relaxed and passively stretched while there is a maximal isotonic contraction of the agonist muscle pulling the extremity further into the agonist pattern. In any synergistic muscle group, a contraction of the agonist causes a reflex relaxation in the antagonist muscle, allowing it to stretch and protecting it from injury. This phenomenon is referred to as *reciprocal inhibition* (Figure 7-7).

Thus with the PNF techniques the additive effects of autogenic and reciprocal inhibition should theoretically allow the muscle to be stretched to a greater degree than is possible with the static stretching or the ballistic technique.

Practical Application

Although all three stretching techniques have been demonstrated to effectively improve flexibility, there is still considerable debate as to which technique produces the greatest increases in range of movement. The ballistic technique is seldom recommended because of the potential for causing muscle soreness.

However, it must be added that most sport activities are ballistic in nature (i.e., they involve kicking or running), and those activities use the stretch reflex to enhance performance. In highly trained individuals, it is unlikely that ballistic stretching will result in muscle soreness. Static stretching is perhaps the most widely used technique. It is a simple technique and does not require a partner. A fully nonrestricted range of motion can be attained through static stretching over time.

PNF stretching techniques are capable of producing dramatic increases in range of motion during one stretching session. Studies comparing static and PNF stretching suggest that PNF stretching is capable of producing greater improvement in flexibility over an extended training period. The major disadvantage of PNF stretching is that a partner is required to help you stretch, although stretching with a partner may have some motivational advantages. More and more athletic teams seem to be adopting the PNF technique as the method of choice for improving flexibility. Figure 7-8 illustrates some guidelines and precautions for stretching, and the box on p. 200 also offers a number of ways one might choose to improve flexibility.

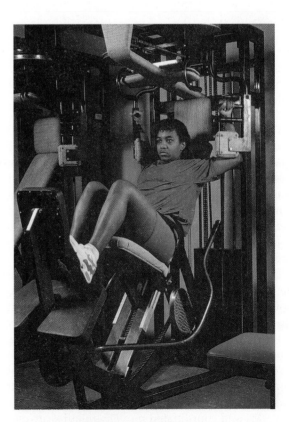

FIGURE 7-7. Reciprocal Inhibition.
A contraction of the agonist muscle will automatically produce relaxation in the antagonist muscle.

FIGURE 7-8. Strength Training.
If strength training is combined with flexibility exercise, a full range of motion may be maintained.

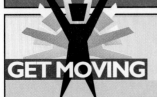

Ways to improve your flexibility

1. Before beginning your stretching program, try to bend over and touch your toes and see how far down you can reach. Make a mental note of where you are starting and then use that as a baseline to monitor improvement.
2. Realize that quite often when you engage in physical activity that you are not used to, you develop some muscle soreness. The more flexible you are, the less chance of soreness.
3. If you are strength training, exercising the muscle through a full range of motion can help improve your flexibility.
4. Losing body fat may help with increasing flexibility.
5. Improving your active range of motion may help your ability to perform an activity. For example, performing a kick in the martial arts may be improved if your flexibility is increased.
6. Your exercise program doesn't necessarily have to concentrate solely on flexibility if you incorporate stretching as part of your warm-up and cool-down.
7. Having good flexibility along with achieving a balance in strength between muscle groups may help you to achieve a better posture.

RELATIONSHIP OF STRENGTH AND FLEXIBILITY

We often hear about the negative effects that strength training has on flexibility. For example, someone who develops large bulk through strength training is often referred to as *muscle bound*. The expression *muscle bound* has negative connotations in terms of the ability of that person to move. We tend to think of people who have highly developed muscles as having lost much of their ability to move freely through a full range of motion.

Occasionally a person develops so much bulk that the physical size of the muscle prevents a normal range of motion. When strength training is not properly done, movement can be impaired. However, there is no reason to believe that weight training, if done properly through a full range of motion, will impair flexibility. Proper strength training probably improves dynamic flexibility and, if combined with a rigorous stretching program, can greatly enhance powerful and coordinated movements that are essential for success in many athletic activities. In all cases a heavyweight-training program should be accompanied by a strong flexibility program (see Figure 7-8).

STRETCHING EXERCISES

Figures 7-9 to 7-20 illustrate recommended stretching exercises that may be safely used to improve flexibility at specific joints throughout the body. The exercises described may be done statically or with slight modification; they may also be done with a partner using a PNF technique.

There are many possible variations to each of these exercises. The exercises selected are those that seem to be the most effective for stretching of various muscle groups. The Safe Tip box on p. 205 provides guidelines and precautions for safe stretching.

There are a number specific stretching exercises that are not recommended because of unnecessary stresses and strains placed on the joints being stretched. Chapter 10 discusses ways to prevent, reduce, and manage injuries that may occur during exercise. Figures 10-22 to 10-33 show stretching exercises that should be avoided.

Text continues on p. 207

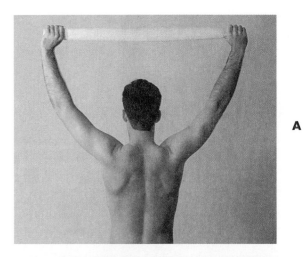

A

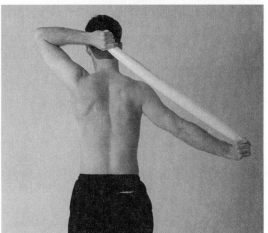

B

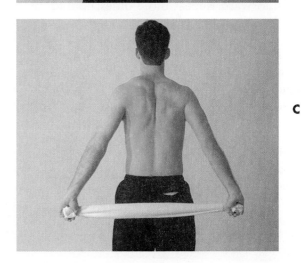

C

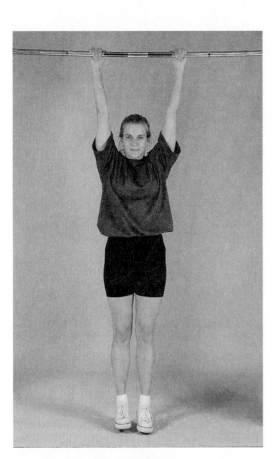

FIGURE 7-9. Arm Hang Exercise.
Muscles stretched: Entire shoulder girdle complex.
Instructions: Using a chinning bar, simply hang with shoulders and arms fully extended for 30 seconds. Repeat five times.

FIGURE 7-10. Shoulder Towel Stretch Exercise.
Muscles stretched: Internal and external rotators.
Instructions: **A,** Begin by holding towel above head shoulder-width apart. **B,** Try to pull towel down behind back, first with left hand and then with right. **C,** You should end up in this position. Reverse order to get back to position in **A.** Repeat five times on each side.

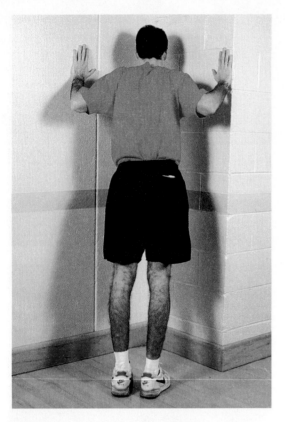

FIGURE 7-11. Chest and Shoulder Stretch Exercise.
Muscles stretched: Pectoralis and deltoid.
Instructions: Stand in a corner, hands on walls, and lean forward. Repeat three times; hold for 30 seconds.

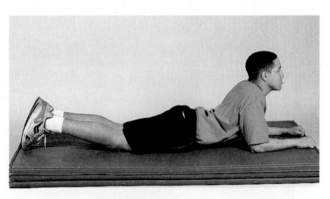

FIGURE 7-12. Abdominal and Anterior Chest Wall Stretch Exercise.
Muscles stretched: Muscles of respiration in thorax and abdominal muscles.
Instructions: Extend upper trunk, support weight on elbows, keeping pelvis on the floor. Repeat three times; hold for 30 seconds.
Caution: Do not use this exercise if you have increased back pain.

A

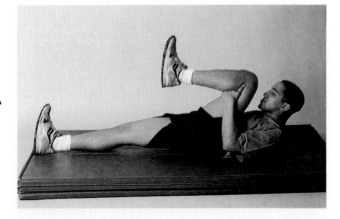

B

FIGURE 7-13. William's Flexion Exercise.
Muscles stretched: Low back and hip extensors. Instructions: **A,** Touch chin to right knee and hold, then to left knee and hold. **B,** Touch chin to both knees and hold. Hold each position for 30 seconds.

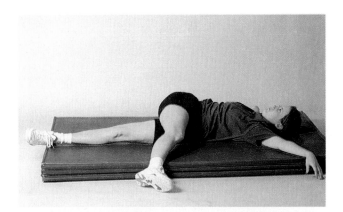

FIGURE 7-14. Low Back Twister Exercise.
Muscles stretched: Rotators of lower back and sacrum and hip abductors.
Instructions: Lie on back on edge of bed or table. Keep shoulders and arms flat on surface. Cross leg farthest from edge over the top and let it hang off the side of bed, keeping knee straight; repeat with other leg. Repeat three times with each leg; hold for 30 seconds.
Caution: If keeping the leg straight produces pain, this exercise may be done with the leg bent. Be sure to exercise caution in returning the leg to the starting position.

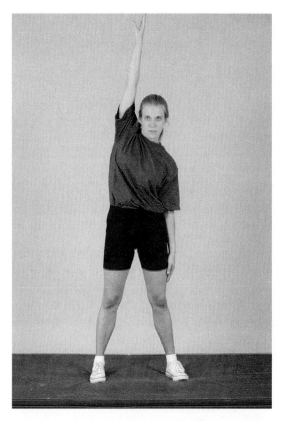

FIGURE 7-16. Lateral Trunk Stretch Exercise.
Muscles stretched: Lateral abdominals and intercostals.
Instructions: Standing with feet spread at shoulder width, hands on hips, drop head toward shoulder and bend trunk in a lateral direction. Hold for 30 seconds and repeat three times on each side.

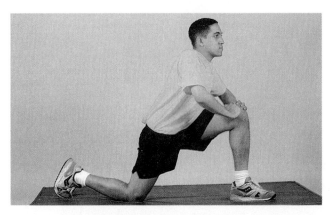

FIGURE 7-15. Forward Lunge Exercise.
Muscles stretched: Hip flexors and quadriceps.
Instructions: In a kneeling position with one knee on the ground, thrust pelvis forward. Repeat three times; hold for 30 seconds.
Caution: Avoid letting the knee extend beyond the foot.

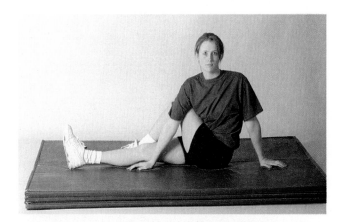

FIGURE 7-17. Trunk Twister Exercise.
Muscles stretched: Trunk and hip rotators.
Instructions: Place one foot over opposite knee. Rotate trunk to bent knee side.

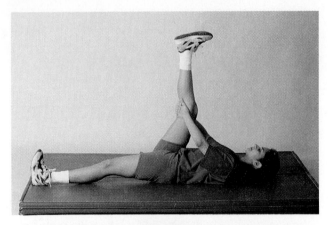

FIGURE 7-18. Hamstring Stretch Exercise.
Muscles stretched: Hip extensors and knee flexors.
Instructions: Lie flat on back. Raise one leg straight
up with knee extended and ankle flexed to 90
degrees. Grasp leg around calf and pull toward
head; repeat with opposite leg. Repeat three times
with each leg; hold for 30 seconds.

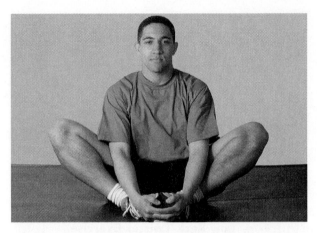

FIGURE 7-19. Groin Stretch Exercise.
Muscles stretched: Hip adductors in groin.
Instructions: Sit with knees flexed and soles of feet
together. Try to press knees flat on the floor; if
they are flat to begin with, try to touch face to
floor. Repeat three times; hold for 30 seconds.

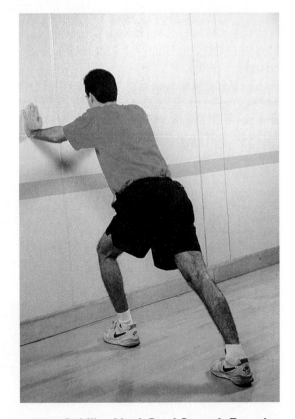

A

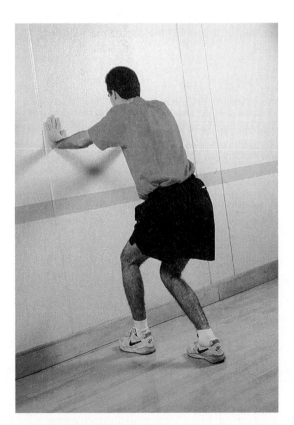

B

FIGURE 7-20.   Achilles Heel Cord Stretch Exercise.
Muscles stretched: Foot plantar flexors. **A,** Gastrocnemius. **B,** Soleus.
Instructions: **A,** Stand facing wall with toes pointing straight ahead and knees straight. Lean forward toward
wall, keeping heels flat on floor. You should feel stretching high in calf. **B,** Stand facing wall with toes pointing straight ahead and knees flexed. Lean forward toward wall, keeping heels flat on floor. You should feel
stretching low in calf. Repeat each position three times; hold each for 30 seconds.

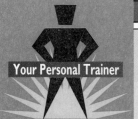

Your Personal Trainer

Rae Soroka, Pre-law student
Age: 19

Scenario

I've been playing tennis off and on with a group of friends all through high school. This year I've gotten more serious with my game and have been playing regularly every other day. I like to stretch and do a few calisthenics before playing. Recently I've had a persistent ache in my lower back. It usually isn't too bad while I'm playing, but by late in the afternoon I can't seem to sit still. It is getting so distracting that it is starting to affect the way I study or even my down time just hanging out in the dorm.

Solution

Low back pain is one of the most common health ailments in the United States. It sounds like you may be experiencing a minor slippage of one of your lumbar vertebrae (spondylolisthesis). This can be caused by the repeated hyperextension of your back while serving.

Initially, rest will help reduce your pain and discomfort. You should limit your physical activity during acute episodes of low back pain, and an antiinflammatory (such as aspirin) may help relieve some of the pressure.

Gentle, passive stretching of the low back region within your level of comfort (don't push it) will help you regain your range of motion. As the pain subsides, start doing exercises to help stabilize the affected region in your lower back. Progressive trunk strengthening exercises such as the abdominal and anterior chest wall stretch and William's flexion exercise will help increase your pain-free range of motion. Paying attention to strengthening your abdominal muscles will also play an important role in your recovery.

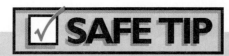

☑ SAFE TIP

GUIDELINES AND PRECAUTIONS FOR STRETCHING

The following guidelines and precautions should be incorporated into a sound stretching program.

- Warm up using a slow jog or fast walk before stretching vigorously.
- To increase flexibility, the muscle must be overloaded or stretched beyond its normal range but not to the point of pain.
- Stretch only to the point of tightness or resistance to stretch (or perhaps until you feel some discomfort). Stretching should not be painful.
- Increases in range of motion will be specific to whatever joint is being stretched.
- Exercise caution when stretching muscles that surround painful joints. Pain should not be ignored because it is an indication that something is wrong.
- Avoid overstretching the ligaments and capsules that surround joints.
- Exercise caution when stretching the low back and neck by avoiding hyperextension and hyperflexion. Exercises that compress the vertebrae and their discs may cause damage.
- Stretching from a seated position rather than a standing position takes stress off the low back and decreases the chance of back injury.
- Stretch the muscles that are tight and inflexible.
- Strengthen the muscles that are weak and loose.
- Always stretch slowly and with control.
- Be sure to continue normal breathing during a stretch. Do not hold your breath.
- Static and PNF techniques are most often recommended for individuals who want to improve their range of motion.
- Ballistic stretching should be done only after static stretching and by those who are already flexible and/or are accustomed to stretching.
- Stretching should be done at least three times per week to see minimal improvement. It is recommended that you stretch between five and six times per week to see maximal results.

ASSESSING FLEXIBILITY

Accurate measurement of the range of joint motion is difficult. Various devices have been designed to accommodate both variations in the size of the joints and the complexity of movements in articulations that involve more than one joint. Of these devices, the simplest and most widely used is the *goniometer* (Figure 7-21).

A goniometer is a large protractor with measurements in degrees. By aligning the two arms parallel to the longitudinal axis of the two segments involved in motion about a specific joint, it is possible to obtain relatively accurate measures of range of movement. The goniometer is useful in a rehabilitation setting, where it is essential to assess improvement in joint flexibility for the purpose of modifying injury rehabilitation programs. Because it is most appropriate to talk about flexibility as being specific to a given joint or movement, there is no doubt that the most accurate method for assessing joint movement is through the use of a goniometer. However, for the average person it is not practical to assess joint movement using goniometry. Lab Activity 7-1 will give you some experience in using a goniometer.

Lab Activities 7-2 through 7-4 will help you assess your existing flexibility. Lab Activity 7-5 will assist you in beginning and monitoring a stretching and flexibility program.

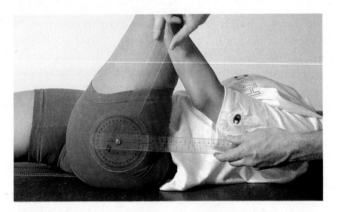

FIGURE 7-21. Goniometric Measurement of Hip Joint Flexion.

SUMMARY

- Flexibility is the ability to move a joint or a series of joints smoothly through a full range of motion.
- Flexibility is specific to a given joint, and the term *good flexibility* implies that there are no joint abnormalities restricting movement.
- Flexibility may be limited by fat or defects in bone structure, skin, connective tissue, ligaments, or muscles and tendons.
- Passive range of motion refers to the degree to which a joint may be passively moved to the end points in the range of motion, whereas active range of motion refers to movement through the midrange of motion resulting from active contraction.
- An agonist muscle is one that contracts to produce joint motion; the antagonist muscle is stretched with contraction of the agonist.
- Ballistic, static, and proprioceptive neuromuscular facilitation (PNF) techniques have all been used as stretching techniques for improving flexibility.

- Each stretching technique is based on the neurophysiological phenomema involving the muscle spindles and Golgi tendon organs.
- PNF techniques appear to be the most effective in producing increases in flexibility.
- Stretching should be included as part of the warm-up period to prepare the muscles for activity and to prevent injury and as part of the cooldown period to help reduce injury. Stretching after an activity may prevent muscle soreness and will help increase flexibility by stretching a loose, warmed-up muscle.
- Strength training, if done correctly through a full range of motion, will probably improve flexibility.
- Measurement of joint flexibility is accomplished through the use of a goniometer.

REFERENCES

Allerheiligren W: Stretching and warm-up. In Baechle T, editor: *Essentials of strength training and conditioning*, Champaign, 1994, Human Kinetics.

Alter MJ: *The science of stretching*, Champaign, 1988, Human Kinetics.

Blanke D: Flexibility. In Mellion M, editor: *Sports medicine secrets*, Philadelphia, 1994, Hanley & Belfus.

Bowden J: Stretching beyond belief: a new twist on flexibility exercise, *Women's Sports Fitness* 17(5):75-78, 1994.

Cornelius WL, Hagemann RW Jr, Jackson AW: A study on placement of stretching within a workout, *J Sports Med Phys Fitness* 28(3):234, 1988.

Godges JJ, MacRae G, Longdon C, et al: The effects of two stretching procedures on hip range of motion and joint economy, *J Orthop Sports Phys Ther* 10(9):350, 1989.

Hendrick A: Flexibility and the conditioning program, *Natl Strength Cond Assoc J* 15(4):62-66, 1993.

McNaught-Davis P: *Flexibility*, London, 1991, Partridge Press.

Ninos J: Guidelines for proper stretching, *Strength Cond* 17(1):44-46, 1995.

Norris C: *Flexibility principles and practices*, London, 1994, A & C Black.

Prentice WE: A review of PNF techniques-implications for athletic rehabilitation and performance, *Forum Medicum* (51):1, 1989.

Schiffer J: Stretching, *New Studies in Athletics* 9(1):67-93, 1994.

Sharkey J: Is ballistic stretching back? *Ultra Fit Australia* 22:22-24, 1995.

Siff M: Using PNF in training, *Fit Sport Rev Int* 22(2):63-64, 1994.

Stamford B: A stretching primer, *Phys Sports Med* 22(9):85-86, 1994.

St George F: *The stretching handbook: ten steps to muscle fitness*, East Roseville, Ill, 1994, Simon & Schuster.

Surburg P: Flexibility: training program design. In Miller P, editor: *Fitness programming and physical disability*, Champaign, 1995, Human Kinetics.

US Department of Health and Human Services, Public Health Services: *Healthy people 2000: national health promotion and disease prevention objectives*, Washington, DC, 1991, USDHHS.

van Mechelen P: Prevention of running injuries by warm-up, cooldown, and stretching, *Am J Sports Med* 21(5):711-719, 1993.

Wessel J, Wan A: Effect of stretching on intensity of delayed-onset muscle soreness, *J Sports Med* 4(2):83-87, 1994.

Worrell T, Smith T, Winegardner, J: Effect of hamstring stretching on hamstring muscle performance, *J Orthop Sports Phys Ther* 20(3):154-159, 1994.

SUGGESTED READINGS

Alter J: *Science of stretching*, Champaign, 1988, Human Kinetics.
Explains the principles and techniques of stretching and details the anatomy and physiology of muscle and connective tissue. Includes guidelines for developing a flexibility program and illustrated stretching exercises and warm-up drills.

Anderson B: *Stretching*, Bolinas, Calif, 1986, Shelter.
An extremely comprehensive best-selling text on stretching exercises for the entire body.

McAtee R: *Facilitated stretching*, Champaign, 1993, Human Kinetics.
Discusses the usefulness of proprioceptive neuromuscular facilitation techniques for improving flexibility and uses illustrations to demonstrate the PNF stretching techniques.

Tobias M, Sullivan JP: *Complete stretching*, New York, 1992, Alfred A Knopf.
A colorful and well-illustrated guide to maximum mental and physical energy, increased flexibility, improved body shape, and enhanced relaxation.

Lab Activity 7-1

Goniometric Measurement

Name _____   **Section** _____   **Date** _____

PURPOSE   This activity is designed to familiarize you with the techniques of goniometric measurement of joint range of motion.

PROCEDURE 1. You will need a goniometer that can measure on a 180-degree scale.
2. Have a partner lie supine on either the floor or a table. Instruct the person to grasp the posterior part of the thigh just above the knee joint and pull the leg upward until tightness or resistance to stretch is present (see Figure 7-21).
3. Line up one arm of the goniometer parallel with the longitudinal axis of the thigh. The other arm should be parallel with the longitudinal axis of the trunk.
4. Read the measurement in degrees from the goniometer.

What is the measurement in degrees of hip joint flexion? _____

How difficult was it to properly align the arms of the goniometer?_____

_____

_____

BP.
120/68

Lab Activity 7-2

Trunk Flexion

Name _____ Section _____ Date _____

PURPOSE   This test measures the flexibility of the lower back muscles and the hip extensors (i.e., the hamstrings and gluteals).

PROCEDURE   Sit with the legs together, knees flat on the floor, and feet flat against some vertical surface. Bend forward at the waist and reach as far forward as possible with the fingers (Figure 7-22).
Your score is determined by measuring the number of inches you can reach either in front of or beyond the vertical surface.
To determine your classification, see Table 7-1.

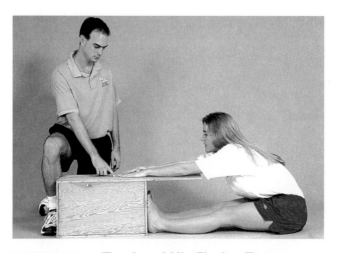

FIGURE 7-22.   Trunk and Hip Flexion Test.
Feet are placed flat against a box, with head up.

TABLE 7-1. Flexibility in Trunk and Hip Flexion (Sit and Reach)		
Classification	**Men**	**Women**
Poor	0 in	0 in
Average	1-3 in	2-4 in
Good	4-6 in	5-7 in
Excellent	7 in	8 in

½ inch!

Lab Activity 7-3

Trunk Extension

Name _____   **Section** _____   **Date** _____

PURPOSE This test measures the flexibility of the abdominal and hip flexor muscles.

PROCEDURE Lie in a prone position on the floor. Have a partner hold your legs and hips to the ground. Grasp your hands behind your neck, inhale, lift your upper trunk as high off the floor as possible, and hold (Figure 7-23).

Your score is determined by measuring the distance from your chin to the floor. To determine your classification, see Table 7-2.

Caution: If a student has back pain this test should be avoided.

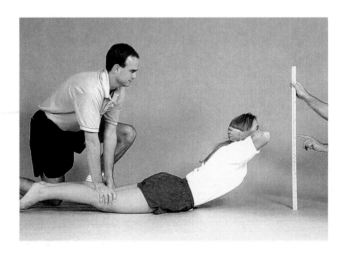

FIGURE 7-23. **Trunk Extension Test.**

TABLE 7-2.	**Flexibility in Trunk Extension**	
Classification	**Men**	**Women**
Poor	16 in	17 in
Average	17-18 in	18-19 in
Good	19-21 in	20-23 in
Excellent	22 in	24 in

18

Lab Activity 7-4

Shoulder Lift Test

Name _____   **Section** _____   **Date** _____

PURPOSE   This test measures the flexibility of the shoulder flexors.

PROCEDURE   Lie prone on the floor with arms extended over the head while holding a stick in the hands. Raise stick as high as possible, with the face and chest kept flat on the floor; hold (Figure 7-24).
Your score is determined by measuring the distance from the stick to the ground. To determine your classification, see Table 7-3.

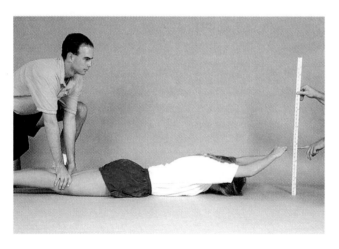

FIGURE 7-24. **Shoulder Lift Test.**

TABLE 7-3. **Flexibility of the Shoulder Joint**		
Classification	**Men**	**Women**
Poor	0-19 in	0-20 in
Average	20-22 in	21-23 in
Good	23-25 in	24-26 in
Excellent	26 in	27 in

12

Summary Worksheet for Flexibility Lab Activities

Name _____   **Section** _____   **Date** _____

Lab Activity 7-1   **Goniometric Measurement**

Degrees of hip joint flexion measured _____

Lab Activity 7-2   **Trunk Flexion**

Total inches measured _____

Flexibility classification _____

Lab Activity 7-3   **Trunk Extension**

Total inches measured _____

Flexibility classification _____

Lab Activity 7-4   **Shoulder Lift Test**

Total inches measured _____

Flexibility classification _____

Lab Activity 7-5

Checklist for an Individualized Stretching Program

Name _____ **Section** _____ **Date** _____

PURPOSE Use this checklist to monitor your stretching program over a period of time.

Exercise	Hold Time (sec)	Repetitions	Day 1	2	3	4	5	6	7	8	9	10	11	12	13	14
Arm hang	30	5														
Shoulder towel stretch	10	5														
Abdominal and anterior chest wall stretch	30	3														
Chest and shoulder stretch	30	3														
William's flexion exercise	30*	3														
Low back twister	30	3														
Pelvic thrust	30	3														
Lateral trunk stretch	30	3														
Quadriceps stretch	30	3														
Hamstring stretch	30	3														
Groin stretch	30	3														
Achilles heel cord stretch	30	3*														
Toe pointer	30	3														

*In each position

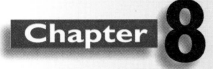

Chapter 8 Assessing Body Composition

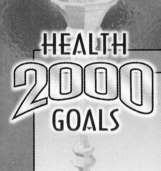

- **Caloric Control and Increased Physical Activity.** Caloric control and increased physical activity are important for attaining a healthy body weight.
- **Overweight.** Reduce overweight to a prevalence of no more than 20% among people age 20 and older and no more than 15% among adolescents age 12 to 19. From 1976 to 1980, 26% of people age 20 to 74 were overweight. *Midpoint Update: currently further from our goal, with 34% of adults overweight.*
- **Sound Dietary Practice.** Increase to at least 50% the proportion of overweight people age 12 and older who have adopted sound dietary practices combined with regular physical activity to attain an appropriate body weight. In 1985, 30% of overweight women and 25% of overweight men age 18 and older were working to improve their dietary intake and increase their frequency of physical activity.

OBJECTIVES

After completing this chapter, you will be able to do the following:

- Describe the problem of being overweight in American society.
- Explain the distinction between body weight and body composition.
- Explain the principle of caloric balance and how imbalances lead to weight gain or loss.
- Assess body composition using skinfold calipers.
- Develop daily logs that chart both energy expenditure and caloric intake.
- Identify various methods for weight loss.
- Explain the importance of lifestyle modification in weight loss.
- Describe methods for losing and gaining weight.
- Develop a program of weight loss or maintenance consistent with your needs.

KEY TERMS

While reading this chapter, you will become familiar with the following terms:

- overweight
- obesity
- body composition
- lean body weight
- adipose cell
- subcutaneous fat
- body mass index (BMI)
- calorie
- kilocalorie
- basal metabolic rate (BMR)
- bulimia
- anorexia nervosa
- bulimia nervosa

It seems that every American at one time or another has been concerned about his or her body weight. Very few people seem to be satisfied with it; some would even like to gain weight. Most look in the mirror and study the "roll" of fat that spreads around their midsection or the dimpled fat on their thighs and wonder how to eliminate it. Wearing a bathing suit becomes an act of courage. Our desire to achieve a more ideal appearance makes us easy targets for those interested in profiting from our concern.

The battle against excess body fat has turned into a multi–billion dollar industry that advertises various diet plans, exercise studios, and countless gimmicks and gadgets guaranteed to help you lose those extra pounds and inches. One thing they don't guarantee is that you will be able to maintain the new, reduced weight. Most people who do lose weight eventually regain it and even some extra pounds. So, why bother to lose weight?

Many people decide to lose weight because they are dissatisfied with their appearance. However, there is little question that being overweight can lead to a number of health-related problems. Well-known exercise physiologist Dr. Herbert deVries has stated, "There are very few, very fat old people around. Your own observations—the national statistics—clearly show that long life does not mean survival of the fattest."

OBESITY

As discussed in Chapter 2, obesity is a risk factor for the development of heart disease, hypertension, and diabetes mellitus. Some terms used to describe degrees of obesity are useful. Being overweight and obese are different conditions. Being overweight implies having excess body weight relative to bone structure and height. This excess could be due to excess fat or to a higher proportion of muscle. Figure 8-1 shows the recently revised categories for healthy weight, moderate overweight, and severe overweight as determined by the U.S. Dietary Guidelines Advisory Committee.

Using the term *overweight* is not very precise. On the other hand, obesity clearly describes a condition of having an excessive amount of fat. It has been estimated that in America about 50 million adult men and 60 million adult women are too fat and need to do something to lose this excess. The problem of having too much body fat has reached epidemic proportions in the United States.

Causes of Obesity

The development of obesity has been attributed to several factors, including heredity, social environment, and a lifestyle that includes poor nutritional habits and sedentary behavior. Many people have a tendency to overeat, but most fail to get enough exercise to "burn up" the energy from food. The excess energy is stored as fat for future energy needs. This chapter will briefly examine some of the major factors that contribute to the development of fat. More emphasis will be given to the impact of our sedentary lifestyle on the development of obesity and how to reduce body fat safely and for a lifetime.

American Lifestyle

It is virtually impossible to do anything socially without having something to eat or drink. We associate food with dating, weddings, birthdays, and funerals. It is difficult to decline food or find something low-fat to eat when in these situations. Furthermore, the topic of food and dieting seems to be very popular, especially among women. For many, overeating in social settings becomes a way of life. As one ages, the extra body fat becomes a threat to health. Instead of becoming concerned about the extra fat's impact on health, most are frustrated with their appearance. They wonder, "Why are my clothes too tight?" and "How did I gain this extra fat?"

People who are concerned about controlling their weight find it difficult because of the quality of life we enjoy. Technology has allowed the American lifestyle to become increasingly sedentary as more "labor-saving" devices are invented. The purpose of devices such as garage door openers and remotes for video and audio equipment is to make life and work easier. These gadgets and machines allow us to have additional leisure time for recreational pursuits. The problem is that instead of becoming more involved in recreational activities that move large muscles, we are sitting around to a greater extent. For example, the golf cart has sped up the game but has taken most of the physical activity out of the sport. Video games are great for improving reaction times and the power of mental concentration, but there are few training effects from pressing a button or moving a joystick. Don't bother to get out of your chair to change channels, just press a button.

Most college graduates accept jobs that involve the use of the mind rather than the muscles. Then,

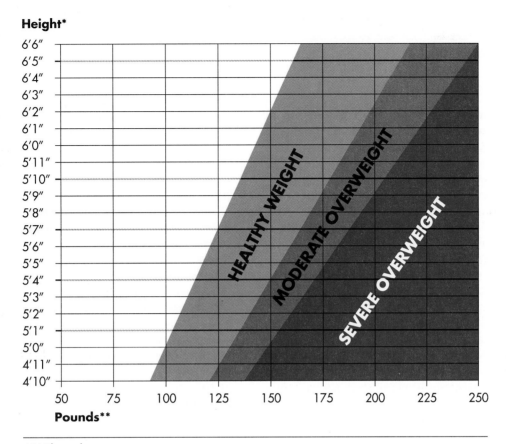

Height*

* Without shoes.
** Without clothes. The higher weights apply to people with more muscle and bone.

FIGURE 8-1. **Height and Weight Chart.**
(Redrawn from Dietary Guidelines Advisory Committee: *Dietary guidelines for Americans*, pp 23-24, 1995 [report]).

we do little in the work environment that increases physical activity levels. We try to park as close to the entrance as possible so we don't waste time and energy walking back and forth. It is easier to hop on an elevator or escalator than to walk up flights of stairs. We go out to lunch with our colleagues (driving to the restaurant) and sit for another hour. Many who gain weight are not eating more than their slimmer friends, they are just not expending as much energy. Most are not aware of how their behavior conserves energy rather than burning it.

What is the best way to control your weight? Most people tend to panic when they realize that they have put on a few extra pounds. They either go on starvation diets or become exercise fanatics, neither of which is particularly enjoyable or provides a long-term solution to the problem.

The key to being able to maintain your weight is to have the motivation to alter your lifestyle in ways that you can "live with." You need to make a commitment to changing your lifestyle so that you burn off extra energy and consume less food. The cumulative effect of these modifications will make weight control an integral part of your lifestyle rather than a behavior you adopt from time to time.

How is ideal body weight determined? It is usually done by consulting age-related height and weight charts such as those published by life-insurance companies. Unfortunately, these charts are inaccurate because they involve data that assesses insurance risk, not ideal body composition. Also, weights are expressed in broad ranges using three general classifications of body types. Often there are no precise instructions given to determine body type. Although these tables are useful as a quick and easy method of assessing degree of overweight, the issue of body

> **overweight** having excess body weight relative to bone structure and height
> **obesity** the condition of having an excessive amount of body fat

composition is not addressed. Therefore health and physical performance is better related to body composition than to body weight.

BODY COMPOSITION

Body composition refers to both the fat and nonfat components of the body. The portion of total body weight that is composed of fat tissue is referred to as the *percentage body fat*. The portion of the total body weight that is composed of nonfat or lean tissue, which includes muscles, tendons, bones, connective tissue, and so on, is referred to as lean body weight. Assessment of body composition is perhaps a bit more difficult than simply stepping on a scale and measuring actual weight. However, body composition measurements are more accurate in attempting to determine precisely how much weight a person may gain or lose.

The average college-age woman has between 20% and 25% of her total body weight made up of fat. The average college-age man has between 12% and 18% body fat. However, it must be indicated that persons who engage in strenuous physical activities on a regular basis tend to have a lower percentage body fat. Male endurance athletes may get their fat percentage as low as 8% to 12%, and female endurance athletes may reach 12% to 18% body fat. It is recommended that body fat percentage not go below 5% in men and 12% in women because a certain amount of body fat is necessary for good health. Table 8-1 summarizes percentage body fat ranges for low, average, overfat, and obese categories.

Body Fat

Fat is found in all of the body's cells. However, a special type, the adipose cell, stores fat. Body fat serves to cushion organs and stores energy for future needs. In general, people tend to have large stores of fat in the abdominal area; women tend to store more fat in their hips and thighs than do men. About half of the body's fat is located under the skin (subcutaneous fat). This fat can be measured in "pinch" tests or more accurately with skinfold calipers. Figure 8-2 provides simple tests for measuring body fat without using

calipers, and the following Health Link box details the health risk of excess fat in the abdominal area.

Adipose Cell Size and Number

Two factors determine the amount of fat found in the body: (1) the number of adipose cells and (2) the size of the adipose cell. The number of adipose cells increases before birth and continues to rise until puberty *(hyperplasia)*. Children who become obese at an early age are believed to have too many fat cells. Also, adolescents who become overweight seem to develop a greater number of fat cells than those of normal weight. It is thought that by early adulthood the number of fat cells becomes fixed. However, some recent evidence suggests that fat cell number may increase under certain conditions during adulthood.

In addition to cell number, cell size is a factor in obesity. The adipose cell stores *triglyceride* (a form of fat), which moves in and out of the cell according to energy needs. The greater the amount of triglyceride contained in the adipose cells, the greater the amount of total body weight that is composed of fat.

The size of the adipose cell depends on the amount of fat stored in it. Fat cell size increases *(hypertrophies)* until early adulthood. In the mature adult, fat cell size

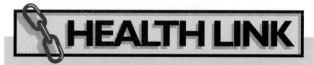

DETERMINING HEALTH RISK WITH A MEASURING TAPE

Recent evidence indicates that excess abdominal fat, the "spare tire," is linked to the development of heart disease, hypertension, and the most common form of diabetes. How can you determine whether your middle is too large? In case you don't have skinfold calipers available a few years from now, you can easily use a cloth measuring tape and some minor math skills to assess your risk.

- Using a flexible cloth measuring tape, measure the circumference of your waist (relax your abdominal muscles and place the tape at the level of your navel). Record the number.
- Measure hip circumference at the widest point around the hips; record the number.
- Divide the waist number by the hip number to obtain the waist-to-hip circumference ratio.
- If the ratio is greater than 0.95 for men or 0.80 for women, you have too much fat around your midsection and are at risk.

TABLE 8-1. Body Composition Classifications of Percentage Body Fat				
	Low	Average	Overfat	Obese
Males	5-11	12-15	15-18	>20
Females	12-18	19-25	26-29	>30

fluctuates as a function of caloric balance. If more calories are consumed than needed, the excess is converted to fat and stored in the adipose cells. Under this condition, adipose cells swell with fat. When the energy from fat is needed to fuel activities, the fat cells lose stored fat and shrink in size.

Body Fat in Children

Contrary to popular belief, a fat baby does not necessarily become a fat child or a fat young adult. However, after age 2 a child begins to adopt the eating behaviors and activity patterns of his or her family members. If this child is still too fat by the time he or she starts school, then it is more likely that he or she will become a fat adolescent and adult. In fact, the chances of this happening are three times greater in the obese child than in children of normal body weight.

In children who become obese at an early age, weight increases are primarily due to increases in the number of fat cells. In adults, weight loss or gain is primarily a function of the changes in fat cell size, not cell numbers. Thus obese adults tend to exhibit a great deal of adipose cell hypertrophy.

Body Fat in Adults

The fat distribution in adults tends to follow particular patterns that are largely inherited or hormonal. Recent evidence indicates that fat deposited in the abdominal area as opposed to the buttocks seems to pose an increased health risk. Many males exhibit a large "pot" belly, with small buttocks and thighs. This is referred to as android or "apple-shaped" obesity.

FIGURE 8-2. Simple Tests for Excess Fat.

Pinch-an-inch test: Using the thumb and index finger, pinch the skin and fat on the hip directly under the armpit, on the back just under the shoulder blade, and on the back of the upper arm over the triceps. If there is more than 1 inch (25 mm) of skin and fat between your fingers, you are probably too fat.

Spare-tire test: Using a tape measure, find the circumference of the chest at the level of the nipples. Then measure the circumference of your waist at the navel. If the waist measurement exceeds the chest measurement, you have too much fat around the abdomen.

Mirror test: Perhaps the best of the three. Simply look at yourself naked in front of a full-length mirror. Now bounce up and down. If parts of your body jiggle that should not, you are overweight. You must be prepared to answer honestly the question, "Am I too fat?"

Risk of developing heart disease, hypertension, and diabetes mellitus has been linked to a waist measurement that is greater than hip measurement. A ratio of waist circumference to hip circumference greater than 0.95 in males and 0.80 in females indicates android obesity. Lab Activity 8-1 will help you calculate your waist-to-hip ratio.

Females more often tend to exhibit gynecoid or "pear-shaped" obesity, in which the fat tends to appear in the buttocks or upper thigh, with moderate fat in the abdomen. This is attributed to high progesterone and estrogen levels in the female, which encourage fat deposition in the lower torso.

The term *cellulite* is often used in magazines and advertisements to identify a type of fat that appears to be dimpled and usually is deposited in the buttocks, upper thighs, and upper arms. Cellulite is a nonmedical term for the ordinary adipose tissue that is found in these sites. Losing weight and exercising will reduce all body fat, including cellulite.

Assessing Body Composition

Among the several methods of assessing body composition are (1) hydrostatic weighing, (2) measurement of bioelectrical impedance, and (3) measurement of skinfold thickness.

Hydrostatic Weighing

Hydrostatic (underwater) weighing involves placing a subject in a specially designed underwater tank to determine body density. Fat tissue is less dense than lean tissue. Therefore the more body fat present, the more the body floats (buoyancy) and the less it weighs in water. Body composition is calculated by comparing the weight of the submerged individual with the weight before entering the tank. If done properly, this technique is very accurate. Unfortunately, the tank and equipment are expensive and generally not available to most coaches and physical educators. In addition, there are other drawbacks with this technique. It is time consuming (especially for large groups), and subjects must exhale completely and hold their breath while underwater. Many students have real problems and fears with this aspect of the technique.

---

body composition   the fat and nonfat components of the body

lean body weight   the portion of total body weight composed of nonfat or lean tissue

adipose cell   type of cell that stores triglyceride, a liquid form of fat

subcutaneous fat   body fat located directly under the skin—approximately half the body's fat is subcutaneous fat

---

Bioelectrical Impedance

The second technique involves the measurement of resistance to the flow of electrical current through the body between selected points. This technique is based on the principle that electricity will choose to flow through the tissue that offers the least resistance or impedance. Fat is generally a poor conductor of electrical energy, whereas lean tissue is a fairly good conductor. Thus the higher the percentage of body fat, the greater the resistance to the passage of electrical energy. Very simply, this method predicts the percentage body fat by measuring bioelectrical impedance. It should be mentioned that bioelectrical impedance measures can be affected by levels of hydration. If the body is dehydrated, the measurement will tend to overestimate percentage of body fat relative to measurements taken when there is normal hydration. The equipment available for taking these measurements is, again, fairly expensive and generally includes the use of computer software.

Measuring Skinfold Thickness

The third technique is based on the idea that about 50% of the fat in the body is subcutaneous (under the skin). By measuring the thickness of this layer of fat, the total percentage of body fat can be calculated. Skinfolds are measured at various body sites using skinfold calipers. Men and women tend to develop fat deposits in different body areas; skinfold measurements must be taken at these specified places. A number of different methods for calculating body fat percentages using skinfold measurements have been developed. The technique proposed by McArdle and co-workers that measures the triceps and subscapular skinfold will be used in Lab Activity 8-2 to determine body fat composition (see Figures 8-11 and 8-12). Although skinfold measurement is a less accurate method than impedance or underwater weighing, most can gain expertise in performing this technique. Furthermore, the calipers are less costly and time consuming to use than the other equipment. Figure 8-3

FIGURE 8-3. Some Common Sources of Error in Taking Skinfold Measurements

- Midpoint incorrectly marked or measured
- Arm not loose at side during measurement
- Caliper placement too deep (muscle is involved)
- Caliper placement too shallow (only skin grasped)
- Caliper reading taken without marks in proper alignment
- Skinfold grasp not maintained at time of caliper reading

---

describes some common errors made when using calipers to measure skinfolds.

Determining Desired Body Weight

Once you have calculated the percentage of your total body weight that is made up of fat tissue, you may determine that you have too much fat. It would be helpful to determine how much weight you have to lose to achieve a normal percentage of body fat. Lab Activity 8-3 will help you calculate your desired body weight.

Determining Body Mass Index

A relatively easy way to determine the extent of overweight or obesity is to use a person's body weight and height measurements to determine body mass index (BMI). BMI is a ratio of body weight to height. This technique represents a method for measuring health risks from obesity using height/weight measurments. Health problems associated with excess body fat tend to be associated with a BMI of more than 25. A BMI of 25 to 30 indicates that a person is overweight. A BMI of 30 or more indicates a state of obesity. Lab Activity 8-4 will help you calculate your BMI.

ENERGY NEEDS
Calories

One pound of body fat tissue is not pure fat, but it represents about 3500 *Calories*. A calorie is simply a measure of the energy value of fat. A calorie by definition is the amount of energy necessary to raise the temperature of 1 gram of water 1° C. However, this unit is too small to be easy to use, so the term kilocalorie is more appropriate. A kilocalorie is equal to 1000 calories. Thus subsequent mention of a specific number of calories in this text refers to kilocalories, which will be denoted as kcal or Calories.

The nutrients in food that provide energy include carbohydrates, proteins, fats, and alcohol. The Caloric content of these energy nutrients is as follows:

Carbohydrate = 4 Calories per gram
Protein = 4 Calories per gram
Fat = 9 Calories per gram
Alcohol = 7 Calories per gram

Proteins and carbohydrates each deliver 4 Calories of energy per gram. One gram of fat delivers 9 Calories of energy. Therefore 1 pound of fat will provide a lot more calories than 1 pound of either protein or carbohydrate. It should also be added that alcohol provides 7 Calories of energy per gram. Any excess of calories, whether it is from alcohol or from foods or supplements that contain protein, carbohydrates, or fat, can be converted to body fat and stored.

Energy Balance

If you have been able to maintain your weight, you are in a state of *energy balance.* That is, the number of calories that you consume in food equals the number that you use for the three energy-requiring processes. If you are trying to gain weight, then you need to consume more calories than you expend. The extra calories will be stored, and you will gain weight (*positive energy balance).* Conversely, if you want to lose weight, you need to expend more energy than you are consuming so that the body has to use its fat stores for energy (*negative energy balance).* Figure 8-4 summarizes the various caloric situations.

It becomes extremely important to consider the implications of caloric values when considering programs for weight loss or gain. The percentage of total body weight that is composed of fat is highly related to the level of physical activity. Persons who have an excess of fat tend to be sedentary and therefore are in a positive calorie situation. In behavioral terms the number of calories in food ingested and the number of calories expended can be modified. You can eat less and exercise more. Caloric expenditure decreases with a decline in physical activity. Basal metabolism declines with aging, usually as a result of a decline in lean muscle mass. It will become necessary to decrease caloric intake by about 2.5% for every 10 years over age 25. Thus as you age it becomes increasingly important to either increase exercise levels or decrease caloric intake to avoid gaining body fat. Adding a moderate level of physical activity to your daily routine will increase your calorie expenditure—so *get moving* (see the box on p. 226 for activities that increase caloric expenditure).

Estimating Caloric Intake

A physically active person needs a sufficient number of calories from food to maintain body weight and composition. Determining caloric intake requires consulting food composition tables such as the ones in Appendix B. These charts identify specific foods and indicate the number of Calories per specified serving size. For example, if you consult Appendix B, you will see that $1\frac{1}{2}$ oz of American cheddar cheese provides 171 Calories. Maintaining a daily food intake log such as in Table 8-2 can determine not only your caloric intake but also your eating patterns and habits. Factors unrelated to nutrition often influence what kinds of foods are selected and how much is eaten. These factors include your mood and social environment at mealtimes. Lab Activity 8-5 will help you calculate your daily caloric intake, and the Health Link box on p. 227 lists suggestions for decreasing your calorie intake.

Estimating Caloric Expenditure

Calories are expended by the body for three different processes: (1) basal metabolism, (2) physical activity or work (work may be defined as any activity that requires more energy than sleeping), and (3) the thermic effect of food (this is the energy that is used after meals to digest food and to absorb and process its nutrients).

For any individual who wants to maintain or alter his or her weight, some estimation of caloric expenditure relative to caloric intake is necessary. The following sections describe how to estimate caloric expenditure.

Determining Basal Metabolic Rate. It is first necessary to determine the amount of Calories (energy) needed to support your basal metabolism. This is the minimal amount of energy required to sustain the body's vital functions such as respiration, heart beat, circulation, and maintenance of body temperature during a 24-hour period. The basal metabolic rate (BMR) is the rate at which calories are spent for these maintenance activities. BMR is most acurately determined in a laboratory through a measurement process known as *indirect calorimetry,* which measures a person's oxygen uptake to predict BMR. Measurement of BMR using this procedure is generally done as soon as the subject awakes; in a quiet, warm environment; and after a 12-hour fast. The term *resting metabolic rate (RMR)* is often used interchangeably with BMR, although the two are measured somewhat differently, with RMR having less stringent measurement restrictions. RMR is usually slightly higher than BMR, which is influenced by the factors listed in the Health Link box on p. 228. Lab Activity 8-6 will help you determine your BMR.

Calories Expended During Physical Activity. Once BMR has been determined, it is necessary to calculate energy requirements of all physical activities done in a 24-hour period. This is the second component of energy needs, referred to as *work.*

---

body mass index (BMI) a method of measuring health risks related to excess body fat using a ratio of body weight to height measurements

calorie a measurement of the energy value of foodstuff

kilocalorie 1000 calories

basal metabolic rate (BMR) based on a 24-hour period, this is the rate at which the body burns calories to maintain vital functions, including respiration, heart beat, circulation, and maintenance of body temperature

FOOD INTAKE   WORK OUTPUT   EFFECT ON WEIGHT

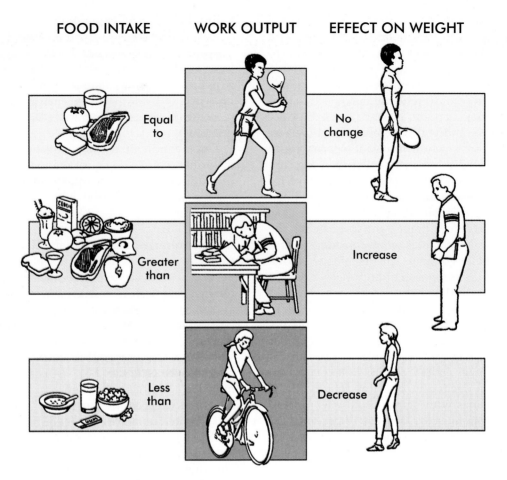

FIGURE 8-4. Caloric Balance
Caloric balance results in weight control. An imbalance leads to weight gain or loss. (Modified from Payne WA, Hahn DB: *Understanding your health,* ed 4, St Louis, 1995, Mosby.)

GET MOVING

Increasing Calorie expenditure through physical activity

Remember to accumulate 30 minutes or more of moderate physical activity on most—preferably all—days of the week.
Examples of moderate physical activities for healthy adults:
1. Walking briskly (3 to 4 miles per hour)
2. Conditioning or general calisthenics
3. Home care, general cleaning
4. Racket sports such as table tennis
5. Mowing lawn, power mower
6. Golf—pulling cart or carrying clubs
7. Home repair, painting
8. Fishing, standing/casting
9. Jogging
10. Swimming (moderate effort)
11. Cycling, moderate speed (10 miles per hour or less)
12. Gardening
13. Canoeing leisurely (2.0 to 3.9 miles per hour)
14. Dancing

Modified from Pate R et al: Physical activity and public health, *JAMA* 273:404, 1995.

TABLE 8-2. Sample Daily Food Intake Log

Time	Food eaten	Amount	Number of Calories	How cooked
Breakfast				
8:00 A.M.	Orange juice	6 oz	80	Frozen
	Milk (whole)	16 oz	300	
	Cheerios	1 1/4 cup	30	
	Sugar	1 tsp	70	
10:30 A.M.	Apple	1	90	
Lunch				
12:30 P.M.	Cheeseburger	1	580	Fried
	French fries	1 sm order	330	Fried
	Fruit punch	16 oz	140	
Dinner				
6:30 P.M.	Pork chop	3 oz	310	Broiled
	Mashed potatoes	1 cup	195	Boiled, buttered
	Butter	2 tsp	200	
	Peas, canned	1/2 cup	90	Boiled
	Milk (whole)	16 oz	300	
	Chocolate cake	1 piece (2 in)	200	
10:00 P.M.	Chocolate cake	1 piece (2 in)	200	
	Milk (whole)	8 oz	150	
		TOTAL	3265	

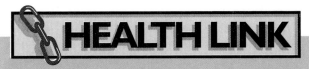

HOW TO DECREASE CALORIE INTAKE

- Eat a variety of foods that are low in calories and high in nutrients.
- Check the Nutrition Facts Label.
- Eat less fat and fewer high-fat foods.
- Eat smaller portions and limit second helpings of foods high in fat and calories.
- Eat more vegetables and fruits without fats and sugars added in preparation or at the table.
- Eat pasta, rice, breads, and cereals without fats and sugars added in preparation or at the table.
- Eat less sugar and fewer sweets (such as candy, cookies, cakes, soda).
- Drink less or no alcohol.

Modified from US Department of Agriculture and US Department of Health and Human Services: *Nutrition and your health: dietary guidelines for Americans,* ed 4, Washington, DC, 1995.

Physical activity, whether it is competitive or recreational, results in an increased need for energy. The goal is to consume enough nutritious foods to meet basic tissue needs while supplying an additional amount to meet increased energy needs for the activity. Generally, people who participate in physical activity need more energy (preferably supplied by starchy foods) but no additional vitamins or minerals. (Chapter 9 will explore the topic of nutrition in greater detail.) As they increase their activity, people usually increase their food intake to meet nutritional needs. If a physically active person's daily energy intake does not match his or her energy expenditure, body weight loss will occur.

There is a wide variation in energy output for work. It is determined by the type, intensity, and duration of a physical activity. Body size is also a factor; heavier people expend more energy in an activity than do lighter people. Specific energy expenditures may be determined by consulting charts that predict energy used in an activity based on (1) the time spent

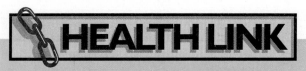

FACTORS INFLUENCING BASAL METABOLIC RATE (BMR)

Body surface area: The greater the amount of body surface area, the higher the BMR. (Like BMI, body surface area is a relationship between body height and weight.) It is important to note that surface area, not body weight, is the influencing factor.

Age: In general, the younger the person, the higher the BMR. As mentioned earlier, for most people, BMR declines with age because of decreases in muscle mass and other tissues. Decreases in muscle mass can be minimized by continuing to engage in physical activity throughout life.

Gender: Men generally have a higher BMR than do women.

Diet: There is a dramatic and sustained reduction in BMR that occurs with very low-calorie dieting.

Exercise: Consistent exercise tends to increase the BMR during the activity and for a period of time after the activity ceases.

in each activity in minutes and (2) the metabolic costs of each activity in kilocalories per minute per pound (kcal/min/lb) of body weight. Table 8-3 lists the number of Calories expended per minute of various activities. For example, by consulting the energy expenditure chart in Table 8-3, a 170-pound man playing basketball for 1 hour will use 642.6 (0.063 kcal/min/lb × 170 lb × 60 min) Calories. If you were to carefully calculate energy costs of all daily activities such as sitting, walking, and studying, you could estimate the amount of energy used in a day. Table 8-4 provides part of a daily activity log that has been used by a male student. Now that you have determined your caloric needs for BMR and daily activities, you can use Lab Activity 8-7 to help calculate your total daily caloric expenditure.

Thermic effect of food. The thermic effect of food represents the amount of energy required to digest, absorb, metabolize, and store the energy nutrients. It is equal to approximately 5% to 10% of the total Calories consumed. Thus 105 to 110 Calories must be consumed to deliver 100 Calories of energy. The thermic effect for a carbohydrate or protein diet is higher than for a fat diet, since more energy is required to absorb and store fat than to metabolize protein or carbohydrate.

Assessing Caloric Balance

If the daily logs for estimating caloric intake and caloric expenditure have been accurately kept (see Lab Activities 8-5 and 8-7), it will be relatively easy to compare the total caloric values to determine whether you are in caloric balance. It is not easy for a college student to maintain caloric balance on a daily basis. One reason is that schedules never seem to be the same from one day to the next. Eating meals and times spent engaged in physical activity may be inconsistent. Estimations of caloric intake for college students range from 1000 to 5000 Calories per day. Estimations of caloric expenditure range from 2200 to 4400 Calories per day for the average student. Energy demands will be higher for those who are physically active and considerably higher for endurance-type athletes, who may require 7000 or more Calories per day. If you desire to lose weight, you must modify your behavior so that you burn more calories for energy than you take in. If you want to gain weight, you must consume more calories than you expend. The Worksheet for Estimating Caloric Balance on p. 259 will determine whether you are in a state of positive or negative caloric balance based on your estimations of caloric intake and expenditure.

SET POINT THEORY OF WEIGHT CONTROL

The set point theory provides an explanation of why it is so difficult to lose or gain weight. The body tends to maintain a certain level of body fat. This theory maintains that the body has a "set point" or some mechanism for maintaining a specific body weight. It operates like a thermostat that is set to control a house's temperature. When the temperature in the house drops below the set point, the furnace turns on. When the temperature warms to the setting, the furnace shuts off. For people, it may be that the body's fat level is set at a particular point, and attempts to reduce this level are met with resistance by the body. It is unclear how this set point is controlled; it may be that the fat cells tend to maintain a certain degree of fat stored within them and resist efforts to reduce their size. If you attempt to lower the set point through dieting alone, metabolic rate decreases to conserve calories. Exercise that elevates metabolism in combination with caloric restriction appears to be the only way to reduce the set point. In any case, the set point theory is just that, a theory that may explain why so many people are unsuccessful at keeping off the fat lost through dieting.

TABLE 8-3.   Energy Expenditure During Physical Activity

To determine the number of calories expended during an activity, multiply the number of calories per minute per pound by your body weight in pounds. Then multiply this figure by the number of minutes you were involved in the activity.

Activity	Cal/min/lb	Activity	Cal/min/lb
Archery	.030	Jumping rope	
Badminton	.044	70 per min	.074
Baseball	.031	80 per min	.075
Basketball	.063	125 per min	.080
Billiards	.018	145 per min	.089
Boxing (sparring)	.062	Lacrosse	.095
Canoeing		Lying at ease	.010
Leisure	.020	Painting (outside)	.035
Racing	.047	Racquetball	.081
Circuit training		Running	
Hydra-Fitness	.060	11.5 min per mile	.061
Universal	.053	9 min per mile	.088
Nautilus	.042	8 min per mile	.095
Free weights	.039	7 min per mile	.104
Climbing hills	.055	6 min per mile	.115
Croquet	.027	5.5 min per mile	.131
Cycling		Cross-country	.074
5.5 mph	.029	Sailing	.002
9.4 mph	.045	Sitting quietly	.009
Racing	.079	Skiing	
Dancing		Cross-country	.074
Aerobic, medium	.047	Downhill	.064
Aerobic, intense	.061	Water	.052
Ballroom	.023	Skindiving	
Eating (sitting)	.010	Considerable motion	.125
Field hockey	.061	Moderate motion	.094
Fishing	.028	Soccer	.059
Football	.060	Squash	.096
Gardening		Swimming	
Digging	.057	Backstroke	.077
Mowing	.051	Breast stroke	.074
Raking	.025	Butterfly	.078
Golf	.039	Crawl, slow	.070
Gymnastics	.030	Crawl, fast	.071
Handball	.063	Side stroke	.055
Hiking	.042	Treading, fast	.077
Horseback riding		Treading, normal	.028
Galloping	.062	Table tennis	.031
Trotting	.050	Tennis	.050
Walking	.019	Volleyball	.023
Ice hockey	.095	Walking (normal pace)	.036
Jogging	.069	Weight training	.032
Judo	.089	Wrestling	.085
		Writing (sitting)	.013

METHODS OF WEIGHT LOSS

There are many weight-reduction techniques available; some are based on sound scientific and nutritional principles, and others are dangerous or a waste of money. Losing weight boils down to creating a situation of negative caloric balance. First, food intake may be decreased by dieting. Second, caloric expenditure may be increased by increasing the amount of physical activity. Finally, a combination of approaches can be attempted.

Weight loss through dieting alone is difficult. Much of what we choose to eat is influenced not by hunger

TABLE 8-4. Sample Daily Activities Log

Clock time	Activity	Total minutes spent in activity	Kcal/min/lb	Total calories expended
5:00–6:00	Basketball	60	0.063	(0.063 x 60 x 170) = 643
6:00–7:00	Studying	60	0.013	(0.013 x 60 x 170) = 133
7:00–7:30	Eating dinner	30	0.010	(0.010 x 30 x 170) = 51
11:00–7:00	Sleeping*	480	0.000	0.000
	TOTAL	630 min or 10.5 hr		

*Sleep is assumed to be at the basal level of activity; therefore it is figured into the basal metabolic caloric needs that you have already calculated.

but by other factors such as customs, advertising, our moods, and the attractiveness and availability of the food supply. Pizza can be delivered to your door with a phone call. Food has meaning to us; we eat sweet, "rich" desserts as rewards for good performances or just to make ourselves feel better. Furthermore, dieting is viewed as the deprivation and punishment one must endure for overindulgence. Every so often, we literally starve ourselves, lose a few pounds, and then promptly return to our "old" eating habits and regain the lost weight. The behavior is repeated without achieving lasting weight control. Thus periodic dieting is ineffective. At best, long-term weight control by dieting alone is successful only 20% of the time. Lab Activity 8-8 will help you to decide if you should consider a weight-loss program.

Losing Body Fat Through Dieting

Obviously, in any weight-loss program the goal is to lose fat, not lean tissue. Unfortunately, many popular diets, the so-called starvation diets, recommend reduction of caloric intake to dangerous levels. It is recommended that the minimum caloric intake for a female not go below 1000 to 1200 Calories per day and for a male not below 1200 to 1400 Calories per day. A minimum level of 1200 Calories may be needed to avoid entering a starvation metabolism. More moderate reductions of total Calories are recommended to lose body fat. Figures 8-5 and 8-6 provide examples of an 1800-Calorie-per-day menu and a moderate 2400-Calorie-per-day menu. Most men will lose weight on 1800 Calories per day; women may have to consume around 1200 Calories per day to lose weight, especially if they are inactive.

Starvation diets that restrict caloric intake below these recommended levels may actually cause a reduction in metabolic rate, thus making weight loss more difficult. The body's metabolic rate goes into "low gear" and conserves calories. The ideal situation is to keep the metabolic rate at normal or raise it to

FIGURE 8-5. 1800-Calorie Sample Meal Pattern.

Breakfast
3/4 c Orange juice
3/4 c Cereal
8 oz Low-fat milk
1 Slice whole wheat toast
    with 1 tsp margarine
Total Calories = 415

Snack
1 Apple
Total Calories = 80

Lunch
1 Chicken sandwich
    (2 slices bread)
5-7 Carrot sticks
1 Peach
8 oz Low-fat milk
Total Calories = 485

Snack
20 Grapes
2 Graham crackers
Total Calories = 155

Dinner
4 oz Lean beef
2 Small rolls
1 c Tossed green salad with 1 Tbsp dressing
4 oz Low-fat milk
1/2 c Low-fat yogurt
Total Calories = 715

Total Calories for day = 1850

burn more calories. The initial weight loss that occurs with severe caloric restriction for the first few days of the diet may be encouraging. However, the majority of this weight loss is not due to the loss of much fat but results from loss of water weight (dehydration) and from some loss of lean tissue.

Losing Body Fat Through Exercise

Clearly, dieting alone is not the answer to long-term weight control. However, the weight lost

FIGURE 8-6. 2400-Calorie Sample Meal Pattern.

Breakfast
3/4 c Orange juice
1 Slice toast with 1 oz cheese
3/4 c Cereal
4 oz Low-fat milk
Total Calories = 420

Snack
1 Banana
Total Calories = 100

Lunch
1 Slice cheese pizza
Tossed green salad with
   1 Tbsp dressing
8 oz Low-fat milk
Total Calories = 425

Snack
1/2 c Raisin-peanut
   mix
1/2 c Apple juice
Total Calories = 360

Dinner
1 c Macaroni and cheese
1/2 c Lima beans
1 c Tomato and cucumber
   slices with 1 Tbsp dressing
1 Dinner roll with 1
   tsp margarine
8 oz Low-fat milk
Total Calories = 895

Snack
1/2 c Sherbet
1 Granola cookie
Total Calories = 185

Total Calories for day = 2385

through exercise involves primarily losses of fat tissue (estimates are as high as 90%) and almost no loss of lean tissue. Establishing new behavior that includes daily physical activity takes a great deal of motivation. For most of us, exercise habits were established early in life. Physical activity in adolescence can prevent the formation of excess adipose tissue and results in an increase in lean body weight. At any age, physical activity when combined with caloric reduction can lead to substantial losses of body fat while preserving lean tissue. Keep in mind that physical activity in the sedentary college student may result in increases in muscle tissue, which is more dense and has greater weight than fat tissue. Thus initial attempts at weight loss through increased activity levels may be frustrating for anyone. You may weigh yourself and see no change or even an increase in weight. Instead of relying on scales that provide no information about changes in body composition, every few weeks you should record tape measurements of your waist, hips, and chest.

Spot Reducing

Many try techniques for "spot reducing." Trying to reduce the level of body fat at specific sites such as the

waist or thighs is useless. During exercise, the energy is supplied from fat stores throughout the body, not just the muscles being moved. However, actively exercising a specific area may increase muscle tone and possibly muscle strength, although the fat in that area will not be reduced. You lose inches off your body, which makes clothing fit more comfortably. Nevertheless, the benefits of aerobic exercise on the entire body are important to overall health.

Weight loss through exercise alone is almost as difficult as losing weight through dieting. People trying to exercise solely for the purpose of losing weight are not likely to stick with an exercise program for long. However, it is essential to realize that physical exercise will not only result in weight reduction but may also enhance cardiorespiratory endurance, improve strength, and increase flexibility. For this reason, exercise has some distinct advantages over dieting in any weight-loss program.

The Key to Losing Body Fat

Undoubtedly the most efficient method of decreasing the percentage of body fat is through some combination of diet and exercise. A moderate caloric restriction combined with a moderate increase in caloric expenditure will result in a negative caloric balance. This method is relatively fast and easy compared with either of the others, especially if it focuses on changing eating habits and activity levels. You don't have to starve and run 6 miles a day. If caloric intake is reduced by 200 to 300 Calories per day and if caloric expenditure is increased by 200 to 300 Calories per day, over a 7-day period this will result in a loss of approximately 3500 Calories, or 1 pound of body fat.

In any weight-loss program, the goal should be to lose 1/2 to 2 pounds per week. The rate of weight loss depends on how much body fat the person has at the start of the period of caloric restriction. In general, the greater the amount of body fat, the more rapidly one loses while on a calorie-reduced diet. This explains why some people lose 4 or more pounds the first week on a low-calorie diet. They had maintained their excess weight on relatively high calorie levels, and the reduction creates a major need for energy from fat stores.

A slower rate of weight loss indicates that the person is making minor lifestyle changes, particularly in regard to eating and physical activity behaviors, that can be maintained over time. The adoption of new behaviors and attitudes takes time. Lab Activity 8-9 will help you to chart your progress.

In any weight-loss program, the "long-haul" approach must be emphasized. It generally took a long time to accumulate that extra weight, and it will take time to lose it safely. This fact is frustrating to the impatient individual who wants results fast. Many of these people starve themselves to lose weight, shed some pounds, then return to their former eating habits and experience weight gain; this is called the "yo-yo" effect. This behavior makes subsequent weight-loss efforts even more difficult, since the body tends to protect its existing fat stores. The following box contains a number of motivational strategies for losing body fat.

Weight-Loss Gimmicks and Fads

Even educated people will resort to almost anything in a desperate effort to lose weight. Each year (especially before the summer months), Americans spend billions of dollars trying to find any method that promises they will lose weight quickly and without much effort. People are willing to spend money and time on diet programs, pills, gadgets, books, and equipment that claim to "melt pounds fast." Claims are made for rubberized suits that are supposed to "sweat" off pounds; mechanical devices to shake, vibrate, or roll off the fat; and pills, creams, and powders to remove "cellulite." Advertisements display physically attractive people who are reported to have lost dozens of pounds while using a device or diet plan. Most weight-loss gimmicks are based on unsound nutritional information and have no basis in scientific fact. Although people may lose weight at first, they become bored with the technique and lose interest. Any weight that was lost is regained.

Starvation Diet Plans

What about the numerous diet plans? It seems that a new diet plan appears in a book that makes the best-seller list monthly. It is not easy to determine whether a diet plan is reliable and safe to follow. Figure 8-7 (pp. 234 to 235) reviews some of the more popular weight-loss plans. The following Safe Tip box also gives some general advice that will help you to judge the quality of approaches to weight control. You will continue to see or hear about unreliable methods as long as people are unable to make the lifestyle changes needed to maintain control over their body weight.

GET MOVING

Ways to lose body fat

1. Take a picture of yourself before you begin your exercise and diet program—enlarge it to an 8 × 10 color glossy and tape it to the door of the refrigerator.
2. Reorient your social life to focus more on activities that involve some form of exercise rather than on eating and drinking.
3. Reward yourself for losing body fat by taking a vacation trip or by going out and buying a new outfit that makes you look really good.
4. Avoid setting short-term goals for losing fat. Setting a long-term goal may help you to permanently change your eating and exercise habits.
5. Use a tape measure to measure your waist and hips. Once a month remeasure to see if there is a difference.
6. If a skinfold caliper is available, have someone take a measurement once a month to check for a decrease in body fat percentage.
7. Participate in discussion groups or counseling sessions with others who are trying to lose weight. Share your commitment to losing body fat with your friends and family so that they can support your effort.
8. If you feel that paying an individual or organization to monitor and oversee your diet and exercise program will help you stick to that program initially—then do it.
9. Pay attention to comments from friends or others when they tell you that you look good or different. We are always harder on ourselves, and it sometimes takes a fresh perspective to notice a positive change.
10. Keep a record or log of the time, setting, reasons, and feelings associated with your eating. Also keep an accurate record of weight loss.
11. Don't totally deprive yourself of enjoyable foods. Eating should be done slowly to savor the taste and aid in digestion.

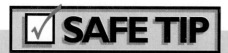

Setting Realistic Goals for Weight Loss

Once you have decided to change your lifestyle to decrease your percentage of body fat, you must set some weight-loss goals. First, determine a desirable weight that is realistic in terms of your age, height, and bone structure. Goals must be reasonable and attainable. If you set too high a goal, you may become dissatisfied with any degree of weight loss that does not meet the goal. Second, use the information determined in **Lab Activity 8-3** to determine a desired body weight based on body fat percentage calculations. Ultimately your goal should be to reach the standards for at least achieving the "good" body fat percentages for your age group as shown in Table 8-5 (p. 246). The third important goal is to determine a reasonable and safe rate of weight loss; it may be as low as ½ pound per week or as high as 2 pounds, depending on how much weight you have to lose. You may lose weight faster at first, but the rate slows and eventually averages out to become close to the goal rate within a few weeks. The Safe Tip box on p. 236 outlines 10 rules of weight control designed to make any weight-loss program safe.

Guidelines for Weight Loss

The American College of Sports Medicine has made the following statements and recommendations regarding weight loss:
- Prolonged fasting and diet programs that severely restrict caloric intake are scientifically undesirable and can be medically dangerous.
- Fasting and diet programs that severely restrict caloric intake result in the loss of large amounts of water, electrolytes, minerals, glycogen stores, and other fat-free tissue (including proteins within fat-free tissues), with minimal amounts of fat loss.
- Mild caloric restriction (500 to 1000 Calories less than the usual daily intake) results in a smaller loss of water, electrolytes, minerals, and other fat-free tissue and is less likely to cause malnutrition.
- Dynamic exercise of large muscles helps to maintain fat-free tissue, including muscle mass and bone density, and results in losses of body weight. Weight loss resulting from an increase in energy expenditure is primarily in the form of fat weight.
- A nutritionally sound diet resulting in mild caloric restriction coupled with an endurance exercise program, along with behavioral modification of existing eating habits, is recommended for weight reduction. The rate of sustained weight loss should not exceed 1 kg (about 2 lb) per week.
- To maintain proper weight control and optimal body fat levels, a lifetime commitment to proper eating habits and regular physical activity is required.

METHODS FOR GAINING WEIGHT

As a society we seem to be preoccupied with losing weight. However, there are people who would like to gain weight. The aim of a weight-gaining program should be to increase lean body mass (muscle) rather than body fat. Muscle mass should be increased only by muscle work combined with an increase in carbohydrate intake (see Chapter 9). It cannot be increased by the intake of any special food or vitamin. Unfortunately, as indicated in Chapter 6, muscle mass and weight may also be increased in an unsafe manner through the use of steroids or growth hormones.

The recommended rate of weight gain is approximately 1 to 2 pounds per week. This can be achieved through positive caloric balance. One pound of fat represents the equivalent of 3500 Calories; lean body tissue, which contains less fat, more protein, and more water than fat tissue, represents approximately 2500 Calories. Therefore to gain 1 pound of muscle, a weekly excess of approximately 2500 Calories is needed. Adding 500 to 1000 Calories daily to the usual diet will provide the energy needs of gaining 1 to 2 pounds per week and fuel the increased energy

FIGURE 8-7. Overview of Diet Plans.

Summary of popular diet approaches to weight control

Approach and examples*	Characteristics and possible negative health consequences
Moderate kilocalorie restriction	
The Setpoint Diet	Usually 1000-1800 kcal/day, with moderate fat intake
Slim Chance in a Fat World	Reasonable balance of macronutrients
Weight Watcher's Diet	Encourages exercise
The American Heart Association Diet	May employ behavioral approach
Mary Ellen's Help Yourself Diet Plan	
The Beyond Diet	Acceptable if vitamin and mineral supplement is used and permission of family physician is granted
Nutripoints	
The Good Calorie diet	
The Callaway Diet	
Fast Food Diet	
50 Ways to Lose Your Blubber	
Macronutrient restriction	
Low carbohydrate	
Dr. Atkins' Diet Revolution	Less than 100 g of carbohydrate per day
Calories Don't Count	
Wild Weekend Diet	Ketosis; poor exercise capacity due to poor glycogen stores in the muscles; excessive animal fat intake
Miracle Diet for Fast Weight Loss	
Drinking Man's Diet	
Woman Doctor's Diet for Women	
The Doctor's Quick Weight Loss Diet	
The Complete Scarsdale Medical Diet	
Four Day Wonder Diet	
Endocrine Control Diet	
Air Force Diet	
Low fat	
The Rice Diet Report	Less than 20% of energy from fat
The Macrobiotic Diet (some versions)	Limited (or elimination of) animal protein sources; also all fats, nuts, seeds
The Pritikin Diet	
The Tokyo Diet	
The Palm Beach Lifelong Diet	Little satiety; flatulence; possibly poor mineral absorption from excess fiber; limited food choices leads to deprivation
The James Coco Diet	
The 35+ Diet	
7-Week Victory Diet	
Fat to Muscle Diet	
T-Factor Diet	
Fit or Fat	
Two Day Diet	
Complete Hip and Thigh Diet	
The Maximum Metabolism Diet	
The Pasta Diet	
The McDougall Plan	
Ultrafit Diet	
Stop the Insanity	
G-Index Diet	
Eat More, Weigh Less	
Outsmarting the Female Fat Cell	
Foods that Cause You to Lose Weight	

Redrawn from Wardlaw GM, Insel PM: *Perspectives in nutrition*, ed 3, St Louis, 1996, Mosby.
*Diets may be listed in more than one category if multiple characteristics apply.

FIGURE 8-7. **Overview of Diet Plans—cont'd.**

Summary of popular diet approaches to weight control

Approach and examples*	Characteristics and possible negative health consequences
Novelty diets	
Dr. Abravanel's Body Type and Lifetime Nutrition Plan (or his other books)	Promotes certain nutrients, foods, or combinations of food as having unique, magical, or previously undiscovered qualities.
Dr. Berger's Immune Power Diet	Malnutrition; no change in habits leads to relapse; unrealistic food choices lead to possible bingeing
Fit for Life	
The Rotation Diet	
The Hilton Head Metabolism Diet	
The Junk Food Diet	
The Beverly Hills Diet	
Dr. Debetz Champagne Diet	
Sun Sign Diet	
F-Plan Diet	
Fat Attack Plan	
Popcorn Plus Diet	
Jean Simpson's Numbers Diet	
Autohypnosis Diet	
The Ultrafit Diet	
The Princeton Plan	
The Diet Bible	
Bloomingdale's Diet	
The Love Diet	
Eat to Succeed	
The Underburner's Diet	
Eat to Win	
Two Day Diet	
Paris Diet	
Very–low-calorie diets (VLCDs)	
Optifast	
Cambridge Diet	Less than 800 kcal/day
The Last Chance Diet	Also known as protein-sparing modified fasts
Genesis	
Medifast	Must be under close physician scrutiny
New Direction	Organ tissue loss—especially from the heart; low serum potassium leads to heart failure; expense; kidney stones; gout
HMR	
Ultrafast	
Thin So Fast	
Formula diets	
U.S.A. (United States of America), Inc.	
Optifast	Can help people who find it easier not to eat whole foods while dieting to lose weight
Genesis	
Cambridge Diet	Based on formulated or packaged products
Herbalife	
The Last Chance Diet	Many are low-kilocalorie diet regimens (see above); no change in habits leads to increased chance of relapse; expense; constipation
Slimfast	
Premeasured diets	
Jenny Craig	Most food supplied in premeasured servings to take much of the decision making out of the process of eating
	Expense; may not allow for easy sound eating later

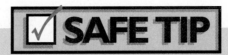

TEN RULES OF WEIGHT CONTROL

1. **"Overweight" is not necessarily "overfat."** Weight isn't fair measurement of fitness or fatness. Measurement of body fat and muscle mass are much better indicators of fitness. Use proven body composition methods to assess the percentage of body fat. Skin fold measurement is the easiest and most inexpensive method to determine percentage of body fat.

2. **So-called "ideal" body fat percentages vary from person to person and sport to sport.** Genetics and training influence individuals' optimal body fat percentages, which vary among men and women.

3. **Intensity and duration of exercise influence the type and amount of fuel burned.** Prolonged, low-intensity exercise promotes fat loss. Short bursts of high-intensity activity burn primarily carbohydrate.

4. **Changes to body composition must be done gradually.** Try either losing or adding one to three pounds per week. Losing fat and gaining muscle take time, and require proper diet and exercise. Rapid weight loss may reduce strength and endurance and result in impaired performance.

5. **Maintain adequate hydration. Drink fluids before, during and after exercise.** Monitor fluid loss by weighing athletes before and after competition.

6. **Carbohydrate is the most important energy source to enhance athletic performance.** Whether trying to gain, maintain or lose weight, high carbohydrate intake is absolutely essential for athletic performance. Carbohydrate storage in the body is accompanied by water storage, which accounts for some fluctuation in weight.

7. **Athletes' protein needs can easily be met through a well-balanced diet.** Current research indicates that special protein or amino acid supplements are not necessary, and will not increase muscle mass.

8. **To decrease calories and promote fat loss, reduce the amount of fat in the diet.** Fat has more than twice as many calories per gram than carbohydrate and protein. Reduce fat intake to help keep body fat down and make more room in your diet for carbohydrate, the most important energy source for athletic performance.

9. **Learn to recognize the signs of eating disorders.** Anorexia and bulimia can seriously affect health as well as athletic performance. The pressure to reach a certain body weight can lead to eating disorders, especially with female athletes. Like any health problem, an athlete with an eating disorder should be referred to the proper medical channels such as a physician, school psychologist or registered dietitian.

10. **Consult an expert.** Work with a health care professional who has the expertise to measure body fat, muscle mass, and determine nutritional requirements for individual athletes, such as a sports nutritionist, physician or athletic trainer.

From Gatorade: *Gatorade Sports Science Institute,* Chicago, 1995, The Quaker Oats Company.

expenditure of the muscle-training program. Serious weight training must be part of the program; otherwise, the excess energy intake will be converted to fat. For recommendations regarding weight training, refer to Chapter 6.

The following suggestions are offered for the college student concerned about a safe weight-gaining program:

- Set a reasonable goal. An exercise program should begin in advance of the competing season. *Rapid weight gain indicates increase in fat, not muscle.*
- Follow an exercise program prescribed by a fitness professional and designed to develop the desired muscles (see Chapter 6).
- Determine the usual caloric intake; then estimate the additional calories needed daily to gain lean weight.

For a young active male college student, an additional 500 to 1000 Calories per day may be needed to gain lean weight. Therefore it is important to plan both the composition and timing of meals and snacks. The diet should be based on the food groups (see Chapter 9), with additional calories obtained from larger portions of foods rich in complex carbohydrates. It is recommended that the diet contain less than 25% of calories from fat. The fat component of the diet should be low in saturated fats and cholesterol. Figure 8-8 (p. 238) is an example of a very

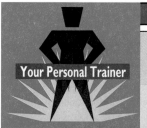

Your Personal Trainer

Roland Meir, American history major
Age: 18

Scenario

I've looked forward to college as a place to reinvent myself. To start with, I planned on losing 15 pounds and getting into shape. I've read a number of magazine articles about low-fat and no-fat diets and have religiously been monitoring my food intake. In addition to my no-fat diet I've been using an exercise bike at the rec center three times a week for 20 minutes. I've been at it for 6 weeks now and haven't had much success.

Solution

It sounds like you have set a realistic plan of action for yourself. However, in terms of weight control the important consideration is the total number of calories that you consume relative to the total number of calories expended.

Monitor both your calorie intake and your fat consumption. Check the nutritional labels of the foods and snacks you eat. Fresh fruits and vegetables are always a good alternative to prepackaged "no-fat" or "low-fat" snacks. Many people eat larger portions of these foods, which are often loaded with high-calorie sweeteners.

A strict no-fat diet is not recommended. Your body needs a certain amount of fat to produce essential enzymes and hormones.

Try adding a bit of diversity to your exercise program. Learning a new skill or trying a new activity is a great way to take your mind off the *work* in working out and is also a great way to meet new people.

Keep at it and you will achieve your goals.

---

high-calorie diet that would sustain the weight of an extremely active young adult. Athletes in training for competition would require very high-calorie diets such as this one.

One should monitor body weight weekly to ensure a gradual weight gain. Measuring skinfold thickness regularly will detect any increases in body fat. An increase in the skinfold thickness indicates a need for a reduction in caloric intake or an increase in training, or both, until it is demonstrated that the percentage of body fat is not increasing. If you are trying to gain weight, you can use the chart in Lab Activity 8-9.

Protein Supplementation

Athletes often believe that more protein is needed to build bigger muscles. Actually, a relatively small amount of additional protein is needed for the muscles developed in a training program. Most Americans consume about twice the amount of protein needed; therefore protein is obtained by eating natural food sources rather than by consuming protein supplements. Furthermore, protein supplements may have undesirable effects on the body.

EATING DISORDERS

Unfortunately for many people in our society, weight loss has become an obsession that poses a

threat to health and well-being. The media bombards the public with an ideal body image that is fashion-model thin. This creates social and internal pressures, especially for young women, to become overly concerned with the relationship of body image to self-image. Pursuing an ideal body image, even one that is unrealistic and unhealthy, becomes an attainable goal. When one believes that a thinner body is the key to becoming more satisfied with one's self, the individual is susceptible to adopting bizarre behaviors in an attempt to find happiness. In some cases, dieting behavior is so extreme that people literally starve themselves to death. Descriptions of some of the more common eating disorders associated with self-image problems follow. Also, Figure 8-9 provides some clues to identifying those with dangerous weight-control behaviors.

Bulimia

Bulimia, believed to be one of the more common eating disorders, involves recurrent episodes of binge-type eating ("pigging-out") followed by purging (vomiting and laxative abuse). Usually the binge con-

> **bulimia** an eating disorder involving recurrent episodes of binge-type eating followed by purging

FIGURE 8-8. A Very High Caloric Sample Meal Pattern (Approximately 6000 Calories).

Breakfast
3/4 c Orange juice
1 c Hot cereal with 2 tsp sugar
1 Egg, fried
1 Slice whole wheat toast
with:
1 tsp Margarine
1 tsp Jelly
8 oz Milk (whole)
Total Calories = 620

Lunch
1 Ham and cheese sandwich:
2 Slices bread
1 oz Cheese

1 oz Ham
1 Tbsp Mayonnaise
1 Serving french fries
1 c Tossed green salad with
2 Tbsp dressing
10 oz Chocolate milkshake
4 Oatmeal cookies
Total Calories = 1440

Dinner
2 Pieces baked chicken (7 oz)
1 c Rice with 1 tsp margarine
1 c Collard greens
(whole)
1/2 c Candied sweet potatoes
2 Pieces cornbread with
1 Tbsp margarine
8 oz Milk (whole)
1 Slice apple pie
Total Calories = 1760

Snack
1 Peanut butter and
jelly sandwich:
2 Slices bread
2 Tbsp Peanut
butter
2 tsp Jelly
1/2 c Raisins
1 c Apple juice
Total Calories = 680

Snack
1 Bagel with:
2 tsp Margarine
2 Tbsp Cream
cheese
1 c Sweetened
applesauce
3/4 c Grape juice
Total Calories = 710

Snack
1 Banana
1/2 c Peanuts
1 c Chocolate milk
Total Calories = 720

Total Calories for day = 5930

FIGURE 8-9. Identifying Behaviors Associated With Eating Disorders.

Reports or observations of the following signs or behaviors should arouse concern:
- Repeatedly expresses concerns about being or feeling fat even when weight is below average.
- Expressions of fear about being or becoming obese that do not diminish as weight loss continues.
- Refusal to maintain even a minimal normal weight consistent with the individual's sport, age, and height.
- Consumption of huge amounts of food not consistent with the person's weight.
- A pattern of eating substantial amounts of food, followed promptly by trips to the bathroom and resumption of eating shortly thereafter.
- Periods of severe calorie restriction or repeated days of fasting.
- Evidence of purposeless, excessive physical activity.
- Depressed mood and expression of self-deprecating thoughts after eating.
- Apparent preoccupation with the eating behavior of other people, such as friends, relatives, or teammates.
- Known or reported family history of eating disorders or family dysfunction.

sists of foods high in calories from fat or sugar, such as bags of cookies, doughnuts, and chips. A typical binge involves the consumption of several thousand Calories during a 1- to 2-hour time period. These binges may occur once a month or in severe cases, several times a day. The behavior is so time consuming, affected college students may have to drop out of school because they have no time for classes or studies.

To avoid gaining weight from the positive caloric situation, the person follows the binge with purging through vomiting, laxatives, or fasting. People who engage in such behavior tend to binge and purge in secret; particularly the purging behavior is hidden from friends and family members.

Persons with bulimia are generally college-age women who are about average or not excessively overfat. Reports of bulimic behavior in young men involve the consumption of large quantities of beer and foods such as pizza, followed by vomiting.

The Bulimic Personality

Although bulimics are often extroverts and socially active, they tend to have problems with interpersonal relationships. They suffer from low self-esteem and feel isolated because of their behavior. Bulimics believe that this behavior is disgusting and beyond their control. They become depressed and anxious, which in turn leads to more bingeing and purging episodes. In severe cases, bulimics become so obsessed with obtaining enough food and laxatives that they have little money for other needs. Sometimes they are arrested in the act of shoplifting these items from stores.

Treatment for Bulimia

If untreated, the purging episodes can damage the body. The depressed bulimic may decide that suicide is the only solution to this abnormal behavior. If you know someone who seems to be able to eat huge amounts of food, is not physically active, yet is not gaining weight, you may suspect this disorder. It often helps to discuss the possibility of bulimia with them and encourage them to obtain counseling.

Treatment should focus on the causes of the behavior, including reasons for the low self-esteem and how to build supportive relationships. Individuals benefit from counseling that teaches how to cope with stress in a more constructive manner than bingeing and purging. Success is often measured in reducing the behavior rather than totally eliminating it. Thus it is essential to be realistic about changing bulimic behaviors; habits take time to change.

Anorexia Nervosa

Anorexia nervosa is a psychological disease in which a person develops an aversion to food and a distorted body image. Over a period of time, the person loses a considerable amount of body weight so that health and life are threatened. Recently, anorexia nervosa has become a more widespread problem, although not as widespread as bulimia. About 90% of the cases involve females, and the disorder usually begins around puberty.

It is usually very obvious that individuals are "anorexic." They are so thin that they appear to have a life-threatening disease such as terminal cancer. The subcutaneous fat layer is nearly absent so that veins can be seen on arms and legs. The typical feminine shape due to body fat deposits is absent. Extreme physical activity behaviors are also characteristic of the illness; the anorexic may jog or work out tirelessly. The normal female hormonal cycle depends on a certain minimum level of body fat; most of these women fail to menstruate.

In certain sports, anorexic behaviors may be apparent, particularly for those athletes who think a thin appearance is important. These sports include gymnastics, dancing, cheerleading, track, and to some degree, tennis. This has been called *anorexia athletica*. These athletes seem to associate a slender appearance with the ability to perform successfully and appear more attractive.

In many instances the condition begins as an attempt to reduce body fat through caloric reduction and increased exercise. Instead of being satisfied with reaching a healthy goal weight, the person becomes obsessed with the ability to control body weight and continues the effort. Anorexics may fast, but often they eat small, precisely measured quantities of food that do not supply enough calories to fuel the high-energy demands of their physical activity or to maintain a reasonable amount of body fat. Reports of a combination of anorexia nervosa and bulimic behaviors are not uncommon. This is often called bulimia nervosa. An estimated 20% of those affected with this psychological disease die from the effects of severe malnutrition or the chemical imbalances created by purging.

Treatment of Anorexia Nervosa

Individuals with anorexia nervosa cannot be convinced that they are "too thin." Their body image is so distorted that even while looking at themselves in a mirror, they think they could lose some more weight. Therefore treating the condition is beyond the abilities of a health or physical educator. Simply referring the person to the campus health clinic is not effective unless specialists are on staff who are qualified to deal with these cases. Anorexics should be referred to licensed psychologists or medical doctors who specialize in treating such cases. In severe cases, long-term hospitalization is necessary. The key to treatment is getting patients to realize that they can gain control over their lives in ways that do not involve dieting. Unfortunately, for many of those who do survive, they do not fully recover but remain underweight and fearful of any future weight gain.

Female Athlete Triad Syndrome

Female athlete triad syndrome is a potentially fatal problem that involves a combination of an eating disorder (either bulimia or anorexia), amenorrhea, and osteoporosis (diminished bone density) and that occurs primarily in female athletes. The incidence of this syndrome is uncertain; however, some studies have suggested that eating disorders in female athletes may be as high as 62% in certain sports, with amenorrhea being common in at least 60%. However, the major risk of this syndrome is that the bone lost in osteoporosis may not be regained.

> **anorexia nervosa**   a psychological disease in which a person develops a distorted body image and an aversion to food
> **bulimia nervosa**   a combination of anorexia nervosa and bulimia that can easily lead to death as a result of severe malnutrition and chemical imbalances

SUMMARY

- Being overweight implies having excess body weight relative to bone structure and height. This excess could be due to excess fat or to a higher proportion of muscle. Obesity clearly describes a condition of having an excessive amount of fat.
- The development of obesity has been attributed to several factors, including heredity, social environment, and a lifestyle that includes poor nutritional habits and sedentary behavior.
- Body composition analysis indicates the percentage of total body weight composed of fat tissue versus the percentage composed of lean tissue.
- The size and number of adipose cells determine percentage body fat. Percentage body fat can be measured by measuring the thickness of the subcutaneous fat with a skinfold caliper at specific areas.
- Changes in body weight are caused almost entirely by a change in caloric balance, which is a function of the number of calories taken in and the number of calories expended.
- Calories are expended by the body for three different processes: (1) basal metabolism, (2) physical activity, and (3) the thermic effect of food. Caloric expenditure may be calculated by maintaining accurate records of the number of calories expended for metabolic needs and in activities performed during the course of a day.

- Weight can be lost either by increasing caloric expenditure through exercise or by decreasing caloric intake through reducing food intake. In general, low-calorie diets don't result in weight loss that can be maintained over time.
- The recommended technique for losing weight involves a combination of moderate caloric restriction and a moderate increase in physical exercise during the course of each day.
- Weight loss should be accomplished gradually over a long period. Realistically, no more than about 2 pounds of actual body weight should be lost during a single week.
- Weight gain should be accomplished by increasing caloric intake and engaging in a weight-training program. It is possible to gain weight and lose fat, thus changing body composition. Equal volumes of muscle weigh more than fat.
- Bulimia is an eating disorder that involves periodic bingeing and subsequent purging.
- Anorexia nervosa is a form of mental illness in which a person reduces food intake and increases energy expenditure to the extent that the loss of body fat threatens his or her health and life.
- Bulimia nervosa is when bulimic behaviors are practiced by the person with anorexia nervosa.
- Female athlete triad syndrome involves an eating disorder, amenorrhea, and osteoporosis.

REFERENCES

Allerheilgen B: How to estimate body fat of college age women, *Strength Cond* 16(6):15-19, 1994.

American College of Sports Medicine: Proper and improper weight loss programs, *Med Sci Sports Exerc* 15:ix, 1983.

Bar-Or O, Baranowski T: Physical activity, adiposity, and obesity, *Pediatr Exerc Sci* 6(4):348-360, 1994.

Barr S, McCargar L: Practical use of body composition analysis in sports, *Sports Med* 17(5):277-282, 1994.

Bemben M, Massey B, Bemben D: Age related patterns in body composition for men age 20-79 years, *Med Sci Sports Exerc* 27(2):264-269, 1995.

Blackburn GL: Weight cycling: the experience of human dieters, *Am J Clin Nutr* 49:1105, 1989.

Bouchard C, Tramblay A, Nadeau A, et al: Long-term exercise training with constant energy intake: effect on body composition and selected metabolic variables, *Int J Obes* 14:57, 1990.

Bray G: Pathophysiology of obesity, *Am J Clin Nutr* 55:488S, 1992.

Champaign BN: Body fat distribution: metabolic consequences and implications for weight loss, *Med Sci Sports Exerc* 22:291, 1990.

Clark N: When thin is not in, *Am Fitness* 13(2):65-66, 1995.

Dengel D, Hagberg J, Coon P: Effects of weight loss by diet alone or combined with aerobic exercise on body composition in older obese men, *Metabolism* 43:867-871, 1994.

Dick R: Eating disorders in NCAA athletic programs, *Athl Train* 26(2):137-140, 1991.

Dietary Guidelines Advisory Committee: *Dietary guidelines for Americans*, pp 23-24, 1995 (report).

Dunbar C, Melahrinides E, Michielli D: The effects of small errors in electrode placement on body composition assessment by bioelectrical impedence, *Res Q Exerc Sport* 65(3):291-294, 1994.

Ellis DL: Sustained depression of resting metabolic rate after massive weight loss, *Am J Clin Nutr* 49:93, 1989.

Freedson P: Body composition. In Costa D, Gutherie S, editors: *Women in sport: interdisciplinary perspectives*, Champaign, 1994, Human Kinetics.

Friedl K, Moore R: Lower limit of body fat in healthy active men, *J Appl Physiol* 77(2):933-940, 1994.

Greene G: Dietary intake and dieting practices of bulimic and non-bulimic college female students, *JAMA* 90:576, 1990.

Gustafson P: The role of diet and exercise in the modification of body composition in obese women, *Clin Kinesiology* 48(2):33-43, 1994.

Haus G, Hoerr S, Mavis B: Key modifiable factors in weight maintenance: fat intake, exercise, and weight cycling, *J Am Diet Assoc* 94:409-413, 1994.

Horswill C: When wrestlers slim to win: what is a safe weight, *Phys Sports Med* 20(9):91-104, 1992.

Ishida Y, Kanehisa H, Carrol J: Body fat and muscle thickness distribution in untrained females, *Med Sci Sports Exerc* 27(2):270-274, 1994.

Jebb S, Elia M: Techniques for measurement of body composition: a practical guide, *Int J Obese Relat Metab Disord* 17:611-621, 1993.

Koenig M, Batra S: Relationship between body fat and anthropometric variability in a large sample of young males, *Int J Sports Med* 15(4):163-167, 1994.

Kuczmarski R: Prevalence of overweight and obesity in the United States, *Am J Clin Nutr* 55:495S, 1992.

Lim C, Lee L: The effects of a 20-week basic military training program on body composition, $\dot{V}o_2$ max, and aerobic fitness of obese recruits, *J Sports Med Phys Fitness* 34(3):271-278, 1994.

McArdle W, Katch F, Katch V: *Exercise physiology, energy, nutrition and human performance*, Philadelphia, 1994, Lea & Febiger.

Nattiv A, Lynch L: The female athlete triad: managing an acute risk to long-term health, *Phys Sports Med* 22(1):60-68, 1994.

Nouton K, Craig N: Assessing body fat of athletes, *Aus J Sci Med Sports* 26(1):6-13, 1994.

Opplinger R, Cassady S: Body composition assessment in women: specific considerations for athletes, *Sports Med* 17(6): 353-357, 1994.

Pate R et al: Physical activity and public health, *JAMA* 273:404, 1995.

Payne WA, Hahn DB: *Understanding your health*, ed 4, St Louis, 1995, Mosby.

Powell J, Tucker L, Fisher A: The effect of different percentages of body fat on exercise and caloric restriction on body composition and body weight in obese females, *Am J Health Promo* 8(6): 442-448, 1994.

Riley E: Eating disorders as an addictive behavior, *Nurs Clin North Am* 26:715, 1991.

Skolnick A: Female athlete triad risk for women, *JAMA* 270:921-923, 1993.

Stout J, Eckerson J, Housh T: Validity of percent body fat estimations in males, *Med Sci Sports Exerc* 26(5):632-636, 1994.

Swoap R, Murphy S: Eating disorders and weight management in athletes. In Murphy S, editor: *Sport psychology intervention*, Champaign, 1995, Human Kinetics.

Thornton JS: Feast or famine: eating disorders in athletes, *Phys Sports Med* 18:116, 1990.

US Department of Agriculture and US Department of Health and Human Services: *Nutrition and your health: dietary guidelines for Americans*, ed 4, Washington, DC, 1995.

US Department of Health and Human Services, Public Health Services: *Healthy people 2000: midcourse review and 1995 revisions*, Washington, DC, 1995, USDHHS.

US Department of Health and Human Services, Public Health Services: *Healthy people 2000: national health promotion and disease prevention objectives*, Washington, DC, 1991, USDHHS.

VanDale D, Saris WH: Repetitive weight loss and weight regain: effects on weight reduction and metabolic rate before and after exercise and/or diet treatment, *Am J Clin Nutr* 49:409, 1989.

Vehrs P, George J, Payne C: Relationship of four methods of body composition assessment, *Med Exerc Nutr Health* 3(1):2-8, 1994.

Wardlaw GM, Insel PM: *Perspectives in nutrition*, ed 3, St Louis, 1996, Mosby.

SUGGESTED READINGS

Bailey C: *Smart exercise: burning fat and getting fit*, Boston, 1994, Houghton Mifflin.
Offers a simple approach to reducing fat. Offers good information about correct body fat levels, exercise, diet, and tracking programs.

Lohman T: *Advances in body composition assessment*, Champaign, 1992, Human Kinetics.
Explores the latest issues, concepts, and controversies in body composition assessment.

Thompson R, Trattner-Sherman R: *Helping athletes with eating disorders*, Champaign, 1993, Human Kinetics.
Discusses the difficult issues of dealing with and treating individuals who have eating disorders.

Lab Activity 8-1

Methods for Calculating Waist-to-Hip Ratio

Name _____   **Section** _____   **Date** _____

PURPOSE   To calculate waist-to-hip ratio.

PROCEDURE 1
1. Using a standard flexible cloth measuring tape, measure the circumference of your waist at the level of the umbilicus with the belly relaxed. Record this measurement on the worksheet below.
2 Next, measure the hip circumference at the widest point around the hips. Record this number on the worksheet.
3. Divide the waist number by the hip number to obtain the waist-to-hip ratio.

WORKSHEET FOR CALCULATING WAIST-TO-HIP RATIO

1. Waist circumference _____ inches
2. Hip circumference _____ inches
3. Waist circumference_____
   ÷ Hip circumference _____ = _____ Waist-to-hip ratio

PROCEDURE 2
1. Using a standard flexible cloth measuring tape, measure the circumference of your waist at the level of the umbilicus with the belly relaxed. Mark this measurement on the left axis of the nomogram (Figure 8-10).
2. Next, measure the hip circumference at the widest point around the hips. Mark this number on the right axis of the nomogram.
3. Place a straight edge between the two marks and determine the waist-to-hip ratio according to where the line crosses the middle axis.

Continued.

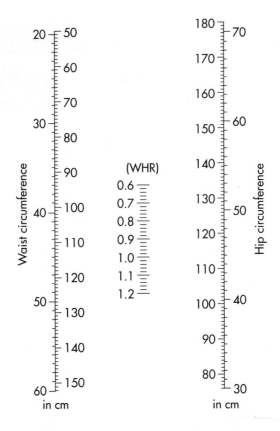

FIGURE 8-10. Nomogram for Determining Waist-to-Hip Ratio (WHR).
Find your waist measurement on the left axis and your hip measurement on the
right axis. Place a straight edge between the two points; where they cross the
center WHR axis determines your ratio.

INTERPRETATION In males, if the waist-to-hip ratio is 0.95 or greater there is too much fat around
the belly and there is increased risk of heart disease, hypertension, or diabetes
mellitus.
In females, if the ratio is 0.80 or greater there is increased risk.

Lab Activity 8-2

Calculating Percentage of Body Fat Using Skinfold Measurements

Name _____   **Section** _____   **Date** _9/23/96_

_– 25 %_

PURPOSE   To calculate percentage body fat using skinfold measures.

PROCEDURE

1. The triceps skinfold is measured over the right arm triceps muscle (back of the upper arm) halfway between the elbow and the tip of the shoulder (Figure 8-11).
   a. Instruct the subject to let the arm hang limply at the side. Grasp the skinfold parallel to the vertical axis of the arm. Lift the skinfold away from the arm, and make sure that no muscle tissue is caught in the fold.
   b. Place the contact surfaces of the calipers $1/2$ inch (12 mm) above the fingers. Release the lever arm on the caliper, and allow pressure from the instrument to bring the two sides together. The caliper pointer then indicates the skinfold thickness in millimeters (mm). Repeat and record the measurement two or three times; then record the average of these measurements on the worksheet provided.
2. The subscapular (below the shoulder blade) measurement site is approximately $1/2$ inch below the inferior angle of the scapula in line with the natural cleavage lines of the skin (Figure 8-12).
   a. Have the subject stand erect with shoulders thrust backward, arm at side. The point of the scapula (shoulder blade) located toward the spine should be obvious. Mark this point, then measure $1/2$ inch below it and place a mark that will be the measurement site.
   b. Standing behind the subject, use the thumb and index fingers and grasp the skinfold in the natural cleavage line (along an imaginary line from elbow to neck). Lift the skinfold away from the scapula, and shake it to make sure no muscle tissue is caught in the fold. Use the caliper to measure as described previously, and record the average on the worksheet.
3. Now that the measurements for the triceps and the subscapular skinfolds are known, percentage body fat can be easily calculated using the following equations.

   Women: Percentage body fat = 0.55(A) + 0.31(B) + 6.13
   Where A = Triceps skinfold (mm)
   B = Subscapular skinfold (mm)

   Men: Percentage body fat = 0.43(A) + 0.58(B) + 1.47
   Where A = Triceps skinfold (mm)
   B = Subscapular skinfold (mm)

4. Consult Table 8-5 to determine the classification of your total percentage body fat.

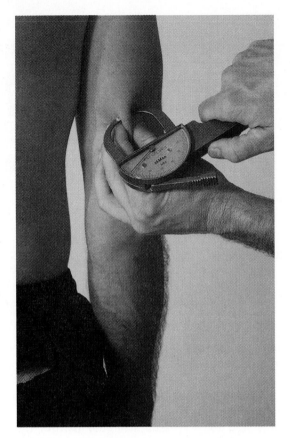

FIGURE 8-11.   Measurement of Triceps Skinfold.

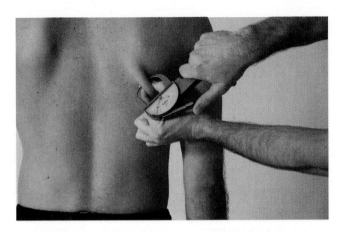

FIGURE 8-12.   Measurement of Subscapular Skinfold.

TABLE 8-5.	**Percentage Fat Based on Skinfolds**								
	Men (9%-17%) Age					**Women (17%-25%)** Age			
Rating	**20-29**	**30-39**	**40-49**	**50+**	**Rating**	**20-29**	**30-39**	**40-49**	**50+**
Dangerously low	<5	<5	<5	<5	Dangerously low	<12	<12	<12	<12
Excellent	5-8.9	5-10.9	5-11.9	5-12.9	Excellent	12-16.9	12-17.9	12-19.9	12-20.9
GOOD	**9-12.9**	**11-13.9**	**12-15.9**	**13-16.9**	**GOOD**	**17-20.9**	**18-21.9**	**20-23.9**	**21-24.9**
Fair	13-16.9	14-17.9	16-20.9	17-21.9	Fair	21-23.9	22-24.9	24-27.9	25-30.9
Poor	17-19.9	18-22.9	21-25.9	22-27.9	Poor	24-27.9	25-29.9	28-31.9	31-35.9
Very poor	>19.9	>22.9	>25.9	>27.9	Very poor	>27.9	>29.9	>31.9	>35.9

INTERPRETATION Ideal body composition consists of low fat and high muscle mass. Height-weight tables only assess one's weight in relation to insurance risk; they do not accurately reflect ideal body composition.

Your percentage body fat can be estimated from skinfold measures. It is recommended that women stay within 17% to 25% fat and men within 9% to 17% fat. Too little body fat may be just as detrimental to your health as too much fat. The critical level for women is no less than 12% and for men is no less than 5%.

WORKSHEET FOR CALCULATING PERCENTAGE OF BODY FAT

1. Triceps skinfold thickness _____ mm
2. Subscapular skinfold thickness _____ mm

Calculation of Body Fat Percentage

1. Use the following formulas to determine percentage of body fat.

Men

$(0.43 \times$ _____ mm$) + (0.58 \times$ _____ mm$) + 1.47 =$ _____ %

Triceps skinfold   Subscapular skinfold   Body fat

Women

$(0.55 \times$ _____ mm$) + (0.31 \times$ _____ mm$) + 6.13 =$ _____ %

Triceps skinfold   Subscapular skinfold   Body fat

2. Using Table 8-5, find your gender and age category. Take the percentage determined above, and determine which health rating you are in. For example, if your percentage is 23 and you are a 22-year-old woman, your health rating is fair.

Calculating Desired Body Weight

Name _____ **Section** _____ **Date** _____

PURPOSE   To determine your desired body weight based on your current body weight and percentage
body fat. This activity is for individuals who want to reduce their percentage of body fat.

PROCEDURE 1. Weigh yourself on a scale, and record the weight in pounds on the worksheet.
2. Record percentage body fat as determined in Lab Activity 8-2 on the worksheet.
3. Indicate your desired percentage body fat on the worksheet.
4. Calculate the percentage body fat to be lost as indicated on the worksheet.
5. Calculate the number of pounds to be lost as indicated on the worksheet.
6. Calculate the desired body weight as indicated on the worksheet.
7. Calculate the desired body weight using the alternative calculation method.

Continued.

WORKSHEET

1. Present body weight   _____ lbs
2. Present percentage body fat   _____ %
3. Desired percentage body fat   _____ %
   (9%-17% for males; 17%-25% for females)

4. _____ % – _____ = _____%
      Present % body fat   Desired % body fat   % body fat to be lost

5. _____ × _____ = _____ lbs
      % body fat to be lost*   Present body weight   Pounds to be lost

6. _____ – _____ = _____
      Present body weight   Pounds to be lost   Desired body weight

Alternative Method

4. _____ lbs × _____ % = _____ lbs
      Present body weight   Percentage body fat*   Present fat weight

5. _____ lbs – _____ lbs = _____ lbs
      Present body weight   Fat weight   Fat-free weight

6. _____ lbs × _____ % = _____ lbs
      Present body weight   Desired % body fat*   Desired fat weight

7. _____ lbs + _____ lbs = _____ lbs
      Fat-free weight   Desired fat weight   Desired body weight

*To perform calculations involving percentages, convert decimals by replacing the percent sign with a decimal point. Then move the decimal point two places to the left.

Calculated desirable weight will often need to be increased by 3 to 5 pounds if either of the following situations is present: (1) if the person has been sedentary or is involved in training to build muscle mass (therefore an allowance must be made for an increase in muscle mass) or (2) if the person is growing.

Lab Activity 8-4

Calculating Body Mass Index (BMI)

Name _____ **Section** _____ **Date** _____

PURPOSE   To determine body mass index (BMI) as a means of examining overweight and obesity.

PROCEDURE
1. Weigh yourself to determine body weight in pounds.
2. Divide your weight in pounds by 2.2 to determine kilograms.
3. Measure your height in inches.
4. Multiply your height in inches by 2.54, and divide by 100 to convert your height to meters.
5. Multiply your height in meters by your weight in meters to get your height in meters squared.
6. Divide your weight in kilograms by your height in meters squared to determine your BMI.

WORKSHEET FOR CALCULATING BMI

1. _____125_____ ÷ 2.2 = _____56.8_____
   Weight (lbs)   Weight (kgs)

2. _____63_____ × 2.54 ÷ 100 = _____1.60_____
   Height (in)   Height (m)

3. _____1.60_____ × _____1.60_____ = _____2.56_____
   Height (m)   Height (m)   Height (m)²

4. _____56.8_____ ÷ _____2.56_____ = _____22.2_____
   Weight (kg)   Height (m)²   Body Mass Index

INTERPRETATION   A body mass index greater than 27.3 for females and 27.8 for males indicates a state of obesity.

Calculating Caloric Intake

Name _____ **Section** _____ **Date** _____

PURPOSE   To determine your daily caloric intake.

PROCEDURE

1. A daily food intake log such as the one in Table 8-2 can be kept over a period of several days to let you know about how many Calories are being consumed on the average each day. College students are notorious for skipping meals and eating multiple snacks. Thus it is important to record everything you consume during the entire 24-hour period. Don't neglect to record extras such as mustard and pickles that you include on a hamburger. The worksheet on p. 254 shows how the daily food intake log should be filled out. Those columns that deal with hunger level and mood may help you to determine what causes you to eat when you do.

2. As with caloric expenditure, adding up the caloric values of all foods consumed during a 24-hour period can give you a reasonably accurate estimate of daily caloric intake.

Continued.

						Hunger level*	Activity and location	Mood†
Time	Food eaten	Amount	Number of Calories	How cooked	Meal or snack	(0-3)	when eating	(1-3)

Worksheet for Calculating Daily Calorie Intake
(Daily Food Intake Log)

Date: _____

Total number of Calories consumed =

*Hunger rating: 0, not hungry; 3, very hungry
† Mood: 1, good/happy; 2, fair/OK; 3, upset.

Determining Your Basal Metabolic Rate (BMR)

Name _____ Section _____ Date _____

PURPOSE   To determine your basal metabolic rate.

PROCEDURE   1. Use Figure 8-13 to determine your body surface area. Using a ruler, draw a straight line from your height to your weight. The point at which that line crosses the middle column shows your surface area in square meters (m²). Record this number beside "Estimated body surface area" on the worksheet. For example, a 20-year-old man whose height is 6 feet (180 cm) and weight is 170 pounds (77.3 kg) would have a body surface area on the nomogram of 1.99 square meters.

Scale I Height	Scale III Surface area	Scale II Weight
in cm	m²	lb kg

FIGURE 8-13. Estimating Total Body Surface Area.
Locate your height on Scale I and then your weight on Scale II. Using a straight edge, connect the two points with a line. The intersection of the line on Scale III is your body surface area.

Continued.

2. Next, use Table 8-6 to find the factor for your sex and age, and multiply your surface area by this factor. Record this number for "BMR factor" on the worksheet below. For example, for a 20-year-old man, the factor is 39.9 kcal per square meter per hour (kcal/m²/h).

TABLE 8-6. Basal Metabolic Rate According to Age and Sex						
	BMR (kcal/m²/h)				**BMR (kcal/m²/h)**	
Age	**Men**	**Women**	**Age**	**Men**	**Women**	
10	47.7	44.9	29	37.7	35.0	
11	46.5	43.5	30	37.6	35.0	
12	45.3	42.0	31	37.4	35.0	
13	44.5	40.5	32	37.2	34.9	
14	43.8	39.2	33	37.1	34.9	
15	42.9	38.3	34	37.0	34.9	
16	42.0	37.2	35	36.9	34.8	
17	41.5	36.4	36	36.8	34.7	
18	40.8	35.8	37	36.7	34.6	
19	40.5	35.4	38	36.7	34.5	
20	39.9	35.3	39	36.6	34.4	
21	39.5	35.2	40-44	36.4	34.1	
22	39.2	35.2	45-49	36.2	33.8	
23	39.0	35.2	50-54	35.8	33.1	
24	38.7	35.1	55-59	35.1	32.8	
25	38.4	35.1	60-64	34.5	32.0	
26	38.2	35.0	65-69	33.5	31.6	
27	38.0	35.0	70-74	32.7	31.1	
28	37.8	35.0	75+	31.8		

3. Next, multiply "Estimated body surface area" by the "BMR factor" and record on the worksheet.
4. Finally, multiply this product by 24 hours per day to find your BMR needs per day.

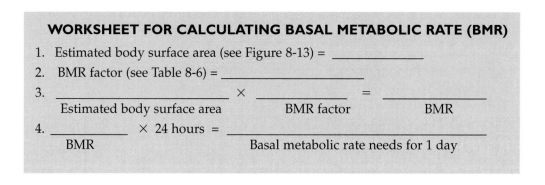

WORKSHEET FOR CALCULATING BASAL METABOLIC RATE (BMR)

1. Estimated body surface area (see Figure 8-13) = _____

2. BMR factor (see Table 8-6) = _____

3. _____ × _____ = _____
   Estimated body surface area   BMR factor   BMR

4. _____ × 24 hours = _____
   BMR   Basal metabolic rate needs for 1 day

Lab Activity 8-7

Calculating Caloric Expenditure

Name _____ **Section** _____ **Date** _____

PURPOSE   To keep a 24-hour log of all activities done during the day: everything from eating breakfast to biking to school or work, recreational activities, and so forth.

PROCEDURE   1. Consult Table 8-3 (p. 229), Energy Expenditure During Physical Activity. Use the guidelines in Table 8-7 below for activities not included in Table 8-3.
2. Record your activities* on the worksheet provided, listing the following:
   a. Clock time—Specify the time of day.
   b. Activity—The type of activity you were involved in.
   c. Total number of minutes spent in the activity.
   d. kcal/min/lb—Locate your nearest body weight in pounds, and use the appropriate column.
   e. Total Calories expended—Multiply total number of minutes by kcal/min/lb
3. To calculate expenditure during sleep, multiply the number of hours you slept by the BMR calculated in **Lab Activity 8-6**.
4. On the worksheet, add the total Calories expended during activities.

TABLE 8-7. **General Guidelines for Energy Expenditure**	
Activity	**kcal/min/lb**
Very light (such as typing, driving)	0.010
Light (such as shopping)	0.021
Moderate (such as dancing, bowling)	0.032
Heavy (such as football, running)	0.062

Continued.

*Every minute of the day should be accounted for.

Clock time	Activity	Total minutes spent in activity	kcal/min/lb	Total calories expended

Worksheet for Calculating Daily Energy Expenditure (Daily Activities Log)   Date: _____

Total Calories expended during activities _____

Add Calories expended in basal metabolism during sleeping only (BMR × number of hours sleeping)_____

Total Calories expended _____

Worksheet for Estimating Caloric Balance

Name _____ **Section** _____ **Date** _____

PURPOSE To help you estimate whether you are in caloric balance, based on your assessment of a day's caloric intake and expenditure.

PROCEDURE 1. Consult **Lab Activity 8-6** for estimated BMR caloric needs. Fill in below. Consult **Lab Activity 8-7** for your estimation of activity caloric needs. Fill in below. Add the two numbers together.

        _____ + _____ = _____ Calories
         BMR Calories   Activity Calories
        (during sleeping)

2. Multiply the sum from step 1 by 0.1 to estimate the number of Calories that are needed for the thermic effect of food (10% of BMR + Activity Calories).

       _____ × 0.1 = _____ Calories

3. Add the sum of Calories from step 1 with the number obtained in step 2 to obtain an estimate of a day's caloric needs.

       _____ + _____ = _____ Total Calories
       Step 1 Calories   Step 2 Calories

4. Consult **Lab Activity 8-5** for an estimation of your caloric intake. Record the number below.

       _____ Calories

5. Compare the total number of energy expenditure Calories obtained in step 3 with the total for intake in step 4.

Check which situation applies:

a. Caloric intake is greater than expenditure   _____

b. Caloric expenditure is greater than intake   _____

c. Caloric expenditure equals intake   _____

Is this day's energy situation in balance, in negative balance, or in positive balance?

_____

Lab Activity 8-8

Should You Consider a Weight-Loss Program?

Name _____ **Section** _____ **Date** _____

PURPOSE   Before you actually begin a weight-loss program you should identify the reasons for your decision.

PROCEDURE   Check all the statements that apply to your situation or beliefs.

	Yes	No
1. I am satisfied with my present body weight	_____	_____
2. My friends and family tell me that I would be more attractive if I lost weight.	_____	_____
3. My doctor has told me that my health is being affected by my weight.	_____	_____
4. Food is not as important to me as my health and appearance.	_____	_____
5. I believe that clothing designed for overweight people is unattractive.	_____	_____
6. I would like to be able to wear clothes that don't feel tight.	_____	_____
7. I am uncomfortable or embarrassed when participating in sports activities.	_____	_____
8. I think that my excess body fat makes me unattractive.	_____	_____
9. I would feel better about myself if I lost some weight.	_____	_____
10. I think that I would be more socially accepted if I had less body fat.	_____	_____

INTERPRETATION   Many people lack the motivation needed to change eating and exercise behaviors that are needed for weight loss. Examine the above statements. If you checked *yes* for number 1, you are satisfied with your body size; if others suggest that you should lose weight, you lack the interest and motivation to be successful. Answering *yes* to statements 2 and 3 indicates that others think you should lose weight, but it is not necessarily your idea too. Health concerns are not always a motivating factor. If you answered *yes* to the rest of the statements, you are probably highly motivated.

Lab Activity 8-9

Monitoring Weekly Weight Loss/Gain

Name _____ Section _____ Date _____

PURPOSE   To help you track your weight loss or gain pattern over a 16-week period.

PROCEDURE 1. Weigh yourself, and record your present weight on the worksheet* on p. 264.
2. On the same day each week, at approximately the same time, reweigh yourself, and place an X in the box that indicates the appropriate number of pounds lost or gained each week from your original starting weight.
3. Connect the Xs by drawing straight lines.

*You may wish to record waist circumferences every 2 weeks, especially if you are increasing your physical activity levels.

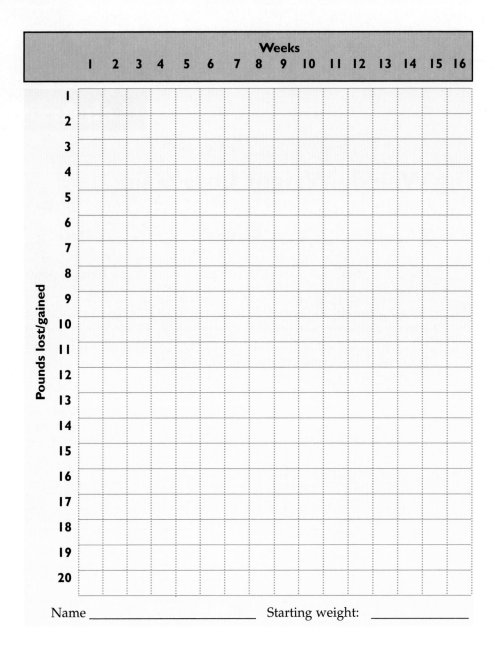

Name _____   Starting weight: _____

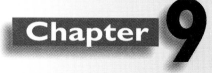

Chapter 9 Eating Healthy

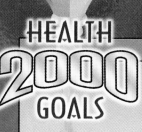

■ **Dietary Fat.** Reduce dietary fat intake to an average of 30% of calories or less and average saturated fat intake to less than 10% of calories among people age 2 and older. From 1976-1980 people age 20 to 74 consumed 36% of their calories from total fat and 13% from saturated fat. *Midpoint Update: headed in the right direction with current statistic of 34%.*

■ **Vegetables, Fruits, and Grain Products.** Increase complex carbohydrate and fiber-containing foods in the diets of adults to five or more servings of vegetables and fruits, and to six or more daily servings of grain products.

■ **Food Labels.** Increase to at least 85% the proportion of people age 18 and older who use food labels to make nutritious food selections. In 1988, 74% of the population used labels to make food selections.

■ **Nutrition Labeling.** Achieve useful and informative nutrition labeling for virtually all processed foods and at least 40% of fresh meats; poultry; fish; fruits; vegetables; baked goods; and ready-to-eat, carry-away foods. In 1988, 60% of sales of processed foods regulated by the FDA had nutrition labeling.

OBJECTIVES

After completing this chapter, you will be able to do the following:

■ Identify common nutrition myths.
■ Identify the six classes of nutrients.
■ Describe the major functions of the nutrients, especially the value of water.

■ Explain how to design a nutritious diet using the Food Pyramid as your guide.
■ Explain the relationship of nutrition to physical performance.
■ Identify your nutritional strengths and weaknesses and establish a program to correct the weaknesses.

KEY TERMS

While reading this chapter, you will become familiar with the following terms:

- diet
- nutrients
- macronutrients
- micronutrients
- nutrient density

- carbohydrates
- fats
- lipids
- proteins
- vitamins

- antioxidants
- minerals
- nutrient requirement
- nutritional recommendation

- vegetarianism
- glycogen supercompensation

People usually think of losing weight when they hear the word *diet*. Actually, **diet** refers to one's usual food selections. What you choose to eat is your diet. Although we have different food likes and dislikes, we all must eat to survive. The relationship of nutrition, diet, and weight control to body composition was briefly described in Chapter 8. This chapter provides an overview of basic nutrition principles, which is important in any discussion of physical fitness. The following information will help you examine your diet and find its strengths and weaknesses.

NUTRITION MYTHS AND MISINFORMATION

All of us are interested in nutrition and perhaps have read popular books about the topic or have listened to the advice of others concerning the use of nutrient supplements designed to enhance performance. Unfortunately, there are more unreliable sources of nutrition information available to the consumer than reliable, fact-filled ones. The typical person is concerned about the value of foods and nutrition to health but cannot tell which sources of information are reliable. Remember that virtually everything you read, see, or hear about nutrition may not be accurate. Usually someone is out to make money from your lack of nutrition knowledge. It is really a "buyer beware" situation. The intent of this chapter is to clear up some of the confusion and make you a more careful consumer of nutrition information.

There are probably more myths associated with the role of nutrition in a well-rounded fitness program than for any other related topic of concern to this motivated group of consumers. People who are interested in achieving a high degree of fitness associate the consumption of special foods or supplements with successful performance. Individuals who are performing well while using these products may attribute their success to the items rather than to their training, skill, or effort. They tell others about their "key" to success. Even when presented with the facts about the worthlessness of most of these products, they defend their behavior and ignore the truth.

There is no doubt that if people really believe that some nutritional powder, pill, or drink is the key to success, they may be successful. Often the belief that an item will have an effect can actually induce the desired effect, even though the item itself really does not have an effect. This is known as a *placebo effect*, which can be very powerful. If under certain circumstances a person is unable to use the supplement, he or she may panic and possibly fail. Thus the supplement provides a psychological boost. In many cases no harm is done. However, many people spend considerable amounts of money on such worthless supplements, and the use of some products can harm the body. For example, excesses of amino acid (protein), vitamin, or mineral supplements can create toxic effects or imbalances in the body. Nutrient imbalances can actually hurt rather than help performance. The levels and mixtures of nutrients are present in foods as balanced biochemistry and are ideal for human consumption, whereas those contained in many supplements are often unlike those found in food because they are not present as balanced biochemistry.

PRINCIPLES OF BASIC NUTRITION
Nutrient Classification

Nutrition is the science of the substances found in food that are essential to life. A substance is essential if it must be supplied by the diet. There are six classes of **nutrients**: carbohydrates (CHO), fats, proteins, vitamins, minerals, and water. These nutrients may be divided into **macronutrients**, which provide energy in the form of calories and include carbohydrates, fat, and protein; and **micronutrients**, which regulate many bodily functions and include vitamins and minerals. Water is an essential nutrient that must be classified separately.

Nutrients are necessary for three major roles:
1. Growth, repair, and maintenance of all tissues
2. Regulation of body processes
3. Providing energy

Most foods are actually mixtures of these nutrients. Some nutrients can be made by the body, but an essential nutrient must be supplied by the diet. Not all substances in food are considered nutrients. Fruits and vegetables and other plant products contain numerous *phytochemicals*, which are currently being investigated for their protective properties against development of premature chronic diseases in humans. There is no such thing as the perfect food; that is, no single natural food contains all of the nutrients needed for health.

Nutrient Density

Nutrient density describes foods that supply adequate amounts of vitamins and minerals in relation to their caloric value. For example, orange juice is nutrient dense when compared to an orange drink that has had vitamin C added to it. The orange juice contains vitamins A and C, folic acid (a B-vitamin), and potassium. The orange drink contains vitamin C but may be made from only 10% orange juice; in addition, the added water and sugar make it a less nutrient-dense choice. The so-called junk foods provide excessive amounts of calories from fat and sugar in relation to vitamins and minerals and therefore are not nutrient dense. If your diet is nutritious and you can "afford" the extra calories, an occasional candy bar or doughnut is acceptable. However, many people live on junk foods that displace more nutrient-dense foods from their diet. This is not a healthy behavior in the long run.

The following section provides an overview of nutrition, including brief descriptions of major food sources and the roles of nutrients in the body.

ENERGY NUTRIENTS (MACRONUTRIENTS)
Carbohydrates (CHO)

The physically active individual has increased energy needs, which should be met mostly with nutrient-dense foods. Carbohydrates are often considered the body's most important source of energy because the brain normally uses 100% carbohydrate for its energy needs. For most individuals, carbohydrates should account for 55% or more of total caloric intake; some recommendations go as high as 60% to 70%. The following sections describe different forms of carbohydrates and their roles in energy production and health maintenance.

Sugars

Carbohydrates are classified as simple (sugars) or complex (starch and most forms of fiber). Simple sugars are further divided into monosaccharides and disaccharides. Monosaccharides, single sugars, are found mostly in fruits, syrups, and honey. Glucose (blood sugar) is a monosaccharide. Milk sugar (lactose) and table sugar (sucrose) are combinations of two monosaccharides and are called *disaccharides*. Table sugar is a disaccharide refined from sugar cane and sugar beets; it is nearly 100% pure CHO. Because it contributes very little in the way of other nutrients, the amount of sugar eaten should account for less than 15% of the total caloric intake. Many Americans eat too much sugar and other sweeteners such as syrups.

Starches

Starches are more complex carbohydrates. A starch is made up of long chains of glucose units. During the digestion process, the starch chain is broken down and the glucose units are free to be absorbed. Food sources of starch, such as rice, potatoes, and breads, often provide vitamins and minerals in addition to serving as the body's principal source of glucose. People think that starchy foods contribute to obesity. However, most of these foods are eaten with fats from butter, margarine, sauces, and gravies that make the food more enjoyable but contribute an excess of calories.

The body cannot use starches and many sugars directly from food for energy. It needs to obtain the simple sugar, glucose (blood sugar). During digestion and metabolism, starches and disaccharide sugars are broken down and converted to glucose. The glucose that is not needed for immediate energy is stored as glycogen in the liver and muscle cells. Between meals, glucose is then released from glycogen as needed. The body, however, can store only a limited amount of glucose as glycogen. Any extra amount of dietary glucose is used for energy needs in preference to dietary and body fat, and limited amounts are converted to body fat. When there is an inadequate intake of dietary carbohydrate, the body has to use protein to make glucose. This is important for maintaining a certain level of blood glucose for the energy needs of the brain. Thus a large amount of protein is diverted from its own important functions. Therefore a supply of glucose must be kept available to minimize the use of protein for energy. This is called the *protein-sparing action* of glucose. Adequate dietary carbohydrate is also important for the cells of many tissues to use fats for energy, and products of incomplete fat metabolism, *ketone bodies*, accumulate when the diet has too little carbohydrate.

---

diet term used when referring to one's usual food selections

nutrients chemical substances in food that nourish the body by providing energy and the building materials needed to regulate chemical reactions in the body

macronutrients provide energy in the form of calories and include carbohydrates, fat, and protein

micronutrients include vitamins and minerals and help to regulate bodily functions

nutrient density foods that contribute more to the nutrient needs of the body rather than the energy needs of the body are classified as having a favorable nutrient density

carbohydrates a primary food substance mainly responsible for providing energy during high-intensity muscular activity

Fiber

In recent years, researchers have given considerable attention to the importance of fiber in the diet. Fiber forms the structural parts of plants and is not digested by humans. Fiber is not found in animal sources of food. At times you may have eaten a stringy piece of meat. Those tough fibers were proteins and not the same material as plant fiber. There are two kinds of dietary fiber: soluble and insoluble. Soluble fiber includes gums and pectins; cellulose is the primary insoluble form. Sources of soluble fiber are oatmeal, legumes, and some fruits. Food sources of insoluble fiber include whole grain breads and bran cereals. Both forms of fiber have healthful properties.

Since it is not digested, fiber passes through the intestinal tract and adds bulk. Fiber aids normal elimination by reducing the amount of time required for wastes to move through the digestive tract. This is believed to reduce the risk of colon cancer. In countries where people consume more fiber than Americans, colon cancer is uncommon. Also, increased fiber intake is thought to reduce the risk of coronary artery disease. Soluble forms of fiber bind to cholesterol passing through the digestive tract and prevent its absorption. Microbial digestion of some fiber sources in the large intestine may result in production of substances that are absorbed and lower cholesterol synthesis in your body. This can reduce blood cholesterol levels. In addition, foods rich in saturated fats (meats, in particular) that are not eaten in moderation, as recommended by the Food Pyramid, often take the place of fiber-rich foods in the diet, thus increasing cholesterol absorption and formation. Also, consumption of adequate amounts of fiber has been associated with lowered incidences of obesity, constipation, colitis, appendicitis, and diabetes.

The recommended amount of fiber in the diet is approximately 25 grams per day. The average American consumes only 10 to 15 grams per day. It is recommended that individuals who consume too little fiber increase the amount of whole grain cereal products and fruits and vegetables in their diets rather than use fiber supplements to increase fiber intake. However, excessive consumption of fiber may cause intestinal discomfort and increased losses of calcium and iron.

Lipids

Fats are the major lipid in the diet and are another essential component of the diet. They are the most concentrated source of energy, providing more than twice the calories per gram when compared to carbohydrates or proteins. Fat is used as a primary source of energy for many body tissues. Some dietary fat is needed to make food more flavorful and for sources of the fat-soluble vitamins. Also, a minimal amount of some types of fat is essential for normal growth and development.

In the United States, dietary fat represents a high percentage of the total caloric intake. For many Americans, a substantial amount of the fat is from saturated fatty acids. This intake is believed to be too high and may contribute to our prevalence of obesity, certain cancers, and coronary artery disease. The recommended intake should be limited to less than 30% of total calories, with saturated fat reduced to less than 10% of total calories.

Saturated Versus Unsaturated Fat

Both plant and animal foods provide sources of dietary fat. Dietary fats exist as triglycerides, which are compounds that consist of three fatty acids attached to glycerol. About 95% of the lipid we eat is fat. Depending on their chemical nature, fatty acids may be saturated or unsaturated. The unsaturated fatty acids can be subdivided into monounsaturates or polyunsaturates. Therefore the terms *saturated*, *monounsaturated*, and *polyunsaturated* are used to describe the chemical nature of the fat in foods. The triglycerides that make up food fats are usually mixtures of saturated and unsaturated fatty acids but are classified according to the type that predominates. For example, canola oil is high in monounsaturated fatty acids and contains smaller amounts of saturated and polyunsaturated fatty acids. Therefore it is classified as a monounsaturated fat.

In general, fats containing more unsaturated fatty acids are from plants and are liquid at room temperature. Vegetable oils from corn, cottonseed, sunflower, and soybean sources are rich in polyunsaturates. Canola, peanut, and olive oil contain large amounts of monounsaturates. Both forms of unsaturated fatty acids may protect against heart disease, especially the monounsaturates. However, saturated fatty acids tend to raise blood cholesterol levels, thus contributing to the development of coronary artery disease. Therefore foods containing more unsaturated fatty acids should be used as substitutes for those containing higher amounts of saturated fats.

Saturated fatty acids are derived mainly from animal sources. These include the fat in meats, such as beef, pork, and lamb, and much of the fat in eggs and dairy products, such as cream, butter, milk, and cheese. Coconut and palm oils, unlike most plant oils, are highly saturated. Initially, highly *un*saturated vegetable fats are used to make margarines, but through the hydrogenation process they become more saturated. This process allows the product to be shaped into sticks, but it also detracts from the benefits of the oil's original unsaturated fatty acid content. With the abundance of processed foods eaten today, it is important to remember that hydrogenated fats and coconut and palm oil are common ingredients in many processed food products.

Other Lipids

Phospholipids and sterols represent the remaining 5% of lipids in our diet. Phospholipids include lecithin; cholesterol is the best known sterol. Cholesterol is consumed in the diet from animal foods, and it is not supplied by plant sources of food. Generally it is wise to avoid eating foods high in cholesterol. Although it is essential for many body functions, the body can manufacture cholesterol from CHO, proteins, and especially saturated fat. Thus there is little if any need to consume additional amounts of cholesterol in the diet. The American Heart Association recommends consuming less than 300 mg/day. Chapter 2 explored the role of cholesterol and the lipoproteins in the development of atherosclerosis.

The omega-3 fatty acids, a group of unsaturated fatty acids, apparently have the capability of reducing the likelihood of diseases such as heart disease, stroke, and hypertension. Also, these fatty acids may improve conditions such as asthma, migraine headaches, and menstrual disorders. These fatty acids are found in cold-water fish such as salmon, herring, tuna, and sardines. Selecting seafood for at least one meal a week is often recommended. However, experts do not recommend the use of fish-oil supplements as a source of the omega-3 fatty acids.

Proteins

Proteins make up the major structural components of the body. They are needed for growth, maintenance, and repair of all body tissues. In addition, proteins are needed to make enzymes, many hormones, and antibodies that help fight infection. In general the body prefers not to use much protein for energy; instead it relies on fats and carbohydrates. Protein intake should be around 12% to 15% of total calories. A summary of current percentages and recommended percentages of calories from carbohydrates, fats, and proteins is shown in Figure 9-1.

The body's need for protein increases during periods of growth, such as during infancy, adolescence, and pregnancy. Also, breastfeeding women have higher needs because proteins are being used to make the protein in their milk. The rapid gain in lean tissue and bone during the adolescent growth spurt is an indication that protein needs are relatively high during this time of life. At this time, about 1 gram of protein is recommended per kilogram of body weight. (One kilogram equals 2.2 pounds.) Both males and

females experience this increase in lean tissue; however, the increase for females is not as great as that for males. By the time the adolescent reaches age 18, the recommended intake for protein drops to 0.8 gram per kilogram. For healthy individuals, protein intake should not exceed 1.6 grams per kilogram.

Amino Acids

The basic units that make up proteins are smaller compounds called *amino acids*. Many of the body's proteins are made up of about 20 amino acids. Amino acids can be linked together in a wide variety of combinations, which is why there are so many different forms and uses of proteins. Most of the amino acids can be produced as needed in the body. The others cannot be made to any significant degree and therefore must be supplied by the diet. These are referred to as the *essential* amino acids. The amount of protein and the levels of the individual essential amino acids in these proteins is important for determining the quality of one's diet. A diet that contains large amounts of protein will not support growth, repair, and maintenance of tissues if the essential amino acids are not available in the proper proportions.

Most of the proteins from animal foods contain all of the essential amino acids (as well as all the nonessential amino acids) that humans require and are called *complete* or *high-quality proteins*. Examples are the proteins found in meat, fish, poultry, eggs, milk, and other dairy products. Incomplete proteins, that is, those sources of protein that do not contain all of the essential amino acids, usually are from plant sources of food. A type of gelatin, which is a product made from animals, is an incomplete protein. Many think that it will improve the growth and appearance of fingernails; this is not true. The protein in nails is different from that in gelatin.

Protein Sources and Need

Fortunately, you do not have to eat all of your food from animal sources of protein. The complete sources of protein can be mixed with the incomplete to form nutritious combinations. For example, rice contains incomplete protein. When mixed with a small amount of chicken (complete protein), the quality of

---

fats primary food substance that can provide energy during long-term endurance activities
lipids include fats, oils, and cholesterol
proteins make up the major structural components of the body and are needed for growth, maintenance, and repair of all body tissues, including the production of enzymes, hormones, and antibodies needed to help fight infection

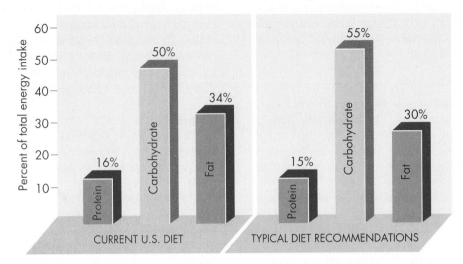

FIGURE 9-1. **Comparison of Calories from Carbohydrates, Fats, and Proteins.**
(From Wardlaw GM, Insel PM: *Perspectives in nutrition,* ed 3, St Louis, 1996, Mosby.)

the protein in the rice is enhanced. Two sources of incomplete proteins, peanut butter and bread, if eaten individually, would not support growth. If eaten as a sandwich, the amounts of the different amino acids complement each other and thus the sandwich is a source of complete protein. Many cultures around the world use such complementary combinations because high-quality animal sources may be less available. Vegetarianism, an alternative eating style for Americans, uses many of the principles of combining various incomplete proteins to obtain more high-quality protein sources. This lifestyle is discussed later in this chapter.

Most North Americans do not have difficulty meeting protein needs, since the typical diet is rich in protein. We tend to consume more than twice the recommended levels of protein. For example, a single day's menu may include ham and eggs with a glass of milk for breakfast; a cheeseburger, baked beans, and a glass of milk for lunch; and chicken with rice and another glass of milk for dinner. This supplies over 100 grams of protein for the day.

Protein Supplementation. There is no advantage to consuming more protein, particularly in the form of protein supplements. Amino acid supplements should be avoided. If more protein is supplied than needed, the body must remove the amino group from the amino acids and excrete it in the urine as urea. The remainder of the amino acid compound must be used for energy instead of fat or carbohydrate. This can create a situation in which excess water is removed from cells, leading to dehydration and possible damage to

the kidneys or liver. Protein supplements may also create imbalances of the chemicals that make up proteins, the amino acids, which is not desirable. A condition of the bones called *osteoporosis* has been linked to a diet that contains too much protein.

Increased physical activity increases one's need for energy and protein, but the increases in muscle mass that result from conditioning and training are associated with only a small increase in protein requirements. These increased protein needs can easily be met with the usual diet. Recent evidence has shown that excessive protein supplementation of 3 to 4 gm/kg of body weight per day can harm the kidneys, increase calcium excretion, and (ironically) inhibit muscle growth and endurance performance. Therefore no protein supplements are needed for the healthy individual who is in a fitness program.

Production of Energy from Carbohydrates, Fats, and Proteins

Energy is obtained from the breakdown of CHO, fats, and proteins to release ATP energy. Glucose is broken down to produce ATP energy in a process referred to as *glycolysis*. Fats and the amino acids from proteins are broken down using related chemical steps. Anaerobic and aerobic conditions that influence the particular amount of energy that can be generated in the breakdown of the energy-supplying nutrients were described in Chapter 5.

The proportions of each of the three energy-supplying nutrients that are used at any one time are a function of the type, duration, and intensity of the activity. During activities with low intensity levels, such as sitting around watching TV or studying, fat is used to provide the bulk of the body's energy needs. Fat is also used primarily in low-intensity, long-duration exercise. Carbohydrates provide the only source of energy for anaerobic situations involving muscle contraction. Carbohydrates are used in high-intensity activities; the harder the work, the greater the use of CHO. The exact role of proteins as an energy source at this point is unclear. Formerly, it was thought that the amino acids from proteins were not used to any appreciable extent for energy. Recent evidence seems to indicate that as much as 10% to 15% of energy needed to sustain endurance activities is from protein. Under conditions in which the activity is sustained over a long duration, all three sources of energy are used. Most sports activities are intermittent in nature, with periods of anaerobic and aerobic situations. Therefore some combination of metabolic processes is used to generate energy from the three sources of calories.

REGULATOR NUTRIENTS (MICRONUTRIENTS)
Vitamins

Although they are required in very small amounts when compared to water, proteins, carbohydrates, and fats, vitamins perform essential roles primarily in the synthesis of regulators of body processes. The need for vitamins was discovered late in the last century. Scientists tried to formulate artificial diets using mixtures of the energy-supplying nutrients and ash, the material that remained after food was burned. Animals fed this synthetic diet did not survive. However, when given a mixture of the artificial food and some natural foods, the animals thrived. Early in this century, scientists recognized that some component of natural foods was necessary for life; these compounds were referred to as vitamins.

In the decades that followed, researchers identified the 13 chemicals found in food that we now know as vitamins and determined their specific roles in the body. Many of these roles are still being explored. Formerly, letters were assigned as names for vitamins. Today, most are known by their scientific names. Table 9-1 lists the different vitamins, their major functions, and their food sources. Vitamins are classified into two groups; the fat-soluble vitamins are dissolved in fats and stored in the body, and the water-soluble vitamins are dissolved in watery solutions and are not stored.

Fat-Soluble Vitamins

Vitamins A, D, E, and K are fat soluble. They are found in the fatty portions of foods and in oils. Since they are stored in the body's fat, it is possible to con-

sume excess amounts and show the effects of vitamin poisoning. The fat-soluble vitamins are less readily excreted and are less likely to be destroyed in cooking than are the water-soluble vitamins.

Vitamin A is important for maintaining vision, for mucus-forming cell activity in the body, for ensuring the health of the immune system, and for various aspects of growth and development. Vitamin A has a precursor or provitamin, beta-carotene. Beta-carotene is the deep yellow/orange pigment found in many fruits and vegetables. In the body, some of the beta-carotene is converted to vitamin A. Because consumption of a diet high in fruits and vegetables is associated with good health, many believe beta-carotene may have important disease-fighting qualities. However, this association may be due to the numerous other phytochemicals present in fruits and vegetables.

Vitamin D is an unusual vitamin in the sense that it may be synthesized by skin cells in the presence of sunlight. Vitamin D is activated in the liver and kidneys to form the hormone calcitriol. Calcitriol increases calcium absorption in the intestine and, along with other hormones, works to maintain calcium metabolism in bones and other organs.

Vitamin E functions to prevent destruction of red blood cells by functioning as an antioxidant (to be discussed later). The likelihood of finding vitamin E deficiencies is low except in smokers or in individuals who have difficulty absorbing fat.

Vitamin K is important in blood clotting. About half of the vitamin K absorbed every day comes from bacterial synthesis in the intestines; the other half comes from the diet. Deficiencies are unlikely. Newborn infants are given an injection of vitamin K because they are born with sterile GI tracts.

Water-Soluble Vitamins

The water-soluble vitamins consist of vitamin C, known as ascorbic acid, and the B-complex vitamins, most now referred to by their scientific names. B-complex vitamins include thiamin (B_1), riboflavin (B_2), niacin (B_3), B_6, folate, B_{12}, biotin, and pantothenic acid. Although vitamins are not metabolized for energy, thiamin, riboflavin, niacin, biotin, and pantothenic acid are used to regulate the metabolism of CHO, proteins, and fats to obtain energy. B_6 regulates the body's use of amino acids. Folate and B_{12} are important in normal blood-cell formation. Vitamin C is used for building bones and teeth, maintaining the

> **vitamins** organic compounds needed in the diet to help support chemical reactions in the body

TABLE 9-1. Vitamins

Vitamin	Major function	Most reliable sources	Deficiency	Excess (toxicity)
A	Maintains skin and other cells that line the inside of the body; bone and tooth development; growth; vision in dim light	Liver, milk, egg yolk, deep green and yellow fruits and vegetables	Night blindness, dry skin, growth failure	Headaches, nausea, loss of hair, dry skin, diarrhea
D	Normal bone growth and development	Exposure to sunlight; fortified dairy products; eggs and fish liver oils	"Rickets" in children—defective bone formation leading to deformed bones	Appetite loss, weight loss, failure to grow
E	Prevents destruction of polyunsaturated fats caused by exposure to oxidizing agents; protects cell membranes from destruction	Vegetable oils, some in fruits and vegetables, whole grains	Breakage of red blood cells leading to anemia	Nausea and diarrhea; interferes with vitamin K if vitamin D is also deficient. Not as toxic as other fat-soluble vitamins
K	Production of blood-clotting substances	Green leafy vegetables; normal bacteria that live in intestines produce K that is absorbed	Increased bleeding time	
B_1 (thiamin)	Needed for release of energy from carbohydrates, fats, and proteins	Cereal products, pork, peas, and dried beans	Lack of energy, nerve problems	
B_2 (riboflavin)	Energy from carbohydrates, fats, and proteins	Milk, liver, fruits and vegetables, enriched breads and cereals	Dry skin, cracked lips	
B_3 (niacin)	Energy from carbohydrates, fats, and proteins	Liver, meat, poultry, peanut butter, legumes, enriched breads and cereal	Skin problems, diarrhea, mental depression, and eventually death (rarely occurs in U.S.)	Skin flushing, intestinal upset, nervousness, intestinal ulcers
B_6	Metabolism of protein; production of hemoglobin	White meats, whole grains, liver, egg yolk, bananas	Poor growth, anemia	Severe loss of coordination from nerve damage
B_{12}	Production of genetic material; maintains central nervous system	Foods of animal origin	Neurological problems, anemia	
Folate (folic acid)	Production of genetic material	Wheat germ, liver, yeast, mushrooms, green leafy vegetables, fruits	Anemia	
C (ascorbic acid)	Formation and maintenance of connective tissue; tooth and bone formation; immune function	Fruits and vegetables	"Scurvy" (rare), swollen joints, bleeding gums, fatigue, bruising	Kidney stones, diarrhea
Pantothenic acid	Energy from carbohydrates, fats, and proteins	Widely found in foods	Not observed in humans under normal conditions	
Biotin	Use of fats	Widely found in foods	Rare under normal conditions	

tissues that hold muscles and other tissues together (connective tissues), and strengthening the immune system. Unlike fat-soluble vitamins, the water-soluble vitamins cannot be stored to any significant extent in the body and should be supplied in the diet each day.

Antioxidant Nutrients

Recently, research information has suggested that a group of nutrients referred to as antioxidants may help to protect the body from a number of potentially harmful chemical reactions and may possibly prevent premature aging, certain types of cancer, heart disease, and other chronic diseases, thus improving long-term health. From normal ongoing physiological processes within the body, chemical reactions occur that produce oxygen molecules called *free radicals*. These free radicals can combine with other chemicals to create compounds that can play a major role in tissue damage. Antioxidants seem able to reduce the free radical mediated oxidative damage to cells by protecting vital cell components from the destructive effects.

Vitamin C, vitamin E, and beta-carotene are antioxidants. Beta-carotene is a plant pigment that is found in dark green, deep yellow, or orange fruits and vegetables. The body can convert beta-carotene to vitamin A. In the early 1980s, researchers reported that smokers who ate large quantities of beta-carotene–rich fruits and vegetables were less likely to develop lung cancer than were other smokers. Since that time, more evidence is accumulating about the benefits of a diet rich in the antioxidant nutrients. In a recent study, supplements of beta-carotene actually increased the rate of lung cancer in long-time male Finnish smokers. This result may have occurred by chance because these Finnish men had been heavy smokers for an average of over 30 years. Many nutritionists believe the benefits of a diet high in fruits and vegetables is associated with the numerous phytochemicals in these foods rather than a single compound.

Some experts believe people should increase their intake of antioxidants, even if it means taking supplements. Others are much more cautious because the long-term safety and efficacy of supplements are unknown. As long as an individual continues to eat a variety of foods, consumption of a nutrient beyond RDA levels is not considered a risk. However, self-prescribed supplements of individual nutrients above RDA levels are often considered a health risk because the nutrient is taken in excess as unbalanced biochemistry. Excessive consumption of beta-carotene causes pigments to circulate throughout the body, which may turn your skin yellow. Use of vitamin C supplements may be dangerous for individuals who

absorb higher-than-normal amounts of dietary iron. Vitamin C increases iron absorption and causes release of iron stores. The result can be a toxic level of iron in the blood. In addition, excesses of vitamin C are not well absorbed; the excess is irritating to the intestines and creates diarrhea. Although less toxic than vitamins A or D, too much vitamin E causes health problems as indicated in Table 9-1.

Vitamin Deficiencies

The illness that results from a lack of any nutrient, especially those needed in such small amounts as the vitamins, is referred to as a *deficiency disease*. Vitamin deficiency diseases are rare in the U.S. However, chronic alcoholics and people consuming bizarre diets often show signs of one or more deficiency diseases. As with the other nutrients, adequate amounts of the different vitamins can be obtained if a wide variety of foods is eaten. For most people, vitamin supplements are a waste of money and can cause toxic effects if too many are taken. Many individuals think that vitamins are "foods" and are safe. However, in large doses, vitamins have druglike effects on the body. Table 9-1 describes some problems associated with both deficiencies and excesses of the different vitamins.

Minerals

Over 20 mineral elements have an essential role in the body and therefore need to be supplied in the diet. These include the minerals listed in Table 9-2. Many other mineral elements are found in the body, although their roles have not been determined. Some of these, such as mercury, lead, gold, and silver, probably have no role but are environmental contaminants that can be measured in body tissues. Mercury and lead are known to be harmful. Most minerals are stored in the body, especially in the liver and bones (which explains why liver usually leads the list of most nutritious foods.) Some minerals perform their roles independently; others play roles along with other minerals or nutrients. For example, magnesium is needed in energy-supplying reactions; sodium and potassium are important for the transmission of nerve impulses. Iron plays a role in energy metabolism but

---

antioxidants a group of nutrients that protect the body from a number of potentially harmful chemical reactions and may prevent premature aging, certain types of cancer, heart disease, and other chronic disease

minerals inorganic compounds, found in small amounts in the body, that are required for normal physiological function

TABLE 9-2.   Minerals of Major Concern

Mineral	Major role	Most reliable sources	Deficiency	Excess
Calcium	Bone and tooth formation; blood clotting; muscle contraction; nerve function	Dairy products	May lead to osteoporosis	Calcium deposits in soft tissues
Phosphorus	Skeletal development; tooth formation	Meats, dairy products, and other protein-rich foods	Rarely seen	
Sodium	Maintenance of fluid balance	Salt (sodium chloride) added to foods and sodium-containing preservatives		May contribute to the development of hypertension
Iron	Formation of hemoglobin; energy from carbohydrates, fats, and proteins	Liver and red meats, enriched breads and cereals	Iron-deficiency anemia	Can cause death in children from supplement overdose
Copper	Formation of hemoglobin	Liver, nuts, shellfish, cherries, mushrooms, whole grain breads and cereals	Anemia	Nausea and vomiting
Zinc	Normal growth and development	Seafood and meats	Skin problems, delayed development, growth problems	Interferes with copper use; may decrease HDL levels
Iodine	Production of the hormone thyroxin	Iodized salt, seafood	Mental and growth retardation; lack of energy	
Fluorine	Strengthens bones and teeth	Fluoridated water	Teeth are less resistant to decay	Damage to tooth enamel

is also combined with a protein to form hemoglobin, the compound that transports oxygen in red blood cells. Calcium has many important functions. It is necessary for proper bone and teeth formation, blood clotting, and muscle contraction.

In general, minerals have numerous roles in various body functions. The section of this chapter that describes mineral supplementation provides information about some of the minerals that are often consumed in limited amounts in the average American diet. If intakes are limited, deficiency diseases can occur.

Vitamins are often confused with minerals. Vitamins are complicated chemical compounds, whereas minerals are often used in their elemental form, such as calcium, phosphorus, or sodium. Some of this confusion is from our familiarity with vitamins and minerals in combination forms known as *nutritional supplements*. The range of safe blood levels for most minerals is very limited, and excesses can lead to toxic effects. Therefore obtaining toxic levels of intake is more likely when one misuses mineral supplements. For example, many small children suffer accidental iron poisoning by taking their mothers' iron pills or overdose themselves on candy-flavored children's vitamin/mineral supplements. As with the vitamins, eating a wide variety of foods is the best way to obtain the minerals needed in the proper concentrations.

Water

Water is the most essential nutrient; one can exist for weeks or even months without protein, vitamins, or minerals. Without water, one perishes in a few days. Most of the body is made up of water, approximately 60% of the adult's weight, although it is interesting to note that in obese individuals the percentage of body water decreases possibly as low as 45%. Water is essential for all body processes because many of the other nutrients are dissolved in water. An adequate supply of water is needed for energy production, digestion, and maintaining the proper environment inside and outside cells.

Water is also necessary for body temperature regulation and for elimination of many waste products from the body. Too little water leads to a condition called *dehydration*; severe dehydration leads to death. The average adult requires a minimum of 2.5 liters of water per day. Water is consumed from beverages and obtained from foods, especially fruits and vegetables.

The healthy body maintains proper internal water levels, conserving or excreting water primarily in urine, but moisture losses from sweat and breath can be substantial. If environmental temperatures are too high and one is sweating excessively, the body's ability to conserve water can be negatively affected. The symptoms of dehydration include fatigue, vomiting, nausea, exhaustion, and fainting. Water must be replaced or death occurs. Therefore water is a critical nutrient for the physically active person, especially when exercise is carried out in hot, humid weather. Failure to consume sufficient quantities of water is often due to being preoccupied with the activity and ignoring the body's thirst signals. Waiting until you become thirsty is often too late in terms of obtaining adequate water replacement during exercise. This is especially true during prolonged exercise in a hot environment. Advice concerning exercising in hot, humid weather was presented in Chapter 4.

NUTRIENT REQUIREMENTS AND RECOMMENDATIONS

A **nutrient requirement** is the amount of the nutrient that is needed to prevent the nutrient's deficiency disease. Determining the precise amounts of nutrients that are needed by individuals is not practical. However, it is known that nutrient needs vary among individuals within a population. Some people may require relatively small amounts of a particular vitamin or mineral. If they don't obtain that level, over time they will start to show the signs of that nutrient's deficiency disease. Fortunately, the levels of nutrients present in foods are adequate to meet the needs of most healthy individuals.

A **nutritional recommendation** for a nutrient is different than the requirement. Scientists establish recommendations for nutrients and calories. First, researchers determine the amount of the nutrient that prevents the deficiency disease for most people. Then an additional amount, referred to as the *margin of safety*, is included. This additional amount ensures that nearly every person, even those who have unusually high needs for the nutrient, will be covered by the recommended level. Most nutrient recommendations are developed in this manner. Every few years, the Food and Nutrition Board of The National Research Council of the Academy of Sciences establishes guidelines called *Recommended Dietary Allowances (RDAs)* that are generally developed by the method described above. These figures are determined by extensive sci-

entific research and assessment of present dietary intakes in the United States, as well as whether or not any deficiencies exist within the population. Other countries have similar standards. Table 9-3 shows the latest RDAs.

Many confuse nutrient recommendations with nutrient requirements. For example, the RDA for ascorbic acid is 60 mg. This does not mean that the *requirement* for ascorbic acid is 60 mg. Recall that for most nutrients, RDAs are set at a level that is higher than the amount needed by the average person to meet the nutrient needs of the majority of the healthy U. S. population. Furthermore, these recommendations were not designed for individuals to use but rather for researchers to determine the nutritional status of a population. For example, if you analyzed your food records from 1 day, you might determine that you are obtaining only 50 mg of ascorbic acid (vitamin C). Although the RDA for vitamin C is 60 mg, you probably don't have to worry about developing scurvy, the deficiency disease. In general, if you are consuming about $2/3$ of the RDA level, it is likely that your diet is adequate. However, if your daily intakes are consistently very low, the likelihood of deficiency symptoms increases.

Food Labels

The USRDAs (United States Recommended Dietary Allowances) were designed to help consumers compare the nutritional value of many food products. For over a decade, the USRDA appeared on nutrient labels. However, this information has been replaced by a new nutrient label format (the Daily Values [DVs]), which uses new standards. These Daily Values include two categories: Reference Daily Intakes (RDIs) (for nutrients with an RDA) and Daily Reference Values (for compounds without an RDA). A sample of the new label is shown in Figure 9-2 (pp. 278 to 279).

Health educators believe that the new format will help consumers make more informed food selections. Concern over the amount of fat, cholesterol, sodium, and fiber in the typical American diet and appropriate health claims on food labels led the drive for a more health-conscious label. A food label presents information in the form of percentages that are based on a

---

nutrient requirement amount of a nutrient required (which varies slightly by individual) to prevent the nutrient's deficiency disease
nutritional recommendation a nutrient requirement plus a "margin of safety;" this is a scientifically determined amount of a nutrient that is slightly above the average amount of a nutrient needed to prevent disease

TABLE 9-3.   Recommended Dietary Allowances[a], Revised 1989

Category	Age (years) or condition	Weight[b] (kg)	(lb)	Height[b] (cm)	(in)	Protein (g)	Fat-soluble vitamins Vitamin A (μg RE)[c]	Vitamin D (μg)[d]	Vitamin E (mg α-TE)[e]	Vitamin K (μg)
Males	15-18	66	145	176	69	59	1000	10	10	65
	19-24	72	160	177	70	58	1000	10	10	70
	25-50	79	174	176	70	63	1000	5	10	80
	51+	77	170	173	68	63	1000	5	10	80
Females	15-18	55	120	163	64	44	800	10	8	55
	19-24	58	128	164	65	46	800	10	8	60
	25-50	63	138	163	64	50	800	5	8	65
	51+	65	143	160	63	50	800	5	8	65
						60	800	10	10	65
Pregnant	1st 6 months					65	1300	10	12	65
Lactating	2nd 6 months					62	1200	10	11	65

[a]The allowances, expressed as average daily intakes over time, are intended to provide for individual variations among most normal persons, since they live in the United States under usual environmental stresses. Diets should be based on a variety of common foods to provide other nutrients for which human requirements have been less well defined. See text for detailed discussion of allowances and of nutrients not tabulated.

[b]Weights and heights of reference adults are actual medians for the US population of the designated age, as reported by NHANES II. The use of these figures does not imply that the height-to-weight ratios are ideal.

standard 2000 Calories and the "percent daily values" shown on the label. For example, a $1/2$ cup serving of a particular food might provide 10% of the recommended daily limit of cholesterol intake of 300 mg. The cholesterol content of other foods that were eaten would have to be added to this to determine whether the day's total cholesterol intake was less than the recommended amount.

Dietary Guidelines

The newest edition of *Nutrition and Your Health: Dietary Guidelines for Americans* (1995) was presented to the nation in the beginning of 1996. This publication includes a list of seven Dietary Guidelines with expanded explanatory text describing the rationale for the individual Dietary Guidelines (Figure 9-3, p. 280). A panel of eminent scientists revised the Dietary Guidelines from the previous edition of 1990. These Dietary Guidelines are basic nutrition advice aimed at the American population with its modern lifestyles. Use of the Food Guide Pyramid (see Figure 9-4) and Nutrition Facts Label on foods (see Figure 9-2) is essential for individuals to follow the Guidelines. The Guidelines provide advice for healthy Americans age 2 and older. To meet the Dietary Guidelines, which should promote health and lower the risk for premature chronic diseases, Americans need to choose a diet with most of the calories from grain products, vegetables, fruit, low-fat milk products, lean meats, fish, poultry, and dry beans. Individuals should also choose fewer calories from fats and sweets.

The Dietary Guidelines continue to emphasize eating a variety of foods (first Guideline). This is best accomplished by choosing a variety of foods from within and across the five food groups from the Food Guide Pyramid. In order to consume a variety of food and eat a nutritious and enjoyable diet, Americans should increase the number of calories burned in daily activities and should choose nutrient-dense foods. Sometimes supplements are necessary, but use of supplements cannot substitute for proper food choices because foods contain many nutrients and other substances that promote health. Most vegetarians eat milk products and eggs and enjoy excellent health. Strict vegetarians (vegans) consume only foods of plant origin and require greater care in meeting their nutritional needs; they must supplement their diets with a source of vitamin B_{12}.

The latest edition of Dietary Guidelines promotes physical activity as critical for energy balance for weight maintenance (second Guideline). In addition, there is no longer an allowance for a higher acceptable weight for adults age 35 and older. The Guidelines advise that a loss of only 5% to 10% of body weight may improve health; they also warn against the practice of unhealthy behaviors such as self-induced vomiting. As found in previous editions, the current edition continues to caution against excessive thinness, losing weight too quickly, and weight-reducing diets for children. Vigorous activity, along with limiting fat intake (but *not* food restriction), is recommended for helping overweight children achieve a healthy

TABLE 9-3.   Recommended Dietary Allowances[a], Revised 1989—cont'd

Water-soluble vitamins							Minerals						
Vitamin C (mg)	Thiamin (mg)	Riboflavin (mg)	Niacin (mg NE)[f]	Vitamin B_6 (mg)	Folate (μg)	Vitamin B_{12} (μg)	Calcium (mg)	Phosphorus (mg)	Magnesium (mg)	Iron (mg)	Zinc (mg)	Iodine (μg)	Selenium (μg)
60	1.5	1.8	20	2.0	200	2.0	1200	1200	00	12	15	150	50
60	1.5	1.7	19	2.0	200	2.0	1200	1200	350	10	15	150	70
60	1.5	1.7	19	2.0	200	2.0	800	800	350	10	15	150	70
60	1.2	1.4	15	2.0	200	2.0	800	800	350	10	15	150	70
60	1.1	1.3	15	1.5	180	2.0	1200	1200	300	15	12	150	50
60	1.1	1.3	15	1.6	180	2.0	1200	1200	280	15	12	150	55
60	1.1	1.3	15	1.6	180	2.0	800	800	280	15	12	150	55
60	1.0	1.2	13	1.6	180	2.0	800	800	280	10	12	150	55
70	1.5	1.6	17	2.2	400	2.2	1200	1200	320	30	15	175	65
95	1.6	1.8	20	2.1	280	2.6	1200	1200	355	15	19	200	75
90	1.6	1.7	20	2.0	260	2.6	1200	1200	340	15	16	200	75

[c]Retinol equivalents. 1 retinol equivalent = 1 μg retinol or 6 μg β-carotene.

[d]As cholecalciferol. 10 μg cholecalciferol = 400 IU of vitamin D.

[e]α-Tocopherol equivalents. 1 mg d-α tocopherol = 1 α-TE.

[f]1 NE (niacin equivalent) is equal to 1 mg of niacin or 60 mg of dietary tryptophan.

weight. However, monitoring of growth by a health professional is strongly advised.

The other five Dietary Guidelines continue to emphasize grain products, fruits, and vegetables as the cornerstone of our diets (third Guideline); the choice of lower-fat products from the milk and meat Food Groups (fourth Guideline); limitation of the use of products with high amounts of sodium or salt (fifth Guideline); moderation in consumption of foods high in simple sugars and no other nutrients (sixth Guideline); and consumption of alcoholic beverages in moderation (if consumed at all).

However, new to the current edition of the Dietary Guidelines is the recommendation of "no more than 30% of total calories" from fat as opposed to the previous recommendation of "30% or less." This revision is intended to downplay the implication that the lower the fat the better. The recommendation also includes replacing higher levels of fat in the diet with grain products, vegetables, and fruits rather than with low-fat, high-sugar foods that are high in calories but have few or no other nutrients. The Dietary Guidelines also have included a statement that says diets high in sugar do not cause diabetes or hyperactivity.

The Health Link and Fit List boxes on pp. 281 and 283 provide some ideas for changing your diet to meet these new dietary guidelines. Since being introduced in the late 1970s, the recommendations have become more accepted by the American public. As a result, the food industry has introduced many new and reformulated products that are low fat, low cholesterol, low sodium, high fiber, or have fewer calories.

FOOD PYRAMID

The RDAs are not practical, and the Dietary Guidelines are too broad to use when trying to plan menus that are nutritious. Not everyone has the time to look up the nutrient content of food selections in food composition tables such as those in Appendix B. Thus food guides were developed as a convenient and easy way to determine the quality of one's diet. Most people are familiar with the "Basic Four Food Groups Plan," which was first introduced in the mid-1950s. More recently, the Basic Four has been redesigned into a *Food Pyramid* concept that is believed to do a better job of educating Americans about the relationship of food choices to health. Figure 9-4 (p. 282) shows the Food Pyramid. For most of the food groupings, a minimum number of servings that should be eaten daily is specified, as are examples of foods from this group. As you can see, carbohydrate-rich foods (the breads and cereals group) form the foundation of the diet. This reflects the recommendations in the Dietary Guidelines that suggest that we need to consume a greater percentage of total calories from this group. The other food groups are shown according to their relative importance in a healthy diet. One major change from the Basic Four plan is that the fruits and vegetables are separated into two distinct groups, each with a specified number of servings. Note that fats and sugars form the small apex of the Pyramid. This indicates that foods rich in fat and sugar should provide the smallest proportion of total calories; no minimum number of servings is suggested, since many Americans consume far too much fat and sugar.

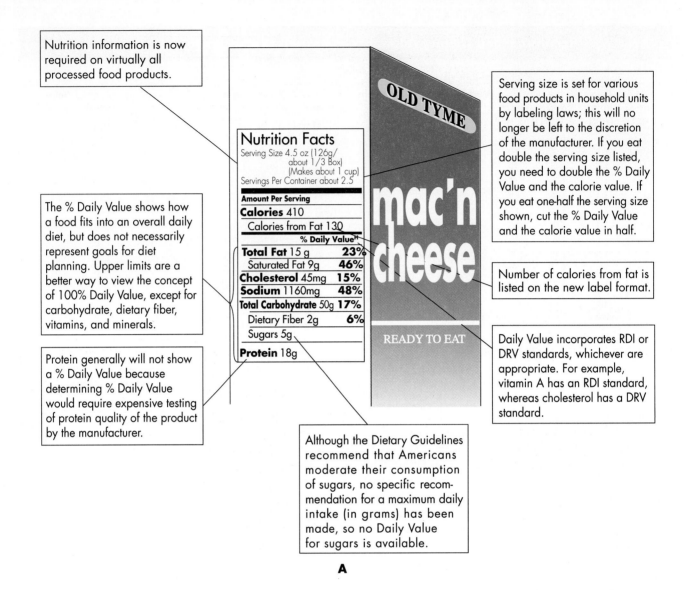

Nutrition information is now required on virtually all processed food products.

The % Daily Value shows how a food fits into an overall daily diet, but does not necessarily represent goals for diet planning. Upper limits are a better way to view the concept of 100% Daily Value, except for carbohydrate, dietary fiber, vitamins, and minerals.

Protein generally will not show a % Daily Value because determining % Daily Value would require expensive testing of protein quality of the product by the manufacturer.

Serving size is set for various food products in household units by labeling laws; this will no longer be left to the discretion of the manufacturer. If you eat double the serving size listed, you need to double the % Daily Value and the calorie value. If you eat one-half the serving size shown, cut the % Daily Value and the calorie value in half.

Number of calories from fat is listed on the new label format.

Daily Value incorporates RDI or DRV standards, whichever are appropriate. For example, vitamin A has an RDI standard, whereas cholesterol has a DRV standard.

Although the Dietary Guidelines recommend that Americans moderate their consumption of sugars, no specific recommendation for a maximum daily intake (in grams) has been made, so no Daily Value for sugars is available.

Nutrition Facts
Serving Size 4.5 oz (126g/ about 1/3 Box) (Makes about 1 cup)
Servings Per Container about 2.5

Amount Per Serving
Calories 410
Calories from Fat 130

% Daily Value**

Total Fat 15 g   **23%**
Saturated Fat 9g   **46%**
Cholesterol 45mg   **15%**
Sodium 1160mg   **48%**
Total Carbohydrate 50g **17%**
Dietary Fiber 2g   **6%**
Sugars 5g
Protein 18g

OLD TYME

mac'n cheese

READY TO EAT

A

FIGURE 9-2. **The Nutrition Facts Panel on a Current Food Label.**
The box is broken into two parts: **A** is the top and **B** is the bottom. The % Daily Value listed on the label is the percentage of the generally accepted amount of nutrient needed daily that is present in one serving of the product. You can use the % Daily Values to compare your diet with current nutrition recommendations for certain diet components.
(From Wardlaw GM, Insel PM: *Perspectives in nutrition,* ed 3, St Louis, 1996, Mosby.)

Many vitamin and mineral amounts no longer need to be listed on the nutrition label. Only vitamin A, vitamin C, calcium, and iron remain. The interest in or risk of deficiencies of the other vitamins and minerals is deemed too low to warrant inclusion.

Some Daily Value standards, such as grams of total fat, increase as energy intake increases. The % Daily Values on the label are based on a 2000 kcal diet.

Labels on larger packages may list the number of calories per gram of fat, carbohydrate, and protein.

Ingredients, listed in descending order by weight, will appear here or in another place on the package. The sources of some ingredients, such as certain flavorings, will be stated by name to help people better identify ingredients that they avoid for health, religious, or other reasons.

Vitamin A 10%	• Vitamin C 0%
Calcium 30%	• Iron 15%

Percent Daily Values are based on a 2,000 calorie diet. Your daily values may be higher or lower depending on your calorie needs:

		Calories:	2,000	2,500
Total Fat	Less than		65g	80g
Sat Fat	Less than		20g	25g
Cholest	Less than		300mg	300mg
Sodium	Less than		2,400mg	2,400mg
Total Carb			300g	375g
Fiber			25g	30g

Calories per gram:
Fat 9 • Carbohydrate 4 • Protein 4

INGREDIENTS: WATER, ENRICHED MACARONI (ENRICHED FLOUR [NIACIN FERROUS SULFATE (IRON), THIAMINE MONONITRATE AND RIBOFLAVIN], EGG WHITE), FLOUR, CHEDDAR CHEESE (MILK, CHEESE CULTURE, SALT, ENZYME), SPICES, MARGARINE (PARTIALLY HYDROGEN-ATED SOYBEAN OIL, WATER, SOY LECITHIN, MONO- AND DIGLYCERIDES, BETA CAROTENE FOR COLOR, VITAMIN A PALMITATE), AND MALTODEXTRIN.

GOOD SOURCE OF CALCIUM SEE SIDE PANEL FOR NUTRITION INFORMATION

Absolute and comparative claims, as well as health claims, can appear on the front panel or on the sides of the package. All must follow legal definitions.

B

FIGURE 9-2. **The Nutrition Facts Panel on a Current Food Label—cont'd.**

- Eat a variety of foods

- Balance the food you eat with physical activity—maintain or improve your weight

- Choose a diet with plenty of grain products, vegetables, and fruits

- Chose a diet low in fat, saturated fat, and cholesterol

- Choose a diet moderate in sugars

- Choose a diet moderate in salt and sodium

- If you drink alcoholic beverages, do so in moderation

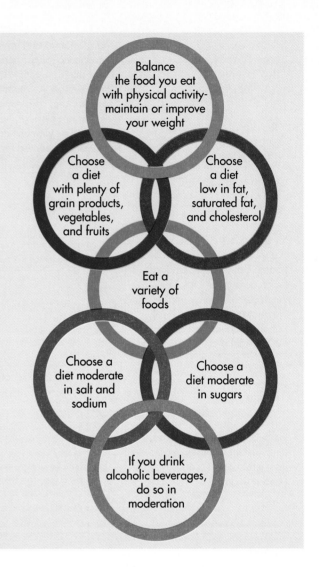

FIGURE 9-3. The 1995 Dietary Guidelines for Americans.
(Redrawn from US Department of Agriculture and US Department of Health and Human Services: *Nutrition and your health: dietary guidelines for Americans*, ed 4, Washington, DC, 1995.)

NUTRITION AND PHYSICAL ACTIVITY

Physically active individuals often believe that exercise increases requirements for nutrients such as proteins, vitamins, and minerals and that it is possible and desirable to saturate the body with these nutrients. There is no scientific basis for ingesting nutrients as supplements unless a medically diagnosed deficiency exists. Exercise increases the need for nutrients, but these needs can be met with dietary food intake. It is necessary to explore some of the more common myths that surround the subject of nutrition's role in physical performance.

Vitamin Supplementation

Many individuals believe that taking large amounts of vitamin supplements (pills) can lead to superior health and performance. A *megadose* of a nutrient supplement is essentially an overdose; the amount ingested far exceeds the RDA levels. The rationale used for such excessive intakes is that if a pill that contains the RDA for each vitamin and mineral makes you healthy, then taking a pill that has 10 times the RDA should make you 10 times healthier. Using that kind of logic is the same as thinking that if one aspirin makes you feel better by reducing soreness, then taking 10 aspirins will make you feel that much better.

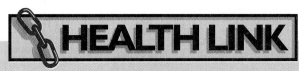

WHAT COUNTS AS A SERVING?*

Grain Products Group (Bread, Cereal, Rice, and Pasta)
- 1 slice of bread
- 1 ounce ready-to-eat cereal
- $1/2$ cup cooked cereal, rice, or pasta

Vegetable Group
- 1 cup raw leafy vegetables
- $1/2$ cup other vegetables—cooked or chopped raw
- $3/4$ cup vegetable juice

Fruit Group
- 1 medium apple, banana, or orange
- $1/2$ cup chopped, cooked, or canned fruit
- $3/4$ cup fruit juice

Milk Group (Milk, Yogurt, and Cheese)
- 1 cup milk or yogurt
- $1 1/2$ ounces natural cheese
- 2 ounces processed cheese

Meat and Beans Group (Meat, Poultry, Fish, Dry Beans, Eggs, and Nuts)
- 2 to 3 ounces cooked lean meat, poultry, or fish
- $1/2$ cup cooked dry beans or 1 egg counts as 1 ounce lean meat
- Two tablespoons peanut butter or 1/3 cup nuts counts as 1 ounce of meat

From US Department of Agriculture and US Department of Health and Human Services: *Nutrition and your health: dietary guidelines for Americans,* ed 4, Washington, DC, 1995.

*Some foods fit into more than one group. Dry beans, peas, and lentils can be counted as servings in either the meat and beans group or the vegetable group. These "cross-over" foods can be counted as servings from either one or the other group, but not both. Serving sizes indicated here are those used in the Food Guide Pyramid and are based on both suggested and usually consumed portions necessary to achieve adequate nutrient intake. They differ from serving sizes on the Nutrition Facts Label, which reflects portions usually consumed.

Also, people think that nutrients are the same as foods and therefore it's safe to consume them in high levels. Excesses of the water-soluble vitamins are excreted in the urine; excesses of minerals can pass through the digestive tract and are eliminated in bowel movements. However, it is possible to flood the digestive tract with these nutrients so that large quantities, far more than the body can handle at one time, are absorbed. These high levels upset the body's natural balance and create toxic effects.

Vitamin C Supplementation
An example of a popular practice among health-conscious individuals is to take megadoses of vitamin C. Such doses have not been shown to prevent the common cold or slow aging. They do cause diarrhea, hyperabsorption of iron in some individuals, and possibly the development of painful kidney stones. Fruits, juices, and vegetables are reliable sources of vitamin C and also supply other vitamins and minerals.

Vitamin E Supplementation
Taking megadoses of vitamin E has become popular among people of all ages. The vitamin functions to protect polyunsaturated fatty acids in cell membranes from being damaged. There is not much evidence to support the notion that this vitamin can extend life expectancy or enhance physical performance. Vitamin E does not enhance sexual ability, prevent graying hair, or cure muscular dystrophy. A person can obtain adequate amounts of vitamin E by consuming whole grain products, vegetable oils, and nuts. However, supplements of vitamin E have been associated with lower levels of oxidized LDL and a lower incidence of heart disease. This is a promising area for medical research and a possible new tool in the fight against atherosclerosis. The medical profession is not recommending supplements of vitamin E but is instead issuing a moratorium on supplement use until long-term safety and efficacy are established.

Vitamin B$_{12}$ Supplementation
The B-complex vitamins that are involved in obtaining energy from CHO, fats, and proteins are often abused by athletes who believe that vitamins provide energy. Any increased need for these nutrients is easily fulfilled when the athlete eats more

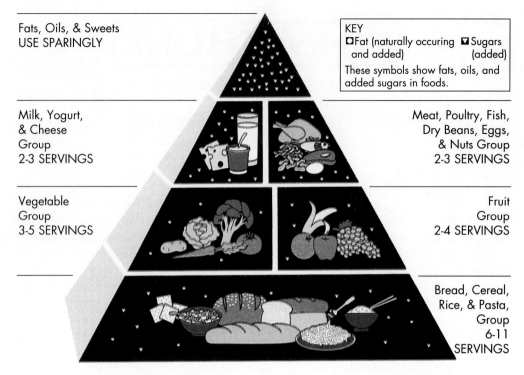

FIGURE 9-4. USDA's Food Guide Pyramid.
Choose foods from each of the five food groups. The Food Guide Pyramid illustrates the importance of balance among food groups in a daily eating pattern. Most of the daily servings should be selected from the food groups that are the largest in the picture and closest to the base of the Pyramid.
- Choose most of your foods from the grain products group (6 to 11 servings), the vegetable group (3 to 5 servings), and the fruit group (2 to 4 servings).
- Eat moderate amounts of foods from the milk group (2 to 3 servings) and the meat and beans group (2 to 3 servings).
- Choose sparingly foods that provide few nutrients and are high in fat and sugars.

NOTE: A range of servings is given for each food group. The smaller number is for people who consume about 1600 calories a day and are sedentary. The larger number is for those who consume about 2800 calories a day and are more active.
(From US Department of Agriculture and US Department of Health and Human Services: *Nutrition and your health: dietary guidelines for Americans*, ed 4, Washington, DC, 1995.)

nutritious foods while training. If athletes do not increase their food consumption, they lose weight because of their high level of caloric expenditure.

Vitamin B_{12} injections are commonly used but would only be effective if they served as a *placebo*. A placebo is a treatment that does not affect the body. However, the person who receives the placebo is told or believes that it will have an impact. The power of the mind is in control; performance often is improved, and the individual swears by the treatment. Under rare conditions, when the person cannot absorb B_{12} from the digestive tract, a B_{12} deficiency occurs and the person becomes quite ill. Furthermore, B_{12} is con-

tained in all animal sources of foods that are widely consumed by Americans.

Mineral Supplementation

Obtaining adequate levels of certain minerals can be a problem for some individuals. Calcium and iron intakes may be low for those who do not include dairy products, red meats, or enriched breads and cereals in their diets. However, one must be careful to first determine whether extra minerals are needed, which will prevent both overdosing and wasting money. The following sections explore some of the minerals that can be lacking in the diet and discuss suggestions for

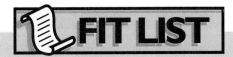

FOOD CHOICES FOR A HEALTHY BODY

- Eat less fat and cholesterol. Eat more lean meats, fish, and poultry. Eat fewer fried foods, chips, and fatty spreads such as margarine and butter.
- When ordering a salad, ask for the dressing "on the side" so that you can control the amount.
- Achieve and maintain a desirable body weight. Chapter 8 addressed this in detail. Eat fewer fatty foods, and exercise more.
- Choose foods that are high in fiber and complex carbohydrates, such as whole grain breads and cereals, rice, tortillas, potatoes, and pasta.
- Eat fewer sugary foods. Drink fewer sugar-sweetened soft drinks.
- Reduce sodium intake by cutting back on salty foods and foods with sodium-containing additives. Read labels for sodium content; don't add salt to foods while cooking; taste foods before adding salt; avoid salty snacks, processed luncheon meats, ham, and pickled foods.
- Use alcohol in moderation, if you choose to drink. Moderation means a limit of two drinks per day. Don't drink and drive or operate other machines. Don't drink if you are trying to become or if you are pregnant.
- Drink fluoridated water. Check with your local water authority to see if fluorine is added to your community's water supply.
- Increase calcium intake by drinking more milk (low-fat) or eating more low-fat yogurt and cheeses.
- Eat more iron-rich foods. Eat food containing vitamin C with vegetable sources of iron to improve the mineral's absorption. Enriched breads and cereals are good sources.

improving the quality of your diet so that supplements may not be necessary.

Calcium

Calcium is the most abundant mineral in the body. It is essential for bones and teeth, muscle contraction, and conduction of nerve impulses. Adequate calcium intake is necessary for infants and growing children.

However, the importance of obtaining adequate calcium supplies throughout life has become more recognized. If calcium intake is too low to meet needs, the body can remove calcium from the bones. Over periods of time, the bones become weakened and appear porous on x-ray films. These bones are brittle and often break spontaneously. This condition is called *osteoporosis* and is estimated to be eight times more common among women than men. The bent-over, humped-back appearance of many older men and women is evidence of the loss of mineral mass in the upper spine, which is no longer able to support the weight of the head. Osteoporosis becomes a serious problem for women after menopause.

It is believed that a lifetime of low calcium intake combined with genetic and hormonal factors affects development of osteoporosis. The RDA for young adults or pregnant and breastfeeding women is 1200 mg; for other adults the RDA is 800 mg (an 8-ounce glass of milk contains about 300 mg of calcium). Physically active amenorrheic women may require as much as 1500 mg, but without resumption of menses and production of estrogen these women continue to risk bone loss. Unfortunately, about 25% of all women in the United States consume less than 300 mg of calcium per day, which is well below the RDA. Also, women who smoke are at greater risk of developing this condition.

High-protein diets and alcohol consumption also increase calcium excretion from the body. Exercise (weight-bearing activity) causes calcium to be retained in bones, so physical activity is beneficial. However, younger women who exercise to extremes so that their normal hormonal balance is upset are prone to develop premature osteoporosis. For women who have a family history of osteoporosis, calcium supplementation, preferably as calcium carbonate or citrate rather than phosphate, may be advisable if they continue to have low intakes of calcium. Check with your doctor before taking any supplements.

Milk products are the most reliable sources of calcium, although other foods, such as fish with edible bones and dried beans and peas, contribute some of the mineral. Many individuals dislike milk, complaining that it "disagrees" with them. They may lack the enzyme *lactase,* which is needed to digest milk sugar, *lactose.* This is referred to as *lactose intolerance* or *lactase deficiency.* The undigested lactose enters the large intestine, where the bacteria that normally reside there use it for energy. The bacteria produce large quantities of intestinal gas, which causes discomfort and cramps. Many lactose-intolerant people also suffer from diarrhea. Fortunately, scientists have produced the missing enzyme, lactase. Lactase is available without prescription in

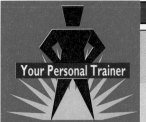

Your Personal Trainer

Phillip Rodriguez, International marketing major
Age: 26

Scenario

I've been in a special work-study program this semester and have had a very easy class load. I've been taking advantage of my extra time by going to the rec center three times a week to swim and weight train. I have also been alternating sessions on the rowing machine and stair stepper. I've never been this fit in my life. I have also had an increased appetite and haven't been holding back in the food department. The problem is even though I'm getting 7 to 8 hours of sleep a night and my workouts have been great, I feel tired and lethargic all the time.

Should I be taking vitamin, mineral, or protein supplements to compensate for my increased physical activity?

Solution

There is a lot of misinformation out there about vitamin and protein supplements that are "designed" to increase performance. Any athlete who is truly consuming anything close to a well-balanced diet will not need vitamin supplementation.

If it is something you really think you need to do, taking a one-a-day multivitamin should not produce negative results. However, the fact that you are getting a fair amount of sleep and eating sufficiently, yet still feel tired, could be related to stress, depression, or even an undiagnosed medical condition like mononucleosis or an iron-deficiency anemia.

It would be wise to consult your physician for a screen of tests to rule out an undiagnosed illness or mineral deficiency.

forms that can be added to foods before eating or taken along with meals.

Iron

Iron deficiency is also a common problem, especially for young females. Lack of iron can result in iron-deficiency *anemia.* Iron is needed to properly form hemoglobin. In this condition, the oxygen-carrying ability of the red blood cells is reduced so that muscles cannot obtain enough oxygen to generate energy. One feels tired and weak. Obviously a person cannot compete at his or her peak level while suffering from an iron deficiency.

Women are more likely to suffer from iron deficiency because they usually eat smaller quantities of food, including those rich in iron, and they experience monthly losses of blood during menstruation. Any time blood is lost from the body, whether it is from blood donation or a serious injury, the body requires a source of iron to form hemoglobin during the production of new red blood cells.

There have been reports that a type of anemia referred to as *sports anemia* often occurs in those involved in training and long-distance running. Whether this is a true anemia is unclear. The bodies of trained athletes undergo an increase in blood volume. If the liquid portion of the blood increases while the number of red blood cells remains the same, it appears as though the red blood cell number is reduced. When their blood is compared to blood from sedentary people, it appears that athletes do not have enough red blood cells and are anemic. However, if the hemoglobin concentration in each red blood cell is normal, the individual is probably healthy.

In general, if a person is mildly anemic and experiences a reduction in performance, it may be reasonable to analyze the diet to determine whether adequate iron-rich foods are being eaten. The person may be able to correct the anemia by consuming iron-rich foods such as red meats, poultry, and enriched breads and cereals. However, if the anemia is serious, performance will be affected. The individual should consult with a physician to determine the source of the problem and obtain advice regarding iron supplementation. Iron supplements should not be taken with coffee or tea because these beverages inhibit iron absorption. It is best to take iron supplements with drinks that are high in vitamin C content because vitamin C causes iron to remain in a more absorbable form.

Sugar and Performance

It has been suggested that ingesting large quantities of glucose in the form of honey, candy bars, or pure sugar immediately before physical activity has a significant impact on performance. As carbohydrates are digested, large quantities of glucose enter the blood. This increase in blood sugar (glucose) levels stimulates the release of the hormone *insulin.* Insulin allows the cells to use the circulating glucose so that blood glucose levels soon return to normal. It was hypothesized that this decline in blood sugar levels was detrimental to performance and endurance. However, recent evidence indicates that for most physically active people, the effect of eating large quantities of carbohydrates is beneficial rather than negative.

Nevertheless, some individuals are sensitive to high carbohydrate intake and experience problems with increased levels of insulin. Also, some people cannot tolerate large amounts of the simple sugar fructose. For these individuals, too much fructose leads to intestinal upset and diarrhea. (Sources of fructose include honey, fruit, and table sugar.) Therefore it is suggested that people test themselves with various high-carbohydrate foods to see if they are affected (but not before a competitive event).

Caffeine

Caffeine is a central nervous system stimulant and was previously discussed in Chapter 3. Most people who consume caffeine in coffee, tea, or carbonated beverages are aware of its effect of increasing alertness and decreasing fatigue. Chocolate contains compounds that are related to caffeine and have the same stimulating effects. However, large amounts of caffeine cause nervousness, irritability, increased heart rate, and headaches. Also, headaches are a withdrawal symptom experienced when one tries to stop consuming caffeinated products.

Although small amounts of caffeine do not appear to harm physical performance, cases of nausea and lightheadedness have been reported. There is evidence that caffeine enhances the use of fat during endurance exercise, thus delaying the depletion of glycogen stores; this would help endurance performance. There is also some evidence that caffeine helps make calcium more available to the muscle during contraction, which would enable the muscle to work more efficiently. However, Olympic officials rightfully consider caffeine to be a drug. It should not be present in an Olympic competitor's blood in levels greater than that resulting from drinking five or six cups of coffee.

Alcohol

Alcohol provides energy for the body; each gram of pure alcohol (ethanol) supplies 7 Calories. However, sources of alcohol provide very little other nutritional value in regard to vitamins, minerals, and proteins. The depressant effects of alcohol on the central nervous system include decreased physical coordination, slowed reaction times, and decreased mental alertness. Also, this drug increases the production of urine, resulting in body water losses (diuretic effect). Therefore use of alcoholic beverages by any individual cannot be recommended before, during, or after physical activity.

Organic, Natural, or Health Foods

Whether or not they are physically active, most people are concerned about the quality of the foods they eat, including both the nutritional value of the food and its safety. Does it contain additives that are dangerous? Should I eat more natural foods and less processed ones? Should I purchase organically grown foods and those described as "health" foods? The following paragraphs examine some of these concerns about the food supply and will help you decide on the need for choosing a more "natural, organic" diet.

Before 1993 there was no legal definition for organic farming methods. Foods grown without the use of synthetic fertilizers and pesticides were described as *organic* and sold in small markets or specialty stores. Those who advocated the use of organic farming methods claimed that these foods were nutritionally superior and safer than the same products grown using chemicals such as pesticides and synthetic fertilizers.

Technically, describing food as organic is meaningless. All foods (except water) are organic; that is, they contain the element carbon. Organically produced foods are often quite expensive compared to the same foods produced by conventional means. For example, organic beef is more costly, but it is supposed to be free of anabolic steroids or growth hormones that may be used by conventional beef producers. However, there is no advantage to consuming organic food products. They are not more nutritious than foods produced by conventional methods. Organic produce often contains small amounts of pesticides because of being grown near farms that use these substances. Nevertheless, for some people the psychological benefit of believing that they are doing something "good" for their bodies justifies the extra cost.

Natural foods have been subjected to very little processing and contain no additives such as preservatives or artificial flavors. However, there is no legal definition for natural, so it is difficult to define how much processing a food can undergo before it becomes "processed" rather than natural. Refined table sugar is a "natural" substance, but it is a pure carbohydrate energy source with no other nutrients. Processing can protect nutritional value. For example, natural foods such as raw fruits and vegetables often lose considerable nutritional value if improperly stored. Preservatives save food that would otherwise spoil and have to be destroyed. Furthermore, many foods in their natural form are quite poisonous. The green layer often found under the skin of potatoes is poisonous if eaten in large amounts. There are poisonous mushrooms and molds in peanuts that could cause liver cancer if their growth were not limited to low amounts.

Both organic and natural foods could be described as *health foods*. However, food experts believe that Americans have the safest and most varied food supply in the world. Our relatively long life expectancy and lack of nutritional deficiencies in comparison to much of the world's population is evidence that our diet is safe and nutritious. Furthermore, even for the athlete no benefit is derived from eating a diet consisting of health foods.

Vegetarianism

Many physically active people are health conscious and try to do things that are good for their bodies. Vegetarianism has emerged as an alternative to the usual American diet. All vegetarians use plant foods to form the foundation of their diet; animal foods are either totally excluded or included in a variety of eating patterns. People who choose to become vegetarians do so for economic, philosophical, religious, cultural, or health reasons. The U.S. Dietary Goals that recommend eating less fat, cholesterol, salt, and sugar while increasing fiber intake easily support a vegetarian eating pattern. As a result, alternative diets such as vegetarianism have become more accepted among Americans. Vegetarianism is no longer considered to be a fad if it is practiced intelligently. However, the vegetarian diet may create deficiencies if nutrient needs are not carefully considered. Physically active people who follow this eating pattern need to plan their diets carefully so that their calorie needs are met. Types of vegetarians include the following:

- *Total vegetarians or vegans:* People who consume plant but no animal foods; meat, fish, poultry, eggs, and dairy products are excluded. This diet has been found to be adequate for most adults if they give careful consideration to obtaining enough calories; sources of vitamin B_{12}; and the minerals calcium, zinc, and iron. It is not recommended for pregnant women, infants, or children because of the difficulty in consuming the quantity of plant foods necessary to meet the caloric and nutritional needs during these life stages.
- *Lactovegetarians:* Individuals who consume milk products along with plant foods. Meat, fish, poultry, and eggs are excluded. Iron and zinc levels can be low in people who practice this form of vegetarianism.

- *Lacto-ovo-vegetarians:* People who consume dairy products and eggs in their diet, along with plant foods. Meat, fish, and poultry are excluded. Again, iron could be a problem.
- *Semivegetarians:* People who consume animal products but exclude red meats. Plant products still form an important part of the diet. This diet is usually adequate.

Preevent Nutrition

The importance and content of the meal eaten before engaging in physical activity has been heatedly debated among coaches, trainers, and physical educators. The trend has been to ignore logical thinking about what should be eaten before competition in favor of upholding the tradition of "rewarding" the athlete for hard work by serving foods that may hamper performance. For example, the traditional steak-and-eggs meal before football games is great for coaches and trainers; however, this is not the best type of meal for the athlete. The important point is that too often people are concerned primarily with the preevent meal and fail to realize that those nutrients consumed over several days before competition are much more important than what is eaten 2 1/2 to 3 hours before an event. The purpose of the preevent meal should be to provide the competitor with sufficient nutrient energy and fluids for competition, while taking into consideration the digestibility of the food and most importantly the eating preferences of the individual athlete. Figure 9-5 gives two examples of preevent meals.

Any physically active person should be encouraged to be conscious of his or her diet. However, there is no experimental evidence to indicate that performance may be enhanced by altering a diet that is basically sound. There are a number of ways that a nutritious diet may be achieved, and the diet that is optimal for one person may not be the best for another. In many instances the individual will be the best judge of what he or she should or should not eat in the preevent meal or before exercising. It seems that a person's best guide is to eat whatever he or she is most comfortable with, within the following basic guidelines:

- Try to achieve the largest possible storage of carbohydrates (glycogen) in both resting muscle and the liver. This is particularly important for endurance activities but may be beneficial for intense, short-duration exercise. More information about specific methods of increasing glycogen storage levels are described later in this chapter.
- A stomach that is full of food during contact sports is subject to injury. Therefore the type of food eaten should allow the stomach to empty quickly. Carbohydrates are easier to digest than fats or pro-

---

FIGURE 9-5. Sample Preevent Meals.

Meal 1

$3/4$ c Orange juice
$1/2$ c Cereal with 1 tsp sugar
1 Slice whole wheat toast with:
   1 tsp Margarine
   1 tsp Honey or jelly
8 oz Skim or lowfat milk
Water
(Approximately 450-500 kcal)

$3/4$ c Orange juice
1-2 Pancakes with:
   1 tsp Margarine
   2 tbsp Syrup
8 oz Skim or lowfat milk
Water
(Approximately 450-500 kcal)

Meal 2

1 c Vegetable soup
1 Turkey sandwich with:
   2 Slices bread
   2 oz Turkey (white or dark)
   1 oz Cheese slice
   2 tsp Mayonnaise
8 oz Skim or lowfat milk
Water
(Approximately 550-600 kcal)

1 c Spaghetti with tomato sauce and cheese
$1/2$ c Sliced pears (canned) on 1/4 c cottage cheese
1-2 Slices (Italian) bread with 1-2 tsp margarine
(avoid garlic)
$1/2$ c Sherbet
1-2 Sugar cookies
4 oz Skim or lowfat milk
Water
(Approximately 700 kcal)

---

teins. A meal that contains plenty of carbohydrates will leave the stomach and be digested faster than a fatty meal. It would be wise to replace the traditional steak-and-eggs preevent meal with a low-fat one containing a small amount of pasta, tomato sauce, and bread.

- Foods should not cause irritation or upset to the gastrointestinal tract. Foods high in cellulose and other forms of fiber, such as whole grain products, fruits, and vegetables, increase the need for defecation. Highly spiced foods or gas-forming foods (such as onions, baked beans, or peppers) must also be avoided because any type of disturbance in the gastrointestinal tract may be detrimental to performance. Carbonated beverages and chewing gum also contribute to the formation of gas.
- Liquids consumed should be easily absorbed and low in fat content and should not act as a laxative. Whole milk, coffee, and tea should be avoided. Water intake should be increased, particularly if the temperature is high.
- A meal should be eaten approximately 2 $1/2$ to 3 hours before the event or before exercising. This allows for adequate stomach emptying, but the individual will not feel hungry during the activity.

- Any food that is disliked should not be eaten. Most important, the individual must feel psychologically satisfied by any preevent meal. Performance may very well be impaired more by psychological factors than by physiological factors.
- Recently, commercially produced, high-calorie liquid meals have been recommended as extremely effective preevent meals. These liquid meals have several advantages: (1) they are generally flavorful and convenient, (2) they contain large quantities of carbohydrates and limited quantities of protein and fat, (3) they generally have high nutritional value, (4) they are liquid and aid in fluid replacement, and (5) they are easily absorbed, leaving little if any undigested material in the intestines by event time. Therefore liquid meals provide an acceptable alternative to traditional preevent meals, but they are an expensive choice.

---

vegetarianism an increasingly popular alternative to the usual American diet, emphasizing the use of vegetables, fruits, legumes, seeds, and nuts to meet the body's food requirements

Glycogen Supercompensation

For endurance events, maximizing the amount of glycogen that can be stored, especially in muscles, may make the difference between finishing first or at the "end of the pack." Glycogen supplies in muscle and liver can be increased by reducing the training program a few days before competing and by significantly increasing carbohydrate intake during the week before the event. Reducing training for at least 48 hours before the competition allows the body to eliminate any metabolic waste products that may hinder performance. The high-carbohydrate diet restores glycogen levels in muscle and the liver. This practice is called glycogen supercompensation. (In the past this has been called glycogen loading.) The basis for this practice is that the quantity of glycogen stored in muscle directly affects the endurance of that muscle.

Glycogen supercompensation is accomplished over a 6-day period divided into three phases. In phase 1 (days 1 to 2), training should be very hard and dietary intake of carbohydrates fairly normal, accounting for about 60% of total Calorie intake. During phase 2 (days 3 to 5), training is cut back, while the individual eats at least 70% or more of the diet in carbohydrates. Studies have indicated that glycogen stores may be increased from 50% to 100%, theoretically enhancing endurance during a long-term event. Phase 3 (day 6) is the day of the event, during which a normal diet must be consumed.

The effect of glycogen supercompensation in improving performance during endurance activities has not yet been clearly demonstrated. It has been recommended that glycogen supercompensation not be done more than two to three times during the course of a year. It must be added that glycogen loading is only of value in long-duration events that produce glycogen depletion, such as in a marathon.

ASSESSMENT OF YOUR NUTRITIONAL AND EATING HABITS

Lab Activity 9-1 helps you calculate carbohydrate, fat, and protein needs. **Lab Activities 9-2** and **9-3** will help you assess both your eating patterns and whether you are currently eating a nutritious diet. **Lab Activity 9-4** helps you follow your eating patterns and food intake over a 7-day period. Are you eating well? **Lab Activity 9-5** tests your knowledge about nutrition. To help you get started eating properly, the following box offers a number of motivational tips.

---

glycogen supercompensation   used by athletes to enhance endurance, this is the practice of decreasing training and increasing carbohydrate intake in the days before a competitive event

---

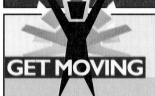

Eating right: things to remember about how and what you eat

1. Remember—it is possible to achieve a balanced diet even though you don't eat something from each of the food groups every day.
2. If taking your "Flintstones vitamin" each day helps you feel better and seems to give you more energy, then by all means—keep taking them. A one-a-day supplement with known required nutrients at RDA levels is usually not necessary, but it is not harmful. Self-prescribing of individual nutrients, especially doses beyond the RDAs, is a concern of nutritionists.
3. Realize that it's OK to occasionally eat a chili dog, pizza, or big juicy steak if you want. The secret is that you can't do this every day—in fact, the less you do it the better off you will be.
4. It is not necessary to avoid fat in your diet. In fact, we need some fat for a number of essential bodily functions, for a palatable diet, and to allow us to follow the Food Pyramid. However, reducing fat intake may help to decrease body fat if we follow the Food Pyramid and are physically active—walking, gardening, exercising, etc. Many people are becoming obese on a low-fat diet because of overconsumption of low-fat snack and dessert products. It is important not to consume more energy than you use. Overeating Calories from any of the three energy nutrients causes weight gain.
5. Write down every type of food that you eat over a 3- to 4-day period to find out how you can better achieve a balanced diet.
6. Eating a healthy diet can help reduce your chances of developing both premature artery disease and cancer.

SUMMARY

- The classes of nutrients are carbohydrates, fats, proteins, vitamins, minerals, and water. Carbohydrates, fats, and proteins provide the energy required for muscular work during activity and also play a role in the function and maintenance of body tissues.
- The energy-providing nutrients are metabolized to provide energy either aerobically or anaerobically (carbohydrate only), depending on the availability of oxygen.
- Vitamins are substances found in food that have no caloric value but are necessary to regulate body processes. Vitamins may be either fat soluble (vitamins A, D, E, and K) or water soluble (B-vitamins and vitamin C).
- The essential minerals are necessary in most physiological functions of the body.
- Water is the most essential of all the nutrients and should be of great concern to anyone involved in physical activity.
- A nutritious diet consists of eating a variety of foods in amounts recommended in the Food Pyramid. If your diet meets those recommended amounts, nutrient supplementation is not necessary.
- Organic or natural foods have no beneficial effect on performance.
- Protein supplementation during weight training is not necessary if a nutritious diet is maintained.
- Many individuals, especially women, need to increase dietary calcium; otherwise they may require calcium supplementation to prevent osteoporosis.
- Individuals with low iron status need to increase their consumption of iron from meat, fish, or poultry, and it also may be necessary to supplement their diet with extra iron to prevent iron-deficiency anemia.
- Vegetarian diets can provide all of the essential nutrients if care is taken and the diet is well thought-out and properly prepared.
- The preevent meal should be (1) higher in carbohydrates, (2) easily digested, (3) eaten $2\,1/2$ to 3 hours before an event, and (4) psychologically pleasing.
- Glycogen supercompensation involves maximizing resting stores of glucose in the muscle, blood, and liver before a competitive event.

REFERENCES

Allred J: Too much of a good thing? An overemphasis on eating low-fat foods may be contributing to the alarming increase in overweight among US adults, *J Am Diet Assoc* 95:417-418, 1995.

Beltz S, Doering P: Efficacy of nutritional supplements used by athletes, *Clin Pharm* 12:900-908, 1993.

Burke L, Read R: Dietary supplements in sport, *Sports Med* 15(1):43-65, 1993.

Clark K: Working with college athletes, coaches and trainers at a major university, *Int J Sports Med* 4:135-141, 1994.

Cole K, Grandjean R, Sobszak R: Effect of carbohydrate composition on fluid balance, gastric emptying and exercise performance, *Int J Sport Nutr* 3:408-417, 1993.

Coleman E: Eating before exercise, *Sports Med Digest* 16(4):6-10, 1995.

Coleman E: Nutritional concerns of vegetarian athletes, *Sports Med Digest* 17(2):1-3, 1995.

Costill D, Hargreaves M: Carbohydrate nutrition and fatigue, *Sports Med* 13(2):86-92, 1992.

Cowart V: Dietary supplements: alternatives to anabolic steroids? *Phys Sports Med* 20(3):24, 1993.

Diplock A: Antioxidant nutrients and disease prevention; an overview, *Am J Clin Nutr* 53:189S, 1991.

Dodd S, Herb R, Powers S: Caffeine and exercise performance: an update, *Sports Med* 15-14-23, 1993.

Food and Drug Administration: Food labeling: reference daily intakes, *Federal Register* 59(2):427-432, 1994.

Food and Nutrition Board, National Academy of Sciences—National Research Council: *Recommended dietary allowances,* ed 11, Washington, DC, 1995, US Government Printing Office.

Grandjean A: Practices and recommendations of sports nutritionists, *Int J Sports Nutr* 3:232-242, 1993.

Grunewald K, Bailey R: Commercially marketed supplements for body building athletes, *Sports Med* 15(2):90-103, 1993.

Hayes AE: United States government policies and programs in nutrition and physical fitness, *Am J Clin Nutr* 49(suppl 5):1039, 1989.

Hennekens C, Buring J, Peto R, editors: Antioxidant vitamins—benefits not yet proved, *New Engl J Med* 330:1080-1081, 1994.

Herbert V: Health claims in food labeling and advertising: literal truths but false messages; deceptions by omission of adverse facts, *Nutr Today* 19:25-30, 1987.

Herbert V: The antioxidant supplement myth, *Am J Clin Nutr* 60:157-158, 1994.

Herbert V: Viewpoint: does mega-C do more good than harm, or more harm than good? *Nutr Today* 28:28-32, 1993.

Holt W: Nutrition and athletes, *Am Fam Physician* 47:1757-1764, 1993.

Horton T et al: Fat and carbohydrate overfeeding in humans: different effects on energy storage, *Am J Clin Nutr* 62:19-29, 1995.

James WP: The role of nutrition and fitness in chronic diseases, *Am J Clin Nutr* 49(suppl 5):933, 1989.

Kirshner E, Lewis R, O'Connor P: Bone mineral density and dietary intake of college gymnasts, *Med Sci Sports Exerc* 24(4):543-549, 1995.

Kleiner S: Nutrition on the run, *Phys Sports Med* 23(2):15-16, 1995.

Kleiner S: The beef on food myths, *Phys Sports Med* 20(10):23-24, 1992.

Kreider R: Amino acid supplementation and exercise performance: analysis of the proposed ergogenic value, *Sports Med* 16(3):190-209, 1993.

Lemon P, Proctor D: Protein intake and athletic performance, *Sports Med* 12(5):313-325, 1991.

Lindamen A: Eating for endurance and ultraendurance, *Phys Sports Med* 20(3):87-101, 1992.

McArdle W, Katch F, Katch V: *Exercise physiology: energy, nutrition, and human performance*, Philadelphia, 1994, Lea & Febiger.

Millard-Stafford M: Fluid replacement during exercise in the heat: review and recommendations, *Sports Med* 13(4):223-233, 1992.

Payne W, Hahn D: *Focus on health*, ed 2, St Louis, 1995, Mosby.

Rauch L, Rodger I, Wilson J: The effects of carbohydrate loading on muscle glycogen content and cycling performance, *Int J Sports Med* 5(1):25-36, 1995.

Reimers K: The role of liquid supplements in weight gain, *Strength Cond* 17(1):64-64, 1995.

Rimm E et al: Vitamin E consumption and the risk of coronary heart disease in men, *New Engl J Med* 328:1450-1456, 1993.

Sherman WM, Peden MC, Wright DA: Carbohydrate feedings 1 hour before exercise improves exercise performance, *Am J Clin Nutr* 54:866, 1991.

Short S: Health quackery: our role as professionals, *J Am Diet Assoc* 94:607-611, 1994.

Sobal J, Marquat L: Vitamin/mineral supplementation use among athletes: a review of the literature, *Int J Sports Med* 4:320-334, 1994.

Springer K, Hager M: Beyond vitamins, *Newsweek* April 25, 1994.

Stampfer M et al: Vitamin E consumption and the risk of coronary disease in women, *New Engl J Med* 328:1444-1449, 1993.

The alpha-tocopherol, beta-carotene cancer prevention study group: The effect of vitamin E and beta-carotene on the incidence of lung cancer and other cancers in male smokers, *New Engl J Med* 330:1029-1035, 1994.

US Department of Agriculture and US Department of Health and Human Services: *Nutrition and your health: dietary guidelines for Americans*, ed 4, Washington, DC, 1995.

US Department of Health and Human Services/Department of Agriculture: *Nutrition and your health: dietary guidelines for Americans*, Washington, DC, 1985, US Government Printing Office.

US Department of Health and Human Services, Public Health Services: *Healthy People 2000: midcourse review and 1995 revisions*, Washington, DC, 1995, USDHHS.

US Department of Health and Human Services, Public Health Services: *Healthy people 2000: national health promotion and disease prevention objectives*, Washington, DC, 1991, USDHHS.

Voelker R: Ames agrees with mom's advice: eat your fruits and vegetables, *J Am Med Assoc* 273:1077-1078, 1995.

Wardlaw GM, Insel PM: *Perspectives in nutrition*, ed 3, St Louis, 1996, Mosby.

Wiita B, Stombaugh I, Bush J: Nutrition knowledge and eating patterns of young female athletes, *JOHPERD* 66(3):33-41, 1995.

Williams C: Diet and endurance fitness, *Am J Clin Nutr* 49(suppl 5):1077, 1989 (review).

Williams M: The use of nutritional ergogenic aids in sports: is it an ethical issue? *Int J Sport Nutr* 4:120-131, 1994.

SUGGESTED READINGS

Barrett S, Herbert V: *The vitamin pushers: how the "health food" industry is selling America a bill of goods*, Buffalo, 1994, Prometheus Books.
Outlines how the health-food companies have created a multi–billion dollar industry, mostly by preying on the fears of uninformed consumers.

Clark N: *Sport nutrition guidebook: eating to fuel your active lifestyle*, Champaign, 1990, Leisure Press.
Contains real-life case studies of nutritional advice given to athletes and provides recommendations for pregame meals.

Cooper K: *Antioxidant revolution*, Nashville, 1994, Thomas Nelson.
Discusses the latest research on antioxidants and tells how they can decrease the risk of cancer and heart disease, delay premature aging, and power the immune system to fight disease.

Crayhorn R: *Nutrition made simple: a comprehensive guide to the latest findings in optimal nutrition*, New York, 1994, M Evans.
Discusses topics including what constitutes a healthy diet, how you can increase your energy, which healthy fats are essential for weight loss and disease prevention, and the role of antioxidants.

Pennington JA: *Food values of portions commonly used*, New York, 1992, Harper Perennial.
Identifies the complete nutrient content, including calories, cholesterol, salt, fats, vitamins, minerals, and fiber of essentially any food that you could eat.

Williams M: *Nutrition for fitness and sport*, Dubuque, 1992, William C Brown.
An excellent and comprehensive guide to the concepts of sound nutrition for individuals engaging in sport or fitness activities.

Yetiv J: *Popular nutritional practices: a scientific appraisal*, Toledo, 1986, Popular Medicine Press.
Comprehensive analysis of nutritional issues and assessment from the perspective of good scientific practice.

Lab Activity 9-1

Calculating Carbohydrate, Fat, and Protein Needs

Name _____ Section _____ Date _____

PURPOSE   To calculate the amount of carbohydrate, fat, and protein you need in your diet.

PROCEDURE   In the space labeled *Calorie Requirement* on the worksheet below, insert your total calories expended as calculated in Lab Activity 8-7 in the previous chapter. Then fill in the
remaining spaces as indicated.

Your Carbohydrate Needs

Carbohydrate Calories = Calorie Requirement × Percent Carbohydrate Recommended (60% to 70%)

_____ × _____ = _____
Calorie Requirement   .60 to .70*   Carbohydrate Calories

Grams of Carbohydrate = Carbohydrate Calories ÷ 4 Calories/gram†

_____ ÷ _____ = _____
Carbohydrate Calories   4 Calories/gram   Grams of Carbohydrate

Your Protein Needs

Body Weight (kg) = Body Weight (lb) ÷ 2.2

_____ ÷ _____ = _____
Body Weight (lb)   2.2   Body Weight (kg)

Protein Requirement (grams) = Body Weight (kg) × .36 to .68 grams/kg

_____ × _____ = _____
Body Weight (kg)   .36 to .68 grams‡   Grams of Protein

---

*If you train for 2 hours or more, use 70%, otherwise 60% should be adequate.
†Consuming more than 600 grams of carbohydrates will not increase glycogen stores further, so if your calculation exceeds 600, target 600
grams.
‡If you engage in intense, endurance exercise daily or are pursuing an aggressive body-building program, use up to 1.5 grams/kg.

Continued.

Your Fat Needs

Fat Calories = Calorie Requirement × Percent Fat Recommended (20% to 25%)

_____ ×	_____ =	_____
Calorie Requirement	.20 to .25	Fat Calories

Grams of Fat = Fat Calories ÷ 9 Calories/Gram

_____ ÷	_____ =	_____
Fat Calories	9 Calories/gram	Grams of Fat

Lab Activity 9-2

Assessing Your Nutritional Habits

Name _____   **Section** _____   **Date** _____

PURPOSE   To identify food-related behaviors.

PROCEDURE   Indicate the number that best describes the frequency of your food-related behavior.

Point Values

0 = never   1 = rarely   2 = occasionally   3 = often   4 = always

2	1. Every day I eat a nutritious breakfast.
2	2. I try to include recommended servings from each of the food groups in my daily diet.
1	3. I eat food without salting it.
2	4. When I snack, I choose fruits, vegetables, low-fat yogurt, or cheese.
2	5. I try to include mostly fresh and less-processed foods in my daily diet.
3	6. I avoid fatty foods and trim off the visible fat from meats.
3	7. I include foods containing fiber, such as fruits, vegetables, whole-grain products, and beans, in my diet.
4	8. I drink skim milk instead of whole or 2% milk.
1	9. I consume fish at least once a week.
2	10. I consume caffeine-free beverages.
1	11. I avoid foods that contain large amounts of honey and sugar.
1	12. For reliable nutrition information, I ask a qualified nutritionist instead of relying on the popular press.
4	13. I do not drink alcoholic beverages.
4	14. I keep my weight within acceptable limits.
4	15. I obtain my nutrients through foods rather than relying on nutritional supplements.
36	TOTAL POINTS

INTERPRETATION

SCORE

50–60	Excellent	Your food-related behavior should contribute to your ability to maintain good health. Keep it up!
45–49	Good	If you make some minor improvements to your food-related behavior, it should be easy to move into the *excellent* rating category.
39–44	Fair	Analyze the statements to determine which had the lowest scores. Then think about actions you can take to improve your nutritional behavior.
<39	Poor	You need to make major changes in your food-related behavior to improve your nutritional status and your overall health. Analyze your responses to the statements and read Chapter 9 carefully.

Modified from Allen R, Hyde R: *Investigation in stress control,* Minneapolis, 1981, Macmillan.

How Does Your Diet Rate?

Name _____ **Section** _____ **Date** _____

PURPOSE   To determine how nutritionally sound your diet is.

PROCEDURE   Answer each of the following questions, and record the appropriate number of points for each answer. Total the number of points after completing all 29 questions.

_____ 1. How many fast-food meals do you have a week? (Salad bar snacks don't count.)

Answers	Score
a. none	a. +3
b. 1	b. 0
c. 2	c. −1
d. 3	d. −2
e. 4 or more	e. −3

_____ 2. How often do you drink? (One serving = 12 oz regular or light beer, 4 oz wine, or 1 oz liquor.)

Answers	Score
a. 1 or less a week	a. +3
b. 2–3 a week	b. −1
c. 4–6 a week	c. −1
d. 1–2 a day	d. −2
e. more than 2 a day	e. −3

_____ 3. How many of your weekly meals include cheese? (Low fat cottage cheese does not count; cream cheese snacks, pizza, cheeseburgers, cheese, and meat dishes do.)

Answers	Score
a. 1 or less	a. −2
b. 2–3	b. +1
c. 4–5	c. −2
d. 6 or more	d. −3

_____ 4. How often weekly do you have fish or shellfish (other than deep-fried entrees or fishsticks)?

Answers	Score
a. none	a. −2
b. 1–2 times	b. +1
c. 3–4 times	c. +2
d. 5 or more times	d. +3

_____ 5. How often do you eat deep-fried foods in a 4-week period (fish, chicken, vegetables, snack foods)?

Answers	Score
a. none	a. +3
b. 1–2	b. 0
c. 3–4	c. −1
d. 5 or more	d. −3

Continued.

_____   6. How often per week are cold cuts or other processed meats (franks, bacon, sausage) on your menu?

Answers	Score
a. none	a. +3
b. 1–2	b. +2
c. 3–4	c. –1
d. 5 or more	d. –3

_____   7. How often per week do you eat freshly prepared red meat (steak, roast beef, beef patties, lamb, pork chops, etc.)?

Answers	Score
a. 1 or less	a. +3
b. 2–3	b. +2
c. 4–5	c. –1
d. 6 or more	d. –3

_____   8. How many times a day do you have vegetables? (One serving = $1/2$ cup; potatoes count.)

Answers	Score
a. none	a. –3
b. 1	b. 0
c. 2	c. +1
d. 3	d. +2
e. 4 or more	e. +3

_____   9. How many servings of the cancer-proofing cruciferous vegetables do you eat per week (broccoli, cauliflower, cabbage, brussels sprouts, greens, kale, kohlrabi, turnips)?

Answers	Score
a. none	a. –3
b. 1–3	b. +1
c. 4–6	c. +2
d. 7 or more	d. +3

_____   10. How many servings of fruits or vegetables do you eat per week to get vitamin A and beta-carotene (vegetable form of vitamin A) (carrots, pumpkins, sweet potatoes, cantaloupe, spinach, winter squash, greens, apricots, broccoli, deep green and yellow fruits and vegetables)?

Answers	Score
a. none	a. –3
b. 1–3	b. +1
c. 4–6	c. +2
d. 7 or more	d. +3

_____   11. Do you eat chicken and turkey without the skin?

Answers	Score
a. yes	a. +3
b. no	b. –3
c. don't eat any	c. +3

_____   12. What do you spread on bread, toast, and muffins?

Answers	Score
a. butter	a. –3
b. cream cheese	b. –3
c. margarine	c. –2
d. diet margarine	d. –1
e. jam	e. 0
f. sugar-reduced spreads or nothing	f. +3

_____ 13. What do you drink most?

Answers	Score
a. fruit juices	a. +3
b. water or club soda	b. +3
c. diet soda	c. −1
d. coffee or tea	d. −1
e. soda or fruit drink	e. −3

_____ 14. How much caffeine do you drink daily? (One serving = 1 cup coffee, 1 cup regular tea, or 12 oz regular cola.)

Answers	Score
a. none	a. +3
b. 1	b. +1
c. 2	c. −1
d. 3	d. −2
e. 4 or more	e. −3

_____ 15. How do you usually season your meals?

Answers	Score
a. garlic or lemon juice	a. +3
b. herbs or spices	b. +3
c. nothing	c. +2
d. soy sauce	d. −3
e. salt	e. −3

_____ 16. Which of these snacks do you eat most?

Answers	Score
a. fruits or vegetables	a. +3
b. low-fat yogurt	b. +2
c. nuts	c. −1
d. chips	d. −2
e. cookies	e. −2
f. granola bar	f. −2
g. candy bar	g. −3

_____ 17. How many times do you have canned or made-from-a-mix soup a week?

Answers	Score
a. none	a. +3
b. 1–2	b. 0
c. 3–4	c. −2
d. 5 or more	d. −3

_____ 18. How many egg yolks do you have weekly? (Include souffles, omelettes, egg puddings, etc.)

Answers	Score
a. 2 or less	a. +3
b. 3–4	b. +2
c. 5–6	c. −1
d. 7 or more	d. −3

_____ 19. Which would you most often select for dessert? (Don't include low-fat, sugar-free versions.)

Answers	Score
a. pie or cake	a. −3
b. ice cream	b. −3
c. yogurt, ice milk, or fruit ice	c. +1
d. fresh fruit or no dessert	d. +3

Continued.

_____ 20. How many calcium-rich foods do you eat a day? (One serving = $2/3$ cup milk or yogurt; 1 oz cheese; 1 $1/2$ oz sardines; 3 oz salmon or 5 oz tofu; 1 cup broccoli.)

Answers	Score
a. none	a. −3
b. 1	b. +1
c. 2	c. +2
d. 3 or more	d. +3

_____ 21. Which of these sandwich fillings would you most often choose?

Answers	Score
a. red meat	a. −3
b. cheese	b. −1
c. peanut butter	c. +1
d. tuna, crab, or salmon	d. +3
e. chicken or turkey	e. +3

_____ 22. What else do you use in sandwiches?

Answers	Score
a. mayonnaise	a. −2
b. low-fat, low-salt mayonnaise	b. −1
c. mustard or ketchup	c. 0
d. nothing	d. +3

_____ 23. Which of these "extras" do you eat at a salad bar?

Answers	Score
a. nothing, lemon, or vinegar	a. +3
b. reduced-calorie dressing	b. +1
c. regular dressings and/or croutons, bacon bits	c. −1
d. cole slaw, pasta salad, potato salad	d. −1

_____ 24. What type of milk do you use?

Answers	Score
a. whole	a. −2
b. 2% lowfat	b. 0
c. 1% lowfat	c. +2
d. $1/2$% or skim	d. +3
e. none	e. 0

_____ 25. How many meals do you have weekly that include dried beans, split peas, or lentils?

Answers	Score
a. none	a. −1
b. 1	b. +1
c. 2	c. +2
d. 3	d. +3

_____ 26. How many whole-grain foods do you eat daily? (Sugar-coated cereal does not count; sugar-free cereals, whole wheat pancakes, cooked cereal, brown or converted rice, bulgur [wheat], rye bread, etc. do.)

Answers	Score
a. none	a. −3
b. 1–2	b. 0
c. 3–4	c. +1
d. 5–6	d. +2
e. 7 or more	e. +3

_____ 27. How many servings of fresh fruit or juice do you have per day? (One serving = 1 piece of fruit or 6 oz juice.)

Answers	Score
a. none	a. –3
b. 1	b. 0
c. 2	c. +1
d. 3	d. +2
e. 4 or more	e. +3

_____ 28. Do you eat lean meats only?

Answers	Score
a. yes	a. +3
b. no	b. –3
c. don't eat meat at all	c. +3

_____ 29. What type of bread do you most often eat?

Answers	Score
a. whole wheat	a. +3
b. rye	b. +2
c. pumpernickel	c. +2
d. white	d. –2

_____ TOTAL POINTS

INTERPRETATION

Score
51 to 85   Excellent
21 to 50   Good. You have a diet to be proud of. Keep it up.
20 and below   You need help. Review the suggestions made in Chapter 9 to improve your diet.

Lab Activity 9-4

Seven-Day Diet Analysis

Name _____ **Section** _____ **Date** _____

PURPOSE   To determine your eating habits during a 7-day period.

PROCEDURE   For a 7-day period, Monday through Sunday, assign yourself the points indicated when each dietary requirement is met. Record your points in the appropriate column for each day. Total your daily and weekly points. Negative points for junk food consumption should be subtracted from your daily and weekly totals.

Food	Points	Maximum Score	Daily Score						
			M	T	W	T	F	S	S
Milk and Milk Products		15							
One cup of milk or equivalent	5								
Second cup of milk or equivalent	5								
Third serving	5								
Vegetables		25							
Three to five servings deep green or yellow	5 each								
Fruits		20							
Two to four servings whole or juices	5 each								
Breads and Cereals		30							
Six or more servings of whole-grain or enriched cereals or breads	5 each								
Protein-Rich Foods		10							
One serving of egg, meat, fish, poultry, cheese, dried beans, or cheese	5								
One or two additional servings of egg, meat, fish, poultry, or or cheese	5								
Junk Foods (or Negative Point Value Foods)									
Sweet rolls	–5								
Fruit pies	–5								
Potato chips, corn chips, or cheese twists	–5								
Candy	–5								
Nondiet sodas	–5								
	TOTAL	100							

Continued.

Point Record

Weekly point total   _____

Negative point total   _____

Adjusted weekly point total   _____

INTERPRETATION

600-700   Excellent dietary practices

450-599   Adequate dietary practices

300-499   Marginal dietary practices

Below 300   Poor dietary practices

Assessing Your Dietary Practices

1. On which day of the week was it most difficult for you to eat a balanced diet? Why? _____

   _____

   _____

   _____

   _____

2. Approximately what percentage of your total points was from foods purchased in a restaurant? _____

   _____

   _____

   _____

3. Approximately how much money did you spend on food during this 7-day period? _____

   _____

4. Was this a typical 7-day period in terms of the types of food eaten? If not, describe how a more typical 7-day period would appear. _____

   _____

   _____

   _____

   _____

5. Your instructor may prepare a dietary profile of the class against which you can evaluate your personal 7-day diet assessment.

Lab Activity 9-5

Nutritional Knowledge Survey

Name _____   **Section** _____   **Date** _____

PURPOSE   To test your knowledge about nutrition.

PROCEDURE   Consider the following statements and answer *True* or *False* in the space to the left of the statement. Answers and an explanation are on the next page, as is information on how to interpret your score.

_____   1.   Butter has more calories than the same amount of margarine.

_____   2.   Carbohydrates are fattening.

_____   3.   Vitamins provide energy for the body.

_____   4.   Excessive amounts of certain vitamins can cause health problems.

_____   5.   Cholesterol is dangerous and should be avoided.

_____   6.   If your serum cholesterol levels are low, you don't have to worry about heart disease.

_____   7.   Millions of Americans suffer from hypoglycemia.

_____   8.   Sugar offers no nutritional value.

_____   9.   Sugar causes hyperactive behavior and attention span disorders in children.

_____   10. Protein supplements are unnecessary for body builders.

_____   11. Zinc supplements will improve your sex drive.

_____   12. Honey is more nutritious than sugar.

_____   13. Meat is essential for a nutritious diet.

_____   14. Fasting removes toxic wastes that build up in your body from dietary sources.

_____   15. Organically grown foods are nutritionally superior to conventionally grown ones.

Answers

1. False   Each has 100 Calories per tablespoon. The nature of the fat is different; butter contains more saturated fat than margarine. Butter also contains cholesterol; margarine does not. However, these differences do not affect the number of calories per serving.

2. False   Carbohydrates contribute 4 Calories per gram, the same as a gram of protein. What is added to the carbohydrate-rich food to make it tasty often piles on the calories. These include fatty spreads, sauces, and gravies.

3. False   Vitamins cannot be broken apart and used for energy. However, many do participate in chemical reactions that extract energy from carbohydrate, protein, and fat.

4. True   Excesses of the fat-soluble vitamins are toxic, and vitamin B_6, niacin, and ascorbic acid can cause health problems if taken in large amounts.

5. False   Cholesterol has many important uses in the body. It is used to make steroid hormones and bile, which is needed for proper fat digestion.

6. False   Although a high serum cholesterol level is associated with the development of heart disease, low serum cholesterol levels are no guarantee of protection. If too much is in the LDL form, the risk of heart disease is higher than someone who has a higher total cholesterol level but more in the HDL form.

7. False   When you haven't eaten, blood sugar drops and you feel hungry. Eating raises blood sugar levels. Hypoglycemia (low blood sugar) associated with metabolic abnormalities is rare. Medical experts consider hypoglycemia a fad disease in most cases.

8. False   Refined white sugar is almost 100% carbohydrate. It is digested into very simple sugars that are used for energy by the body.

9. False   Despite many personal reports, sugar does not cause behavioral problems in children or adults. As the answer to #8 explains, it is a simple chemical that is broken down and used for energy. Often, sugar-laden foods also contain caffeine and related stimulants, which may explain the association of sugar with hyperactive behavior.

10. True   Protein supplements are unnecessary because most Americans obtain plenty of protein in their normal diet. Exercise, not extra protein, builds muscles. More protein than needed is processed by the body and used for energy or converted to fat.

11. False   Severe zinc deficiency leads to poor growth and failure to develop sexually. However, this is extremely rare in the United States.

12. False   Honey contains large amounts of the simple sugar fructose. Fructose is one of the components of table sugar. The body converts fructose to glucose irrespective of the source. Considering how much honey is used and the tiny amounts of nutrients it contains, honey is just a more expensive choice as a sweetener.

13. False   The iron in red meat is more easily absorbed than that in plant foods. However, fish and chicken contribute iron too. Thus red meat is not essential as a food.

14. False   Fasting actually creates metabolic wastes that must be eliminated, since more body fat is burned for energy than under fed conditions. There are no health benefits derived from fasting.

15. False   Studies have demonstrated no nutritional superiority of foods grown with natural fertilizers and without pesticides.

Scoring: Give yourself one point for each correct response and total your points.

Total: _____

Score	Rating	Comments
13-15	Superior	You have sound knowledge of the subject.
9-12	Good	Good start; you may want to read reliable nutrition books to enhance your knowledge.
6-8	Fair	Read Chapter 9 again for more information.
<5	Poor	You have accumulated some misinformation about nutrition; try locating some reliable reading material and study Chapter 9.

Chapter 10 Preventing Injury

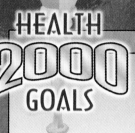

HEALTH 2000 GOALS

■ **Protective Equipment.** Extend requirements of the use of effective head, face, eye, and mouth protection to all organizations, agencies, and institutions sponsoring recreation and sporting events that pose risk of injury.

• Few intramural sports and organized leagues require protective gear.
• Organizations with recreation and sports programs, as well as those that provide space, equipment, or facilities for sports, can reduce traumas by requiring the use of appropriate protective gear.

OBJECTIVES

After completing this chapter, you will be able to do the following:

■ Realize that participation in physical activity creates situations in which injury is likely to occur.
■ Discuss the principles and guidelines of injury prevention.
■ Differentiate between acute and chronic injury.
■ Describe acute traumatic injuries, including fractures, contusions, ligament sprains, and muscle strains.
■ Define and differentiate between muscle strain and muscle soreness.

■ Discuss chronic overuse injuries involving tendinitis and bursitis in relation to the inflammatory process.
■ Identify the causes of low back pain and explain how it can best be avoided.
■ Describe the most common overuse injuries that occur in physical activity.
■ Describe the RICE approach to the initial treatment of injuries.
■ Identify exercises that may be dangerous or contraindicated.

KEY TERMS

While reading this chapter, you will become familiar with the following terms:

• acute injuries
• chronic injuries
• fractures

• contusion
• sprain
• strain

• muscle soreness
• tendinitis
• bursitis

• low back pain
• RICE

articipation in any type of physical activity places you in situations in which injury can occur at any given moment. Although some of these injuries are serious, and a few are life threatening, most sport-related injuries are not serious and lend themselves to rapid rehabilitation.

The bones of the skeletal system provide the primary structural support mechanism. In addition to support, the skeletal system serves as the point of attachment for the musculotendinous units. When contracted, the muscles produce angular movements of the skeletal bones that allow us to walk, run, throw, twist, and turn. Unfortunately, the skeletal and muscular systems were not designed to meet all the demands that strenuous physical activity often places on them. Sooner or later the forces become too great for them to handle, and injury occurs.

PREVENTION OF INJURIES

We often engage in physical activities for the purpose of promoting health. There is no reason to think that physical activities have the capacity to impair health. In fact, fitness programs such as those described in previous chapters reduce the possibility of injury. The overload demands placed on the body during training enable it to handle added stresses and strains that occur during physical activity. Thus the first step in preventing injuries associated with physical activity involves designing a well-planned fitness program based on the basic principles discussed in Chapter 4: overload, gradual progression, consistency, specificity, individuality, and safety.

Ironically, the nature of participation in any type of physical activity increases the possibility that injury will occur. Therefore much of this book discusses principles that reduce the chance of injury during physical activity. Injuries are to a large extent preventable, and paying attention to some simple guidelines can make exercise safer and more enjoyable.

Perhaps the biggest mistake that people make when beginning a fitness program is starting at a level that is too advanced and then trying to progress too quickly. Sedentary persons must begin at a much lower level and gradually increase their level of activity. Moreover, people stop exercising temporarily for a variety of reasons; when they start exercising again, there is a tendency to try to begin where they left off. They do too much, too fast, and too soon.

What to Do If Injury Occurs

Have you ever had problems with an injury? Lab Activity 10-1 will help you think about how the injury occurred and what could have been done to prevent it. In Chapter 4 it was mentioned that one of the essentials of any type of training is safety. If you are involved in a physical activity and realize that a specific part of your body is causing discomfort or pain that affects your performance, it is strongly recommended that this problem be evaluated immediately. The sooner an injury is diagnosed and treatment begun, the less chance there is that continued activity will make the problem worse.

The popular quote "no pain, no gain" holds no credibility with regard to an activity program. Pain indicates that something is wrong. You should stop the activity immediately and determine what is producing the pain. There is a great difference between overloading the system while you are working hard during training and pushing yourself to train when you are hurt. When one is dealing with injuries, common sense is of prime importance.

Who Should Evaluate an Injury?

It is important to remember that caution must be exercised when trying to evaluate an injury. A considerable amount of experience and training is required to determine accurately not only what may have caused an injury but also exactly what the injury is. These evaluation skills are far beyond the capabilities of most college students. Injuries should be evaluated by persons experienced in dealing with these sport-related problems. Physicians, athletic trainers, and physical therapists all have strong evaluation skills. However, the physician makes the injury diagnosis, whereas the athletic trainer or physical therapist assumes responsibility for injury rehabilitation.

ACUTE VERSUS CHRONIC INJURIES

No matter how much attention is directed toward the general principles of injury prevention, it is still likely that some physical problems will occur that may be classified as either *acute* or *chronic*. Acute injuries are caused by trauma; chronic injuries can result from overuse. In this chapter we will discuss some of the more generalized traumatic and overuse injuries that are likely to occur during physical activity.

ACUTE TRAUMATIC INJURIES

Fractures

Fractures (broken bones) occur as a result of extreme stresses and strains placed on bones. They generally can be classified as being either *closed* or *open*. A closed fracture is one in which there is little or no displacement of the bones. Conversely, in an open fracture there is enough displacement of the fractured ends that the bone actually breaks through surrounding tissues, including the skin. Both types of fractures can be serious if not managed properly. With an open fracture there is an increased possibility of infection.

Several different varieties of fractures can occur, and in most instances the fracture of a bone requires immobilization for some period of time in a cast. In general, fractures of the long bones of the arm and leg require approximately 6 weeks of casting, and the smaller bones may require as little as 3 weeks of either casting or splinting. In some instances, immobilization may not be required for healing. For example, breaks of the four small toes are difficult to splint or cast. Of course, complications such as infections may lengthen the time required for both casting and rehabilitation.

For a fracture to heal, bone-producing cells must lay down a bony formation called a *callus* over the fracture site during the immobilization period. Once the cast is removed, the bone must be subjected to normal stresses and strains so that tensile strength may be regained before the healing process is complete.

The only definitive technique for determining if a fracture exists is to have it x-rayed. If a fracture occurs, it should be managed and rehabilitated by a qualified orthopedist, athletic trainer, or physical therapist.

Stress Fractures

Perhaps the most common fracture that results from physical activity is a stress fracture. Unlike the other types of fractures that have been discussed, the stress fracture results from overuse rather than acute trauma. Common sites for stress fractures include the weight-bearing bones of the leg or foot. In either case, repetitive forces transmitted through the bones produce irritations at specific spots on the bone. The pain usually begins as a dull ache, which becomes progressively painful day after day. Initially, pain is most severe during activity. However, when a stress fracture develops, pain becomes worse after the activity is stopped.

The biggest problem with a stress fracture is that often it will not show up on an x-ray until the bone-producing cells begin laying down bone. At that point, a small white line apears on the x-ray. If a stress fracture is suspected, it is best to stop the activity for a period of at least 14 days. Stress fractures do not usually require casting; however, if they are not handled correctly, they may become true fractures that must be immobilized.

Contusions

A contusion is another word for a bruise. We are all very familiar with the mechanism that produces a bruise. A blow from some external object causes soft tissues (i.e., skin, fat, and muscle) to be compressed against the hard bone underneath. If the blow is hard enough, capillaries will be torn, which allows bleeding into the tissues. If the bleeding is minor, it will often cause a bluish-purple discoloration of the skin that persists for several days. The contusion may be very sore to the touch, and if damage has occurred to muscle, pain may be experienced on active movement. In most cases the pain will cease within a few days and discoloration will disappear usually in a few weeks.

The major problem with contusions occurs where an area is subjected to repeated blows. If the same area, or more specifically, a muscle, is bruised over and over again, small calcium deposits may begin to accumulate in the injured area. These pieces of calcium may be found between several fibers in the muscle belly, or calcium may build up to form a spur, which projects from the underlying bone. These calcium formations may significantly impair movement and are referred to as *myositis ossificans*.

The key to preventing myositis ossificans occurring after from repeated contusion is to protect the injured area with padding. If the area is properly protected after the first contusion, myositis may never develop. Protection and rest may allow the calcium to be reabsorbed, eliminating any need for surgery.

The two areas that seem to be the most vulnerable to repeated contusions during physical activity are the quadriceps muscle group on the front of the thigh and the biceps muscle on the front of the upper arm. The formation of myositis ossificans in these or any other areas may be detected by x-rays.

---

acute injuries sharp or severe injuries caused by trauma

chronic injuries long-term injuries caused by overuse

fractures broken bones caused by stress and/or strain

contusion another term for a bruise, which is an injury that does not break the skin

Ligament Sprains

A **sprain** involves damage to a ligament that provides support to a joint. A ligament is a tough, relatively inelastic band of tissue that connects one bone to another. The main structural support and stability of a joint is provided by the ligaments, which may be either thickened portions of a joint capsule or totally separate bands. The positioning of the ligaments partly determines what motions a joint is capable of making.

If a joint is forced to move beyond normal limits or planes of movement, injury to the ligament is likely to occur. The severity of the damage is subject to many different classifications; however, the most commonly used system involves three degrees of sprain.

- *First-degree sprain.* There is some stretching and separation of the ligamentous fibers, with moderate instability of the joint. Mild to moderate pain, localized swelling, and joint stiffness should be expected.
- *Second-degree sprain.* There is some tearing and separation of the ligament fibers, with moderate instability of the joint. Moderate to severe pain, swelling, and joint stiffness should be expected.
- *Third-degree sprain.* There is total tearing of the ligament, which leads to major instability of the joint. Initially, severe pain may be present, followed by little or no pain as a result of total disruption of nerve fibers. Swelling may be great, and the joint tends to become very stiff some hours after the injury. Usually a third-degree sprain with marked instability requires surgical repair. Frequently, the force producing the ligament injury is so great that other ligaments or structures surrounding the joint may also be injured. Rehabilitation of third-degree sprains involving surgery is a long-term process.

The greatest problem in the rehabilitation of first- and second-degree sprains is restoring stability to the joint. Once a ligament has been stretched or partially torn, inelastic scar tissue forms, preventing the ligament from regaining its original tension. Thus to restore stability to the joint, the other structures surrounding that joint, primarily muscles and their tendons, must be strengthened. The increased muscle tension provided by strength training can improve stability of the injured joint.

Muscle Strains

The musculotendinous unit was described and diagrammed in Chapter 6. Basically the muscle is composed of separate fibers that are capable of simultaneous contraction when stimulated by the central nervous system. Each muscle is attached to bone at both ends by strong, relatively inelastic tendons that cross over joints.

If a muscle is overstretched or forced to contract against too much resistance, separation or tearing of the muscle fibers occurs. This damage is referred to as a **strain** (Figure 10-1). Muscle strains, like ligament sprains, are subject to various classification systems. The following is a simple system of classification of strains:

- *First-degree strain.* Some muscle fibers have been stretched or actually torn. There is some tenderness and pain on active motion. Movement is painful, but full range of motion is usually possible.
- *Second-degree strain.* A number of muscle fibers have been torn, and active contraction of the muscle is extremely painful. Usually a depression or divot can be felt somewhere in the muscle belly at the place where the muscle fibers have been torn. Some swelling may occur because of capillary bleeding; therefore some discoloration is possible.
- *Third-degree strain.* There is a complete rupture of a muscle in the area of the muscle belly where muscle becomes tendon or at the tendinous attachment to the bone. There will be significant impairment to or perhaps total loss of movement. Initially, pain is intense but quickly diminishes because of complete nerve fiber separation.

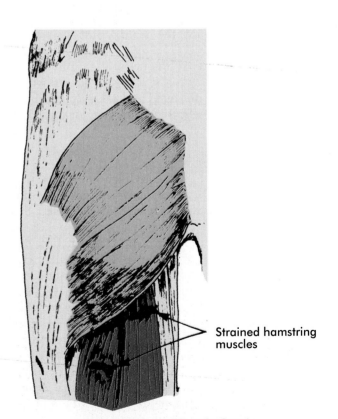

Strained hamstring muscles

FIGURE 10-1. Muscle Strain.

Muscle strains can occur in any muscle and usually result from some uncoordinated activity between muscle groups. Third-degree strains are most common in the biceps tendon of the upper arm or in the Achilles heel cord in the back of the calf. When either of these tendons tears, the muscle tends to bunch toward its attachment at the bone site. Third-degree strains involving large tendons that produce great amounts of force must be surgically repaired. Smaller musculotendinous ruptures such as those that occur in the fingers may heal by immobilization with a splint.

Regardless of the severity of the strain, there is no question that the time required for rehabilitation is fairly lengthy. In many instances muscle strains are incapacitating, making rehabilitation time for a muscle strain even longer than for a ligament sprain. Incapacitating muscle strains occur most frequently in the large, force-producing hamstring and quadriceps muscles of the lower extremity. The treatment of hamstring strains requires a healing period of 6 to 8 weeks and a considerable amount of patience. Trying to return to activity too soon often causes reinjury to the area of the muscle that has been strained, and the healing process must begin again.

Muscle Soreness

It is well known that overexertion in strenuous muscular exercise often results in muscular pain. All of us at one time or another have experienced muscle soreness, usually resulting from some physical activity to which we are unaccustomed. You will find that the older you get, the more easily muscle soreness seems to develop.

There are two types of muscle soreness. The first type of muscle pain is acute and accompanies fatigue. It is transient and occurs during and immediately after exercise. The second type of soreness involves delayed muscle pain that appears approximately 12 hours after injury. It becomes most intense after 24 to 48 hours and then gradually subsides so that the muscle becomes symptom-free after 3 or 4 days. This second type of pain is described as a syndrome of delayed muscle pain leading to increased muscle tension, swelling, increased stiffness, and resistance to stretching.

This delayed-onset muscle soreness is thought to result from several possible causes. It may occur from very small tears in the muscle tissue, which seems to be more likely with eccentric or isometric contractions. It may also occur because of disruption of the connective tissue that holds muscle tendon fibers together. Delayed-onset muscle soreness may also be caused by localized muscle spasm resulting from reduced oxygenated blood supply to the muscle.

Muscle soreness may be prevented by beginning at a moderate level and gradually progressing the intensity of the exercise over a period of time. Treatment of muscle soreness usually also involves static or PNF stretching activity. As for other conditions discussed in this chapter, ice applied within the first 48 to 72 hours is important as a treatment for muscle soreness.

CHRONIC OVERUSE INJURIES
Importance of Inflammation in Healing

For most people, the word *inflammation* has negative connotations. However, it is important to understand that inflammation is an essential part of the healing process. Once a structure is damaged or irritated, inflammation must occur to initiate the healing process. Symptoms of inflammation include pain, swelling, warmth, and perhaps redness. During the inflammatory process, affected cells release chemicals that facilitate the healing process. Inflammation is supposed to be an acute process that ends when its role in the healing process has been accomplished. However, if the source of irritation (i.e., the repetitive movements that cause stress to the tendon) is not removed, then the inflammatory process becomes chronic rather than acute. When this occurs, an acute condition may become a chronic disabling problem.

Tendinitis

Of all the overuse problems associated with physical activity, tendinitis is probably the most common. Any term ending in the suffix *itis* means there is inflammation present. Tendinitis means inflammation of a tendon. During muscle activity a tendon must move or slide on other structures around it whenever the muscle contracts. If a particular movement is performed repeatedly, the tendon becomes irritated and inflamed. This inflammation is manifested by pain on movement, swelling, possibly some warmth, and usually crepitus. *Crepitus* is a crackling sound. It is usually caused by the tendon's tendency to stick to the surrounding structure

---

sprain injury that damages a ligament or joint capsule surrounding a joint

strain separation or tearing of muscle fibers due to the muscle being overstretched or forced to contract against too much resistance

muscle soreness can be acute (occurring during or immediately after exertion) or delayed (occurring approximately 12 hours after exertion) and is experienced after participation in physical activity to which one is not usually accustomed

tendinitis inflammation of a tendon that occurs as a result of trauma or overuse

while it slides back and forth. This sticking is caused primarily by the chemical products of inflammation that accumulate on the irritated tendon.

The key to the treatment of tendinitis is rest. If the repetitive motion causing irritation to the tendon is eliminated, chances are the inflammatory process will allow the tendon to heal. Unfortunately, if you are seriously involved with some physical activity, you may find it difficult to totally stop what you have been doing and rest for 2 or more weeks while the tendinitis subsides. It is desirable to substitute some form of activity, such as bicycling or swimming, that will allow you to maintain your present fitness level while avoiding continued irritation of the inflamed tendon. Tendinitis most commonly occurs in runners in the Achilles tendon in the back of the lower leg or in swimmers in the muscle tendons of the shoulder joint. However, it can flare up in any activity in which overuse and repetitive movements occur.

Bursitis

Bursitis occurs around joints, where there is friction between tendons and bones, skin and bone, or muscle and other muscles. If there were not some mechanism of protection in these high-friction areas, it is very likely that chronic irritation would exist.

Bursae are small sacs with a lining (synovial membrane) that contains a small amount of fluid (synovial fluid). Just as oil lubricates a hinge, these small bags of fluid permit motion of these structures without friction.

If excessive movement or perhaps some acute trauma occurs around the bursae, they become irritated and inflamed and begin producing large amounts of synovial fluid. The longer the irritation continues or the more severe the acute trauma, the more fluid is produced. As fluid continues to accumulate in the limited space available, pressure tends to increase, causing pain in the area. Bursitis can be an extremely painful condition that has the capability of severely restricting movement, especially if it occurs around a joint. Synovial fluid will continue to be produced until the movement or trauma producing the irritation is eliminated.

Occasionally, a bursa sac completely surrounds a tendon, allowing more freedom of movement in a tight area. This type of sac is referred to as a *synovial sheath*. Irritation of this synovial sheath may restrict tendon motion. All joints have many bursae surrounding them. The three bursae that are most commonly irritated as a result of various types of physical activity are the subacromial bursa in the shoulder joint under the clavicle; the olecranon bursa on the tip of the elbow; and the prepatellar bursa on the front surface of the patella. All three of these bursae produce

large amounts of synovial fluid, affecting motion at their respective joints.

MANAGING BACK PAIN

There is no question that low back pain is one of the most annoying and disabling ailments known to man. Many causes and cures for low back pain have been proposed. However, there are so many different things that can cause pain in the low back, no single incriminating cause or absolute cure can be identified. This discussion of low back pain will concentrate on some of the most common causes.

Certainly, the older you get, the more problems you tend to have in the low back. Although low back pain does not become a major problem for most people until their middle twenties, many people have minor congenital defects that are not realized until they experience pain as a result of faulty body mechanics, poor posture, or inflexibility.

Spine

The human spine is composed of 24 vertebral bodies, each separated from the others by a fibrocartilaginous disk. There are 7 cervical vertebrae in the neck region, 12 thoracic vertebrae in the thorax, and 5 lumbar vertebrae in the low back. The sacrum, another part of the spine, is a large triangular bone located below the small of the back in the pelvis (Figure 10-2, *A*). The function of the spine is twofold: to provide structural support for an upright posture and to protect the spinal cord and the spinal nerves where they exit from the spinal column to provide motor and sensory functions. The position of the vertebrae in the spinal column is maintained by a number of strong ligaments and muscles that attach to each vertebra. The vertebral disks that separate each segment serve as shock-absorbers in the spinal column.

Causes of Low Back Pain

Muscle Imbalance in Low Back Pain

Of all the causes of low back pain, none is more common than imbalances between the strength and flexibility of the various muscle groups associated with the low back. Structurally, the vertebral column (including the sacrum), the bones of the pelvis, and the femur (bone of the upper leg) are all important with regard to low back pain. As indicated in Figure 10-2, *B*, the abdominal muscles attach to the pelvis in the front of the trunk, the erector muscles attach the vertebral column to the pelvis in the back of the trunk, and the hamstring muscles of the leg attach to the lower portion of the pelvis slightly toward the back.

In most cases, the abdominal muscles are weak and stretched out, the erector muscles are tight and inflex-

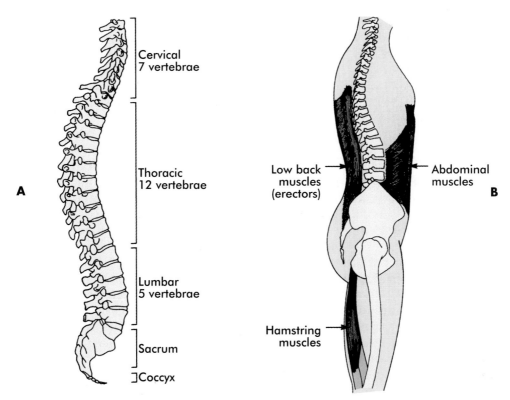

FIGURE 10-2. The Spine and Its Muscles.
A, The spinal column has five regions of vertebrae. **B,** The muscles of the low back, the abdominal muscles, and the hamstring muscles all attach to the vertebrae or pelvis and can play a major role in back pain.

ible, and the hamstring muscles are also tight. Because each of these muscle groups attaches to and affects the movement of the pelvis relative to the vertebral column, it is essential to maintain some balance in terms of strength and flexibility between the groups. In many cases an exercise program that attempts to increase the strength and therefore the tone of the abdominal muscles, improve the flexibility of the erector muscles in the low back, and stretch out the tight hamstring muscles may alleviate many complaints of low back pain. Low back strengthening exercises are described later in this chapter.

Herniated Disk

It is widely believed that disk degeneration and rupture is one of the more common causes of low back pain. This hypothesis has been challenged recently, but it is true that disk-related problems produce many low back complaints.

A vertebral disk is similar to the type of chewing gum that has a liquid center. A sudden twist or jerking movement can cause the liquid center (nucleus) of the disk to protrude to one side, resulting in pressure on the spinal nerve at that segment. Pressure will usually cause pain to radiate down the leg. The most common

areas for disk-related problems are in the disks between the fourth and fifth lumbar vertebrae and between the fifth lumbar vertebra and the sacrum. This condition is commonly referred to as a *herniated disk.* A disk herniation should definitely be treated by a qualified physician (Figure 10-3).

Lumbosacral Sprains

Not all low back pain results from problems related to the vertebral disks. A more contemporary explanation of low back pain involves a sprain of the intervertebral ligaments resulting from sudden rotation of the vertebrae. This type of injury is most common in the lower lumbar and sacral areas and is often referred to as a *lumbosacral sprain.*

Rotation of a vertebra can be caused by forces incurred from sudden twisting movements or bend-

---

bursitis inflammation of the bursae, the connective tissue structures surrounding a joint
low back pain one of the most annoying and disabling ailments resulting from a number of conditions including muscle imbalances in the lower back, herniated disk, and sprains of ligaments in the lower back

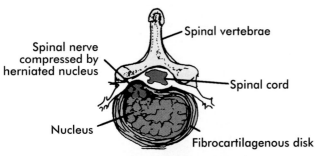

Spinal nerve compressed by herniated nucleus

Spinal vertebrae

Spinal cord

Nucleus

Fibrocartilagenous disk

FIGURE 10-3.   **Vertebral Disk Herniation.**

ing over to pick up an object while the spine is twisted. The force from one of these motions can cause a vertebra to rotate out of its normal alignment.

A vertebra that is rotated tends to impinge on the spinal nerve in much the same manner as a herniated disk does, thereby causing pain. When pain is present because of a change in position of one vertebra, the muscles surrounding the area of pain in the vertebral column tend to go into spasm to protect the area and prevent additional injury. This muscle spasm only tends to pull the rotated vertebra further out of line, increasing the spinal nerve impingement and pain. Any type of movement is painful and is at best restricted.

Sacroiliac Sprains

Two strong ligaments on each side of the sacrum connect this portion of the vertebral column to the pelvic bone known as the *ilium*. A sprain of either of these sacroiliac ligaments usually results from stepping off a curb or into a hole, thus causing one sacroiliac joint to forcefully rotate either forward or backward with respect to the other and stretching at least one of the ligaments.

Stretching of the ligament produces pain, and once again the muscles in the surrounding area go into spasm to protect the injured ligament. The spasm pulls one sacroiliac joint further out of line with respect to the other. Pain will be felt directly over the sacroiliac joint that has been sprained.

Many treatment and rehabilitation techniques involving mobilization and manipulation have been proposed for treatment of both lumbosacral and sacroiliac sprains. Treatment by qualified professionals who possess a sound understanding of these treatment techniques is highly recommended.

Prevention of Low Back Pain

To treat the injury, some knowledge of the source of low back pain is important, but it is more important to understand how low back pain can be avoided. To prevent low back pain, the practice of avoiding unnecessary stresses and strains should be integrated into your daily life. The back is subjected to these stresses and strains when one is standing, lying, sitting, working, and exercising. Care should be taken to avoid postures and positions that can cause injury.

Standing and Leaning Posture

If standing posture is correct, it should be possible to draw a straight line from the ear, through the tip of the shoulder, over the middle of the hip bone, just behind the knee cap, and just in front of the ankle bone on the lateral side (Figure 10-4).

The major problems associated with standing posture are rounded shoulders and excessive curve in the lumbar area (Figure 10-5). To get an idea of what good posture should feel like, back up against a wall. Press your shoulders and low back flat against the wall and tighten all the muscles (Figure 10-6). Then walk away from the wall in that position. When bending over and leaning on an object, the knees should be flexed rather than straight or hyperextended (Figure 10-7). Lab Activity 10-2 will help you assess your standing posture.

Lying Posture

The back is subjected to many stresses and strains while a person is lying down. Most of us spend

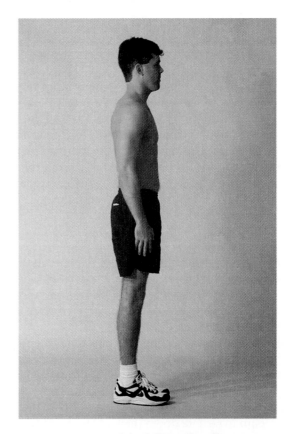

FIGURE 10-4.   **Ideal Standing Posture.**

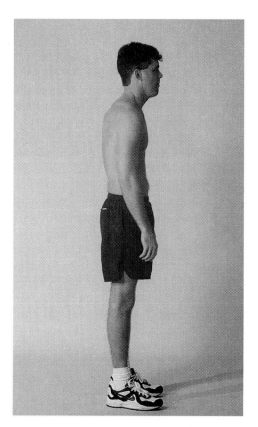

FIGURE 10-5.   **Poor Standing Posture.**
Poor standing posture can increase low back pain.

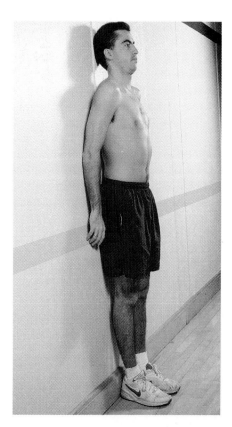

FIGURE 10-6. **Test for Correct Standing Posture.**
Standing with the low back pressed firmly into the wall will give some indication of what correct posture should feel like.

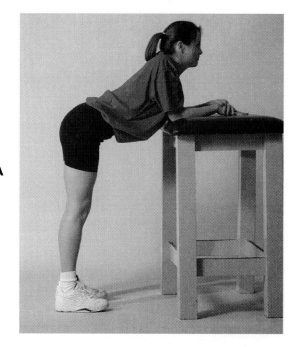

A

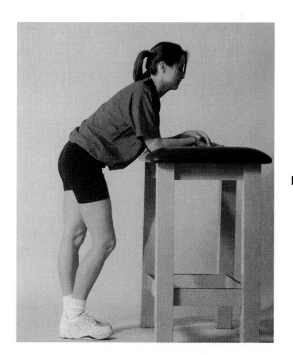

B

FIGURE 10-7. **Correct Way to Lean.**
Always lean on an object with your knees bent. **A,** Incorrect. **B,** Recommended.

between 7 and 10 hours each day sleeping. Improper positions during sleep can cause chronic low back pain. It is essential to have a good, firm mattress. Sleeping on a bed that is too soft can increase the tendency toward swayback.

Swayback can also result from sleeping flat on your back with no pillow. It is more correct when sleeping on the back to place a pillow under the knees or under the head so that the low back will flatten (Figure 10-8). This position is also recommended for resting or just lying around. It must be added that sleeping on your back while using a pillow under your head may cause

some additional problems with rounded shoulders and a head-forward position.

Lying on the stomach face down also tends to enhance a swayback (Figure 10-9). Bending the knee and the hip on one side does not take pressure off the low back (Figure 10-10). The best position for sleeping is to sleep on your side, with your knees flexed and your head on a pillow for support (Figure 10-11). This flattens the low back and almost totally eliminates stress.

Sitting Posture

Of the postural positions discussed to this point, it is likely that the sitting posture causes the greatest stress and strain to the low back. The slumping posture many of us use when watching television or while sitting on a soft sofa produces significant stress to the shoulders and neck (Figure 10-12).

When sitting, you should slide all the way up against the back of the chair so that the low back has

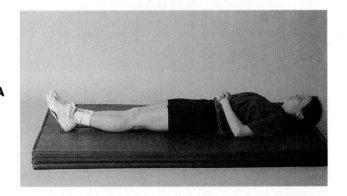

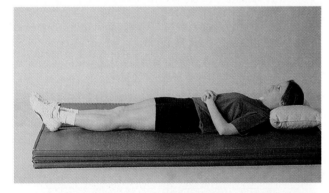

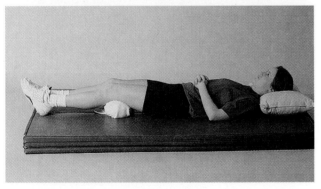

FIGURE 10-8. Sleeping on Back.
Sleeping on the back is safe only when the head and both knees are supported. **A,** Incorrect. **B,** Incorrect. **C,** Recommended.

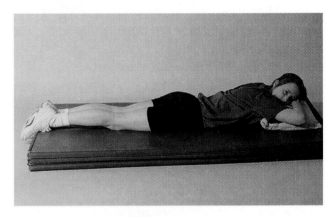

FIGURE 10-9. Sleeping on Stomach.
Sleeping on the stomach exaggerates swayback position.

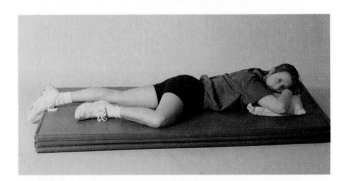

FIGURE 10-10. Sleeping on Stomach with Bent Knee.
Sleeping on the stomach with one knee flexed does not eliminate pressure on the low back.

some support. The neck and back should be held erect in a straight line. The feet may be propped up to further flatten out the low back (Figure 10-13). The knees should be slightly above the hips.

Any variation in the recommended correct sitting position will add stress to the low back. When sitting or driving for a long time, some type of support should be placed behind the low back, and the position of the backrest should be changed periodically (Figure 10-14). Leaning forward away from the back support while driving is not recommended.

Working Posture

When lifting objects from the ground, it is important to remember to use the legs rather than the back to lift. Always turn and face the object you are going to lift. Bend at the knees, and keep your low back straight rather than trying to keep your legs straight

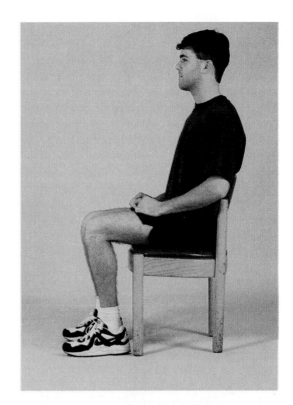

FIGURE 10-13. Ideal Sitting Position.
Ideal sitting position is erect, with the low back flattened against a support.

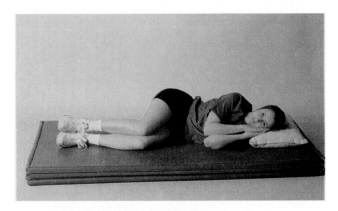

FIGURE 10-11. Sleeping on Side.
The side-lying sleeping position flattens the low back. A pillow should support the head.

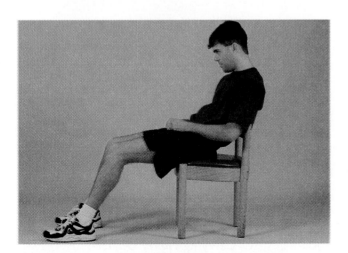

FIGURE 10-12. Poor Sitting Position.
Slumping in a chair strains the neck and shoulders.

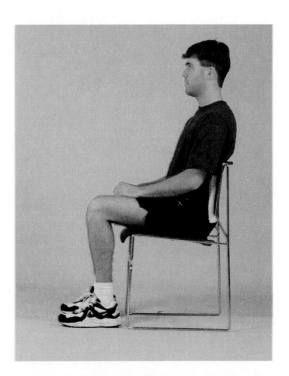

FIGURE 10-14. Support for Lower Lumbar Area.
It may help to place a support behind the lumbar area when sitting or driving for long periods of time.

and bending at the waist (Figure 10-15). Don't try to lift the object higher than your waist. When carrying heavy objects, hold them close to you with your elbows locked at your sides (Figure 10-16). It is best to remember that when you are working, it pays to take a little extra time to position yourself properly for lifting and carrying heavy objects to avoid repeated stress to the low back.

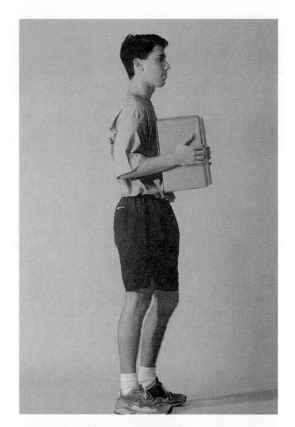

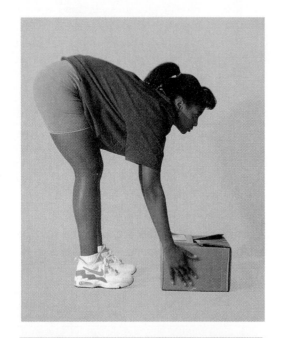

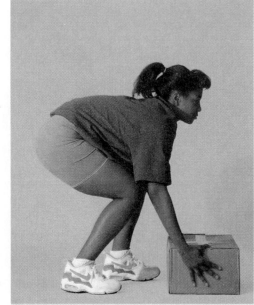

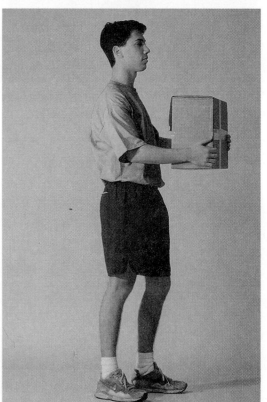

FIGURE 10-15. **Lifting Heavy Objects.**
A, Incorrect. Do not keep the low back straight.
B, Recommended lifting position.

FIGURE 10-16. **Carrying Heavy Objects.**
Heavy objects should be carried close to the body.
A, Correct. **B,** Incorrect.

Low Back Exercises

For the average person the major problem in low back pain is that the muscles in the low back are too tight and the abdominal muscles are relatively weak. Preventive exercises should be directed toward improving flexibility of the low back muscles while increasing the strength and tone of the abdominal muscles. Figure 10-17 indicates an exercise for improving low back flexibility.

Curl-ups are the best exercise for strengthening the abdominal muscles. Curl-ups must be done with the knees flexed to 90 degrees to eliminate the curve in the low back. The abdominal muscles should be contracted. The head should be lifted off the floor, and the trunk should curl into the sit-up position. Alteration of this technique may cause additional strain to the low back (Figure 10-18). It is necessary only to do a partial curl-up to provide maximal benefit to the abdominal muscles. A full curl-up may place additional stress on the low back.

The pelvic tilt exercise may also be used to strengthen abdominal muscles and loosen low back muscles to eliminate swayback. It is done by lying on the back on the floor and pressing the low back flat against the floor (Figure 10-19). It is also important to stretch the hamstring muscles. Having good flexibility

A
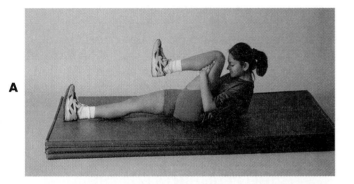

B
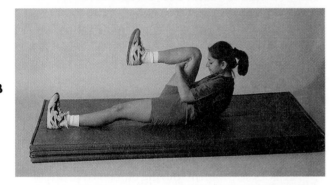

C
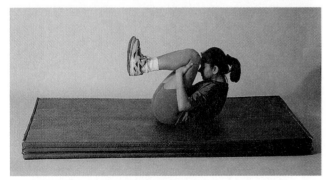

FIGURE 10-17. **Low Back Stretch Exercise.**
Muscles stretched: Extensors of lumbar and sacral vertebrae.
Instructions: Lie flat on back. **A,** Bring right knee up and touch chin to knee; **B,** bring left knee up and touch chin to knee; **C,** bring both knees up and touch chin to knees. Repeat entire sequence three times; hold each position for 30 seconds.

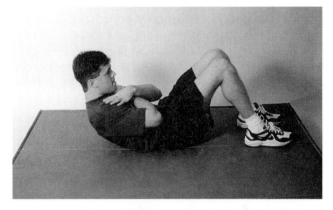

FIGURE 10-18. **Curl-Ups.**
Curl-ups should be done with knees flexed and neck curled to prevent low back strain. It is necessary only to do a partial curl sit-up, lifting the shoulder blades off the ground.

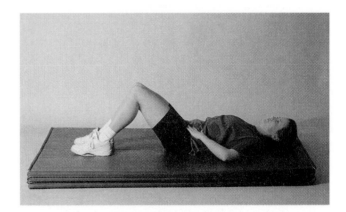

FIGURE 10-19. **Pelvic Tilt Exercise.**
Pelvic tilt exercise is used to correct swayback by contracting the abdominal muscles and intervertebral joints of the low back.

in the hamstrings reduces the tendency for the pelvis to rotate backward, thus affecting the curve in the lumbar area (see Figure 7-18). "Cat-stretch" exercises involve arching the back, which places the low back muscles in a stretched position. These exercises are excellent for stretching both the muscles and the joints between the vertebrae of the low back (Figure 10-20). Exercises that should be avoided to reduce the risk of low back pain include straight-leg sit-ups, straight-leg lifts, bent-over rowing exercise, back hyperextension, donkey kicks, and bench press with feet on the floor.

Additional helpful hints and recommendations for preventing low back pain are provided in the following Safe Tip box.

ADDITIONAL INJURIES COMMONLY ASSOCIATED WITH PHYSICAL ACTIVITY

In addition to those discussed previously, there are many injuries of both the acute and chronic variety that can occur with participation in physical activity. There are a few injuries that seem to occur frequently with physical activity. Table 10-1 provides a brief description of the causes and signs of the more common injuries.

TAKING CARE OF INJURIES

Initial first aid and management techniques for most musculoskeletal injuries associated with physical activity are fairly simple and straightforward.

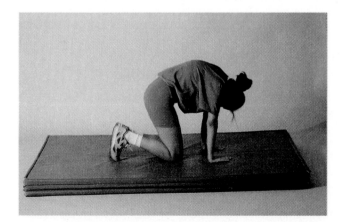

FIGURE I0-20. **Cat-Stretch Exercise.**
Cat-stretch exercises involve arching the back and are excellent for stretching back muscles and intervertebral joints of the low back.

Limiting Swelling

Regardless of which type of injury we are talking about, there is one problem they all have in common—swelling. Swelling may be caused by any number of factors, including bleeding; production of synovial fluid; an accumulation of inflammatory byproducts; *edema*, which is nothing more than an accumulation of body fluid; or a combination of several factors. No matter which mechanism is involved, swelling produces increased pressure in the injured area, and increased pressure causes pain. Swelling is most likely during the first 72 hours after an injury. Once swelling has occurred, the healing process is significantly retarded. The injured area cannot return to normal until all the swelling is gone. **Thus first-aid management should be directed toward controlling**

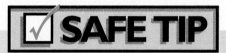

HELPFUL HINTS FOR THE PREVENTION OF LOW BACK PAIN

- Avoid wearing high-heeled shoes, which can increase the curvature in the low back. All your shoes should have the same heel height.
- When carrying heavy objects, try to balance the load, and carry the weight as close to your body as possible.
- Don't try to lift or move objects that are too heavy for you. Find someone to help you.
- Avoid sudden straining-type movements. This is a problem during athletic participation; however, if the low back and abdominal muscles have been properly conditioned, the chances of injury are significantly reduced.
- Avoid always carrying a heavy book bag on the same shoulder. Switch sides periodically.
- Avoid buying soft mattresses or chairs. Even though they may feel comfortable initially, they can cause significant low back pain over time.
- If low back injury occurs, consult a professional who is highly trained in the treatment of low back pain. Many people who have low back pain seem to be turning to chiropractors for treatment. There are good and bad chiropractors just as there are good and bad physicians, athletic trainers, massage therapists, and physical therapists. It pays to talk to people about the skill of the person you choose to treat you. Remember that getting a second opinion is always a good idea.

TABLE 10-1.   Summary of Common Injuries Associated With Physical Activity

Injury	Condition
Achilles tendinitis	A chronic tendinitis of the "heel cord" or muscle tendon located on the back of the lower leg just above the heel. It may result from any activity that involves forcefully pushing off with the foot and ankle such as in running and jumping. This inflammation involves swelling, warmth, tenderness to touch, and pain during walking and especially running.
Ankle sprains	Stretching or tearing of one or several ligaments that provide stability to the ankle joint. Ligaments on the ouside or lateral side of the ankle are more commonly injured by rolling the sole of the foot downward and toward the inside. Pain is intense immediately after injury, followed by considerable swelling, tenderness, loss of joint motion, and some discoloration over a 24- to 48-hour period.
Athlete's foot	A fungal infection that most often occurs between the toes or on the sole of the foot and that causes itching, redness, and pain. If the skin breaks down, a bacterial infection is possible. It may be prevented by keeping the area dry; using powder; and wearing clean, dry socks that do not hold moisture. It is best treated using over-the-counter medications that contain the active ingredient miconazole (MicaTin).
Blisters	Friction blisters can occur anywhere on the skin where there is friction or repetitive rubbing, but they most often occur on the hands or feet. The blister takes on a reddish color, becoming raised and filling with fluid. It can be quite painful, and if it occurs on the foot it may be disabling. Taking measures to reduce friction, such as wearing gloves, breaking in new footwear, and wearing appropriately fitting socks, is helpful in preventing blisters.
Groin pull	A muscle strain that occurs in the muscles located on the inside of the upper thigh just below the pubic area and that results from either an overstretch of the muscle or from a contraction of the muscle that meets excessive resistance. Pain will be produced by flexing the hip and leg across the body or by stretching the muscles in a groin-stretch position (see Figure 7-19).
Hamstring pull	A strain of the muscles on the back of the upper thigh that most often occurs while sprinting. In most cases severe pain is caused simply by walking or in any movement that involves knee flexion or stretch of the hamstring muscle. Some swelling, tenderness to touch, and possibly some discoloration extending down the back of the leg may occur in severe strains.
Patellofemoral knee pain	Nonspecific pain occurring around the knee, particularly the front part of the knee, or in the knee cap (patella). Pain can result from many causes, including improper movement of the knee cap in knee flexion and extension; tendinitis of the tendon just below the knee cap, which is caused by repetitive jumping; bursitis (swelling) either above or below the knee cap; and osteoarthritis (joint surface degeneration) between the knee cap and thigh bone. It may involve inflammation with swelling, tenderness, warmth, and pain associated with movement.
Plantar fasciitis or arch pain	Chronic inflammation and irritation of the broad ligament that runs from the heel to the base of the toes, forming part of the long arch on the bottom of the foot. It most often occurs in runners or walkers. It is frequently caused by wearing shoes that do not have adequate arch support. At first, pain is localized at the attachment on the heel; it then tends to move more onto the arch. It is most painful when you first get out of bed and in the evening when you have been on your feet for long periods.
Quadriceps contusion "charlie horse"	A deep bruise of the muscles in the front part of the thigh caused by a forceful impact or by some object that results in severe pain, swelling, discoloration, and difficulty flexing the knee or extending the hip. Without adequate rest and protection from additional trauma, small calcium deposits may develop in the muscle.

TABLE 10-1.	Summary of Common Injuries Associated With Physical Activity—cont'd
Injury	**Condition**
Racquetball or golfer's elbow	Similar to tennis elbow, except the pain is located on the medial or inside surface of the arm just above the elbow at the attachment of the wrist and finger flexor muscles. It occurs in those activities that involve repeated, forceful flexion of the wrist, such as hitting a forehand stroke in racquetball. Golfers also develop this inflammation in the trailing arm from too much wrist flexion in a golf swing.
Shin splints	A "catch-all" term used to refer to any pain that occurs in the front part of the lower leg or shin, most often caused by excessive running on hard surfaces. Pain is usually caused by strain of the muscles that move the ankle and foot at their attachment points in the shin. It is usually worse during activity. In more severe cases it may be caused by stress fractures of the long bones in the lower leg, with the pain being worse after activity is stopped.
Shoulder impingement	Chronic irritation and inflammation of muscle tendons and a bursa underneath the tip of the shoulder, which results from repeated forceful overhead motions of the shoulder such as in swimming, throwing, spiking a volleyball, or serving a tennis ball. Pain is felt when the arm is extended across the body above shoulder level.
Sunburn	An extremely common problem for anyone who exercises outside. Overexposure to the sun can ultimately cause certain types of skin cancer. It is critical to protect yourself from the sun by applying sunscreens and paying attention to the SPF (sun protection factor). Wearing a hat and other protective clothing to cover the skin can further help to minimize overexposure to ultraviolet light.
Tennis elbow	Chronic irritation and inflammation of the lateral or outside surface of the arm just above the elbow at the attachment of the muscles that extend the wrist and fingers. It results from any activity that requires forceful extension of the wrist. Typically occurs in tennis players who are using faulty techniques hitting backhand ground strokes. Pain is felt above the elbow after forcefully extending the wrist against resistance or applying pressure over the muscle attachment above the elbow.

the swelling. If the swelling can be controlled initially in the acute state of injury, it is likely that the time required for rehabilitation will be significantly reduced.

To control and severely limit the amount of swelling, the RICE principle can be applied. RICE stands for **R**est, **I**ce, **C**ompression, and **E**levation. Each factor plays a critical role in limiting swelling, and all four methods should be used simultaneously.

Rest

Rest after any type of injury is an extremely important component of any treatment program. Once a body part is injured, it immediately begins the healing process. If the injured part is not rested and is subjected to external stresses and strains, the healing process never really gets a chance to do what it is supposed to do. Consequently, the injured part does not

heal, and the time required for rehabilitation is markedly increased. The number of days necessary for resting varies with the severity of the injury. Parts of the body that have experienced minor injury should rest for approximately 72 hours before a rehabilitation program is begun.

Ice

It is widely agreed that initial treatment of acute injuries should employ cold. Therefore ice is used for most conditions involving strains, sprains, and contusions. It is most commonly used immediately after injury to decrease pain and promote local constriction of the vessels (vasoconstriction), thus controlling hemorrhage and edema. It is also used in the acute phase of inflammatory conditions such as bursitis, tenosynovitis, and tendinitis conditions in which heat may cause additional pain and swelling. Cold is also used to reduce the reflex muscle spasm and spastic conditions that accompany pain. Its pain-reducing (analgesic) effect is probably one of its greatest benefits. One explanation of the analgesic effect is that cold slows the speed of nerve transmission, so the pain sensation is reduced. It is also possible that cold bombards pain receptors with so many cold impulses that pain impulses are lost. With ice treatments, the patient usually reports an uncomfortable sensation of cold, followed by burning, then an aching sensation, and finally complete numbness.

Because the subcutaneous fat (under the skin) slowly conducts the cold temperature, applications of cold for short periods of time will be ineffective in cooling deeper tissues. For this reason, longer treatments of approximately 20 minutes are recommended. It is generally believed that cold treatments are more effective in reaching deep tissues than are most forms of heat. Cold applied to the skin is capable of significantly lowering the temperature of tissues at a considerable depth. The temperature to which the deeper tissues can be lowered depends on (1) the type of cold that is applied to the skin, (2) the duration of its application, (3) the thickness of the subcutaneous fat, and (4) the region of the body to which it is applied. Ice packs should be applied to the area for at least 72 hours after an acute injury. With many injuries, regular ice treatments may be continued for several weeks.

Compression

Compression (pressure) is equally as important as ice for controlling swelling. The purpose of compression is to reduce the amount of space available for swelling by applying pressure around the injured area. The best way of applying pressure is to use an elastic wrap (such as an Ace bandage) to apply firm but even pressure around the injury.

Because of the pressure built up in the tissues, it may become painful to leave a compression wrap in place for a long time. However, there is no question that it is essential to leave the wrap in place even though there may be significant pain, because it is so important in the control of swelling. The compression wrap should be left in place for at least 72 hours after an acute injury. In many chronic overuse problems, such as tendinitis, tenosynovitis, and particularly bursitis, the compression wrap should be worn until the swelling is almost entirely gone.

Elevation

The fourth factor that assists in controlling swelling is elevation. The injured part, particularly an extremity, should be elevated to eliminate the effects of gravity on blood pooling in the extremities. Elevation assists the veins, which drain blood and other fluids from the injured area, returning them to the central circulatory system. The greater the degree of elevation, the more effective the reduction in swelling. For example, in an ankle sprain (Figure 10-21) the leg should be placed in a position so that the ankle is virtually straight up in the air. The injured part should be elevated as much as possible during the first 72 hours.

The appropriate technique for initial management of the acute injuries discussed in this chapter, regardless of where they occur, is the following:

- Apply a compression wrap directly over the injury. Wrapping should start at a point that is farther away from the trunk of the body and end closer to it. Tension should be firm and consistent. It may be helpful to wet the elastic wrap to facilitate the passage of cold from ice packs.
- Surround the injured area entirely with ice packs or bags, and secure them in place. The ice should be left on for 20 minutes initially and then 1 hour off and 30 minutes on as much as possible over the next 24 hours. During the following 48-hour period, ice should again be applied as often as possible.
- The injured part should be elevated for most of the initial 72-hour period after injury. It is particularly important to keep the injury elevated while sleeping. This also allows the damaged part to rest after the injury. The initial management of an injury is extremely important to reduce the length of time required for rehabilitation.

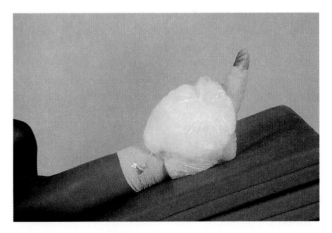

FIGURE 10-21. RICE.
Rest-ice-compression-elevation technique for treatment of a sprained ankle.

RICE acronym for a way to control and limit swelling by using rest, ice, compression, and elevation

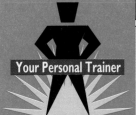
Your Personal Trainer

Pat O'Donnel, Spanish teacher
Age: 28

Scenario

I was playing a pick-up game of basketball at lunch a few days ago and twisted my right ankle going for a rebound. I didn't think much of it at the time, and simply left the game. I stayed off it as much as possible. Yesterday it was red, puffy, and quite tender. This morning it has turned a blackish-blue, and I have a severe limp and even less mobility.

Solution

Proper initial management of the injury could have prevented a great deal of the swelling. Remember this for next time.

For now, to help facilitate the healing process you should use the RICE principle of *r*est, *i*ce, *c*ompression, and *e*levation.

Keep your ankle wrapped in an elastic-type bandage. Be sure not to cut off blood circulation to your ankle and foot. Progression to a full–weight-bearing load and a normal stride will decrease your recovery time.

When the pain and swelling subside, you will need to work on improving the strength and mobility of your injured ankle. Two or three times a day you should do ankle circles (circling your ankle in the air) 10 to 15 times in each direction. The Achilles tendon stretch, toe raises, and shifting your body weight between the injured and noninjured ankle will also help you recover from this injury.

LONG-TERM REHABILITATION

Although initial treatment will be virtually the same for everyone, long-term plans for rehabilitation are variable and will be affected by many factors. The goal of rehabilitation should be to return the person to his or her usual physical activities as quickly and as safely as possible. Most persons involved in physical activity, whether recreational or competitive, are interested in a speedy return to activity after injury. Thus the rehabilitation program philosophy should be extremely aggressive. Early movement involving both flexibility and strength training is important. It is important to remember that for a structure to heal properly, it must perform the function for which it was designed. In the case of an injured muscle, it must be made to contract against resistance and produce movement. Strength training through a full range of motion is essential.

Long-term rehabilitation programs require the supervision of a trained professional if they are going to be safe and effective. Persons highly trained in the area of injury rehabilitation, such as athletic trainers or physical therapists, should be contacted to supervise rehabilitation programs. An injury that is not properly rehabilitated may continue to cause many problems with a person's increasing age.

EXERCISES TO BE AVOIDED

Throughout this text, but in particular in Chapters 6 and 7, an effort is made to recommend specific exercises that are both effective and safe. Over the years, a number of exercises that place abnormal stresses, strains, and compression forces on particular muscles or joints have been recommended and widely used that potentially predispose these structures to injury. Appropriate stretching, strengthening, conditioning, and in some cases corrective exercises are described in detail within individual chapters. Figures 10-22 through 10-33 identify a series of exercises that for one reason or another are *not* recommended as being safe and may potentially result in injury. For each of the potentially dangerous exercises in Figures 10-22 through 10-33, a suggestion is given for an alternative and safe exercise that has been previously recommended. The following box provides a number of guidelines that will decrease your chance for injury in whatever fitness activity you pursue.

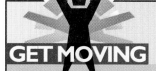

Ways to avoid injury

1. Always warm up properly before engaging in any activity.
2. Do not neglect the cool-down period after exercise.
3. Make certain that muscles are stretched sufficiently. Use full range-of-motion static stretching during an active warm-up period, and use total body stretching during the cool-down period.
4. Avoid passive overstretching to reduce the possibility of injury to the ligaments or joint capsule.
5. Avoid any movements, exercises, or activities that produce compression or impingement of joint motion.
6. Begin at a low intensity, and progress within your individual limits to higher intensities. Do not try to do too much too soon.
7. Avoid holding your breath and straining too hard during intense activity.
8. Choose a level of intensity that is compatible with your abilities in terms of strength, power, and endurance.
9. Select the appropriate clothing for exercising in hot or cold environments.
10. Make sure you are acclimated to the environment in which you are exercising, regardless of whether it is extremely hot or cold.
11. Select and use high-quality equipment when engaging in any physical activity. Breakdown of cheap or low-quality equipment may prove to be more expensive in the long run should injury occur.
12. Listen to what your body is telling you. If you experience pain during activity, stop immediately.
13. Do not engage in any activity that you think may have the potential to result in injury.
14. Receive a doctor's OK to begin physical activity, especially if you are over age 40 and have any history of heart disease.

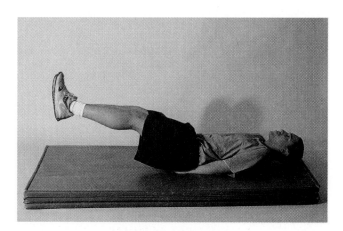

FIGURE 10-22. Straight-Leg Lifts.
Used for strengthening abdominal muscles and hip flexors. Tends to tilt the pelvis forward, thus causing hyperextension of the low back, which compresses the intervertebral disks.
Safe alternative exercise: Curl-ups, bent-knee leg lifts, sitting tucks (see Figures 6-37, 6-27, and 6-41).

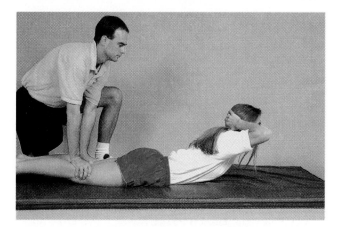

FIGURE 10-23. Back Hyperextensions.
Used to strengthen low back muscles and stretch abdominal muscles. Causes compression of intervertebral disks with possible disk herniation or spinal nerve impingement.
Safe alternative exercise: Reverse leg lifts (see Figure 6-28).

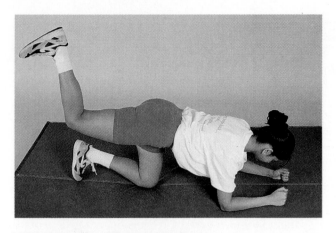

FIGURE 10-24. **Donkey Kicks.**
Used to develop extensor muscles of the low back. Involves a ballistic backward and upward kick with the leg and an extension of the neck. Causes compression of intervertebral disks and possible disk herniation or spinal nerve impingement.
Safe alternative exercise: Leg lifts (see Figure 6-43).

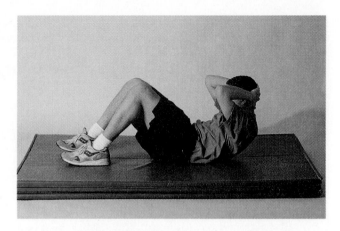

FIGURE 10-26. **Curl-Ups With Hands Behind Neck.**
Used for strengthening abdominal muscles. Pulls head and neck into hyperflexed position, stretching the intervertebral joint ligaments of the cervical spine.
Safe alternative exercise: Curl-ups (see Figure 6-37).

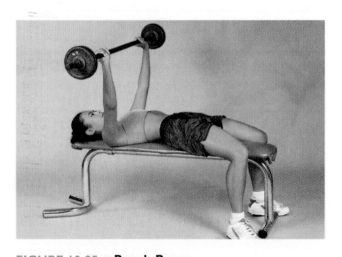

FIGURE 10-25. **Bench Press.**
Used for strengthening pectoral and triceps muscles. This lift, done with the feet on the floor and an arched back, hyperextends the low back.
Safe alternative exercise: Bench press (see Figure 6-13).

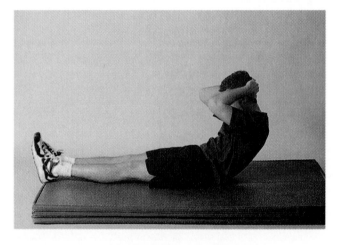

FIGURE 10-27. **Straight-Leg Sit-Ups.**
Causes a forward tilt of the pelvis, placing the low back in a hyperextended position, thus adding unnecessary compression forces.
Safe alternative exercise: Curl-ups (see Figure 6-37).

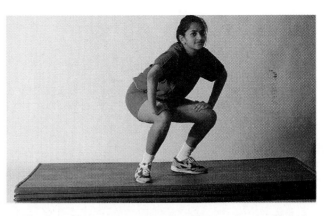

FIGURE 10-30. **Deep Knee Bends.**
Used for strengthening hip and knee extensors.
Places extreme compressive forces on the knee
joint, stressing ligaments, joint capsule, and cartilage
(menisci).
Safe alternative exercise: Forward lunge exercise
(see Figure 7-15).

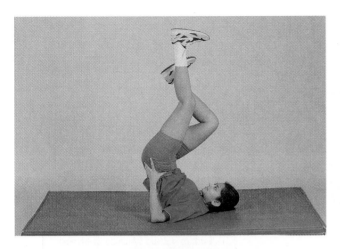

FIGURE 10-28. **Upright Bicycling.**
Used for strengthening abdominal muscles. Places
the cervical and upper thoracic regions of the
spine in a hyperflexed position, creating increased
compression forces on intervertebral disks and
stretching intervertebral ligaments.
Safe alternative exercise: Supine bicycle (see
Figure 6-42).

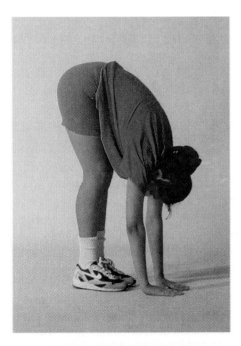

FIGURE 10-29. **Standing Toe Touches.**
Used to stretch the hamstring muscles. Causes
hyperextension of the knees and pressure in the
low back, especially if the hamstring muscles are
tight.
Safe alternative exercise: Hamstring stretch exercise (see Figure 7-18).

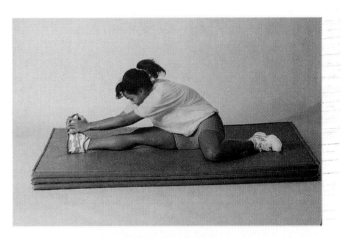

FIGURE 10-31. **Hurdlers' Stretch.**
Used for stretching the quadriceps muscle.
Rotation of the tibia with compression of the knee
joint causes stress to the medial ligaments and
compression of the medial cartilage.
Safe alternative exercise: Forward lunge exercise
(see Figure 7-15).

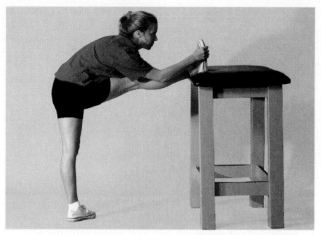

FIGURE 10-32. Bar Stretch.
Used for stretching hamstring muscles.
Hyperextends the knee, placing stress on the posterior joint capsule and ligaments. Also stretches and may irritate the sciatic nerve, which innervates most of the muscles in the posterior leg.
Safe alternative exercise: Hamstring stretch exercise (see Figure 7-18)

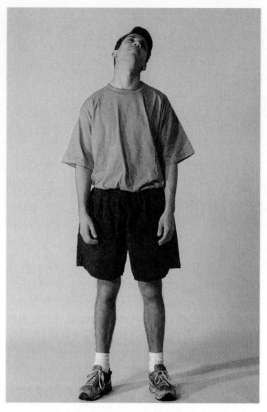

FIGURE 10-33. Neck Circles.
Used for range of motion in the cervical spine. Requires hyperextension of the cervical spine, which causes unnecessary compression of the cervical intervertebral disks.

SUMMARY

- Injuries associated with a physical training program most often can be avoided by designing a well-planned program based on the principles of overload, progression, consistency, specificity, individuality, and safety.
- Listen to what your body is telling you. The "no pain, no gain" mentality will likely worsen an existing injury. The best way to prevent injury is to begin at low levels of intensity and gradually progress at your own speed.
- Injuries can be classified as being either *acute traumatic injuries* or *chronic overuse injuries*. Acute injuries include fractures, contusions, muscle strains, ligament sprains, and muscle soreness. Overuse injuries that can become chronic include tendinitis and bursitis.
- Low back pain can have many causes, but the most common are herniated disks, lumbosacral

strains, sacroiliac sprains, excessive tightness of the hamstrings, and weak abdominal muscles.
- Low back pain can be prevented by paying attention to standing, lying, sitting, and working posture to prevent the low back from being placed in potentially injurious positions.
- All injuries should be initially managed using rest, ice, compression, and elevation to control swelling and thus reduce the time required for rehabilitation.
- Injuries that occur during physical activity should be diagnosed by a physician, and rehabilitation should be supervised by an athletic trainer or physical therapist.
- There are several exercises that are not recommended because of increased potential for injury.

REFERENCES

American Academy of Orthopaedic Surgeons: *Athletic training and sports medicine,* Park Ridge, Ill, 1991, American Academy of Orthopaedic Surgeons.

American Orthopaedic Society for Sports Medicine: *Sports-induced inflammation,* Park Ridge, Ill, 1990, American Academy of Orthopaedic Surgeons.

Anderson M, Hall S: *Sports injury management,* Baltimore, 1995, Williams & Wilkins.

Armstrong R, Warren G, Warren J: Mechanisms of exercise induced muscle fiber injury, *Sports Med* 12:184-207, 1991.

Arnheim D, Prentice WE: *Principles of athletic training,* St Louis, 1997, Mosby.

Gallaspie J, May D: *Signs and symptoms of athletic injuries,* St Louis, 1996, Mosby.

Gould J, Davies G: *Orthopedic and sports physical therapy,* St Louis, 1990, Mosby.

Herring S: Exercise therapy for patients with acute low back pain, *Clin J Sports Med* 4(2):142, 1994.

Morris A: *Sports medicine: prevention of athletic injuries,* Dubuque, 1992, WC Brown.

O'Donoghue D: *Treatment of injuries to athletes,* Philadelphia, 1984, WB Saunders.

Pfeiffer R, Magnus B: *Concepts of athletic training,* Boston, 1995, Jones & Bartlett.

Prentice W: *Rehabilitation techniques in sports medicine,* St Louis, 1994, Mosby.

Prentice W: *Therapeutic modalities for sports medicine,* St Louis, 1994, Mosby.

Press J, Young J: Low back pain. In Mellion M, editor: *Sports medicine secrets,* Philadelphia, 1994, Hanley & Belfus.

Saunders D: *Evaluation, treatment and prevention of musculoskeletal disorders,* Bloomington, Minn, 1985, Educational Opportunities.

Scoppa F, Massara G: Back school: an interdisciplinary approach to low back pain, *J Int Council Health Phys Educ Rec Sport Dance* 30(2):30-33, 1994.

Strauss R: *Sports medicine,* Philadelphia, 1992, WB Saunders.

US Department of Health and Human Services, Public Health Services: *Healthy people 2000: national health promotion and disease prevention objectives,* Washington, DC, 1991, USDHHS.

Whitehead R: Finding a source of low back pain, *Phys Sports Med* 23(5):49-50, 1995.

SUGGESTED READINGS

Arnheim D, Prentice W: *Principles of athletic training,* St Louis, 1997, Mosby.
Currently in its ninth edition; generally considered to be the "Bible" for the athletic training profession, with comprehensive coverage of all facets of sports medicine.

Hage M: *The back pain book: a self-help guide for daily relief of neck and back pain,* Atlanta, 1992, Peachtree Plaza.
Well-illustrated text that discusses how to protect and care for your back while performing normal daily activities such as sleeping, sitting, and standing; also shows exercises for srengthening and maintaining flexibility of the back.

Micheli L: *The sports medicine bible,* New York, 1995, Harper Perennial.
A clearly written basic text that explains how to recognize and prevent injuries from occuring. Also discusses prinicples and management of injuries that do occur.

Sammann P: *YMCA healthy back book: a proven program from the world leader in back care education,* Champaign, 1994, Human Kinetics.
Discusses and demonstrates a series of exercises to maintain a healthy back.

Schatz M: *Back care basics,* Berkeley, Calif, 1992, Rodmell Press.
Provides the reader with an approach to back care and rehabilitation without the use of drugs or surgery.

Lab Activity 10-1

Fitness and Injury Record

Name _____   **Section** _____   **Date** _____

PURPOSE   To apply the information in this chapter to your own fitness program. This information may help you to create a safe and protective fitness program.

PROCEDURE Circle the appropriate response and answer the following questions.

1. Have you ever had an injury to the following body parts from participating in physical activity?

Neck	Yes	No
Upper back	Yes	No
Lower back	Yes	No
Shoulder	Yes	No
Elbow	Yes	No
Hand or wrist	Yes	No
Hip	Yes	No
Knee	Yes	No
Ankle	Yes	No
Foot	Yes	No

2. Have you ever had a fracture?   Yes   No
3. Have you ever had a dislocation?   Yes   No
4. Have you ever had heat exhaustion or heatstroke?   Yes   No
5. Have you ever had surgery?   Yes   No

Continued.

6. If you answered *yes* to any of the above, describe the injury.

_____

_____

7. How did the injury or injuries occur? _____

_____

_____

8. How was the injury treated? _____

_____

_____

9. How could it have been prevented?_____

_____

_____

10. How could a better fitness program have prevented this injury?

_____

_____

11. Have you modified your fitness program because of the injury? How? _____

_____

_____

_____

Lab Activity 10-2

Postural Screening Test

Name _____   **Section** _____   **Date** _____

PURPOSE   To analyze standing posture to determine normal postural alignment.

PROCEDURE 1. With a partner, drop a plumb line (string with a fishing weight) from the ceiling
(Figure 10-34).
2. Have your partner stand sideways, and line up the anatomical points to see whether
they fall in a straight line.

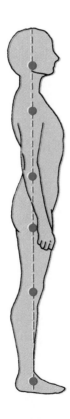

FIGURE 10-35. **Good Standing Posture.**
Good standing posture should be assessed by determining whether a
series of anatomical points falls along a straight line.

Do all the landmark points line up along the plumb line? If not, which ones are not in line?

_____
_____
_____
_____

What can be done to correct these postural abnormalities?

_____
_____
_____

Do you currently have episodes of low back pain? If yes, describe the pain.

_____
_____

How do you think this pain may be related to postural abnormalities?

_____
_____

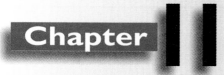

Chapter 11 Handling Stress

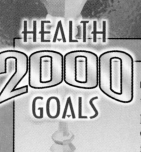

HEALTH 2000 GOALS

■ **Adverse Health Effects.** Reduce to less than 35% the proportion of people age 18 and older who have experienced adverse health effects from stress within the past year. In 1985, 42.2% of people age 18 and older reported a possible stress-induced, health-related illness. *Midpoint Update: headed in the right direction with current statistic of 39.2%.*

■ **Stress Control.** Decrease to no more than 5% the proportion of people age 18 and older who report experiencing significant levels of stress and who do not take steps to reduce or control their stress. In 1985, 21% of the population reported that they experienced stress and did nothing to control it.

■ **Stress Management.** Increase to at least 40% the proportion of work sites employing 50 or more people that provide programs to reduce employee stress. In 1985, 26.6% of work sites offered stress-reduction programs to their employees.

OBJECTIVES

After completing this chapter, you will be able to do the following:

■ Define the terms *stress, stressor, eustress,* and *distress.*
■ Identify warning signs of stress.
■ Describe various kinds of psychological, physiological, and sociological stressors.
■ Explain how stress can be either beneficial or harmful.
■ Describe how the body responds to stress both physiologically and psychologically.

■ Describe Selye's general adaptation syndrome.
■ Explain various acceptable ways of coping with stress, and explain how the use of defense mechanisms can be counterproductive.
■ Describe the role of physical activity in coping with stress.
■ Identify various relaxation techniques for coping with stress.
■ List general guidelines for coping with stress.

KEY TERMS

While reading this chapter you, will become familiar with the following terms:

- stress
- stressor
- eustress
- distress
- arousal
- anxiety
- general adaptation syndrome
- coping
- defense mechanism
- stress management
- relaxation techniques

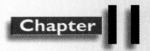

t is important for the health-conscious, physically active individual to understand the potential impact of stress on the body. Stress has been linked to many diseases. It may also interfere with performance or the attainment of one's goals. Most importantly, stress that is poorly managed greatly reduces the quality of one's life.

WHAT IS STRESS?

The term **stress** comes from the Latin word *stringere,* meaning "to draw tight." The term refers to the responses that occur in the body as a result of what is called a **stressor,** or *stimulus.* Stress occurs when the internal balance or equilibrium of the body systems is disrupted.

Everyone experiences stress, and some stress is needed to perform the daily tasks of life and more importantly to stimulate growth and development. Stress can be beneficial. However, too much stress, especially when it exists for a prolonged period of time and is unrelieved, can result in physical and mental illness.

Dr. Hans Selye, biologist and endocrinologist, defined stress as the "nonspecific response of the body to any demand made upon it to adapt, whether that demand produces pleasure or pain." He further points out that stress is caused or triggered by stressors that may be physical, social, or psychological and that may be negative or positive in nature.

Selye called human reactions to positive stressors **eustress,** that is, stress that is beneficial, and he used the term **distress** to describe detrimental responses or negative stressors. Often there is a fine line between whether something produces eustress or distress. For example, moderate physical training is a stressor that can make you become stronger and more fit. However, if you do too much too soon, it can produce distress in the form of soreness or injury.

Sometimes the difference between eustress and distress is only a matter of interpretation; do you interpret the stressor as a threat or a challenge? Although we may habitually respond in ways that seem automatic and beyond our control, we can choose to examine the way we think and then work on changing counterproductive thinking or beliefs.

Stress should not, however, be considered solely as a physiological phenomenon. Stress has also been viewed from a psychological or cognitive perspective. Current research suggests that the stress response is not a simple biological response to nonspecific stressors but is instead an interrelated process that includes the presence of a stressor, the circumstances in which the stressor occurs, the interpretation of the situation by the person, his or her typical reaction, and the resources available to deal with the stressor. For example, one person may find downhill skiing fun and exciting, looking forward to taking winter vacation to ski the slopes. Another person may have tried to ski, but dislike of cold weather and fear of injury makes skiing a distressing activity. Therefore the stress response in a given situation is dependent upon the individual's perceptions.

TYPES OF STRESSORS

There are many different types of stressors. Each day individuals encounter stressful situations that may be insignificant or great, pleasant or painful, physical or emotional. Stressors in college may be tests or dislikes for a subject, professor, or classmate. Most have experienced problems with family members, concern over money, or arguments with loved ones. Exposure to heat, cold, noise, and other environmental conditions such as pollutants are physiological stressors, as are illnesses, injuries, and allergies. Family problems, dealing with overcrowding, loneliness, and boredom are psychological stressors. Furthermore, one type of stressor can create the other. For example, worry over a final (psychological stress) can be so preoccupying that a person fails to obtain enough sleep (physiological stress). Figure 11-1 lists specific sources of stressors.

Significant changes that occur during a person's lifetime are major stressors. Holmes and Rahe have developed a life-change scale to show how various life events can cause stress as they change a person's lifestyle. The scale was developed after noting increased frequency of illness after many major life stressors. Subsequently this scale has been adapted to look at life changes within the college population. **Lab Activity 11-1** will help you assess your major life stressors.

PSYCHOLOGICAL OR COGNITIVE RESPONSE TO STRESS

Once the initiation of the stress process is stimulated by the presence of a stressor, psychological or

FIGURE 11-1. Specific Sources of Stressors.

Physical Stressors

Heat
Cold
Pain
Hunger
Exercise
Lack of sleep
Disease
Physical aches and pains
Sexual arousal

Psychosocial Stressors

Family expectations
Loss of friend

Troubles with a significant other
Isolation
Unemployment
Loneliness
Depression
Fear

Environmental Stressors

Noise
Pollution
Floods
Inclement weather
Overcrowding

cognitive processes take over, determining the manner in which the stressor is perceived. An individual's perceptions of a particular situation can elicit a response that may vary from arousal to anxiety. Arousal is the body's heightened awareness that a stressor is present and is a signal to higher centers in the brain to respond (physiological). Anxiety, on the other hand, is described by Speilberger as feelings of tension, apprehension, nervousness, and worry. He maintains that these are cognitive rather than biological responses.

The degree to which a particular situation elicits an emotional response depends to a great extent on how the individual appraises the situation and how well prepared he or she feels to handle it. Those individuals who are prone to stress tend to make extreme, absolute, global judgments and engage in cognitive distortions in which they overemphasize the most negative aspects of a given situation. Our thought processes seem automatic, but we need to emphasize the necessity of examining our beliefs and working on changing them when they are erroneous or counterproductive.

Certainly there are both biological and cognitive responses to stressors. Even though we talk about them as two separate processes, they are interrelated and occur simultaneously.

PHYSIOLOGICAL RESPONSE TO STRESS

Every organ system in the body is affected by the stress response. There are two physiological regulatory systems in the body that govern the stress response: the nervous system and the endocrine system. There are differences between the nervous and endocrine systems in terms of how quickly they respond to a stressor and how long their responses

are sustained. The endocrine system secretes hormones that prepare the body to deal with a stressful situation. These hormones may remain in the bloodstream for several weeks. The endocrine system's responses to stress endure, whereas the nervous system's responses are short-lived. This suggests that the endocrine system is most important for any connection between stress and disease. Figure 11-2 summarizes the effects of stress on various physiological systems.

General Adaptation Syndrome

Selye described the body's physiological response to stress as the general adaptation syndrome (GAS). His research showed that the response to stressors follows a three-stage pattern of alarm, resistance, and exhaustion.

During the alarm stage the body undergoes physiological changes that are collectively referred to as the *fight-or-flight syndrome* (e.g., increased heart rate, blood pressure, and respiratory rate). These responses

---

stress a term that comes from the Latin word *stringere*, meaning "to draw tight"—a response that occurs in the body, causing tension

stressor a stimulus that causes stress in the body

eustress term for the human reaction to a positive form of stress

distress term for the human reaction to a negative form of stress

arousal a heightened biological awareness by the body that a stressor is present

anxiety cognitive responses to stress, including feelings of tension, apprehension, nervousness, and worry

general adaptation syndrome Selye's description of the physiological response to stress that follows a three-stage pattern of alarm, resistance, and exhaustion

---

FIGURE 11-2. Stress and Specific Physical Disorders.

Heart Disease Personality: Having the characteristics of a Type A personality is a risk factor for coronary artery disease (see Chapter 2).

High Blood Pressure: Individuals who are under stress are more likely to have high blood pressure. This may have some relationship to personality type.

Immune System: Chemicals released during the stress response suppress the immune system, which involves a network of organs, tissues, and white blood cells that fight disease.

Digestive System: Stress can cause heartburn, diarrhea, gastritis, and gas. Stress will not cause an ulcer but can make an ulcer feel worse.

Headaches: Tension headaches and migraine headaches are both more likely to occur with increased stress.

Skin Problems: Certain skin conditions such as acne, herpes simplex, psoriasis, hives, and eczema are likely to appear or worsen with increased stress.

Muscles: Stress causes increased tension, particularly in the muscles of the neck and upper back, that can lead to the development of painful trigger points.

Respiratory Problems: Stress can worsen asthma, especially the type of asthma that is exercise-induced.

Diabetes: Stress can affect blood sugar levels, which is a potentially dangerous problem for a diabetic.

---

are the body's normal physiological reactions to danger and prepare a person to "fight" against a hostile stressor or "flee" from danger. These physiological changes are primarily a nervous system response to prepare the body for vigorous muscular action.

In the resistance stage, the body adjusts to stress and appears to return to its normal state of internal balance. An example of the effects of prolonged stress would be your boss at work who makes your life miserable. You must control your emotions so that you can still perform your job in the presence of this stressor. Since changes in the endocrine system are maintained during this resistance stage, the effects continue for several weeks, months, years, or even decades, depending on the vitality of the person affected. However, sustained resistance can result in a strain on the body's adaptive resources.

If stress persists for a long time, exhaustion sets in. The person becomes less able to resist stress. Research has indicated that stress is highly correlated to a breakdown of various physiological systems. Sustained stress can affect various body systems so that illness and even death may result. For example, the cardiovascular system is affected by stress. Some experts believe that emotional stress is one of the leading contributing factors in the development of heart disease. Other systems of the body are also affected. The muscular system may respond to stress with uncontrolled spasms called *tics* or *bracing*, which involve muscles remaining tense in a chronic, unhealthy manner. It has been suggested that more research needs to be conducted to see if there is any relationship between stress and problems affecting the bones and joints (such as arthritis), skin eruptions (hives and acne), headaches, and the breakdown of the body's immune system. When this natural form of defense against disease breaks down, the person can become more susceptible to illnesses.

Personality and Stress

In identifying people who are at risk for developing cardiovascular disease, researchers believed that there was a connection between behavior pattern and risk of heart disease. People were classified as being either "type A" or "type B" personalities. The type A person is always "on the go," never satisfied with his or her level of achievement, appears tense, suffers from a sense of time urgency, and is competitive and impatient. In contrast, the type B person is more easy-going and relaxed, more patient and satisfied with his or her level of achievement. The type A person was believed to have a higher risk of developing cardiovascular disease. Recent research suggests that only those individuals who have *hostile* or *angry* behavior patterns are at risk. Therefore identifying the sources of anger and hostility in these people and helping them with behavior modification may allow them to cope more effectively with stress. Figure 11-3 lists questions that will enable you to determine how you feel about yourself. The Health Link box on p. 337 provides some ideas to help you cope with anger. **Lab Activity 11-2** will help you determine whether you exhibit stress-related behaviors.

FIGURE 11-3. The Way You Feel About Yourself May Indicate Stress.

Are you:
- Impatient?
- Easily angered?
- Frequently frustrated?
- In need of recognition?
- Obsessed with being a winner?
- A worrier?
- A person who fears failure?
- Viewing the future with trepidation?
- Upset when subjected to criticism?
- Indecisive?
- Interested in controlling others?
- Possessed with a guilt complex when you make mistakes?
- Overwhelmed by responsibility?

NOTE: If you answer *yes* to any of these conditions, it may indicate that the way you feel about yourself is causing stress in your life.

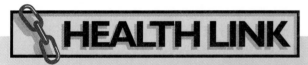

HEALTH LINK

COPING WITH ANGER

- Anger may be a major factor in ulcers, headaches, loss of self-esteem, and cardiovascular disease, although certainly these problems may result from causes other than anger. To cope with anger, take charge of your own feelings. Resolve not to let somebody else make you angry. One way to deal with anger is by expressing it early on rather than letting it build up.
- When you get angry in a particular situation, ask yourself the question, "Is it helping or hurting me?" If it is hurting you, use the experience as a way to prevent such situations from occurring again.
- Keep a daily record of the times you exhibit anger—why it occurred, how long it lasted. Such a record will increase your awareness of such behavior.
- When angry, take time out before the feeling becomes too intense. This will give you time to cool down and rethink your behavior. If possible, do something physical during the time out. It will help you to release your anger arousal.
- Since tension is one of the first signs of anger, when it occurs, practice relaxing by such means as deeper and slower breathing and stretching.

WARNING SIGNS OF STRESS

Persons under stress tend to display certain warning signs and symptoms that vary from one person to the next. Selye lists 27 detectable signs of danger (Figure 11-4). If you experience one or more of these symptoms, you are experiencing some degree of negative stress. You should also determine if your stress level is too high. If it is, try to reduce your negative stress level to avoid developing physical or emotional problems.

Physical Signs

You can see from Selye's list that some physical and emotional signs of distress affect certain organ systems. Heart palpitations are cardiovascular in nature, vomiting is gastrointestinal in nature, and breathlessness is respiratory in nature. Some signs reflect muscular tension, such as frequent headaches, fatigue, and trembling hands. Pain in the back or neck may be experienced while one is studying for long periods of time and maintaining the same position. Other signs reflect the psychological responses to stress. Conscious feelings such as being fearful, apprehensive, confused, or disoriented are often reported.

Anxiety and Depression

Anxiety and depression are two common signs of stress. Anxiety can reflect a feeling of dread and apprehension, perhaps of some anticipated danger or lack of proper plans and strategies for coping with an anticipated danger. Going into an exam unprepared can lead to feelings of apprehension. There may be worry about many things that can go wrong in accomplishing future plans. Depression can be characterized by loss of interest in usual activities, sadness, lack of energy, and poor concentration abilities. These feelings can result from the negative interpretation of events. For example, breaking up with a boyfriend or girlfriend may be perceived as negative for one of the partners. This individual may report feeling rejected and very depressed. However, another individual may perceive the situation in a more positive light. He or she may determine that the relationship was not a healthy one and that breaking up represents an opportunity to learn from the experience and find a more suitable partner.

Sleep Disturbance

Insomnia is a common sign of stress that drains a person's energy. The reason for insomnia may be that you are anxious or excited about future events. Losing sleep because you are concerned and worried about an upcoming paper or exam is a sign of stress. Although missing a night or two of sleep may be a normal thing for some people, for others it can be a symptom of stress.

FIGURE 11-4. Signs of Stress.

Selye lists stress symptoms that may represent danger signs. Do you ever experience one or more of these symptoms?

Irritability and depression	Stuttering or other speech problems
Heart palpitations	Insomnia
Dryness of throat and mouth	Breathlessness
Impulsive behavior	Sweating
Inability to concentrate	Frequent urination
Feelings of weakness or dizziness	Diarrhea and indigestion
Crying	Migraine headaches
Anxiety	Premenstrual tension or missed menstrual cycles
Emotional tension	Pain in back
Nervous tics	Increased smoking
Vomiting	Loss of appetite
Easily startled by small sounds	Nightmares
Nervous laughter	Fatigue
Trembling hands	

Sexual Dysfunction

Sexual dysfunction can be a sign of stress. Furthermore, such a condition can lead to further stress if the condition continues to exist as a result of worry. Because sexual release is one method of alleviating stress, lack of this ability creates further problems. Concerns over the possibility of becoming pregnant or contracting a sexually transmitted disease through sexual contact can contribute to stress.

Lowered Self-Esteem

The way you feel about yourself can produce stress in your life. People with low self-esteem may perceive situations as being more negative and more difficult to deal with. They may be less able to find effective solutions to their problems and thus become depressed with their lives. Being comfortable with who you are and with your perceptions of how others feel about you can help you reduce stress levels.

COPING WITH STRESS

Life is filled with many challenges, some of which represent potential obstacles in the path of your career and life goals. Coping is an attempt to effectively manage or control stress so that it does not dominate your life. By coping with stress, you use techniques that alter the physiological and psychological consequences of stress. Some of these methods are useful in the short run but are harmful because the source of the stress has not been properly handled. Other methods of coping are beneficial because they allow people to achieve self-fulfillment. They learn to manage conflicts, sources of pressure, and frustration without experiencing harm to their bodies. The box on p. 339 offers a number of ways you can effectively deal with stress in your personal life.

Negative Coping Behaviors

There are many examples of negative or harmful ways of coping with stressful situations. Some people under stress experience a change in appetite. The result may be overeating or undereating. Others increase the number of cigarettes they smoke, feeling that relief comes with every puff on the cigarette. However, the chances are that the more you smoke, the more you are stressed, because nicotine increases heart rate and acts on the body to temporarily raise blood pressure, levels of cholesterol, and the hormone *norepinephrine*. An increase in the consumption of alcohol may also be a sign of stress. Drinking permits a person to relax and forget some of the things that are causing stress, but it may result in dependence on alcohol to experience additional psychological relief. Thus increased drinking can lead to further problems, including alcoholism.

Some people increase their caffeine intake when under stress. The average cup of coffee contains 100 to 150 mg of caffeine, and consumption of caffeine can cause insomnia, headaches, and nervousness. Caffeinated soft drinks can have the same stimulating effects. It is recommended that you gradually decrease the amount of caffeinated beverages consumed to avoid the discomfort of withdrawal symptoms. Lab Activity 11-3 will help you determine how well you cope with stress.

Ways to deal with stress

GET MOVING

1. First try to be honest with yourself about all the things that are going on in your life, and then share your worries with someone you love, trust, or respect.
2. When you are feeling hassled and little things upset you that shouldn't, take a deep breath, count to 10, and then put everything in perspective. Ask yourself, "Is this the worst thing that is ever going to happen to me? Has anyone I love been hurt or affected? Will this still make me mad tomorrow?"
3. Become a better time manager. Keep a prioritized list of things to be done each day. Break down large, time-consuming projects into small chunks and reward yourself when you complete each part. Accept the fact that there is only so much time each day and that as long as you're working consistently, what you don't get done today you can finish tomorrow.
4. Work on developing healthy lifestyle habits that will enhance your resistance to stress (e.g., exercise), and avoid negative addictions such as smoking and drinking.
5. Keep a diary of things that seem to cause you stress so that over a period of time you can identify patterns or situations that cause problems. Then figure out how you can eliminate these stress-inducing situations.
6. Try to be positive and optimistic. If you constantly look for what's wrong with you or others around you, you will always find something, which often makes you feel even worse. Instead, focus on the positive aspects of all situations and try to find a little something that is good about each situation.
7. Laugh at yourself and try to maintain a sense of humor no matter what the situation.
8. Accept the fact that you can't control everything in your life and realize that your way is not always going to be the best way. Try to relax and accept other ways of doing things.
9. Develop a network of people—both family and friends—whom you love and trust, and put a degree of faith in their support when things get tough. Live your life for the good times that you share with these people, but make sure they will be there for you when things aren't so good.
10. Try to constantly focus on the pleasant aspects of your life and on the things that you can do to improve your situation.
11. Don't procrastinate. If you constantly put off things that you don't want to deal with or that are unpleasant, and you know that sooner or later you are going to have to address them, your level of frustration escalates and you feel more stressed. Deal with every situation as soon as you can.

Coping With Stress Through Defense Mechanisms

In a very broad sense, every behavior or thought that satisfies a particular need can be a defense mechanism. However, in psychology these mechanisms are defined and categorized as therapists interpret the meaning behind everyday behavior. Essentially, these mechanisms protect the ego; they preserve the harmony within a person and provide some sense of adequacy. Normally these defense mechanisms are positive responses. For example, they can help a person cope with anxiety.

We all use defense mechanisms, but if these mechanisms are allowed to become a habitual pattern of behavior or provide excuses for individuals to avoid responsibility for their actions, the behavior can become counterproductive. For example, a commonly used defense mechanism is projecting blame on some-

---

coping an attempt to effectively manage or control stress so that it does not dominate one's life

defense mechanism a psychological device that is designed to protect the ego, preserve inner harmony, and provide a sense of adequacy

one or something for failure. The person rationalizes that the reason they failed a test is because the professor used "trick" questions or that his or her test was "unfair." However, the student may have missed several classes and failed to spend enough time studying. Denial is another form of defense mechanism. Many alcoholics deny that they have a drinking problem rather than accept the reality of their dependency.

The particular defense mechanism that is operating at a given moment depends on the particular situation and the past history of reinforcement. Reinforcement occurs when the individual has successfully used a defense mechanism in the past. He or she will tend to use this mechanism in subsequent situations. A word of caution: these mechanisms are often deceptive devices; that is, they are not necessarily the most effective way to deal with stress. They may bolster the ego, but they can also circumvent real problems. If this is the case, they are being used to evade dealing with reality and responsibility. Figure 11-5 lists some of the major forms of defense mechanisms. The Fit List box on p. 341 provides some ideas to help cope with the stress of studying.

REDUCING STRESS WITH PHYSICAL ACTIVITY

Although there are several methods and techniques to control stress, physical activity is one of the most helpful. It is believed that exercise burns up stress hormones. Activity helps to release the physical and emotional tension that can accumulate when you are under stress. A lifestyle in which stress is successfully managed is thought by some to provide a balance between work, play, rest, and exercise.

Michael, in *Stress Adaptation Through Exercise*, found that physical activity provides a low type of stress for the endocrine system's adrenal glands, which allows them to more effectively counter severe stress. Increased adrenal activity as a result of exercise appears to result in the creation and formation of reserves of the steroid hormones that counteract stress. deVries found that activities such as jogging, bicycling, walking, and benchstepping for durations from 5 to 30 minutes and with target heart rates of 30% to 60% of maximum rate resulted in significant relaxation for tense persons.

Selye suggests that the person who exercises regularly is able to resist stressors better and that situations that are stressful do not represent as much harm to the trained person as to the sedentary person. Thus exercise appears to provide a mental diversion from problems and activities that can cause stress.

Matteson and Ivancevich, in their book *Managing Job Stress and Health*, indicated that the general benefits of exercise include the following:

- Greater strength and endurance, leading to more efficient use of energy
- Improved cardiovascular function, including lowering of blood pressure and a lower heart rate
- Less fatty tissue in the body

FIGURE 11-5. Defense Mechanisms.

Rationalization:	A mental mechanism that is used to avoid facing a loss of self-esteem or to prevent feeling guilty. For example, a student who flunks out of college remarks, "Who needs it?"
Projection:	Attribution of unacceptable personal qualities to other people, as when the inability to make friends evokes the response, "The people are all unfriendly."
Compensation:	Substitution of an attainable goal for one that may be unattainable. For example, the physically inadequate student who wants to be a star athlete, but cannot, puts all his energies into journalism, at which he can excel.
Sublimation:	Change of direction of a basic drive toward a new goal when the original goal is impossible to obtain. For example, a student with a basic drive of aggression directs it to playing football rather than taking it out on classmates by picking fights with them.
Repression:	Removal from consciousness of memories that are painful and desires that produce strong guilt feelings. For example, a student fails to keep an appointment with a professor who failed him in another subject. This mechanism can be harmful when it creates stress and behavioral problems.
Fantasy:	Type of daydreaming involving substitution of imagination for reality. For example, a student imagines she is the top student in the class or the star athlete on the team.
Identification:	Identification with another person such as a professor, a coach, or a famous personality. This mental mechanism becomes harmful when it interferes with the development of a person's real self and identity.

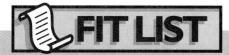

COPING WITH STRESS WHILE STUDYING

- After each class, find the time to review your notes. If you wait until just before the exam, some of the information may be unclear, and you may not have time to check with the instructor or others in the class.
- List the study tasks that need to be performed, and organize the materials that you need to study.
- Break large tasks into smaller ones, and concentrate on one task at a time.
- Select a place to study where there will be a minimum of interruption.
- If background music is desired and helpful, keep the volume low and make selections relaxing, not loud and brassy.
- Take periodic breaks. Go for a walk or do something different to relax.
- Get adequate sleep. It is difficult to study when you are tired.
- Do not expect too much of yourself. Set practical goals for each of your courses. Concentrate on the most challenging courses.
- If poor grades and long assignments are a source of stress, talk to your professors. You may want to seek help from the school's health clinic. Remember, too much stress can make you miserable and ill.

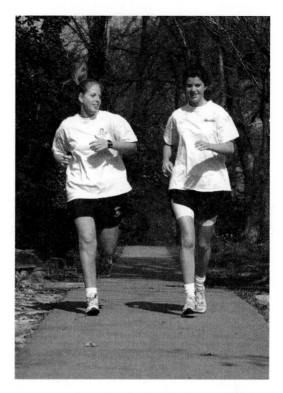

FIGURE 11-6. **Exercise Is Conducive to Relaxation.**

- Better appearance and a more positive self-concept
- Better muscle tone and posture
- Better use of food
- Greater cardiac output
- Increased number of red blood cells, furthering oxygen delivery to cells
- Better sleeping pattern
- Less consumption of drugs, including alcohol and tobacco
- Better control of body fat
- Lower cholesterol levels in the blood

According to Anderson, physical exercise provides three benefits for humans: (1) maintenance of good muscular tone, which makes it possible to engage in a variety of physical activities; (2) creation of a healthy cardiovascular system; and (3) a sense of well-being as a result of reduced stress. Consequently individuals are more relaxed after exercising (Figure 11-6).

Charlesworth and Nathan point out that the human body and the image of the body that is held by some persons is a stressor, whether because of too much weight, poor muscular development, or poor posture. Exercise can improve your body development and thus improve your self-image. They also point out that when problems confront you and appear difficult to solve, physical activity can provide a mental release and an opportunity to arrive at solutions in a more relaxed manner.

The values of exercise are not limited to the physical; exercise also contributes to sound mental health. Many who exercise regularly state that exercise makes them feel better. Results of research on muscle tension and brain-wave activity suggest that exercise lowers arousal levels and anxiety/tension. Psychiatrist William Menninger pointed out that physical activity provides an outlet for instinctive aggressive drives by enabling a person to "blow off steam," providing relaxation and supplementing daily work and study. He stressed that "recreation, which is literally recreating relaxation from regular activity, is a morale builder."

Matteson and Ivancevich provide some major explanations of the influence of physical activity on stress:

- Changes that are psychological in nature result from physiological and biochemical changes that come from exercise.

• The awareness of physiological changes taking place as a result of activity by the person exercising may lead to lower stress.
• Regular exercise may condition stress adaptation mechanisms in the body, causing an increased reserve of steroids to counter stress.
• The challenges offered by physical activity and meeting those challenges successfully may result in more positive responses to stress-provoking situations.

Coping With Stress Caused by Physical Activity

Although physical activity is usually thought of as one of the most effective ways to manage stress, for some individuals physical activity is a stressor. Following the guidelines in the Safe Tip box below will increase the chance that your participation in physical activity is associated with eustress rather than distress.

Effects of Stress on Performance

J. B. Oxendine has developed what is called the *Inverted-U Theory*, which relates stress to performance (Figure 11-7). The theory suggests there is an optimal level of stress that results in better performance as a result of added motivation, such as the performance of a player in a sport contest. When there is too little stress, however, the needed motivation is not present, and as a result the performance or accomplishment of a task is minimal or does not occur. Furthermore, if there is too much stress, performance may be disrupted and the task poorly accomplished or not done at all. The amount of stress needed to have optimum performance will depend on the task to be accomplished and the individual involved.

Life Stress and Sport-Related Injury

Williams and Anderson have proposed a model for stress and injury related to activity. The actual stress response comes about as a result of the athlete's consideration of the demands posed by the stressor, the resources for dealing with it, and the consequences imposed by the stressor. The physiological responses that affect and are affected by this cognitive appraisal include muscle tension, narrowing of the field of vision, and increased distractibility. The effects of all of these responses can lead to athletic injury. It is hypothesized that if the stress response is too strong to be handled by the individual's available resources, injury is likely to occur.

Thus it appears that a relationship exists between a high degree of life stress and the incidence of sport-related injuries. Furthermore, recent studies have also indicated that individuals who have a high degree of social support tend to have a lower incidence of injury. Activity-related stress may be

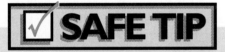

PREVENTING STRESS FROM INTERFERING WITH YOUR WORKOUT

• Before beginning a physical fitness program, get a thorough physical examination from your family physician. Take a physical stress test if it is recommended.
• There is no shortcut to fitness. Recognize that it takes time. Do not try to cut corners to get in shape in 1 or 2 days.
• Engage in warm-up and cool-down exercises before and after a vigorous physical workout.
• Do not exercise if you feel ill.
• Observe such warning signs as dizziness, nausea, breathlessness, and pain.
• Check your heart rate after exercising. It should return to near normal resting rate within 10 minutes after you stop. If it does not, the activity may have been too vigorous or may have been performed for too long a time.
• Drink plenty of water.
• Do not perform heavy exercises immediately after eating a heavy meal.

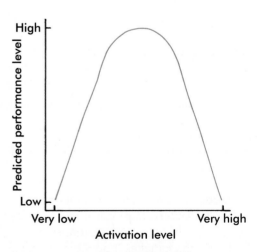

FIGURE 11-7. Inverted-U Diagram.
The Inverted-U Theory shows that optimal level of stress will result in the highest level of performance.

reduced by intervention techniques including imagery, biofeedback, and progressive relaxation, which will be discussed later.

STRESS MANAGEMENT

It is important for you to develop and incorporate into your lifestyle any techniques that will help you effectively reduce stress. Figure 11-8 lists some general guidelines for reducing stress. However, stress management involves more than simply reducing the total quantity of stress in your life; it also means being able to change the quality of stress in your life. Uncontrolled stress can result in physical and psychological disorders that pose a real threat to well-being. To manage stress effectively you must realize that you are responsible for your own emotional and physical well-being. Your perception of events, if not the events themselves, is under your control. You need not allow other people's behavior to affect your ability to maintain a relatively stable emotional and physical condition. Besides using physical activity, learning to control thought processes can be an effective method of managing stress. Collectively referred to as relaxation techniques, these methods have been demonstrated to be very helpful. A few of the more common relaxation techniques are presented on the next few pages.

RELAXATION TECHNIQUES

Relaxation is essentially a mental phenomenon concerned with the reduction of tensions that could originate from muscular activity but are more likely to result from psychological responses to our hectic lifestyles. Relaxation techniques may be broadly classified as either mind-to-muscle techniques that control the level of stimulation along the nerve pathways coming from the brain to the muscles (yoga, meditation, imagery, and autogenic training) or muscle-to-mind techniques that control the level of stimulation going to the brain from the muscles (progressive relaxation, massage, and biofeedback).

The Jacobson Technique

Dr. Edmond Jacobson, who made the first objective investigation of the relationship of exercise and relaxation, developed a technique that has two basic steps.

1. *The person learns to recognize muscle tension in subtle as well as in gross forms.* Gross tension is easily identified. With fists tightly clenched, hold your arms outstretched to the side at shoulder height for 1 minute. Note the feeling of exertion and discomfort in the forearms and shoulders. Drop your arms to the side and relax the muscles of the arms and hands completely. Note the effort-

---

FIGURE 11-8. General Guidelines for Stress Reduction.

Selye set forth several suggestions for stress reduction, including:

- Try not to be a perfectionist. Instead, perform and work within your capabilities.
- Spend your time in ways other than trying to befriend those persons who don't want to experience your love and friendship.
- Enjoy the simple things of life.
- Strive and fight only for those things that are really worthwhile.
- Accent the positive and the pleasant side of life.
- On experiencing a defeat or setback, maintain your self-confidence by remembering past accomplishments and successes.
- Do not delay tackling the unpleasant tasks that must be done; instead, get at them immediately.
- Evaluate people's progress on the basis of their performance.
- Recognize that leaders, to be leaders, must have the respect of their followers.
- Adopt a motto that you will live in a way that will earn your neighbor's love.
- Try to live so that your existence will be useful to society.
- Clarify your values.
- Take constructive action to eliminate a source of stress.

Other suggestions

- Maintain good physical and mental health.
- Accept what you cannot change.
- Serve other people and some worthy cause.
- Share worries with someone you can trust.
- Pay attention to your body.
- Balance work and recreation.
- Improve your qualifications for the realistic goals you aspire to.
- Avoid reliance on things such as drugs and alcohol.
- Don't be narcissistic.
- Manage your time effectively.
- Laugh at yourself.
- Get enough rest and sleep.
- Don't be too hard on yourself.
- Improve your self-esteem.

---

stress management reducing the total quantity of stress and changing the quality of stress in your life to decrease the physical and psychological threat of stress on your well-being

relaxation techniques controlling thought processes to effectively manage stress

less relaxation, which Dr. Jacobson calls the "negative of exertion." Subtle tension, involving less muscle effort than that just illustrated, is sometimes difficult to detect. It takes concentration and practice to learn to recognize minor tension in the trunk, neck, face, throat, and other body parts. However, it is important to learn to recognize subtle muscle tension to be able to relax.

2. *The person learns to relax completely.* Complete relaxation is accomplished using techniques of progressive relaxation. Progressive relaxation involves alternately tensing (5 to 10 seconds) and relaxing (45 seconds) the muscles, moving through the body in a systematic fashion to tense and relax all major muscle groups. Concentrate first on the large muscle groups in the arms, legs, trunk, and neck. Then the forehead, eyes, face, and even the throat have tension eased through a program of progressive relaxation. Carried out in the fashion outlined by Jacobson, the program teaches the person to relax his or her whole body to the point of negative exertion. The result is a release of tension, an antidote to fatigue, and also an inducement to sleep.

Over the years Jacobson's techniques have been altered and adapted to the needs of the particular individual teaching the exercises. The exercises described in Figure 11-9 provide examples of a progressive relaxation technique.

Exercises to Further Relaxation

The following exercises are also designed to help reduce tension. They are best practiced alone and in quiet surroundings.

- Choose a particular time of day when interruptions are unlikely, and make an effort to sit quietly for a few minutes each day at that time.
- Sit in a comfortable position, and rest your hands in your lap or on your knees. Gently close your eyes, and concentrate on a single thing. Choose something pleasant to think about. If your mind is distracted, refocus your thoughts on the object of your concentration.
- While sitting quietly with your eyes closed, tighten your fists and focus on the feeling of tension in your hands. Slowly release the hands, studying the feeling of relaxation. Practice this several times until you are able to identify the feeling of relaxation as it happens. Try this with different parts of your body.
- Find a comfortable position lying on the floor. Try lying on your back with your head turned to one side, your arms away from your body, and

your feet and ankles loose. Turn your palms up, and tighten your hands into a fist. Slowly let your hands relax. Concentrate on the feeling of relaxing your hands. Send the release up through your arms, and relax the entire body.
- Lying on the floor, roll to one side and curl up, bringing your knees to your chest. This is a position familiar to us as children. Turn your thoughts back to a day when you were a child and full of adventure and curiosity. As you return to the present, bring back with you that sense of wonder, and open your eyes to the adventures that lie ahead.
- Find a relaxing position. As you slowly close your eyes, let your thoughts wander, and think of pleasant experiences that you have had such as sitting on a beach or watching a sunset with a cool breeze in your face.
- Sitting quietly or lying down, empty your mind of unhappy thoughts—anger, irritation, resentment, disappointment—and adopt a positive outlook. Concentrate on being positive!
- Think of yourself as a rag doll, and collapse your body. Practice completely loosening every muscle you have.
- Practice releasing the muscles in the different areas of your face—cheeks, temples, lips, and chin. Your face should be blank of all expression.

As described above, these techniques sound easy. However, it is essential to understand that few if any stress-management techniques bring instant relief from distress. To learn how to relax, regular practice is essential, as is trying several different techniques. Practice each a number of times until you find those techniques that work best. Everyone is different, and we all have to determine what works best for us.

Yoga

Yoga originated in India approximately 6000 years ago. Its basic philosophy is that most illness is related to poor mental attitudes, posture, and diet. Practitioners of yoga maintain that stress can be reduced by a mixture of mental and physical approaches. Through yoga it is possible for some to cope with such stress-induced responses as overeating, hypertension, and smoking. Yoga's meditative aspects help, it is believed, in alleviating psychosomatic illnesses. It aims to unite the body and mind to reduce stress; for example, Dr. Chandra Patel, a yoga expert, has found that persons who practice yoga can reduce blood pressure indefinitely as long as they continue to practice yoga. Various body postures and breathing exercises are used in this activity.

Hatha-yoga uses a number of positions through which the practitioner may progress, beginning with

FIGURE 11-9. Jacobson's Progressive Relaxation Exercises.

Relaxation of the face, neck, shoulders, and upper back (4 or 5 minutes)

Let all your muscles go loose and heavy.
Just settle back quietly and comfortably.
Wrinkle up your forehead now, wrinkle it tighter.
And now stop wrinkling up your forehead.
Relax and smooth it out . . .
Picture the entire forehead and scalp becoming smoother, as the relaxation increases . . .
Now frown and crease your brows and study the tension.
Let go of the tension again . . .
Smooth out the forehead once more.
Now, close your eyes.
Keep your eyes closed, gently, comfortably, and notice the relaxation.
Now clench your jaws, push your teeth together.
Study the tension throughout the jaws.
Relax your jaws now . . .
Let your lips part slightly . . .
Appreciate the relaxation.
Now press your tongue hard against the roof of your mouth.
Look for the tension.
All right, let your tongue return to a comfortable and relaxed position.
Now purse your lips, press your lips together tighter and tighter.
Relax your lips . . .
Notice the contrast between tension and relaxation . . .
Feel the relaxation all over your face, all over your forehead, and scalp, eyes, jaws, lips, tongue, and throat . . .
The relaxation progresses further and further.
Now attend to your neck muscles.
Press your head back as far as it can go and feel the tension in the neck.
Roll it to the right and feel the tension shift . . .
Now roll it to the left.
Straighten your head and bring it forward.
Press your chin against your chest.
Let your head return to a comfortable position and study the relaxation . . .
Let the relaxation develop.
Shrug your shoulders right up.
Hold the tension.
Drop your shoulders and feel the relaxation . . .
Neck and shoulders relaxed.
Shrug your shoulders again and move them around.
Bring your shoulders up and forward and back.
Feel the tension in your shoulders and in your upper back.
Drop your shoulders once more and relax . . .
Let the relaxation spread deep into the shoulders right into your back muscles.
Relax your neck and throat, and your jaws and other facial areas, as the pure relaxation takes over and grows deeper
. . . deeper . . . even deeper.

the simplest and moving to the more complex. The purpose of the various positions is to increase mobility and flexibility of the body. However, many of the recommended positions are potentially dangerous.

Slow, deep, diaphragmatic breathing can help in alleviating stress. Many people breathe in a shallow fashion. However, deep breathing, fully expanding your chest as you inhale, helps to lower blood pres-

sure and heart rate. Deep breathing has a calming effect on the body. It also increases production of endorphins, the body's own natural, morphinelike pain-killing substances.

Breathing Exercises

Some people just use deep breathing as relief from stress. These persons maintain that as the body takes in more oxygen, they feel better and experience less stress. Also, by concentrating on the breathing, the source of stress often is forgotten. A typical deep-breathing exercise for relaxation involves sitting, closing the eyes, inhaling slowly and deeply through the nose to expand the diaphragm and the abdomen, and then exhaling slowly through the mouth. When inhaling, you could say, "I am," and then during each exhalation, say the word "relaxed." This process should be repeated eight or ten times or as long as you wish and are comfortable. After this routine, you should breathe normally and rest quietly in a relaxed condition. Whenever you find yourself in a stressful situation, such as before taking a final exam or standing in front of an audience, use deep breathing to relax.

Benson's Technique

Herbert Benson, a Harvard cardiologist, has also developed a system of relaxation through the use of breathing exercises combined with muscular relaxation efforts. His technique calls for closing your eyes, relaxing all muscles beginning with the feet and then progressing to the face, and breathing through the nose and saying, "one in," and then exhaling and saying, "one out." This is continued for 10 to 20 minutes. The technique should be done once or twice daily, but not within 2 hours after any meal because it may interfere with digestion.

Meditation

Meditation uses mental focusing exercises to control or concentrate one's attention. In most forms, meditation involves sitting quietly for a period of time, usually 15 to 20 minutes, and concentrating on a single word or image while breathing slowly and rhythmically. Utmost concentration is important in this process.

The response that underlies this process is sometimes called the *relaxation response*. Bringing about the relaxation response, meditation advocates say, helps the body to counteract the biochemical changes that cause stress. The goal of this technique is to elicit the relaxation response whenever the individual confronts stressful situations. The relaxation response, it is believed, causes beneficial physiological changes such as a decrease in respiratory rate, heart rate, blood pressure, and muscle tension.

Transcendental Meditation

Transcendental meditation (TM), the most widely used of the various forms of meditation, was popularized by the Maharishi Mahesh Yogi, an Indian teacher. In this technique the meditator silently chants a mantra (a monosyllabic word or sound) for 20 min-

utes, twice a day, morning and evening. The word *transcendental,* meaning "going beyond," is used to illustrate that with this technique, one goes beyond a wakeful state to a state of restfulness that is characterized by a greater state of alertness. The mantra that a person uses is supposedly chosen for that person alone and is kept secret to enhance attentiveness and calm the conscious mind.

Imagery

Imagery can be used as a means of relaxation to cope with stressful situations. Images are pictures formed within the mind. The procedure is to sit relaxed, close your eyes, and concentrate on a particular image. You may imagine being in a very peaceful environment such as in a quiet forest. With practice and by paying attention to precise details such as colors, shapes, smells, and sounds, a very realistic picture can be quickly created in your mind. With more practice, you can learn to project your own body image into this picture and ultimately to perform various tasks within the mind. For example, you visualize how you will deal with a stressful situation such as participation in a competitive event. By creating various scenarios, you can learn to cope with all possible variations of a situation that may be stress producing before confronting them in real life. The imagery can be continued as long as you wish. Following this process may help you relax your mind and body and thus relieve stress. Also, it may prepare you to cope with an anticipated stressful situation more effectively.

Massage

Massage is a mechanical stimulation of the tissues by means of rhythmically applied pressure and stretching. Massage can be very relaxing as a stress-reducing technique. Slow, gentle, superficial stroking may relieve tension and soothe, rendering the muscles more relaxed. Massage causes an increase in skin temperature and in circulation to the underlying muscles. It is also used to decrease pain associated with spasm or tension. The psychological effects of massage may be as beneficial as the physiological effects. Placing your hands on another person helps them feel that someone is helping them. Massage can reduce anxiety, which can lead to increased relaxation. You can massage your neck, face, head, and shoulders. To many, touch is a useful form of nonverbal communication and can be reassuring.

Autogenic Training (Hypnosis)

This technique was developed by Johannes H. Schultz, a German psychiatrist, after observing that patients who were hypnotized had less fatigue and tension than those not in this state of mind. Therefore he designed this technique to enable other persons to obtain the same benefits without having to experience hypnosis therapy. It involves a series of specific exercises and autohypnosis that is designed to accomplish a deep mental and physical state of relaxation. The individual experiences two physical sensations while progressing through the six different stages that are involved with this technique. First, one experiences a feeling of warmth as he or she concentrates on a psychological perception that the arteries are dilating. This perception results in a relaxed state. Second, he or she concentrates on the feeling of heaviness in the torso. This results in the actual relaxation of the muscles.

Biofeedback

Biofeedback is a common form of stress management and relaxation therapy. Its main goals are to teach concentration, relaxation, awareness, and self-control. A machine monitors various body functions and relays the information to the subject in the form of either sounds or lights. Some body functions, for example, those controlled by parts of the nervous system, are often imperceptible to us. Biofeedback develops awareness of changes in basic body functions and enables a person to actively control the responses and processes. For example, muscle biofeedback enables the subject to become aware of his or her level of muscular tension by observing the monitoring equipment. As a result of becoming more aware of the feelings associated with relaxation, individuals can learn how to control muscle tension. Thus biofeedback helps people to become aware of tensions they had not previously perceived and learn to reduce them, eventually without relying on the monitoring machines.

SUMMARY

- Everyone experiences stress, and some stress is needed to perform the daily tasks of life for growth and development. Stress involves physiological and psychological responses. Selye described the body's physiological response to stress as the *general adaptation syndrome.*
- There are many different types of stressors that can be broadly classified as *psychological stressors* and *physiological stressors.*
- Each day in college life, students encounter many stressors of varying magnitudes. Stress is not always harmful; some stress is needed for personal growth.
- The way you feel about yourself may result in stress.
- Uncontrolled stress can result in physical and mental disorders.
- Persons who are under stress tend to display certain danger signs and experience symptoms that indicate the body's malfunctioning.
- Coping skills to ward off stress are those procedures that allow a person to deal with reality in a positive way.

- Ways to cope with stress include exercise, proper rest, relaxation, and setting realistic goals.
- People sometimes try to cope with stress by using techniques called *defense mechanisms.*
- The better you understand your own behavior and motives, the better able you are to cope with stress and develop into a productive human being.
- Physical activity is one of the best ways to resist stressors and to relax.
- Physical activity provides benefits such as a healthy cardiovascular system, a sense of well-being, mental release, and a better self-concept.
- Physical activity can contribute to better body composition and thus prevent some forms of stress.
- There are several relaxation techniques for coping with stress, including the Jacobson relaxation technique, yoga, breathing exercises, meditation, imagery, massage, autogenic training, and biofeedback.

REFERENCES

Allen RJ, Hyde DH: *Investigations in stress control,* Minneapolis, 1981, Burgess.

Anderson RA: *Stress power,* New York, 1978, Human Sciences.

Beck A: Cognitive approaches to stress. In Woolfolk R, Lehrer P, editors: *Principles and practice of stress management,* New York, 1984, Guilford Press.

Charlesworth EA, Nathan RG: *Stress management: a comprehensive guide to wellness,* Houston, 1984, Behavioral Press.

Cooper KH, Gallman JS, McDonald JL: Role of aerobic exercise in reduction of stress, *Dent Clin North Am* 30(suppl):S133, 1986.

Crocker P: Managing stress in competitive athletes, *Int J Sports Psych* 23(2):161-175, 1992.

Cronin SD, Pencak M: Exercise may evoke rather than reduce stress, *J Nurs Adm* 19(7):3, 1989.

DeBenedette V: Getting fit for life: can exercise reduce stress? *Sports Med* 16(6):185, 1988.

deVries HA: Physical education, adult fitness programs: does physical activity promote relaxation? *J Phys Educ Rec* 46(7):53, 1975.

Farmer K: Biofeedback and visualization for peak performance, *J Sports Rehab* 4(1):59-64, 1995.

Friedman M, Rosenman RH: *Type A behavior and your heart,* Greenwich, Conn, 1974, Fawcett.

Giermek K, Osiadlo G: Psychological responses for selected relaxation techniques, *Biol Sport* 11(2):109-114, 1994.

Gould D: Psychological skills for enhancing performance: arousal regulation strategies, *Med Sci Sports Exerc* 26(4):478-485, 1994.

Hardy CJ, Riehl R: An examination of the life-stress injury relationship among noncontact sport participants, *Behav Med* 14:113, 1988.

Holmes TH, Rahe TE: The social readjustment rating scale, *J Psychosom Res* 11:213, 1967.

Jacobson E: *Progressive relaxation,* Chicago, 1938, University of Chicago Press.

Matteson MT, Ivancevich JM: *Managing job stress and health,* New York, 1982, The Free Press.

McGuigan F: The contribution of basic science to stress management, *Int J Stress Manag* 1(3):247-248, 1994.

Meichenbaum D: *Stress innoculation training,* New York, 1985, Pergamon Press.

Meirer K: Physical activity and stress; the road not taken and implications for society, *Quest* 46(1):136-145, 1994.

Michael ED: Stress adaptation through exercise, *Res Q Exerc Sport* 28:50, 1957.

Oxendine JB: Emotional arousal and motor performance, *Quest* 8:23, 1970.

Pargman D: *Stress and motor performance: understanding and coping,* Ithaca, NY, 1986, Movement Publications.

Pullig-Schatz M: Stressed out? *Phys Sports Med* 22(11):87-89, 1994.

Samples P: Does "sports massage" have a role in sports medicine? *Phys Sports Med* 15:3, 1987.

Selye H: *The stress of life,* ed 2, New York, 1978, McGraw-Hill.

Seward B: *Managing stress,* Boston, 1994, Jones & Bartlett.

Speilberger CD: *Anxiety: current trends in theory and research,* New York, 1972, Academic Press.

US Department of Health and Human Services, Public Health Services: *Healthy people 2000: midcourse review and 1995 revisions,* Washington, DC, 1995, USDHHS.

US Department of Health and Human Services, Public Health Services: *Healthy people 2000: national health promotion and disease prevention objectives,* Washington, DC,1991, USDHHS.

Williams JM, Anderson MB: *The relationship between psychological factors and injury occurrence.* Paper presented to the North American Society for Psychology of Sport and Physical Activity, Scottsdale, Ariz, 1986.

SUGGESTED READINGS

Benson H: *Beyond the relaxation process,* New York, 1984, Berkley Books.
Discusses techniques of stress reduction and how stress may be related to other ailments.

Eliot R: *From stress to strength: how to lighten your load and save your strength,* New York, 1994, Bantam Books.
Written by a physician who discusses how stress can cause a heart attack or stroke.

Meichenbaum D: *Stress innoculation training,* New York, 1985, Pergamon Press.
Presents a systematic study of stress innoculation, a treatment modality aimed at the reduction and prevention of stress; based on Meichenbaum's earlier theories on cognitive behavior modification as a means of influencing and controlling stress.

Murray, M: *Stress, anxiety, and insomnia,* Rocklin, Calif, 1995, Prima Publishing.
Discusses how stress, anxiety, and insomnia can be controlled by natural dietary choices and a relaxing exercise routine.

Pargman D: *Stress and motor performance: understanding and coping,* Ithaca, NY, 1986, Movement Publications.
Deals with the relationship between performance and stress; concentrates primarily on sport skill performers, but the theories may be applied to anyone who engages in any form of competition.
Techniques and strategies for managing and coping with stress are presented in detail.

College Schedule of Recent Experience

Name _____   Section _____   Date _____

PURPOSE   To predict your chances of developing a stress-related illness.

PROCEDURE   On the answer sheet on the following page, indicate the number of times during the last 12 months that each of the following life-change events has happened to you.

1. Entered college.
2. Married.
3. Had either a lot more or a lot less trouble with your boss.
4. Held a job while attending school.
5. Experienced the death of a spouse.
6. Experienced a major change in sleeping habits (sleeping a lot more or a lot less or a change in part of the day when asleep).
7. Experienced the death of a close family member.
8. Experienced a major change in eating habits (a lot more or a lot less food intake or very different meal hours or surroundings).
9. Made a change in or choice of a major field of study.
10. Had a revision of your personal habits (friends, dress, manners, associations).
11. Experienced the death of a close friend.
12. Have been found guilty of minor violations of the law (traffic tickets, jaywalking, etc.).
13. Had an outstanding personal achievement.
14. Experienced pregnancy or fathered a pregnancy.
15. Had a major change in the health or behavior of a family member.
16. Had sexual difficulties.
17. Had trouble with in-laws.
18. Had a major change in the number of family get-togethers (a lot more or a lot less).
19. Had a major change in financial state (a lot worse off or a lot better off than usual).
20. Gained a new family member (through birth, adoption, older person moving in, etc.).
21. Changed your residence or living conditions.
22. Had a major conflict in or change in values.
23. Had a major change in church activities (a lot more or a lot less than usual).
24. Had a marital reconciliation with your mate.
25. Were fired from work.
26. Were divorced.
27. Changed to different line of work.
28. Had a major change in the number of arguments with spouse (either a lot more or a lot less than usual).
29. Had a major change in responsibilities at work (promotion, demotion, lateral transfer).
30. Had your spouse begin or cease work outside the home.
31. Had a marital separation from your mate.
32. Had a major change in the usual type and/or amount of recreation.
33. Had a major change in the use of drugs (a lot more or a lot less).
34. Took a mortgage or loan *less* than $10,000 (such as purchase of a car, TV, school loan, etc.).
35. Had a major personal injury or illness.
36. Had a major change in the use of alcohol (a lot more or a lot less).
37. Had a major change in social activities.
38. Had a major change in the amount of participation in school activities.

39. Had a major change in the amount of independence and responsibility (e.g., for budgeting time).
40. Took a trip or a vacation.
41. Were engaged to be married.
42. Changed to a new school.
43. Changed dating habits.
44. Had trouble with school administration (instructors, advisors, class scheduling, etc.).
45. Broke or had broken a marital engagement or a steady relationship.
46. Had a major change in self-concept or self-awareness.

Answer and Scoring Sheet

First, for the number corresponding to each of the life events listed, indicate the number of times (1, 2, 3, etc.) that the particular event has occurred in your life during the past 12 months. Then multiply each item by the indicated weight, and total the scores.

1.	_____	$\times$ 50 =	_____	24. _____	$\times$ 58 =	_____
2.	_____	$\times$ 77 =	_____	25. _____	$\times$ 62 =	_____
3.	_____	$\times$ 38 =	_____	26. _____	$\times$ 76 =	_____
4.	_____	$\times$ 43 =	_____	27. _____	$\times$ 50 =	_____
5.	_____	$\times$ 87 =	_____	28. _____	$\times$ 50 =	_____
6.	_____	$\times$ 34 =	_____	29. _____	$\times$ 47 =	_____
7.	_____	$\times$ 77 =	_____	30. _____	$\times$ 41 =	_____
8.	_____	$\times$ 30 =	_____	31. _____	$\times$ 74 =	_____
9.	_____	$\times$ 41 =	_____	32. _____	$\times$ 37 =	_____
10.	_____	$\times$ 45 =	_____	33. _____	$\times$ 52 =	_____
11.	_____	$\times$ 68 =	_____	34. _____	$\times$ 52 =	_____
12.	_____	$\times$ 22 =	_____	35. _____	$\times$ 65 =	_____
13.	_____	$\times$ 40 =	_____	36. _____	$\times$ 46 =	_____
14.	_____	$\times$ 68 =	_____	37. _____	$\times$ 43 =	_____
15.	_____	$\times$ 56 =	_____	38. _____	$\times$ 38 =	_____
16.	_____	$\times$ 58 =	_____	39. _____	$\times$ 49 =	_____
17.	_____	$\times$ 42 =	_____	40. _____	$\times$ 33 =	_____
18.	_____	$\times$ 26 =	_____	41. _____	$\times$ 54 =	_____
19.	_____	$\times$ 53 =	_____	42. _____	$\times$ 50 =	_____
20.	_____	$\times$ 50 =	_____	43. _____	$\times$ 41 =	_____
21.	_____	$\times$ 42 =	_____	44. _____	$\times$ 44 =	_____
22.	_____	$\times$ 50 =	_____	45. _____	$\times$ 60 =	_____
23.	_____	$\times$ 36 =	_____	46. _____	$\times$ 57 =	_____

Subtotal = _____   Subtotal = _____

Total life-change score = _____

INTERPRETATION

The number of life changes that a person experiences each year may be classified as mild, moderate, or excessive. An increased number of life changes is associated with an increase in the incidence of illness and accidents during the following 12-month period. It is estimated that people experiencing only mild life changes over the past year have an estimated 30% chance of becoming ill or having an accident. Those having an excessive number of life changes are at a much higher risk of developing significant health problems. The higher the score in life-change units, the greater the potential for significant illness or accident.

Category	Scoring range
Mild	0-499
Moderate	500-999
Excessive	1000 or above

Lab Activity 11-2

Your Personal Stress Inventory

Name _____   **Section** _____   **Date** _____

PURPOSE
To manage stress effectively, you need to learn about your unique patterns of stress: what factors promote it, how you experience it, and how you cope with it. Understanding your patterns and becoming more aware of early signs of stress are important first steps in managing stress.

This personal inventory will help you beome more aware of your responses to stress, life events that may impact your stress level, and how you cope with stess. There are no right or wrong answers; instead, the scoring system is designed to give a general indication of stress levels and to help you focus on those unhealthy responses that could be changed through improved stress-management techniques.

PROCEDURE
1. Circle the appropriate response for each question.
2. Total your score.

Response	Never	Rarely	Some-times	Often	Very often
Physical Responses to Stress					
1. I have frequent headaches.	N	R	S	O	A
2. I get stomachaches or experience discomfort.	N	R	S	O	A
3. My back aches.	N	R	S	O	A
4. I have stiffness in my shoulders or upper back.	N	R	S	O	A
5. My blood pressure is elevated.	N	R	S	O	A
6. I get palpitations or a rapid heartbeat.	N	R	S	O	A
7. I get short of breath and breathe rapidly.	N	R	S	O	A
8. I feel dizzy or shaky.	N	R	S	O	A
9. I'm fatigued, tired, or unrested.	N	R	S	O	A
10. I feel "wound up" and tense inside.	N	R	S	O	A
Total Number O's and A's Circled:				_____	_____
Behavioral Responses to Stress					
1. I eat compulsively or too fast.	N	R	S	O	A
2. I light up a cigarette.	N	R	S	O	A
3. I drink alcohol or use mood-altering drugs.	N	R	S	O	A
4. I grind my teeth.	N	R	S	O	A
5. I clench my fists.	N	R	S	O	A
6. I pace, walk rapidly, or rush.	N	R	S	O	A
7. I tap my feet.	N	R	S	O	A
8. I sleep a lot or have trouble falling asleep.	N	R	S	O	A
9. I sulk and don't talk to people.	N	R	S	O	A
10. I snap back or get angry with others.	N	R	S	O	A
Total Number O's and A's Circled:				_____	_____

Response	Never	Rarely	Some-times	Often	Very often
Cognitive (Thinking) Responses to Stress					
1. I can't concentrate on what I'm doing.	N	R	S	O	A
2. I forget things or I get confused.	N	R	S	O	A
3. My thoughts seem to race.	N	R	S	O	A
4. This isn't where I want to be in my life.	N	R	S	O	A
5. I worry a lot.	N	R	S	O	A
6. I have recurring, troublesome thoughts.	N	R	S	O	A
7 I can't turn off my thoughts at night and relax.	N	R	S	O	A
8. I have trouble sleeping because of things on my mind.	N	R	S	O	A
9. Things must be perfect.	N	R	S	O	A
10. I must do it myself.	N	R	S	O	A
Total Number O's and A's Circled:				_____	_____
Emotional (Feelings) Responses to Stress					
1 I feel depressed, sad, and unhappy.	N	R	S	O	A
2. I can't say no without feeling guilty.	N	R	S	O	A
3. I feel worthless, disappointed in myself and life.	N	R	S	O	A
4. I don't get a sense of accomplishment most days.	N	R	S	O	A
5. I feel trapped.	N	R	S	O	A
6. I can't seem to share my feelings with my family/friends.	N	R	S	O	A
7. I feel exploited, used by others.	N	R	S	O	A
8. I'm afraid of things that once didn't bother me.	N	R	S	O	A
9. I feel cynical and disenchanted.	N	R	S	O	A
10. I feel agitated, irritated, short-tempered, impatient.	N	R	S	O	A
Total Number O's and A's Circled:				_____	_____

INTERPRETATION

Total the number of circled responses in the columns indicating frequent reactions to stress (O: Often and A: Always). Those reactions will most likely be the first to alert you that you are experiencing excessive stress.

Notice which category (physical, behavioral, cognitive, or emotional) has the most O's and A's. For example, if you have more frequent reactions in the physical category, you may want to become aware of those tension spots and learn about relaxation or biofeedback techniques to reduce stress.

By simply becoming aware of your signs of stress, you'll be taking a major step toward better managing your stress level.

Lab Activity 11-3

Coping With Stress

Name _____ **Section** _____ **Date** _____

PURPOSE To determine how well you cope with stress.

PROCEDURE Ask yourself, "How often do I use this as a means to cope with stress?" Then circle the letter that most appropriately applies to you.

Response	Never	Rarely	Some-times	Often	Very often
1. Take tranquilizers, sleeping pills, aspirin, or other medications.	N	R	S	O	A
2. Try to relax by deep breathing, taking a short break, or sitting in a quiet place.	N	R	S	O	A
3. Eat compulsively or drink alcohol or caffeine.	N	R	S	O	A
4. Look more lightly at the situation.	N	R	S	O	A
5. Light up a cigarette.	N	R	S	O	A
6. Try to use time well. Prioritize my needs.	N	R	S	O	A
7. Go out and buy something. Spend money inappropriately.	N	R	S	O	A
8. Call up a good friend and share my feelings or concerns.	N	R	S	O	A
9. Click on the television and try to divert my attention.	N	R	S	O	A
10. Take a walk or get some other exercise.	N	R	S	O	A
11. Not bother anyone else and dwell on the problem until I can solve it.	N	R	S	O	A
12. Begin a new project or work on my hobby.	N	R	S	O	A
13. Throw something or snap back at someone.	N	R	S	O	A
14. Seek spiritual counseling or consult with a therapist.	N	R	S	O	A

Total Number O's and A's Circled
(Odd Numbers Only): _____ _____

Total Number O's and A's Circled
(Even Numbers Only): _____ _____

INTERPRETATION

Compare the odd- to the even-numbered responses. Did you have more O's and A's for the odd- or even-numbered items? If you tend to use the even-numbered techniques more often, you're using more effective coping methods.

The odd-numbered items are generally less effective ways of coping with stress. Overeating, smoking, or using medication or alcohol to relax are particularly counterproductive techniques. Diverting your attention by watching TV may be partially effective as a means of managing stress, but you may wish to strive for more effective and productive responses such as talking with a friend, exercising, or using a relaxation technique.

Select one or two of your less-effective methods and try to substitute more effective means of managing stress. Experiment for a few weeks with some new methods of managing stress, and evaluate how they work for you. Take a personal inventory in a few months, and see if your use of stress-management techniques has shifted to include some more effective methods.

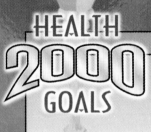

HEALTH 2000 GOALS

■ **Physical Activity and Fitness Programs.** Increase to at least 85% the proportion of workplaces with 50 or more employees that offer health-promotion activities. In 1985, 65% of work sites with 50 or more employees offered at least one health-promotion activity; in 1987, 63% of medium and large companies had wellness programs. *Midpoint Update: headed in the right direction with 81% of companies offering a health-activity or wellness program.*

■ **Leisure-Time Activity.** Of people age 18 and older 24% report no leisure-time physical activity. Increase to 85% the proportion of people age 6 and older who engage in leisure-time physical activity. In 1985 only 76% of people age 18 and older participated in active leisure-time activities.

OBJECTIVES

After completing this chapter, you will be able to do the following:

■ Describe the advantages and disadvantages of a walking or running program.
■ Describe the advantages and disadvantages of a swimming program.
■ Describe the advantages of cycling as an activity for improving cardiorespiratory fitness.
■ Describe the advantages of rope skipping as an aerobic activity.
■ Describe the advantages of aerobic dance exercise as a means of improving cardiorespiratory endurance.
■ Develop a personal physical fitness program that incorporates all the key elements of health-related fitness.

KEY TERMS

While reading this chapter, you will become familiar with the following terms:

- walking
- running
- swimming
- cycling
- rope skipping
- aerobic dance exercise
- aquatic aerobics
- step aerobics

In previous chapters you have been given the basic principles, guidelines, and techniques for becoming physically fit. This chapter applies this information to specific fitness activities, each of which can help you improve cardiorespiratory endurance, muscular strength and endurance, flexibility, and body composition. These activities primarily involve aerobic-type exercises. Remember that aerobic exercise is any physical activity that uses large-muscle, whole-body, rhythmic movements performed at least three times per week, for a minimum of 20 minutes, at an intensity level of 50% to 85% of your maximum oxygen uptake or heart rate reserve (see Chapter 5). See the following box for a number of tips on how to stay motivated in your aerobic fitness program.

WALKING*

If **walking** is your primary form of exercise, you're part of a large club that has become the fitness phenomenon of the 1990s. More than 60 million Americans now walk for exercise, making it the number one participation sport in the country. Including walk-a-thons and competitive race walks, it is estimated that there are more than 10,000 walking events annually. When it comes to success, studies show higher rates of adherence to walking than to any other exercise program.

*Reprinted with permission of *The Walking Magazine*, 711 Boylston Street, Boston, MA 02116, © 1989.

GET MOVING

Ways to help motivate you to exercise aerobically

1. Pick a minimum distance you'll walk, run, swim, or bicycle: 2 miles, 30 minutes, 20 telephone poles. When you reach your goal, pat yourself on the back. Walk to where you'll meet a friend, shop, or go to the movies. Keep a positive attitude—don't wake up asking yourself *if* you'll exercise today, but *when* you'll exercise.
2. One of the greatest enemies of exercise is boredom—the monotony of the same old routine. The solution is simply variety: different companions, new routes, other times, or simple games. Walk or jog up hills or stairs (be ready for a more vigorous workout, however). Try different speeds. Go mall walking. Take a turn on your high school track; walk backwards. Anything that will break the monotony will keep you going and make your exercise program fun.
3. Exercise with a friend, spouse, partner, neighbor, or fellow worker—it doesn't matter. Having a companion not only makes the activity social and more fun but also gives you a commitment to another person—a strong motivator.
4. Community centers, YMCAs, health clubs, hospitals, and malls across the country are forming walking, jogging, cycling, and swimming clubs to promote these activities' benefits and enjoyment. Besides the opportunity to meet new friends, membership generally offers everything from use of health clinics to the participation in organized events. Considerations for joining a health club are discussed in Chapter 13.
5. Train for an event. Organized exercise events are becoming increasingly popular. For example, in 1994 it was estimated that over 12,000 noncompetitive, family-oriented walks occurred. These events attract participants of all ages and fitness levels who want to walk just for the health and fun of it.
6. Keep a logbook of your progress. Once you've started a program, you may want to keep track of your mileage, time, pace, heart rate, and perhaps even feelings about yourself. Jotting down progress is motivational; it's also rewarding to watch your distance and speed go up while your weight, waistline, and heart rate go down.

Reasons for Walking

There are several reasons why people are walking for fitness. It is an activity that can be pursued at almost any time, anywhere, with anyone, at no cost. Besides being fun, a walking regimen can be started easily at any age and can be worked into almost anybody's daily schedule. Although some techniques are better than others, walking demands little skill or practice. It does require a pair of comfortable shoes, but no other specialized clothing or equipment is really necessary. As long as you're in relatively good health, the activity presents few, if any, health hazards. As with any program involving your health, just check with your physician before you begin.

Walking for Exercise

How well does walking stack up as a form of exercise? The answer depends on what you want from a fitness program—your goals for getting in shape and staying fit. Certainly, walking may not provide the same results as more strenuous activities. It won't tone or sculpt your muscles as strength training and weight training will, nor will it provide the same short-term aerobic benefits that hill climbing or cross-country skiing will. However, you may be surprised to discover how beneficial it can be and how high walking ranks when compared to other popular exercise activities.

For example, walking at a pace of 1 mile in 15 minutes is equal to bicycling at 1 mile in 6 minutes. Striding at a more leisurely rate of 1 mile in 20 minutes requires the same energy as cycling at 1 mile in 12 minutes. Such figures indicate that walking can expend a lot of energy. There is, however, even more tangible evidence of the fitness benefits that walking offers. Numerous studies show that it can be a very effective component of a weight-loss program. An average (150 lb) male, for example, will metabolize (burn) about 540 Calories walking briskly up a slight incline for 45 minutes. That's more calories than he would burn if he were to run for the same length of time at an 11-minute per mile pace.

Briskly walking up even a slight hill can be very strenuous. But even walking at a fitness pace of 1 mile per 15 minutes on a level surface provides enough exercise to burn 261 Calories in 45 minutes. That's more than the average male would use cycling at a pace of 1 mile in 11 minutes for the same amount of time. The principle is the same for women, although on average they burn 20% fewer calories for the same activity.

Getting the most out of walking requires some attention to technique, a few reasonable goals, and a little self-assurance that walking for fitness is not only fun but can also be your ticket to a lifetime of good health. Sometimes the thought of starting a regular activity seems overwhelming. Such a feeling is not unusual. Most people feel they have little energy to spare in a day, especially after performing tiresome mental tasks. Engaging in a little exercise such as walking gives you more energy to tackle your busy day.

Walking for Relaxation

One of the most important benefits of fitness walking comes from simply taking time off from the strains of everyday life. Universally, walkers report that their fitness programs help them deal with daily stresses. With few exceptions, they note such exercise brings not only contentment but also clarity and focus to their thinking. Regardless of your age or fitness level, you can enjoy the same experience. Just set aside some time in the next day or so and take a walk. The following pointers will help you get maximum benefits from an activity that can reward you with a lifetime of fitness.

Walking Technique

Walking's greatest value as a fitness activity is that you can just go out and walk. Like other physical activities, technique becomes a factor in developing a more effective program. In walking, the development of proper technique involves correct stride, arm swing, posture, and a steady pace (Figure 12-1). Although it's fun to experiment with techniques, it's by no means mandatory in walking. You know how to put one foot in front of the other, and there's no reason to complicate a simple activity. First and foremost, walking should be pleasurable. If you want to try it with slightly different twists, here are several tips.

Stride

Your stride should be natural and comfortable. Don't make the mistake of taking too long a stride (the average is 2.6 ft)—you'll feel awkward and quickly exhausted. Instead, simply lean forward at your ankles (not your waist), relax, and let your body pick its own stride. This self-selected stride will be most efficient for you.

Arm Swing

Walking can be a total body activity if you don't let your arms dangle at your sides. For a sense of how important arm motion is, try keeping your hands in

> **walking** more than a simple means of locomotion, this is a very safe and easy form of exercise that is the number one participation sport in the United States

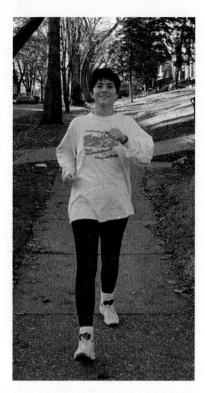

FIGURE 12-1. Walking Is the Most Popular Aerobic Fitness Activity.

your pockets when walking briskly. It's possible, but it will quickly feel awkward and tiring because it disrupts your body's natural balance. Swinging your arms serves like a pump that aids the distribution of oxygen throughout the body. Furthermore, swinging your arms faster tends to make you walk faster. To increase your speed, increase your arm swing. As a result, your stride will be more efficient, your breathing will be better, and you'll be able to walk longer without getting tired. Relax your shoulders and keep your elbows relaxed and bent at about 90 degrees. You'll find that arm swing also improves upper-body muscles.

Posture

Without adopting a stiff marching stance, you should walk with your head erect, stomach pulled in, and back straight. As speed increases there should be a slight forward lean to the body. Look up or straight ahead, not down. Besides improving the scenery, it will help ensure that your head and torso are aligned over your lower body, facilitating circulation of blood and oxygen. Once you get into walking regularly, you'll find that it helps you retain an erect and confident posture throughout your day.

Pace

All walking is good for you, but maintaining a steady, brisk pace will maximize its benefits. The normal pace for most people is 1 mile every 15 to 20 minutes. An easy way to check your speed is by counting paces per minute. A good base rate is 120 paces per minute, although this varies depending on terrain. As a rule, to avoid overdoing it you should always be able to carry on a normal conversation while logging your distances. If you're out of breath and feeling strained, slow down. Also, if you can't repeat the same distance at the same pace the very next day, give yourself a break—you're walking too far, too fast, too soon.

Racewalking

Racewalking is one of the fastest growing sports of the 1990s. There are two main principles involved in racewalking: (1) your lead foot must make contact with the ground before your rear foot leaves the ground; and (2) when the supporting leg is directly under your body, your knee must be momentarily straight. This distinguishes racewalking from normal walking or jogging. Straightening the knee creates the racewalker's trademark, the "hip-wiggle." Some tips for racewalking are as follows:

- Maintain a slight forward leaning posture.
- Keep the upper body loose.
- Swing the arms close to your body.
- Increase the rotation in your hips by walking with the inside of each foot landing on the same straight line and avoiding a swayback position.
- The knees should be straight but not stiff.
- The supporting knee must be straightened when it passes under the body center.
- The toe of the rear foot must not leave the ground until the heel of the advancing foot has made contact, and the lead foot should skim the ground when it passes under the supporting leg.

The Rockport Walking Program

Lab Activity 5-5 on pp. 137 to 141 provides a detailed presentation of the Rockport Fitness Walking Test and Exercise Programs. Outlined in Table 12-1 are suggested guidelines for a sample 10- to 20-week walking program for beginning, intermediate, and advanced walkers. It is progressive in nature and should include a warm-up and cool-down. It is not intended that the program be etched in stone. If you find a particular week's workout tiring, slow down. You do not have to complete the program in 10 weeks. Take longer if you wish. The program calls for engaging in a minimum of three exercise periods each week. You may want to follow the program daily.

TABLE 12-1. The Exercise Program

You can improve your aerobic capacity and promote life-long health with the walking program outlined here. Your designated program is designed specifically for your current fitness level.

At the end of the 20-week period, retake the Rockport Fitness Walking Test™ to determine your new fitness level and exercise program.

On each program there are columns labeled "pace" and "heart rate." Pace is only an approximation. Your walking speed should be determined by the pace that keeps your heart rate at the percentage of maximum listed. For your percentage of maximum heart rate use the chart provided.

% of Maximum Heart Rate Chart (10-Second Count)

Age	60%	70%	80%
20-29	19-20	22-23	25-27
30-39	18-19	21-22	24-25
40-49	17-18	20-21	23-24
50-59	16-17	19-20	21-23
60+	14-16	16-18	19-21

BRONZE PROGRAM

Week	1-2	3-4	5	6	7-8	9	10	11	12-13	14	15-16	17-18	19-20
WARM-UP/COOL-DOWN (stretches before and after walk in min.)	5-7	5-7	5-7	5-7	5-7	5-7	5-7	5-7	5-7	5-7	5-7	5-7	5-7
MILEAGE	1.0	1.25	1.5	1.5	1.75	2.0	2.0	2.0	2.25	2.5	2.5	2.75	3.0
PACE (mph)	3.0	3.0	3.0	3.5	3.5	3.5	3.75	3.75	3.75	3.75	4.0	4.0	4.0
HEART RATE (% of max)	60	60	60	60-70	60-70	60-70	60-70	70	70	70	70	70-80	70-80
FREQUENCY (times per week)	5	5	5	5	5	5	5	5	5	5	5	5	5

GREEN PROGRAM

Week	1-2	3-4	5-6	7	8-9	10-12	13	14	15-16	17-18	19-20
WARM-UP/COOL-DOWN (stretches before and after walk in min.)	5-7	5-7	5-7	5-7	5-7	5-7	5-7	5-7	5-7	5-7	5-7
MILEAGE	1.5	1.75	2.0	2.0	2.25	2.5	2.75	2.75	3.0	3.25	3.5
PACE (mph)	3.0	3.0	3.0	3.5	3.5	3.5	3.5	4.0	4.0	4.0	4.0
HEART RATE (% of max)	60-70	60-70	60-70	70	70	70	70	70-80	70-80	70-80	70-80
FREQUENCY (times per week)	5	5	5	5	5	5	5	5	5	5	5

TABLE 12-1.   The Exercise Program—cont'd

BURGUNDY PROGRAM

Week	1	2	3-4	5	6-8	9-10	11-12	13-14	15	16-17	18-20	Maintenance
WARM-UP/COOL-DOWN (stretches before and after walk in min.)	5-7	5-7	5-7	5-7	5-7	5-7	5-7	5-7	5-7	5-7	5-7	5-7
MILEAGE	2.0	2.25	2.5	2.75	2.75	3.0	3.0	3.25	3.5	3.5	4.0	4.0
PACE (mph)	3.0	3.0	3.0	3.0	3.5	3.5	4.0	4.0	4.0	4.5	4.5	4.5
HEART RATE (% of max)	70	70	70	70	70	70	70-80	70-80	70-80	70-80	70-80	70-80
FREQUENCY (times per week)	5	5	5	5	5	5	5	5	5	5	5	3-5

GOLDENROD PROGRAM

Week	1	2	3-4	5	6	7	8	9-10	11-14	15-20	Maintenance
WARM-UP/COOL-DOWN (stretches before and after walk in min.)	5-7	5-7	5-7	5-7	5-7	5-7	5-7	5-7	5-7	5-7	5-7
MILEAGE	2.5	2.75	3.0	3.25	3.25	3.5	3.75	4.0	4.0	4.0	4.0
PACE (mph)	3.5	3.5	3.5	3.5	4.0	4.0	4.0	4.0	4.5	4.5	4.5
HEART RATE (% of max)	70	70	70	70	70-80	70-80	70-80	70-80	70-80	70-80	70-80
FREQUENCY (times per week)	5	5	5	5	5	5	5	5	5	3	3-5

BLUE PROGRAM

Week	1	2	3	4	5	6	7-20	Maintenance
WARM-UP/COOL-DOWN (stretches before and after walk in min.)	5-7	5-7	5-7	5-7	5-7	5-7	5-7	5-7
MILEAGE	3.0	3.25	3.5	3.5	3.75	4.0	4.0	4.0
PACE (mph)	4.0	4.0	4.0	4.5	4.5	4.5	4.5	4.5
HEART RATE (% of max)	70	70	70	70-80	70-80	70-80	70-80	70-80
FREQUENCY (times per week)	5	5	5	5	5	5	3	3-5

At week 7 in the Goldenrod and Blue programs, begin incorporating hills into your walks.

RUNNING

Perhaps no other physical fitness activity has become as much a part of our American way of life as walking or running. Running has long been accepted as an essential training component for the competitive athlete in almost every sport. But within the last 20 years, millions of people have taken to the streets and now run or jog on a regular basis. More than 26,000 men and women began the 1995 New York Marathon, and it was estimated that more than 89% of these people completed the 26-plus–mile run.

The running phenomenon doesn't seem to be restricted to any one segment of the population. Young children, college students, office personnel, laborers, elderly persons, people of all backgrounds, and both sexes regularly put on their running shoes and go for a run.

Reasons for Running

Why has running attracted such widespread attention? Different people offer different reasons, but it seems that most people run for two major reasons, either for the effects that a regular running program can have on physical appearance or for some important health-related reason. Running is an aerobic exercise that involves whole-body, large-muscle activities performed repetitively. This muscular activity requires energy, so calories are expended during the activity. Thus many people run as a means of controlling weight and burning off additional calories.

Burning Calories During Running

The number of calories expended during running depends on the intensity and the duration of the activity. Regardless of whether you walk, jog, or run 1 mile, it is estimated that an average-size adult will burn off approximately 100 to 120 Calories. Of course, the actual number of Calories used is determined by the size of the individual and to some extent the running speed. The person who runs for 30 minutes at a 6-minute per mile pace will burn off considerably more calories than another who walks for the same 30-minute period but at a 12-minute per mile pace. (The runner will cover 5 miles in 30 minutes, while the walker covers 2 1/2 miles.)

The 100 to 120 Calorie-per-mile figure is a bit misleading. Assuming that 1 pound of fat contains approximately 3500 Calories, persons who run a 26-mile marathon would only burn off 2600 to 3120 Calories, far less than 1 pound of body fat. However, the fact that the metabolic rate is increased during activity and remains elevated while slowly returning to normal during a several-hour period after the activity accounts for the expenditure of a large amount of a few additional calories (see Chapter 8).

Health Benefits of Running

Although many people run to control their weight and to attain a healthful physical appearance, some people run for other physiological benefits a running program offers. The effects of a sedentary lifestyle on the cardiovascular system have been previously discussed. Physically active persons are less prone to cardiovascular disease than are those who are sedentary. Running increases the efficiency of the cardiovascular system and alters the buildup of cholesterol in the arterial walls.

Running for Relaxation

Many people report that running (or jogging) is relaxing and alleviates stress, tension, and depression. They express feelings of greater self-worth and enthusiasm toward life after a run. The euphoric feeling has been called a "runner's high," and although most people agree that this is a psychological phenomenon, there is a physiological explanation for this "high." The brain releases opiate-like substances called *endorphins*, which are thought to be responsible for this effect. Regardless of the underlying mechanisms, running seems to produce an escape from daily pressures.

Perhaps the biggest advantage of running is that, unlike swimming and cycling, the only equipment it requires is a pair of running shoes and some shorts. Many people choose to invest large sums of money on expensive running outfits and warm-up suits; however, these are not necessary to get started on a jogging program. Running offers the advantages of low cost, flexibility of time, year-round availability, and a relatively high level of benefit in return for time and effort.

Disadvantages to Running

There are some disadvantages to running. Because the feet and legs are subjected to repetitive pounding on the running surface, overuse injuries are very likely. Most of these injuries involve the muscles, tendons, ligaments, and occasionally bones of the lower extremity. Proper running and training techniques and properly fitted running shoes can reduce the number of injuries associated with running.

Running Technique

Running is a skill that most of us learn at an early age. Because no two persons are anatomically exactly the same, each person will have a slightly different

running enjoyed by people of all ages, backgrounds, and sexes, running (jogging) has long been accepted as the essential training component for competitive athletes.

running style or form. However, there are certain things that all runners should pay attention to in terms of running style and proper form to help make running more efficient and reduce the possibility of injury: (1) foot strike and stride length, (2) proper body position, (3) arm movement, and (4) breathing pattern.

Foot Strike and Stride Length

Foot strike and stride length vary according to running speed. The faster the running speed, the longer the stride length. The knee should always be slightly flexed to absorb the impact of the foot strike. These two factors can significantly reduce the forces being transferred through the ankle, knee, and hip joints, reducing the possibility of injuries resulting from overuse (Figure 12-2).

The point of impact on the sole of the foot depends on the running speed (Figure 12-3). During sprinting, the ball of the foot should contact the ground first, with the heel never coming in contact. When running at a moderate speed, the contact is almost flat-footed, with most of the pressure in the midfoot area. In long-distance running, the heel should strike first, followed by the side border of the foot and the push-off from the ball of the great toe. The biggest mistake made by a runner is taking too much impact on the toes and not enough on the heels.

Proper Body Position

By far the most comfortable posture is one in which the shoulders are relaxed and the trunk leans slightly forward. The elbows should be at about 90 degrees, with the hands and fists relaxed. The pelvis should be rotated slightly forward. The head and face should be held upright, the runner looking a short distance in front and occasionally at the ground. The most critical factor is to be relaxed. If you are tense while running, you tend to be stiff, and this results in fatigue.

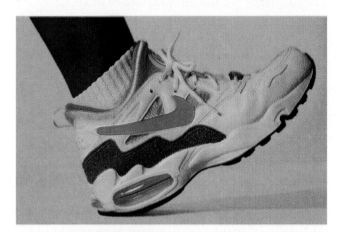

A

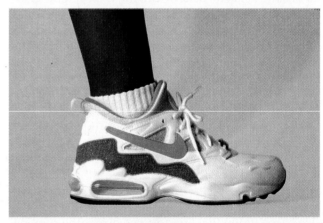

B

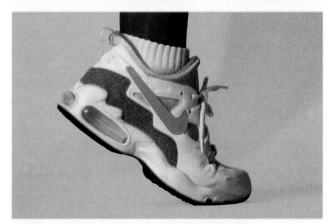

C

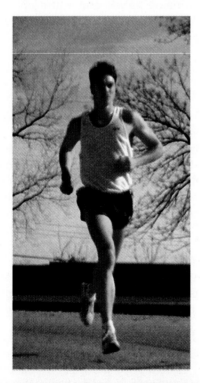

FIGURE 12-2. **Proper Running Technique.**
The heel should strike the ground in front of the knee, which should be flexed to absorb impact.

FIGURE 12-3. **Foot Contact in Running.**
A, Heel; **B,** foot flat; **C,** toe.

Arm Movement

The faster you run, the more the arms tend to move. Some arm movement is necessary to maintain balance. But in slow, long-distance running, arm swing should be kept at a minimum. The arms should be held slightly away from the trunk, with the forearms parallel to the ground. The fists should not be clenched, and the fingers and thumb should be slightly flexed. Again, the arms and hands should be relaxed and swing rhythmically with foot strike. Excessive arm motion results in trunk rotation, which over an extended period of time causes fatigue and an unnecessary expenditure of energy. Occasionally the arms should be totally relaxed and dropped to the side momentarily.

Breathing

Adequate breathing while running is essential; if sufficient oxygen is not supplied to the working muscles, activity cannot be continued for very long. In short sprint races, such as the 60- to 110-yard dash, many sprinters do not breathe at all and rely on anaerobic metabolism to provide sufficient oxygen. However, in long-distance running, which is aerobic, oxygen must be supplied continuously to working muscle. Breathing is best accomplished using the abdominal rather than diaphragmatic (chest) muscles. Diaphragmatic breathing is a more shallow type of breathing and is usually associated with breathing through the nose. Abdominal breathing is deeper and is accomplished by breathing through the mouth.

Abdominal breathing may prevent the so-called *stitch in the side* that is more likely to occur with diaphragmatic breathing. The cause of the stitch in the side is unknown but is most often associated with lack of oxygen in the diaphragm muscle due to a lack of blood flow.

Breathing should be rhythmic, and you should try to breathe primarily through the mouth to facilitate abdominal breathing. Concentrating on breathing often allows you to "lose yourself" and become more attuned to your body functions during a period of strenuous exercise.

Running Shoes

We stated earlier that the only equipment you really need to become involved in a running program is a pair of running shoes. This makes the process of buying an appropriate running shoe sound very simple, when in fact the purchase of running shoes may be a confusing experience. It is not uncommon for a shopper to enter a sporting goods store and be confronted by an entire wall filled with different types of running shoes. The logical question in this situation is where do you begin? Recommendations for purchas-

ing different types of fitness shoes are made in Chapter 13.

Runner's World magazine publishes a yearly study that critically analyzes all current brands and models of running shoes. For the more serious runner it is recommended that this source be consulted for detailed information, because the more you run, the more critical it is that a running shoe be built precisely for your foot. Running shoes should be used only for running, to extend the life of the shoe and thereby maximize the runner's investment. Since a different gait pattern is used for walking than for running, the walking shoe may tend to break down in such a way that injuries may result from switching to a running gait.

Running Guidelines

In Chapter 5 we indicated that you should begin at your own level and progress at your own rate by gradually increasing the amount of training time and intensity (as indicated by monitoring heart rate changes). Table 12-2 indicates recommended training sessions for beginning, intermediate, and advanced college-age runners. Figure 12-4 provides you with a sample of a 16-week jogging program.

SWIMMING

Like running, swimming is an excellent method of developing cardiorespiratory fitness. Like running, it has broad appeal; we find all types of people engaging in swimming fitness programs (Figure 12-5).

Reasons for Swimming

The physiological benefits of swimming are similar to those of running; however, there are several differences that should be addressed. The first difference is that in swimming not only must the arms and legs be used to propel the body through the water but also some energy must be expended to keep the body afloat. The drag of the water, the extent of which is determined by the size, shape, and speed of the person moving through it, provides an excellent form of resistance for improving muscle strength and endurance. For these reasons it has been estimated that the amount of energy required to swim a given distance is approximately four times as great as running an equal distance. Exercise heart rates are gener-

swimming increases muscular strength and endurance while reducing stress and strain on weight-bearing joints; swimming 1 mile can require burning up to four times the amount of energy as running the same distance

TABLE 12-2. Recommended Training Sessions for College-Age Runners

Level	Activity	Time for 1 mile (min:sec)	Speed (mph)	Approximate HR intensity	Approximate distance covered (20 min)
Beginner	Slow jog	12:00	5 mph	60%	1.66 miles
	Intermediate jog	10:00	6 mph	65%	2.00 miles
Intermediate	Brisk jog	8:34	7 mph	70%	2.33 miles
	Slow run	7:34	8 mph	75%	2.66 miles
Advanced	Intermediate run	6:40	9 mph	80%	3.00 miles
	Fast run	6:00	10 mph	85%	3.33 miles

FIGURE 12-4. A Gradual Jogging Program Progression.

	Warm-up	Target zone exercising	Cool-down	Total time
Week 1				
Session A	Stretch and limber up for 5 min	Then walk 10 min. Try not to stop.	Walk slowly 3 min, and stretch 2 min	20 min
Session B	Repeat above pattern			
Session C	Repeat above pattern			

Continue with at least three exercise sessions during each week of the program.

	Warm-up	Target zone exercising	Cool-down	Total time
Week 2	Stretch and limber 5 min	Walk 5 min, jog 1 min, walk 5 min, jog 1 min	Walk slowly 3 min, stretch 2 min	22 min
Week 3	Stretch and limber 5 min	Walk 5 min, jog 3 min, walk 5 min, jog 3 min	Walk slowly 3 min, stretch 2 min	26 min
Week 4	Stretch and limber 5 min	Walk 4 min, jog 5 min, walk 4 min, jog 5 min	Walk slowly 3 min, stretch 2 min	28 min
Week 5	Stretch and limber 5 min	Walk 4 min, jog 5 min, walk 4 min, jog 5 min	Walk slowly 3 min, stretch 2 min	28 min
Week 6	Stretch and limber 5 min	Walk 4 min, jog 6 min, walk 4 min, jog 6 min	Walk slowly 3 min, stretch 2 min	30 min
Week 7	Stretch and limber 5 min	Walk 4 min, jog 7 min, walk 4 min, jog 7 min	Walk slowly 3 min, stretch 2 min	32 min
Week 8	Stretch and limber 5 min	Walk 4 min, jog 8 min, walk 4 min, jog 8 min	Walk slowly 3 min, stretch 2 min	34 min
Week 9	Stretch and limber 5 min	Walk 4 min, jog 9 min, walk 4 min, jog 9 min	Walk slowly 3 min, stretch 2 min	36 min
Week 10	Stretch and limber 5 min	Walk 4 min, jog 13 min	Walk slowly 3 min, stretch 2 min	27 min
Week 11	Stretch and limber 5 min	Walk 4 min, jog 15 min	Walk slowly 3 min, stretch 2 min	29 min
Week 12	Stretch and limber 5 min	Walk 4 min, jog 17 min	Walk slowly 3 min, stretch 2 min	31 min
Week 13	Stretch and limber 5 min	Walk 2 min, jog slowly 2 min, jog 17 min	Walk slowly 3 min, stretch 2 min	31 min
Week 14	Stretch and limber 5 min	Walk 1 min, jog slowly 3 min, jog 17 min	Walk slowly 3 min, stretch 2 min	31 min
Week 15	Stretch and limber 5 min	Jog slowly 3 min, jog 17 min	Walk slowly 3 min, stretch 2 min	30 min

Week 16 on

Check your pulse periodically to see if you are exercising within your heart rate target zone. As you become fit, try exercising within the upper range of your heart rate target zone. Remember that your goal is to continue getting the benefits you are seeking and to enjoy your activity.

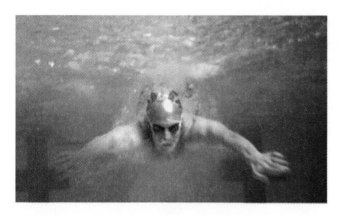

FIGURE 12-5. Swimming for Cardiorespiratory Endurance.

ally lower in swimming due to a lowered body temperature and the buoyancy of the water.

Energy expenditure and heart rates vary with the type of stroke. For both trained and highly skilled swimmers swimming at any given speed, the breaststroke seems to require the greatest amount of energy, followed by the backstroke, with the front crawl being the least taxing.

Advantages of Swimming

Swimming also eliminates a lot of stresses and strains on the weight-bearing joints that are commonly caused by running. Although the shoulder joint receives a significant amount of overuse-type stress, the ankle and knee joints are spared the trauma of the foot repeatedly banging into a hard surface. It is common for athletic trainers and physical therapists to recommend swimming as a substitute activity for a runner who has sustained some injury to the lower extremity. A runner who continues to train via running may make the injury worse, whereas the swimming used in the injury rehabilitation process will maintain cardiorespiratory conditioning until the injured person can return to training on the track.

Swimming Equipment

A swimsuit and perhaps a pair of goggles for persons whose eyes are irritated by chlorine are all that are necessary to begin a swimming program. For many the biggest drawback of using a swimming program for cardiorespiratory conditioning is the unavailability of a swimming pool. However, there are more than 2.5 million public and private swimming pools in the United States. If a pool is available, finding a free lane to swim in can be frustrating. There are usually a number of outdoor pools available during the summer months; however, in many areas, when the weather turns cold it becomes difficult to find an indoor pool. Indoor pools are typically available at a YMCA, on most college campuses, at some

high schools, and at many private health clubs or spas. In many cases, membership is required.

Swimming Technique

Although almost everyone can go out and run with little or no training, not everyone can jump into a pool and begin to swim. Simply being able to propel yourself through the water is a skill that must be learned, and swimming efficiency may only be considered once the basic skills have been mastered. Specific techniques of the crawl or freestyle stroke are discussed. The techniques for the backstroke, sidestroke, breaststroke, and butterfly are somewhat similar. Several books on swimming are recommended at the end of this chapter.

Water Entry Phase

When the hand is out of the water, the elbow should be bent at about 90 degrees and held high. The palm should be tilted outward so that the thumb enters the water first. The hand should enter the water at a point directly in line with the ear and about a foot in front of the head as if you were trying to catch the water.

Power Phase

After the hand has entered the water the palm turns toward the centerline of the body and forcefully pulls the water underneath the body as the elbow begins to bend once again until the arm is directly under the chest. At this point the hand continues to push water away, straightening the arm while the palm rotates inward toward the thigh. The little finger leads as the hand exits the water.

Recovery Phase

During the recovery phase the elbow exits the water first and continues to bend until it reaches 90 degrees. The hand moves upward along the body as the palm rotates outward and the elbow extends and once again reaches out to catch the water.

Kicking

When kicking the power comes almost totally from the hips. The knees should be kept almost straight, with the toes pointed. The feet should be about a foot apart and should only break the surface of the water with the heel.

Breathing

You may choose to breath bilaterally or on one side only. If breathing bilaterally, breathe every third stroke. As the hand breaks the surface of the water, begin rolling the body toward that hand and turn the head in the same direction, making sure to bring the mouth and nose just slightly out of the water. As the hand reenters the water, roll the body and turn the

TABLE 12-3. Guidelines for a Swimming Program

Level	Swimming distance*	Time Required (min)	Approximate HR intensity
Beginner	300-400 yards (12-16 lengths)	15	60%-70%
Intermediate	700-800 yards (28-30 lengths)	30	70%-80%
Advanced	1200-1600 yards (48-64 lengths)	40	80%-90%

*1 length = 25 yards.

head simultaneously in the opposite direction and exhale air as the hand and arm are completing the power phase.

Table 12-3 indicates recommended training sessions for beginning, intermediate, and advanced college-age swimmers.

CYCLING

Cycling is another aerobic activity that is excellent for improving cardiorespiratory endurance. It is also enjoyed by people of all ages, primarily because of the ease with which anyone can learn to ride without formal training (Figure 12-6).

Reasons for Cycling

Like running and swimming, cycling produces some very desirable physiological responses in terms of strength, endurance, and weight control. There are few data that suggest that cycling produces any overuse-type injuries; therefore cycling is frequently used by trainers and therapists as an alternative training method for the injured athlete.

There are numerous considerations for cycling, including selection of a bicycle, adjusting it to fit your body, maintaining it in good condition, and safety while cycling. It is strongly recommended that you purchase a cycling helmet made of some lightweight polystyrene material to protect yourself from head injury should an accident occur. Before getting started, we recommend that you consult some of the texts for bicyclists listed in the references at the end of the chapter.

Bicycling Equipment

Bicycles come in thousands of different makes and models, with countless numbers of available accessories and options. Prices range anywhere from a minimum of $90 for a standard three-speed bike all the way up to several thousand dollars for professional touring or racing bikes. For the average person the cost of getting involved in some type of cycling activity is not much more than for a pair of good running shoes.

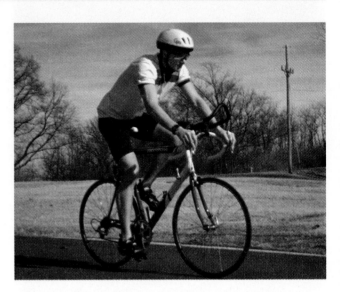

FIGURE 12-6. Cycling.
Cycling can be enjoyed by people of all ages.

Stationary Exercise Bicycles

Perhaps the biggest problem with cycling is locating a safe place to ride. No matter how safety conscious you are on the bicycle, there is always a danger posed by traffic. For this reason, stationary exercise bikes, or ergometers, have become popular. Prices for stationary bikes range from about $70 to about $3500. The stationary bike allows you to gain all the cardiovascular benefits of cycling without having to worry about dealing with traffic safety. Additionally, you can exercise in privacy, regardless of outdoor conditions, and you can read, watch TV, or listen to music at the same time. However, for many, sitting in one place and pedaling is extremely boring. Most people enjoy the changes in scenery experienced while biking. Also, you can change routes as a way of maintaining interest.

Regardless of which cycling method you choose, the same principles of continuous training apply as indicated in Chapter 5. The intensity must be great enough to elevate the heart rate to between 50% and 85% of maximal oxygen uptake, and this activity should be sustained for at least 20 minutes. This training level will ensure improvement of cardiorespiratory endurance over a period of time (Table 12-4).

TABLE 12-4. Guidelines for a Cycling Program			
Level	Cycling distance (miles)	Time required (min)	Approximate HR intensity (%)
Beginner	4	20	60-70
Intermediate	6	30	70-80
Advanced	9-10	40	80-90

Proper Seat Adjustment

Perhaps one of the most important considerations in cycling is the proper adjustment of the seat. When sitting on the seat, with one pedal as close to the ground as possible and with the toe on the pedal, you should have your knee bent very slightly (less than 10 degrees). With your heel on the pedal the knee should be fully extended. You should not be able to touch the ground with your feet if the seat is adjusted to the appropriate height. Adjusting the seat too low can produce soreness in the front part of the thigh.

ROPE SKIPPING

Rope skipping has many advantages for someone looking for an inexpensive and convenient form of exercise. Nearly everyone can learn to rope skip. It contributes to all the components of physical fitness, particularly in the area of cardiorespiratory endurance.

If you have been sedentary or have had health problems, you should see a physician and get a physical evaluation before beginning rope skipping as a fitness activity. It is also wise to do some warm-up exercises to increase blood flow, heart rate, flexibility, and respiration rate. Jumpers should be cautioned that rope jumping is an extremely vigorous activity and should be started gradually. In the beginning you should jump for just a few seconds, then walk to catch your breath, then jump again. Gradually, increase the time you jump. Ultimately you should be able to jump for 15 to 20 minutes. Alternating jumping with walking is a good way to develop cardiovascular fitness.

Advantages of Rope Skipping

Rope skipping raises the heart rate, and as you continue to use this activity in your fitness program, it improves not only cardiorespiratory endurance but also muscular endurance. These qualities enable the muscular system to perform the activity for prolonged periods of time with less strain and fatigue. Because rope skipping requires a degree of coordination, speed, and agility, it can also have a beneficial effect in improving these areas.

Rope skipping can expend as much energy as running. Another advantage is the relatively short time it takes to perform the activity. Some people rope skip intermittently for 20 minutes, which is almost equivalent to jogging for 30 minutes, at least in terms of energy expenditure. An added advantage of rope skipping for many students is that they do not have to skip on hard surfaces. Some students find jogging difficult because of the need to run on hard surfaces. Rope skipping, however, may be performed indoors or outdoors on a hard or soft surface. Rope skipping can be done almost anywhere at any time, provided there is space enough for the rope to make a complete revolution.

Rope-Skipping Equipment

The equipment needed for rope skipping is inexpensive. The cost of a jump rope ranges from $3.50 to $20, depending on type. There are various types of jump ropes: sash, cord, plastic, and plain rope. Handles may be wooden or plastic. Weighted handles are available, or the participant may choose not to use handles but instead to tie a knot at the ends of the rope. To be sure the rope is of a proper length, bring the handles up to the side of the body. The handles should be at armpit height. Also, it is helpful to wear proper clothing. The ideal outfit would include a pair of gym socks, a pair of comfortable shorts, a T-shirt or blouse, and shoes with adequate cushioning to reduce the force of repetitive impact and the risk of injury to the lower extremity. Other clothes may be worn as long as they do not interfere with the rope-skipping activity.

Rope-Skipping Techniques

Rope skipping can be done alone or in pairs. The ends of the rope are held loosely in the fingers. Elbows should be close to the sides and the arms pointed

cycling whether recreational, competitive, or somewhere in between, cycling improves cardiorespiratory endurance, muscular strength, and muscular endurance; cycling is rarely known to produce overuse injuries and is often used as an alternative training method for injured athletes

rope skipping an inexpensive and convenient form of exercise that develops each of the components of physical fitness while improving coordination, speed, and agility

away from the body. The arms and shoulders move in a circular motion; as the rope follows a circular motion, further momentum can be provided by rotating the wrists. Jump by pushing off from the toes just high enough to allow the rope to pass under your feet.

Rope-skipping routines should be designed to help you progress from a short series of workouts to extended workouts. Your program development plan should be flexible and take into consideration your goals and level of fitness; otherwise the activity could become boring or too physically difficult. Figure 12-7 shows rope-skipping techniques as recommended by the American Heart Association.

AEROBIC DANCE EXERCISE

A number of different activities that have been identified in this chapter are aerobic in nature. In today's terminology the word *aerobics* is primarily used to refer specifically to aerobic dance exercise, which may well be the country's largest, most widespread organized fitness endeavor. The growth in aerobic dance exercise during the past decade has been truly phenomenal. Referred to as a "sport" by the National Sporting Goods Association, in 1985 aerobics was found to be the third-fastest growing sport in the United States. It is estimated that more than 30 million Americans, both males and females, now participate

---

FIGURE 12-7. Rope-Skipping Stunts.

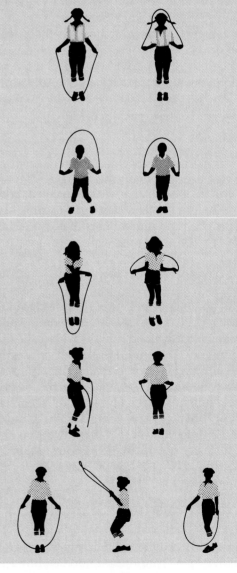

Basic Single Short Rope Skills

1. Basic Jump
   1. Jump on both feet.
   2. Land on balls of feet.
   3. Jump once for each revolution of rope.
      Hint: Keep feet, ankles, and knees together.

2. Side Straddle
   1. Jump to a straddle position.
   2. Return to basic jump.
      Hint: Spread feet shoulder width apart.

3. Criss Cross
   1. Cross arms until elbows touch, and jump over rope.
   2. Keep arms crossed while turning rope.
   3. Open rope and perform basic jump.
   4. Cross right arm over left or cross left arm over right.
      Hint: Keep hands down low on the cross.

4. Forward 180
   1. Swing rope to left, half turn of body to left.
   2. Jump over backward turning rope.
      Hint: The body turns to follow the rope; the skill may be performed to the left or the right.

5. Backward 180
   1. Jump a backward turning rope.
   2. Half turn of body left (keeping rope in front of face).
   3. Jump rope forward.
      Hint: Turn the body to follow the rope; the skill may be performed to the left or the right.

Illustrations from American Heart Association: *Jump for the health of it*, Dallas, 1983, AHA.

in aerobic exercise. Aerobics is a combination of choreographed fitness routines set to music. In other words, it is movement to music that contributes to physical fitness by improving cardiorespiratory endurance, strength, flexibility, and muscular endurance.

Almost anyone can do aerobic exercise; your physical condition will determine at what pace you should work. It is recommended that the target heart rate be maintained for at least 20 minutes during the aerobics or cardiorespiratory conditioning portion of the workout. Aerobics uses various stretching, strength, and other exercises to achieve the target heart rate and produce a vigorous workout.

Aerobics is a vigorous physical activity that can provide an inexpensive and practical workout for most people. It increases the working capacity of the cardiovascular and pulmonary systems. If done on a regular basis, it should result in increased energy and stamina and better ability to handle life's stresses and tensions. It contributes to weight control and can be a source of fun and relaxation.

Very little equipment is needed for aerobics. Comfortable clothing includes items such as leotards, shorts, T-shirts, and shoes designed especially for aerobics. There are literally thousands of aerobics classes offered throughout the United States each day at local health clubs, universities, recreational centers, and so on. Many television stations feature aerobics classes, and there are countless aerobics videos available so that viewers can exercise in the privacy of their own living rooms. Aerobics can be performed almost anywhere, since very little space is needed to perform the range of motion involved in the exercises.

High-Impact Versus Low-Impact Aerobics

As a rapidly developing participation sport, aerobics is undergoing an evolutionary process. Different styles of aerobics have been advocated over the last few years. High-impact aerobics is the more traditional form, in which the cardiorespiratory conditioning component consists of running, jumping, and hopping movements set to music. High-impact aerobics has produced a significant number of musculoskeletal injuries as a result of the repetitive pounding of the lower extremity against a hard surface. In low-impact aerobics, the impact to the lower extremity is reduced by eliminating excessive jumping and by keeping one leg slightly bent and in constant contact with the floor throughout the conditioning phase of the workout. Traveling movements rather than stationary steps are used, with an emphasis on maintaining proper body alignment at all times. Arm movements are often exaggerated to elevate heart rate, and in certain cases wrist weights may also be added.

However, arm movements should be kept under control, with the arms in a state of partial contraction. You should avoid flailing the arms uncontrollably.

Low impact does not mean low intensity. Even though the approach is a bit different, the goal of low-impact aerobics is the same as for high-impact aerobics: to improve cardiorespiratory endurance by elevating and maintaining heart rates at training levels. Low-impact aerobics are most appropriate for those individuals who are beginners, older, overweight, pregnant, or who have a history of injuries. In certain cases, nonimpact aerobics, in which neither of the feet ever leaves the floor, may be recommended.

Aquatic Aerobics

Many aerobics instructors are now advocating aquatic aerobics, done in water to eliminate any jarring of the weight-bearing body parts while using the water's resistance to movement during the conditioning component. Of all the types of aerobics, water aerobics is likely to be the safest. The stresses and strains exerted on the musculoskeletal system while exercising on land are virtually nonexistent in the water. In fact, the application of aquatic exercise is rapidly becoming a standard in injury rehabilitation.

Water aerobics has become a popular form of exercise, because it can be done in the water in an upright position but it does not require swimming skill. Again, the principles and guidelines relative to intensity, duration, and frequency of exercise apply to aquatic aerobics. It is estimated that 2.5 million people routinely engage in aquatic aerobics.

Step Aerobics

Step aerobics or "stepping," which is one of the hottest new trends in fitness, offers a high-intensity, low-impact workout (Figure 12-8). It uses a bench ranging between 4 and 8 inches high and slower music that makes it appropriate for all age groups. The intensity of the workout can be modified by changing the height of the bench. Important consider-

aerobic dance exercise a series of movements and exercises combined with music that contributes to physical fitness by improving cardiorespiratory endurance, strength, flexibility, and muscular endurance

aquatic aerobics a variation of aerobic dance exercise performed in water to increase resistance and eliminate jarring of the weight-bearing parts of the body; a very safe form of exercise, aquatic aerobics is rapidly becoming a standard in injury rehabilitation

step aerobics a popular trend in fitness that offers the benefit of a high-intensity, low-impact workout

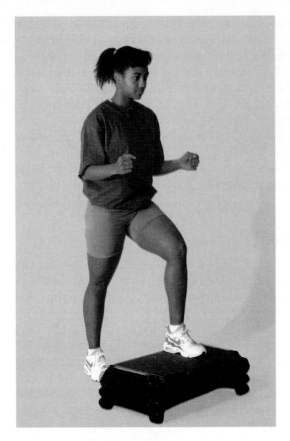

FIGURE 12-8. Step Aerobics.
One of the hot new fitness activities sweeping the country.

ations and guidelines for engaging in step aerobics include the following:

- A fairly erect posture should be maintained while stepping, with the head forward, chest out, and a slight forward bend at the waist. An exaggerated bend at the waist can lead to back problems.
- Tall people may need a slightly higher step. The knee should never be flexed more than 90 degrees.
- You should try to strike the entire foot in the center of the step when ascending.
- You should learn to gently lower yourself off the step, striking the ground with the ball of the foot first. As fatigue sets in, you tend to not use muscular control to lower yourself, increasing the force of the impact.
- Avoid stepping off of the front of the step. This action increases the stress on many of the joints in the body.
- Wear shoes designed for aerobics classes. They should be relatively new and provide good cushioning and side support.

Slide Aerobics

Perhaps the newest variation of aerobic dance exercise is slide aerobics. This is an activity that involves sliding back and forth from side to side in a rhythmical manner on a slick surface made of polyurethane or Teflon while wearing socks that slip on over shoes (Figure 12-9). The technique is similar to an ice skating movement.

Circuit Aerobics

Circuit aerobics combines the use of resistance equipment with an advanced aerobic dance exercise class. Approximately 30 minutes is devoted to aerobic dance and 30 minutes to resistance training at various stations. The two components may be performed separately or in combination with an aerobic dance routine between resistance training stations.

Hand and Wrist Weights

Holding light hand weights or wearing banded wrist weights is a common practice in various forms of aerobic exercise. Addition of these light weights increases energy expenditure during activity. It is necessary to swing or pump the arms to achieve this increase in energy expenditure. Simply carrying the weight has little or no effect.

Several precautions should be considered when using hand or wrist weights, because their use increases both systolic and diastolic blood pressures; gripping hand weights causes an increase in diastolic blood pressure. Thus people with heart disease and hypertension should avoid their use. Shoulder pain may develop or be aggravated with the use of weights. To avoid this problem, do not lift weights above shoulder level.

Guidelines and Precautions for Aerobic Dance Exercise

If you have not been active physically or if you have had health problems, see a physician before beginning an aerobics program. Persons who are overweight or have a family history of heart disease should have a physician's approval or a stress test before beginning an aerobic fitness program. Periodically during an aerobic fitness class, you should stop and check your heart rate to be certain that it is within the limits for safe exercise.

A warm-up program of stretching exercises is recommended. Warm-up could include exercises such as trunk stretching, trunk circles, half-knee bends, twists, and reaches. Follow a developmental sequence by going from simple tasks at the beginning of the program to more complex tasks later on. At the end of each workout, take time for cool-down. Cool-down exercises should be done in a relaxed manner at a comfortable speed and strength.

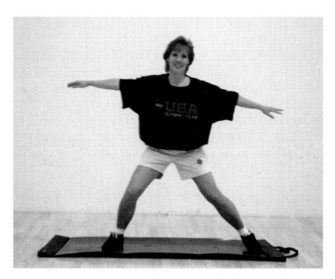

FIGURE 12-9. **Slide Aerobics.**
Slide aerobics is the newest variation in aerobic exercise

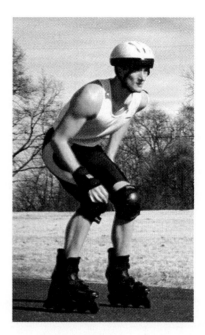

FIGURE 12-10. **Rollerblading.**
Rollerblading or in-line skating is an extremely popular activity on college campuses

Program development should be flexible to allow you to engage in activities appropriate for your interest and level of ability. Programs will vary according to each person's needs, interests, and physical condition. The object in most cases is to structure the aerobics program so that the intensity and length of the activity are gradually increased.

IN-LINE SKATING (ROLLERBLADING)

In-line skating or rollerblading is another "hot" fitness and recreational activity that is quickly gaining popularity throughout the United States (Figure 12-10). However, rollerblading is not a new activity. Rollerblading is essentially "high-tech" rollerskating. A pair of rollerblades looks similar to ice skates that have had the blade replaced with a series of 4 to 6 small wheels. These polyurethane wheels are made for gliding on hard, smooth surfaces. Prices for a pair of rollerblades range from about $60 to several hundred dollars. Rollerbladers are capable of speeds approaching 25 miles per hour. For this reason it is essential that pads be worn to protect elbows, knees, and hands. It is also recommended that protective headgear, such as a cycling helmet, be worn to minimize the likelihood of injury.

The motion used with rollerblading is similar to ice skating, which requires pushing with the legs from side to side and using a side-to-side swinging motion of the arms for balance. Rollerblading uses gross movements of both the arms and the legs, making it an excellent aerobic activity.

Guidelines and Precautions for In-Line Skating

Safety in rollerblading is of critical importance. It is essential that you wear the appropriate protective equipment, including elbow and knee pads and wrist guards. A helmet is also recommended. Perhaps the most difficult thing about rollerblading is learning how to stop. The brake is most often located on the heel of the right skate. To stop you should keep your left foot forward and lean back slightly to contact the ground with the the brake pad. You should not venture out into either vehicle or pedestrian traffic until you have mastered some degree of control on rollerblades.

SKILL-RELATED LIFETIME FITNESS ACTIVITIES

In this chapter, activities have been emphasized that are considered to be primarily aerobic in nature. These activities are more oriented toward the maintenance or improvement of the health-related components of fitness, in particular, cardiorespiratory endurance. Although these activities are effective in promoting and maintaining good health, it must be stressed that **any physical activity in which you choose to participate can contribute to optimal health.** Like the aerobic activities, skill-related activities such as golf, tennis, volleyball, softball, racquetball, and handball are sports in which individuals can choose to participate throughout their lifetime. In these sport activities, the motor skill–related components of fitness discussed in Chapter 1 become very important to performance. To a large extent, power, speed, agility, balance, neuromuscular coordination, and reaction time contribute to success or failure in a particular sport. Practice and repetition of that activity can, over a period of time, improve and enhance these skill-related components. It must be reemphasized that the health-related fitness components, muscular strength and endurance, flexibility, and cardiorespiratory endurance, may also be critical to

sport performance. These components form the basis for most of the skill-related activities.

Certainly, there may be a number of reasons for choosing to engage in a particular physical activity: relaxation, competition, or socialization. Obviously the best reason to choose a particular physical activity is for the pure enjoyment that it provides for you. **Lab Activity 12-1** helps you look at the patterns of physical activity in which you engage during an entire week. Based on what you have learned from the previous chapters, does your lifestyle include a sufficient amount of exercise?

SUMMARY

- Walking is a convenient, inexpensive activity that contributes to one's health and fitness. It has become the most popular form of exercise in American society.
- Running is also a popular aerobic exercise. Many people run to control their weight and to attain a healthful appearance, whereas others run for the many physiological benefits. Running also produces a psychologically stimulating effect.
- Proper running technique requires that you pay attention to the way your foot strikes the ground, your body position, your arm movement, and your breathing pattern.
- Swimming offers physiological benefits similar to running; however, the physical stresses and strains to the lower extremity that occur with running are eliminated.
- Swimming requires approximately four times more energy to cover a given distance than does running.
- Both swimming and cycling may be used as substitute activities for an injured person who is incapable of running.
- Cycling is an aerobic activity that offers physiological benefits similar to swimming and running.

- Rope skipping has many advantages for a person looking for an inexpensive and convenient form of exercise.
- Rope skipping raises the heart rate, and as a person continues to use this activity in his or her fitness program, it improves not only cardiorespiratory endurance but also muscular endurance.
- Aerobic dance exercise is movement to music for fitness. Aerobic dance exercise contributes to physical fitness through improvement of cardiorespiratory endurance, balance, strength, flexibility, and muscular endurance.
- Aerobic exercise uses various stretching, strengthening, and other exercises to achieve the target heart rate and produce a vigorous workout.
- Aerobic dance exercise may be high impact or low impact. Aquatic aerobics, circuit aerobics, and step aerobics are variations of traditional aerobic dance exercise that are all gaining popularity.
- The lifetime fitness activity that you choose to participate in doesn't necessarily have to be aerobic in nature. Any activity that you select will contribute to improving overall health.

REFERENCES

American Heart Association: *Jump for the health of it,* Dallas, 1983, AHA.

Austin G, Noble J: *Swimming for fitness,* London, 1994, AC Black.

Bicycling and cycling, *Clin Sports Med* 13(1):1-129, 1994.

Dolgener F, Hensley L, Marsh J: Validation of the Rockport fitness walking test in college males and females, *Res Q Exerc Sport* 65(2):152-158. 1994.

Ewing A: Effect of exercise with light hand weights on strength, *J Orthop Sports Phys Ther* 8:553, 1987.

Forester J: *Effective cycling,* Cambridge, 1993, MIT Press.

Graves JE: The effects of hand held weights, wrist weights, and ankle weights, *Med Sci Sports Exerc* 20:265, 1988.

Hawkins J, Hawkins S: *Walking for fun and fitness,* Englewood, Colo, 1996, Morton Publishing.

Hoyt C, Hoyt J: *Cycling,* Dubuque, Iowa, 1984, William C Brown.

International Dance Exercise Association: *Aerobic dance-exercise instructors' manual,* San Diego, 1987, International Dance Exercise Association Foundation.

Koenig J, Jahn D: The effect of bench step aerobics on muscle strength, power, and endurance, *J Strength Cond Res* 9(1):43-49, 1995.

Mazzeo K: *Fitness through aerobics and step training,* Englewood, Colo, 1996, Morton Publishing.

McArdle W, Katch F, Katch V: *Exercise physiology: energy, nutrition and human performance,* Philadelphia, 1994, Lea & Febiger.

Mellion M: Bicycling. In Mellion M, editor: *Sports medicine secrets,* Philadelphia, 1994, Hanley & Belfus.

Meyers C: *Walking: the complete guide to complete exercise,* New York, 1992, Random House.

Munnings F: The walking message: have people heard it? *Med Exerc Nutr Health* 3(1):56-59, 1994.

Noakes T: *Lore of running,* Champaign, 1991, Leisure Press.

Normansell K: Aerobic dance exercise. In Miller P, editor: *Fitness programming and physical disabilities,* Champaign, 1995, Human Kinetics.

Ounpuus S: The biomechanics of walking and running, *Clin Sports Med* 13(4):843-863, 1994.

Pickett B: Stepping up fitness can be fun, *J Int Council Health Phys Educ Recreat Sport Dance* 31(3):46-47, 1995.

Powell M, Swanson J: *In-line skating: the skills for fun and fitness on wheels,* Champaign, 1993, Human Kinetics.

Rippe J, Ward A: *The Rockport walking program,* New York, 1986, Prentice-Hall.

Runner's World 1995 Shoe Buying Guide 30(4):49-73, 1995.

Sloane E: *The all new complete book of cycling,* New York, 1988, Simon & Schuster.

Stamford B: Mall walking, burning calories in the great indoors, *Phys Sports Med* 22(12):101-102, 1994.

Stokes L: Walking with hand-held weights, *Hughston Health Alert* 6(3):1-3, 1994.

US Department of Health and Human Services, Public Health Services: *Healthy people 2000: midcourse review and 1995 revisions,* Washington, DC, 1995, USDHHS.

US Department of Health and Human Services, Public Health Services: *Healthy people 2000: national health promotion and disease prevention objectives,* Washington, DC, 1991, USDHHS.

Webb T: *Step fitness workout,* New York, 1994, Workman Publishing.

White T: *The wellness guide to lifelong fitness,* New York, 1993, Rebus.

Whitten P: *The complete book of swimming,* New York, 1994, Random House.

Wilford HN, Blessing D, Olson M: Is low impact aerobic dance an effective cardiovascular workout? *Phys Sports Med* 17(3):95, 1989.

SUGGESTED READINGS

Austin G, Noble J: *Swimming for fitness,* London, 1994, AC Black.
A guide to exercising in water. Explains through photographs and drawings how to perform swimming techniques and how muscular strength, cardiovascular endurance, and well-being can be improved.

Freid-Cassorla A: *In-line skating: the ultimate how-to guide,* Rocklin, Calif, 1995, Prima Publishing.
Includes tips for getting started, choosing equipment, basic and advanced techniques, safety gear, equipment maintenance, and recommended workouts.

Gutman B: *Blazing bladers,* New York, 1992, Tom Doherty Assoc.
A complete guide for the rollerblader. Discusses equipment, clothing, safety tips, stunts, and sports of the new activity.

Meyers C: *Walking: the complete guide to complete exercise,* New York, 1992, Random House.
A basic "how-to" on walking. It is comprehensive yet concise and well written. Discusses basic techniques of a walking program and emphasizes the effectiveness of combining a sensible eating program.

Noakes T: *Lore of running,* Champaign, 1991, Leisure Press.
A physician/runner discusses the physiology of running, the medical considerations of your health history, and practical guidelines for running.

Perry D: *Bike cult,* New York, 1995, Four Walls Eight Windows.
A guide to bicycling as a way of life. Includes tips on equipment, tours, books, movies, art, etc.

Plevin A: *Cycling: a celebration of the sport and the world's best places to enjoy,* New York, 1992, Byron Priess/Richard Ballantine.
Discusses cycling relative to equipment, riding clubs, touring, and the future of the sport.

Rippe J, Ward A: *The Rockport walking program,* New York, 1986, Prentice-Hall.
A program designed to help you lose weight and maintain better health regardless of age. Based on research from Rockport, it presents information on a combination walking and diet program.

White T: *The wellness guide to lifelong fitness,* New York, 1993, Rebus.
An excellent, extremely well-illustrated and colorful text that addresses walking, running, swimming, cycling, and aerobic dance all in significant detail; this is a valuable resource.

Whitten P: *The complete book of swimming,* New York, 1994, Random House.
A comprehensive book on swimming written for both the experienced swimmer who wants to improve and for rookies who aren't sure where to begin.

Physical Activity Record

Name _____   **Section** _____   **Date** _____

PURPOSE   To determine your patterns of physical activity during a 7-day period.

PROCEDURE   Using the Activity Record, record your activity during the next week. Each day record the number of hours or partial hours that you were engaged in a particular activity. If the activity you were engaged in is not listed, try to approximate the activity to one that is included on the Activity Record. Multiply the number of hours by the weighted value (quality points). Do this each day for 7 consecutive days. Total the quality points and divide by 7 to obtain a daily average.

Activity Record

Activity	Mon.	Tues.	Wed.	Thur.	Fri.	Sat.	Sun.	Total for Week	Weighted Value	Total Quality Points
SLEEPING									$\times 1.0 =$	
SITTING ACTIVITIES										
Eating										
Reading/ studying										
Sewing/ typing										
Desk work										
Driving/ riding										
Watching TV										
Other similar activities										
Sitting Activities Total									$\times 1.5 =$	
STANDING ACTIVITIES										
Showering										
Dressing										
Strolling										
Light house-work										
Job-related standing										
Other similar activities										
Standing Activities Total									$\times 2.0 =$	
WALKING ACTIVITIES										
Slow walking (to and from classes or around home or office)									$\times 3.0 =$	
Fast walking (late to class or appoint-ments)									$\times 4.0 =$	
Climbing stairs									$\times 6.0 =$	

Activity Record—cont'd

Activity	Mon.	Tues.	Wed.	Thur.	Fri.	Sat.	Sun.	Total for Week	Weighted Value	Total Quality Points
MILD ACTIVITIES										
Cycling (8 mph)										
Badminton										
Tennis (beginner)										
Tennis (doubles)										
Rapid calisthenics										
Volleyball										
Gardening										
Softball										
Golf (walking and carrying clubs)										
Other										
Mild Activities Totals									x 6.0 =	
MODERATE ACTIVITIES										
Cycling (11 mph)										
Tennis (singles)										
Racquetball										
Slow running										
Swimming (laps)										
Touch football										
Soccer										
Hiking										
Swimming (beginner)										
Other										
Moderate Activities Totals									x 8.0 =	

Continued.

Activity Record—cont'd

Activity	Mon.	Tues.	Wed.	Thur.	Fri.	Sat.	Sun.	Total for Week	Weighted Value	Total Quality Points
STRENUOUS ACTIVITIES										
Cycling (13 mph)										
Handball (competitive)										
Racquetball (competitive)										
Squash (competitive)										
Running (6 mph)										
Vigorous basketball										
Swimming (competitive)										
Strenuous Activities Totals									x 10.0 =	

Total number of Quality Points for all activities during 7-day period = _____

Divide total number of Quality Points by 7 to obtain a daily average.   _____

INTERPRETATION

If your average score is below 40 points, you probably are living a very sedentary life. An average score of 41 or above would suggest that you are probably enjoying many of the benefits derived from regular physical activity.

1. How would you characterize your current exercise program in terms of the quantity and quality of physical activity?
2. What form of physical activity do you enjoy the most?
3. Given your current level of activity, how would you describe how you physically feel at this time?
4. Describe your attitude toward participating in regular physical exercise.
5. How would you like to change your current exercise program, and what could you do to implement this change? Also, outline your goals in relation to the benefits of exercise.

Modified from Allen RJ, Hyde DH: *Investigations in stress control,* Minneapolis, 1981, Macmillan.

Chapter 13 Buying Fitness Products

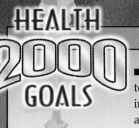

HEALTH 2000 GOALS

■ **Public Education.** Efforts need to address specific barriers that inhibit the adoption of physical activity by different population groups.

• Individuals of all socioeconomic levels need information on the availability of group activities in the community; appropriate footwear; safe walking, biking, and fitness trails; and available swimming pools and tennis courts. In 1988 only 46% of municipal and county park and recreation departments provided fitness trails, 29% provided hiking trails, 21% provided biking trails, and 15% provided snow trails.

OBJECTIVES

After completing this chapter, you will be able to do the following:

■ Describe what is necessary to be a careful consumer of health and fitness products.
■ Discuss the various types of exercise equipment that may be used in a health and fitness program.

■ Explain how clothing should be selected for exercising in hot or cold environments.
■ Discuss what you should look for in health and fitness books and magazines.
■ Identify special considerations for selecting a health or fitness club.

KEY TERMS

While reading this chapter, you will become familiar with the following terms:

• consumerism
• fitness and exercise equipment
• exercise clothing
• fitness books and magazines

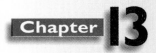

THE CONSUMER IN THE HEALTH AND FITNESS MARKET

To say that the emphasis on health and fitness in American society has increased significantly during the past decade is a gross understatement. The consumer of health and fitness products has become the target of an unprecedented media advertising blitz. The stereotypical image of the healthy and fit body appears in countless magazines at newsstands, on television, and in newspaper ads. Advertising includes everything from health foods and vitamins to exercise equipment, fitness centers, and weight-loss centers.

Further evidence of the magnitude of the interest in fitness and exercise is seen in the expenditures for sporting goods and exercise equipment; these expenditures have reached an all-time high. The sale of sporting goods has become big business. In 1983 sporting goods' sales reached $13.6 billion. Sales of about $20 billion were recorded in 1990. The athletic shoe business alone has become a $2 billion-a-year business. Recent sales figures show that close to $4 billion is being spent on athletic clothing annually. Sales of home exercise equipment have skyrocketed from $723 million in 1982 to about $3 billion today as individuals seek the convenience of being able to work out at home. Stationary bicycles, rowing machines, treadmills, stair climbers, and weight systems are the most popular items. Sales of diet and exercise books continue to rise. Corporate fitness programs and commercial health clubs have attracted a record number of members. The number of athletic and recreational programs in schools and communities has also shown a substantial increase. The list goes on and on. There is little doubt that a significant amount of misinformation is being disseminated in an effort to merchandise a lucrative health and fitness industry.

Marketing experts are extremely sensitive to the vulnerability of American consumers when it comes to buying products that promise to make them look and feel better. How can the consumer separate fact from hype? It is essential for consumers to educate themselves by taking a critical look at a product or service to be purchased. For example, if you are going to buy a new automobile, perhaps you begin by looking at advertisements. You may wish to consult an independent consumer magazine to look at performance specifications, maintenance record, and so on. Then you go to the dealers to find who can offer the best price along with a reputation for good service. Chances are that you will buy your new car from that dealer. The point is that most people shop around and are careful when making a choice about a large purchase such as an automobile. They take the time necessary to learn everything they can about the product. The wise consumer will take a similar approach when buying health and fitness products. You should realize that it is easy to be "taken in" by advertisements that project an image that seems to be in demand by consumers. Practicing consumerism means that wise consumers will take the time to analyze the entire product and to decide if the outlay of money is necessary to reap the benefits they desire.

SELECTING FITNESS EQUIPMENT

The extent and variety of fitness and exercise equipment available to the consumer is at times mind boggling. Prices of equipment can range from between $2 for a jump rope or frisbee to $60,000 for certain computer-driven isokinetic devices. It is certainly not necessary to purchase expensive exercise equipment to see good results. You will achieve many of the same physiological benefits from using a $2 jump rope that result from running on a $10,000 treadmill. The following sections identify and discuss some of the more popular pieces of exercise equipment.

Free Weights Versus Weight Machines

There are various types of exercise equipment that can be used with progressive resistive exercise, including free weights (barbells and dumbells) or exercise machines such as Cybex, Universal, Nautilus, Eagle, DP, Soloflex, and Body Master. Dumbells and barbells require the use of iron plates of varying weights that can be easily changed by adding or subtracting equal amounts of weight to both sides of the bar. Most of the exercise machines have a stack of weights that are lifted through a series of levers or pulleys. The stack of weights slides up and down on a pair of bars that restrict the movement to only one plane. Weight can be increased or decreased simply by changing the position of a weight key.

Advantages and Disadvantages

There are advantages and disadvantages to both the free weights and exercise machines. The machines are relatively safe to use in comparison with free weights. For example, if you are doing a bench press with free weights, it is essential to have someone "spot" you (help you lift the weights back onto the support racks if you don't have enough strength to complete the lift); otherwise you may end up dropping the weight on your chest. With the exercise machines you can easily and safely drop the weight without fear of injury.

It is also a simple process to increase or decrease the weight by moving a single weight key with the weight machines, although changes can generally be made only in increments of 10 or 15 pounds. With free weights, iron plates must be added or removed from each side of the barbell.

Costs of purchasing free weights are substantially lower than the exercise machines. Regardless of which type of equipment is used, the same principles of isotonic training may be applied.

Stationary Exercise Bikes

Many different exercise bikes are available to the consumer (Figure 13-1). Bicycle companies such as Schwinn or Ross and companies such as Lifecycle, Cybex, Tunturi, Vitamaster, and Proform, which specifically manufacture exercise equipment, are well-known name brands. Exercise bikes priced below $150 tend to be somewhat unstable. Most good models range between $200 and $800. Computerized exercise bikes used in health clubs may cost between $1500 and $3500.

There are essentially three types of exercise bikes: single action, dual action, and recumbent. When you pedal a "single-action" model, resistance is created from a device such as a flywheel. A bike that has a flywheel that weighs at least 50 pounds will generally last longer and will be a bit more expensive. With the flywheel you can change the resistance with a twist of a knob.

The "dual-action" models also let you pump the handlebars back with your arms. Most of these bikes use a fan to create resistance, which can be increased by pumping the arms and legs faster. The dual-action models allow you to rest your feet on coaster pedals and exercise only your arms. Obviously, those models that work both the upper and lower extremities require a higher energy expenditure.

Most stationary bikes have you sitting on a bicycle seat in a standard position. There are some relatively new design variations that allow you to sit in a recumbent position. This position exercises the hamstring muscles to a greater degree and is useful for individuals who have back problems or poor balance.

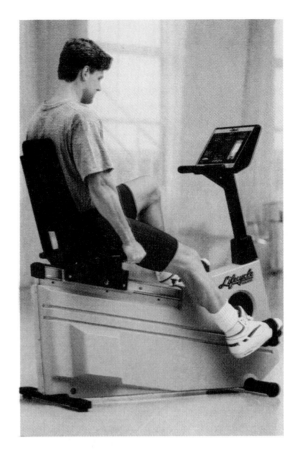

FIGURE 13-1. Stationary Exercise Bike.
Many are reasonably priced; people can choose to exercise at any time in the privacy of their homes.

Training stands hook a resistance device to your regular bicycle, allowing you to convert it to a stationary bike at relatively low cost. Features that are important to look for include a comfortable padded seat and some type of monitor that tells you how far you have pedaled or the time elapsed. Models with pedal straps will work your legs on the upstroke and the downstroke.

Treadmills

An exercise treadmill is a belt stretched between two rollers (Figure 13-2). The belt may be driven man-

---

consumerism weighing the pros and cons of a product to decide if the outlay of money is necessary to reap the benefits desired

fitness and exercise equipment the market for machines, equipment, and devices designed to improve physical fitness has grown at a mind-boggling rate; you can achieve many of the same physiological benefits from using a $2 jump rope as you can from running on a $10,000 treadmill

ually in the least expensive models or by a motor in more expensive ones. Sears, Tunturi, Vitamaster, Voit, DP, Precor, and Proform are among the more common brands of treadmills manufactured for home use. Costs range from $300 to $2200. More expensive machines have a bigger motor, a wider belt, and a faster top speed up to about 5 mph. It is difficult to find a good motor-driven treadmill for under $500. Treadmills subjected to high usage in health clubs cost between $1000 and $12,000. Most of the more expensive motor-driven treadmills allow you to adjust both the speed of the belt and the incline angle to alter intensity.

Machine motors vary in both type and size. The type of motor can be either AC or DC. AC motors run at full speed all the time, relying on a transmission-like pulley system to regulate speed. This means most models start up at full speed and can be somewhat dangerous when getting on. Treadmill motors that are DC can be run at different speeds; thus start-up is not much of a problem. All models come with some type of speed control. Motor size varies from 1/2 horsepower to more than 1 horsepower. Bigger motors can handle heavier loads and higher speeds. The treadmill must be able to go at least 5 mph to run. It is important to make sure that the length of the belt is long enough to accommodate your stride length. Handrails increase the safety of the unit.

Stair Climbers

Stair climbers have become one of the more popular types of exercise machines (Figure 13-2). They are essentially a set of levers attached to some resistance device. Your legs pump the levers as if you were climbing stairs. Models that allow you to push the steps straight down are generally safer and reduce the chance of developing tendinitis in your heel. Models vary in how they apply resistance, using a flywheel, hydraulic piston, drive train, or wind resistance. In some models the stairs are linked. As one goes down, the other automatically goes up. Dual-action models allow you to work both the arms and the legs simultaneously. The more expensive models have a series of stairs that rotate as if you were climbing the wrong direction on an escalator. Monitors on many models display information such as time, steps per minute, and energy expenditure. Some may be programmed to vary both the speed and amount of resistance during the course of a workout.

Sears, Tunturi, DP, and Precor are brand names of the typical home models. Stairmaster and Lifestep make most of the more expensive units for commercial use. Stair-climbing machines cost between $200 and $3000. Most of the home models are around $500. Programmable units cost a minimum of $800.

Rowing Machines

Rowing machines are designed to mimic the action of rowing a boat or sculling (Figure 13-3). Most brands have some type of movable handles, which are similar to oars, and a sliding seat. Exercise involves pressing against stationary footplates with the legs while sliding backward on the seat and simultaneously pulling on the handles to create a rowing motion. Rowing machines are similar to stair climbers in terms of their resistance mechanisms, which may include a flywheel, hydraulic piston, or wind resistance.

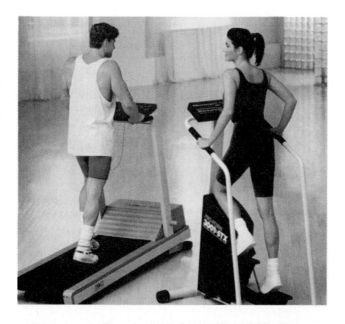

FIGURE 13-2. **Treadmill** *(left) and* **Stair Climber** *(right).*

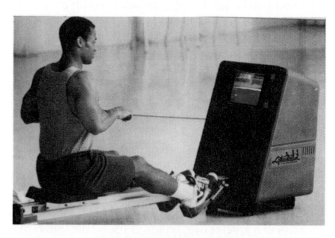

FIGURE 13-3. **Rowing Machine.**

Sears, DP, and Tunturi are the most common home models of rowing machines. Costs range between $200 and $800 for home models. Rowing machines for health clubs range between $1000 and $3000.

Ski Machines

A ski machine offers many of the aerobic benefits of cross-country skiing without having to worry about the snow (Figure 13-4). These machines have two flat boards, one for each foot, that slide back and forth in a groove on rollers. The arms are also involved, using either telescoping poles or a rope and pulley instead of the ski poles. The design of these machines allows you to simultaneously exercise both the upper and lower extremity.

Ski machines have either dependent or independent leg motion. With a dependent machine the leg boards are connected. As one goes forward, the other goes backward. On independent machines the leg boards slide independently, making them somewhat more difficult to master but also affording you a better workout. Resistance on the ski machine comes from either an electromagnetic flywheel or from a belt wrapped around a flywheel that provides friction. Some models do not have variable resistance. More expensive models may also incline, increasing the stress on the quadriceps muscles in the front of the thigh. Most machines have some type of monitor that can show heart rate, resistance, speed, calories expended, etc. Most of these machines can be folded and require little space for storage.

There are several manufacturers of ski machines, including NordicTrack, Precor, Proform, DP, Vitamaster, and Tunturi. Ski machines range in price from $300 to as high as $2000 for health club models.

How to Decide

None of the machines previously described will meet all of your fitness needs. As discussed earlier in the text, it is important to vary your workout to keep your fitness program new and exciting. You can use Table 13-1 as a reference to help you pick the aerobic exercise machine that will best meet your needs at the gym or in deciding what to purchase to supplement your home program.

Passive Exercise Devices and Techniques

Unfortunately, many consumers of health and fitness products are lured into thinking that there is some easy way to achieve physical fitness with little or no physical effort. The marketing of a variety of devices such as rubberized suits that let you sit around and sweat off weight; electrical devices that make muscles contract; and mechanical devices that shake, vibrate, or roll fat off can be very appealing as shortcuts to getting fit. There are, however, no shortcuts.

Passive Motion Machines

These machines have only been introduced into the health and fitness market in recent years. Passive motion machines are designed to exercise individual body parts by moving them for you with no effort on your part. You are simply required to lie or sit still while the machine does all the work. For example, one machine is designed to flex and extend your trunk and low back, while another may flex and extend your hip and your knee. Manufacturers claim that these machines will help improve muscular endurance since a particular body part is moving repeatedly, improve flexibility by using slow continuous movement, and burn off fat while reducing cellulite in the exercised areas. All of these claims are totally ludicrous. The only potential benefit offered to healthy individuals by these machines is relaxation. However, similiar passive exercise devices referred to as *constant passive motion (CPM)* machines are widely and effectively used in rehabilitation for postsurgical patients to minimize development of scar tissue.

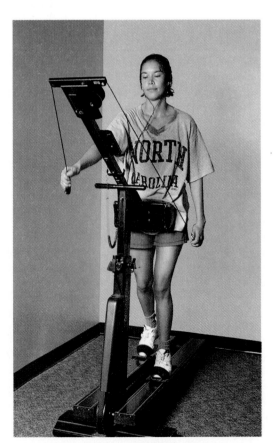

FIGURE 13-4. Ski Machine.

TABLE 13-1. Comparing Aerobic-Exercise Machines

Machine	What it does	What to look for	Comments
Exercise bicycle	Most models work only the lower body, but some have pumping handlebars for arms and shoulders. Some can be programmed for various workouts, such as climbing hills.	Smooth pedaling motion. Comfortable seat. Handlebars that adjust to your height. Pedal straps to keep your feet from slipping and to make your legs work on the upstroke too. Easy-to-adjust work load. Solid construction. Some models let you pedal backward, which enhances working your hamstring muscles.	Puts less strain on joints than running. Adjust the seat so that your knee is only slightly bent when the leg is extended. To prevent knee problems, don't set the resistance too high: you should be able to pedal at least 60 rpm. Recumbent models let you sit back in a chairlike seat; this puts less strain on back, neck, and shoulders.
Bicycle trainer	This stand allows you to convert your regular bike for indoor use. Rear wheel typically rests on a roller.	One that is easy to mount your bike on; some don't require removal of front wheel. Wind-resistance designs simulate outdoor conditions.	Since this uses your regular outdoor bike, it is likely to be comfortable. The stand is less expensive than stationary bikes.
Treadmill	Some machines have adjustable inclines to simulate hills and make workouts more strenuous. Some can be programmed for various preset workouts.	Easily adjustable speed and incline. Running surface that is wide and long enough for your stride and that absorbs shock well. A strong motor, which can handle high speeds, and a heavy load.	Many models have side or front hand rails: some people like them for balance. To prevent a mishap, straddle the machine before starting it; slow it down gradually before you get off.
Stair climber	Some larger models simulate real stair climbing. But most home models have pedals that work against your weight as you pump your legs; this puts less strain on your knees since you don't take real steps.	Smooth stepping action, large comfortable pedals and no wobble. Easily adjustable resistance. Comfortable handlebars or rails for balance. Some people prefer pedals that remain parallel to the floor, others like pivoting pedals. Models with independent pedals provide a more natural stepping motion.	Beginners shouldn't overexert themselves, since blood pressure and heart rate may rise quickly. Start with short steps and a slow pace. Put your entire foot on the pedal, not just the ball. Try to keep your knees aligned over your toes. Leaning on the rails or front monitor will reduce your energy expenditure.
Rowing machine	Provides a fuller workout than running or cycling; tones muscles in upper body. Most have hydraulic pistons to provide variable resistance; many larger models use a flywheel. One new model actually has a flywheel in a water tank to mimic real rowing.	Piston-type models have hydraulic arms and are cheaper and more compact than flywheel models, which have smoother action that's usually more like real rowing. Check that seat and oars move smoothly to reduce friction. Foot rests should pivot.	Proper rowing technique and cadence put little strain on body. If you have a back problem, consult your physician first. Make sure your legs, not your back, power your rowing motion. In early part of stroke, your arms should move forward before you bend your knees. When using a flywheel model, pull the bar into your abdomen, not to your chin.
Cross-country ski machine	Works most muscle groups. Simulates outdoor sport: feet slide in tracks, hands pull on cords or poles, either independently or in synchronized movements.	A base long enough to accommodate your stride. Adjustable leg and arm resistance. Smooth action. Machines with cords rather than poles may provide an especially strenuous upper-body workout.	Provides perhaps the best all-around workout. It may take some practice to coordinate your movements. Puts little strain on body; shouldn't aggravate knee problems.

From White T, Editors of the University of California at Berkeley Wellness Letter: *The wellness guide to lifelong fitness,* New York, 1993, Random House.

Motor-Driven Exercise Bikes

Stationary exercise bikes or rowing machines that are motor driven may have some value in increasing circulation, particularly around joints. However, they are totally ineffective in elevating heart rate and thus stressing the cardiovascular system.

Vibrating Belts and Rolling Machines

Vibrating belts placed around the trunk or the extremities to shake fat and muscle tissue or rolling machines that use movable wooden rollers to compress fat and muscle tissue in a rolling fashion have been promoted to break up fat tissue, thus making it easier to burn off. They also claim to increase muscle tone and improve posture. The truth is that they do not "break up" fat, but they may damage connective tissue around joints and within a muscle. The rollers may also cause bruising of the skin and fat from repeated compression. Use of these machines should definitely be avoided by people with low back pain and by pregnant women.

Massage

Massage can be an extremely effective therapeutic technique. It is most typically used for stimulating circulation, for inducing relaxation, and for loosening up muscles. However, as in the case of rolling machines, it will not selectively rub fat away from a specific spot.

Rubberized Inflatable Suits

Rubberized inflatable suits are also called *sauna shorts* or *sauna sleeves*. Promoters claim that the pressure created by the garment will help to break down fat tissue by squeezing it and that the rubber garment will help you to "sweat off" fat. Once again these claims are ridiculous. Fat cannot be "squeezed off." Furthermore, sweating does not burn off a significant amount of fat.

Wearing rubberized suits may help you lose body weight fairly quickly, but the weight loss represents the water weight of perspiration rather than that of fat tissue. Elevation of body core temperature by wearing rubberized suits may predispose an individual to various forms of heat stress, which was discussed in Chapter 4.

Electrical Stimulating Devices

In general, electrical stimulating devices use low amperage electrical current of sufficient intensity to cause involuntary muscle contraction. The technique involves connecting the electrodes to specific areas of the body and generating a weak electrical current to contract the muscles. (Promoters claim that the muscle contraction requires energy, thus calories will be used from stored fat to supply energy.) Once again, there is no credibility to the value of this technique for weight loss or fitness.

Electrical stimulating currents are routinely used by qualified rehabilitation specialists for treating many different musculoskeletal and neurological problems. When appropriate treatment limits are selected, electrical currents can be effectively used for pain control and muscle reeducation after injury, as well as to decrease muscle spasm and to reduce muscle atrophy. The indiscriminate use of electric currents by untrained individuals is strongly discouraged and in many states is against the law.

Spas, Steam Baths, and Saunas

In the health and fitness industry, the use of spas (hot tubs), steam baths, and saunas is widespread. Most health and fitness clubs offer the use of at least one form of these to their members. Hot tubs and whirlpool baths are increasingly being installed in private homes. Of all their therapeutic benefits, perhaps none is more important than the relaxation factor. Relaxation seems to be the primary reason why so many people are interested in using them. However, claims that sitting in either water or air at high temperatures will cause fat loss are again totally unfounded. Whatever weight is lost is due to a loss of water. Water loss should be immediately replaced through proper rehydration from beverages.

Saunas are likely to produce the greatest amount of body water loss, because the air is hot and extremely dry. Thus significant amounts of water will be lost through the rapid evaporation of sweat. Temperatures in a sauna should not be higher than 180° F. You should limit yourself to no more than 15 minutes in the sauna at that temperature.

Steam baths have a much lower temperature than saunas and should be no higher than 120° F. However, the humidity in a steam bath is 100%; thus individuals will appear to be sweating more heavily. Under humid conditions, sweat cannot evaporate to dissipate body heat, and body temperature rises rapidly. It is necessary to limit time in a steam bath to no longer than 10 minutes.

Spas or hot tubs involve full body immersion in a whirlpool at a temperature that should be no higher than 100° F for no longer than 10 minutes.

Certain precautions should be taken when using any of these units; if you have a heart condition, skin infection, or are pregnant you should avoid their use. Furthermore, do not use any of these without cooling down after exercise; wash off all oils or lotions before use; never drink alcohol before use; if you feel faint for any reason, get out immediately; and always have someone with you when using any of these.

Tanning Beds

For years, having a deep golden brown tan was associated with being fit and healthy. During the past decade, artificial tanning beds have become very popular in the health and fitness club industry. These tanning salons, beds, and booths usually consist of an array of long tubes that produce ultraviolet light. The lights are positioned in some type of frame that allows for exposure of the entire body.

We now know beyond any doubt that prolonged or continuous exposure to ultraviolet light rays predisposes an individual to the development of skin cancer. Manufacturers of artificial tanning devices claim the ultraviolet light produced by tanning devices is safe. The Food and Drug Administration (FDA) has warned the public that sunlamps are dangerous. Besides the risk of skin cancer, long-term exposure to a form of ultraviolet light (UVA) causes premature aging of the skin with wrinkling and sagging. Production of UVA tanning beds is largely unregulated. Furthermore, there is generally no standard of training for people who operate these machines. Their knowledge of the tanning process and the danger of exposure to ultraviolet radiation may be limited at best. Therefore extreme caution should be exercised whenever you are exposed to ultraviolet radiation either from sunlight or artificial sources.

SELECTING APPROPRIATE CLOTHING AND SHOES FOR EXERCISE

Nothing is more frustrating than attempting to complete a task without the right equipment. At times even the most dedicated fitness fanatics will cancel a workout if they don't have the right equipment to safely and efficiently complete their program. Having the right exercise clothing (shirt, shoes, shorts, socks, sweats, or suit) designed for the activity you choose to participate in will make it easier for you to adhere to your exercise program. Once you get properly outfitted, plan ahead. Keeping an extra set of clothes in your locker or the trunk of your car will prevent you from using this as an excuse for not working out.

Clothing for Exercising in Hot, Humid Weather

Guidelines for selecting clothing for exercising in hot, humid weather are relatively simple and straightforward. Clothing chosen should allow for maximal dissipation of body heat while minimizing the heat gained from the environment. By far the most effective means of heat loss involves the process of evaporation. If sweat remains on the skin, it will not produce heat

loss. Thus the material worn must be lightweight and must dry very quickly by permitting sweat to evaporate. The body area that has the greatest number of sweat glands is the upper back and shoulders. Consequently a tank top will allow for greatest exposure for evaporation. Radiation of heat from the sun or other hot surfaces such as pavement will cause the body to gain heat. Clothing should be a light color to reflect as much radiant heat energy as possible.

It is also advisable to wear a hat, which will help block some of the radiant heat energy from the sun. It is critical that the hat be made of some type of mesh fabric to allow heat to dissipate from the head. As indicated in Chapter 4, about 40% of the heat lost from the body is from the head.

Clothing for Exercising in Cold Weather

In situations where the weather is cold the goal of wearing clothing is to create a "semitropical microclimate" for the body and prevent chilling. The clothing should not restrict movement and should be as lightweight as possible. Also, the material should permit free passage of sweat and body heat. Otherwise sweat would accumulate on the skin or in the clothing and provide a chilling effect when activity ceases. This dampness, in combination with cold and wind, plays a critical role in the development of hypothermia. Individuals should routinely dress in thin layers of clothing that can be easily added or removed when the temperature increases or decreases. Constant adjustment of these layers will reduce sweating and the likelihood that clothing will become damp or wet.

Before exercise, during activity breaks, and after exercise, a warm-up suit or sweat clothes should be worn to prevent chilling. Activity in cold, wet, or windy weather poses some problem because such weather reduces the insulating value of the clothing. Consequently, the individual may be unable to achieve a level of metabolic heat production sufficient to keep pace with body heat loss. In cold weather, a hat should be worn to minimize excessive heat loss from the head.

Shoe Selection

The athletic and fitness shoe manufacturing industry has become extremely sophisticated and offers a number of options when it comes to purchasing shoes for different activities. Terms like *forefoot varus support* or *rear foot valgus wedge* are confusing to a person who simply wants to buy a pair of good running, aerobic, or court shoes. Most people are simply interested in finding a long-lasting shoe that will provide good

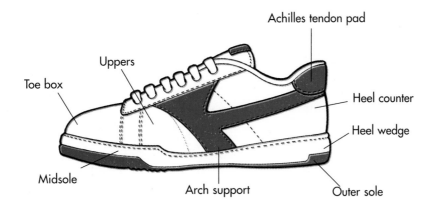

FIGURE 13-5. Parts of a Well-Designed Shoe.
(Modifed from Payne WA, Hahn DB: *Understanding your health,* ed 4, St Louis, 1995, Mosby.)

support and comfort. Figure 13-5 shows the major parts of a shoe. For the average individual, the following guidelines can help you select the most appropriate shoe to fit your needs.

• *Toe box.* There should be plenty of room for your toes in the fitness shoe. Most experts recommend a $1/2$- to $3/4$-inch distance between the longest toe and the front of the shoe. A few fitness shoes are made in varying widths. If you have a very wide or narrow foot, most shoe salespersons can recommend a specific shoe for your foot. The best way to make sure there is adequate room in the toe box is to have your foot measured and then try on the shoe.

• *Sole.* The sole should possess two qualities. First, it must provide a shock absorptive function; second, it must be durable. Most shoes have three layers on the sole: a thick spongy layer, which absorbs the force of the foot strike under the heel; a midsole, which cushions the midfoot and toes; and a hard rubber layer, which comes in contact with the ground. The average runner's feet strike the ground between 1500 and 1700 times per mile. Thus it is essential that the force of the heel strike be absorbed by the spongy layer to prevent overuse-type injuries from occurring in the ankles and knees. "Heel wedges" are sometimes inserted either on the inside or outside surface of the sole underneath the heel counter to accommodate and correct for various structural deformities of the foot that may alter normal biomechanics of the running gait. A flared heel may be appropriate for running shoes but is not recommended in aerobic or court shoes. The sole must provide good traction and must be made of a tough material that is resistant to wear. Most of the better-known brands of shoes tend to have well-designed, long-lasting soles.

• *Heel counters.* The heel counter is the portion of the shoe that prevents the foot from rolling from side to side at heel strike. The heel counter should be firm but well fitted to minimize movement of the heel up and down or side to side. A good heel counter may prevent ankle sprains and painful blisters.

• *Shoe uppers.* The upper part of the shoe is made of some combination of nylon and leather. The uppers should be lightweight, capable of quick drying, and well ventilated. The uppers should have some type of extra support in the saddle area, and there should be some extra padding in the area of the Achilles tendon just above the heel counter.

• *Arch support.* The arch support should be made of some durable yet soft supportive material and should smoothly join with the insole. The support should not have any rough seams or ridges inside the shoe, which may cause blisters.

• *Price.* Unfortunately, for many people price is the primary consideration in buying running shoes. Both running shoes and court shoes range between $40 and $160 per pair. Aerobic shoes tend to be less expensive, in the $30 to $80 range. When buying fitness shoes, remember that in many fitness activities, shoes are important for performance and prevention of injury. Thus it is worth a little extra investment to buy a quality pair of shoes. Figures 13-6 and 13-7 provide additional information to help you choose the best athletic shoe for your needs.

> **exercise clothing** the right exercise clothing (shirt, shoes, shorts, socks, sweats, or suit) designed for the activity you choose to participate in will make it easier for you to adhere to your exercise program

---

FIGURE 13-6. **Choosing an Appropriate Athletic or Fitness Shoe.**

Tennis
Flexibility: more rigid than running type, firm sole
Uppers: leather or leather with nylon
Heel flare: none
Cushioning: less than running types
Soles: polyurethane
Tread: flattened

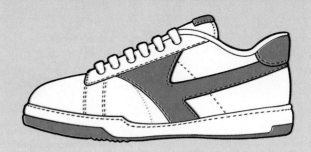

Aerobic

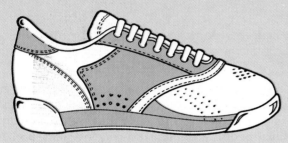

Flexibility: rates in between running and tennis types
Uppers: leather or leather with nylon
Heel flare: very little
Cushioning: rates in between running and tennis types
Soles: rubber or polyurethane
Tread: needs to be flat, may have pivot dot

Running
Flexibility: ball of foot is flexible
Uppers: nylon or nylon mesh
Heel flare: flared for greater stability
Cushioning: heel and sole well-padded
Sole: made of carbon-based material for greater durability
Tread: grip is enhanced by deep grooves

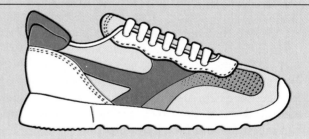

Illustrations modified from Payne WA, Hahn DB: *Understanding your health,* ed 4, St Louis, 1995, Mosby.

Using a Shoe Orthotic

An orthotic is a device that some people use for correcting biomechanical problems that exist in the foot that can potentially cause an injury. The orthotic is a plastic, rubber, or leather support that is placed in the shoe as a replacement for the existing insert. Ready-made orthotics can be purchased in sporting goods or shoe stores. Some people need to have orthotics that are custom made by a physician, podiatrist, or physical therapist. These will be more expensive but can be well worth the expense if your feet cause you pain and discomfort especially when you are exercising.

JOINING A HEALTH CLUB

It is easy to get caught up in a desire to join a health club. You walk in the front door and may immediately be greeted by an attractive, energetic receptionist who quickly introduces you to an attractive, energetic "fitness consultant," which is the term frequently used in fitness centers to label the salesperson. You may be escorted into a large exercise room with plush carpeting on the floor, mirrors on every wall, chrome-plated exercise equipment, and high-energy music coming from the stereo system. Your eyes tend to ignore the overweight gentleman or the frail lady working on machines in the corner and go straight to the Adonis or Aphrodite working out in the center of the room. It is easy to think, "Hey, this place is beautiful, and if it can make me feel comfortable and look like that at the same time, I want to join—NOW." Unfortunately, in this situation the consumer has already decided to purchase the hype without investigating the facts.

Certainly it is possible to find health clubs that offer good quality instruction and guidance in addition to an aesthetically pleasing environment in which to work out. The following guidelines are important for

FIGURE 13-7. **Tips For Purchasing Fitness Shoes.**

The following suggestions can help you when selecting the most appropriate athletic shoes to meet your fitness needs.

Tennis
- Choose a shoe that provides adequate cushioning in the heel counter.
- Select one with good side support and snug fit in the back of the heel.
- Make certain that the toe box fits comfortably.
- Select a shoe with less tread.

Aerobic
- Select a shoe width that is as wide as the widest part of the foot.
- Choose leather or nylon uppers (canvas does not provide enough support).
- Purchase a shoe that has a flattened tread in the front part of the foot and a rubber sole.

Running
- Examine the shape of your feet, including the depth of the arches. Proper shoe fit is critical to comfort and safety; check with other runners for suggestions and shop carefully.
- Determine how your running style affects the wear pattern by analyzing the soles of your old running shoes. (Some runners wear out the soles along the inner and outer edges of the foot; they need a shoe with better support features. Others tend to wear out the tread along the outer foot; they need a shoe that provides more padding than support.)

those individuals who are considering joining a health or fitness club.

Types of Facilities

Familiarize yourself with the many different types of facilities available, that is, spas, gyms, YMCAs, and facilities at universities or high schools. Many times local schools or colleges will offer excellent facilities for public use at little or no cost. You can most often find a listing of facilities in the telephone book. It is important to contact all the available sources to get the most detailed information.

Location of Facility

Certainly the location of the facility is an important factor in deciding whether to join. Be sure to consider the following:
- Is it close or easily accessible to your house or apartment?

- Will you be stopping to exercise on your way to or from work or school?
- What is the traffic like near the facility at the times of day you are most likely to go?

Equipment Available

Check the type of equipment available. Ask yourself the following questions:
- Do they have weight equipment (free weights, exercise machines)?
- Is there a pool, whirlpool, sauna, steam room, running track, racquetball court, and aerobic exercise room?
- Is there sufficient available locker space, with showers and changing areas?
- Do they have the type of equipment necessary for your fitness program?

Programs Offered

Check the type and quality of programs offered, such as individualized and supervised weight training, aerobic exercise classes, jogging classes, yoga, weight-control programs, and cardiac rehabilitation programs.

Hours of Operation

It is important that the place where you plan on working out fits into your personal schedule. Be sure to verify:
- What are the hours of operation of the facility?
- Are they open 7 days per week?
- Is it a coed facility?
- Can both males and females work out there 7 days a week?
- What are the most crowded times?

Qualifications of Personnel

You must be careful to consider the qualifications of the instructors. Many health and fitness clubs employ attractive, fit individuals whose primary function is to sell memberships to the club. Ask the salesperson the following questions:
- What is the background of the personnel who will be supervising your program?
- Do they have a background in physical education, exercise physiology, athletic training, or physical therapy?
- Are they certified by the American College of Sports Medicine as fitness instructors?
- Do they have aerobics instructor's certification from the American College of Sports Medicine, the International Dance Exercise Association, or the Aerobics and Fitness Association of America?
- Do they have a background in applied physiology of exercise?

Membership Contracts

Health and fitness clubs tend to offer a wide range of membership contract options ranging from pay-by-the-visit to lifetime memberships. It is a good idea to avoid long-term contracts, especially in the beginning. Health clubs sell a lot of memberships because people tend to get caught up by the aesthetics of the facility and are manipulated by some very good salespeople. The firm commitment to consistently use the facility three to four times per week that is made in the sales office tends to become less important for most people over time. If all the people who bought memberships in a club were to show up at one time, it is likely that you would not be able to get in the door. If you do decide to join, check on various payment options that best suit your budget. Also check on additional fees that you may have to pay for extras such as reserving racquetball courts or enrolling in aerobics classes.

Trial Periods

Before signing a contract, it is a good idea to spend several sessions working out at the club, talking with the instructors and with other club members. Current members can answer specific questions about the quality of the facility and can identify its deficiencies. If there is some objection to doing this on the part of the management, then you should exercise extreme caution about signing a contract.

Be Knowledgeable About Fitness

It is probably wise to avoid the clubs or organizations that advertise programs, classes, equipment, or techniques that claim to result in "overnight" strength gains, weight loss, or improvements in appearance. You must realize that reaching your fitness goals requires selecting an activity you enjoy. The activity should not overload the body but progress within your individual limitations. Furthermore, by being consistent in your training program, you will accomplish your goals safely by paying attention to the basic principles outlined within this text.

READING FITNESS MAGAZINES AND BOOKS

As with the various types of exercise equipment, consumer demand for fitness books and magazines dealing with health and fitness issues makes publication in this area an extremely lucrative enterprise. It is difficult, if not totally impossible, to pick up a popular magazine that does not contain at least one article about health and fitness. It is reasonable to assume that the majority of people in the United States obtain most of their health and fitness information while standing in line at the grocery store. This is certainly not to say that grocery store sources of health and fitness information are unreliable, but there is a tremendous amount of misinformation relative to health and fitness issues routinely spread through the popular media. Often the articles in magazines are written by individuals with little or no health or fitness expertise who may interview fitness experts. Occasionally you will find experts writing the articles. The same is true for so-called experts who appear on TV or radio talk shows. These people have charming personalities but often lack reliable credentials.

A trip to the local bookstore or public library to locate books dealing with health, wellness, fitness, exercise, sports, diet, and nutrition can be overwhelming. Many excellent, accurate books are available. These books are written by health and fitness experts. Unfortunately, many of the best-selling and certainly the best-marketed books are written by celebrities who look fit and attractive. Some of these books contain excellent information. Others include some facts along with misinformation and border on being dangerous.

How do you know whether information presented in the popular literature is reliable? Simply by being an informed consumer. The information presented in this text is accurate and up-to-date. College textbooks are reviewed several times by people who are recognized as experts in the field of health and fitness. The knowledge you have obtained from this text and your fitness coursework should make you a more informed consumer.

BOTTOM LINE FOR THE CONSUMER

Regardless of the type of exercise equipment, the aesthetics of a health club, or the claims of nutritional products, the bottom line is that the responsibility for getting fit and healthy ultimately lies with you. The following box is designed to help clarify a number of situations that you, as the consumer, will be faced with when deciding to purchase fitness products or services. Remember, a commitment to a fitness program is first and foremost a commitment to yourself. Being cautious, asking a number of questions, and being well informed will help you make the best choice possible.

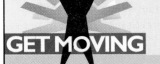

The benefits of choosing the right exercise equipment

1. Some people find that buying a piece of exercise equipment and paying their hard-earned money helps keep them motivated to use it.
2. Some people prefer exercising in the privacy of their own home; having home exercise equipment may allow you to read, watch TV, or listen to music that you enjoy while working out.
3. A health club is a very social place. There are all types of people who join health clubs, and going there on a regular basis is a great way to get to know other people who share similar interests.

4. Reward youself for staying faithful to your exercise program by buying yourself a nice-looking outfit to exercise in.
5. Most health clubs have spas, saunas, and steam rooms, and some still have rollers and vibrating machines. If you want to use these for relaxation or because they feel good, by all means—do so. But remember that they will not help you lose body fat.
6. Even though forking out big bucks to buy the most appropriate pair of shoes for your exercise progam hurts the pocketbook, it may help to reduce the chance of injury.

How, where, or what you choose to do or use to get yourself fit and healthy is of little consequence as long as you pay attention to the basic principles that have been detailed in earlier chapters in this text. Basing your fitness program on the facts rather than on marketing techniques is the way to get fit. If you find that joining a health club or buying expensive exercise equipment in some way motivates you to adhere to your program, then by all means, do so. But never neglect the basic principles.

fitness books and magazines we are bombarded with fitness, health, and nutrition information from radio, TV, newspapers, and even while in line at the grocery store; be sure to check the credibility of any source before acting on advice

SUMMARY

- Practicing consumerism means that wise consumers will take the time to analyze the entire product and to decide if the outlay of money is necessary to reap the benefits they desire.
- There is an incredible amount and diversity of exercise equipment available to the consumer. Deciding on what type of equipment is best for you to use or purchase should be based primarily on individual interests and the goals of your physical activity program.
- It is not necessary to spend a lot of money to buy expensive exercise equipment. If you understand the principles of exercise, you can achieve excellent results using a little or no equipment.
- Various types of exercise equipment can be used with progressive resistive exercise, including free weights (barbells and dumbbells) and exercise machines.
- Stationary bicycles, treadmills, rowing machines, stair climbers, and ski machines are all useful machines for exercising. Cost is an important consideration in purchasing these pieces of equipment and can range from several hundred to several thousand dollars.
- Passive motion machines are designed to exercise individual body parts by moving them for you with no effort on your part. Manufacturer's claims relative to any physical benefit other than relaxation have little or no merit.
- Spas, saunas, and steam baths should be used for relaxation and are not effective in reducing percentage body fat.
- The use of tanning beds and tanning booths generally is not recommended.
- Selecting appropriate clothing for exercising in hot or cold weather is important and can help to prevent heat-related illnesses or hypothermia.
- Buying shoes for exercising can be confusing and expensive, yet it is essential that you select the most appropriate shoe for the activity in which you will participate. Choosing the appropriate shoe can help to minimize injury.
- You must "do your homework" when choosing a health club, making sure to ask all the right questions and finding out about the qualifications of health club personnel. Don't be afraid to ask questions and fully investigate a health and fitness club before joining.
- Fitness books and magazine articles should be critically analyzed by the informed and educated consumer of health and fitness products.
- Regardless of the type of exercise equipment, the aesthetics of a health club, or the claims of nutritional products, the bottom line is that the responsibility for getting fit and healthy ultimately lies with you.

REFERENCES

Bryant C, Peterson J: Warm soothing safety: making saunas, steam rooms and hot tubs safe, *Fitness Manag* 8(10): 26-29, 1992.

Cardinal B: Six steps to selecting exercise equipment, *Athl Bus* 18(9):39-47, 1994.

Cohen A: Fitness equipment: the next generation, *Athl Bus* 19(3):26-36, 1995.

Consumer Reports: *Consumer Reports 1996 buying guide,* New York, 1996, Consumer Reports.

Cornacchia H, Barrett S: *Consumer health,* St Louis, 1993, Mosby.

DeBenedette V: Health club tanning booths: risky business, *Phys Sports Med* 15:59, 1987.

Duda M: The medical risks and benefits of sauna, steam bath and whirlpool use, *Phys Sports Med,* 15:170, 1987.

Franklin M, Smith L, Inscoe L: The metabolic costs of continuous passive motion exercise, *Med Exerc Nutr Health* 3(4):180-184, 1994.

Gautier MM: Continuous passive motion: the no exercise exercise, *Phys Sports Med* 15:142, 1987.

Hata O, Umezawa N: Use of fitness facilities, equipment, and programs, *J Sports Manag* 9(1):78-84, 1995.

Healthy Hearts: No fitness center is complete without the latest in cardiovascular exercise equipment, *Athl Bus* 19(3):69-87, 1995.

Howley E, Colacino D, Swenson T: Factors affecting the oxygen cost of stepping on an electronic stepping ergometer, *Med Sci Sports Exerc* 24:1055-1058, 1992.

Huegli R, Mannie K, Peterson D: The importance of exercise machines in strength training: round table, *Natl Strength Cond Assoc* 15(5):18-19, 1993.

Kardong D: Oldies but goodies: these time-tested workout machines have become indoor classics, *Runner's World* 29(12):68-73, 1994.

Khazei D: Treadsetters: treadmills are almost as easy to buy as they are to use, *Men's Fitness* 10(7):50, 1994.

McKeon M: Equipment purchasing: how to get the best deal, *Ultrafit* 49:52-53, 1993.

New shades of risk at tanning salons, *Consumer Reports,* p 73, Feb 1986.

Nicholas J: Equipment review: Stair Master, *Ultrafit* 17:56-57, 1994.

Payne WA, Hahn DB: Understanding your health, ed 4, St Louis, 1995, Mosby.

Peterson C, Bryant J: *The Stair Master fitness handbook,* Indianapolis, 1992, Masters Press.

Prentice W: *Therapeutic modalities in sports medicine,* St Louis, 1994, Mosby.

Research reveals Nordic Track most closely simulates the motions of cross country skiing, *J Orthop Sports Phys Ther* 15(4):195, 1992.

Runner's World 1995 shoe buying guide 30(4):49-73, 1995.

Shafran J: Homework: heart-pumping hardware, fitness equipment to give you an aerobic edge, *Women's Sport Fitness* 17(1):57-60, 1995.

Shea S, Brunick T: Tenth annual shoe review, *Walking Mag* 10(2):61-76, 1995.

Stamford B: Saunas, steam rooms, and hot tubs, *Phys Sports Med* 17:188, 1989.

US Department of Health and Human Services, Public Health Services: *Healthy people 2000: national health promotion and disease prevention objectives*, Washington, DC, 1991, USDHHS.

Webb D, Stevenson M: Life expectancy costing of exercise equipment, *J Natl Intramural Rec Sports Assoc* 18(2):28-30, 1994.

White T, Editors of the University of California at Berkeley Wellness Letter: *The wellness guide to lifelong fitness*, New York, 1993, Random House.

Young L: Health and fitness equipment: the best buys, *Fitlink* 2:67, 1993.

Zawatsky P: Stair machines: climbing to peak fitness, *Hughston Health Alert* 7(2):1-4, 1995.

SUGGESTED READINGS

Hirsch J: *The spa book,* New York, 1988, Perigee Books.
A guide to selecting and choosing health spas.

Kane WN: *Test your health and fitness IQ,* New York, 1987, Berkley Books.
Contains a number of health, nutrition, and fitness assessments.

Levy M, Shafran J: *Gym psych: the insider's guide to health clubs,* New York, 1986, Fawcett Columbine.
A consumer guide that offers guidance in choosing a health and fitness club.

COLLEGE FITNESS RESOURCES

This appendix is intended to make you aware of college and university physical fitness and health programs that are available to most college students. The lack of students' knowledge or use of services that are provided by many colleges and universities may result in low levels of fitness among the student population. College resources to enhance and protect the health and fitness of students commonly include a health center that not only provides immediate care to sick students but also offers health-related educational programs that provide seminars and training sessions relating to such things as smoking cessation, cardiorespiratory function, medical self-help, and childbirth. Physical education programs offer a broad range of activities for all students. Most colleges and universities also sponser intercollegiate and intramural athletic programs. Some larger institutions offer sports medicine and health education clinics.

For the most part these programs are cost effective for the student who has already paid tuition and fees to attend academic classes. They also have the advantage of convenience, since they are generally located on campus.

Physical Education Programs

The physical education program in most colleges and universities provides a basic instructional class or service program, an adapted physical education program, and an intramural and extramural athletic program. In some cases the intercollegiate athletic program is also a part of the total physical education program.

Physical Education Instructional Service Program

The instructional service program in physical education provides the skills, strategies, understandings, and essential knowledge concerning the relation of physical activity to physical, mental, emotional, and social development. Participants are also provided with some ways to develop and maintain an optimal state of physical fitness. The instructional service program is available to all students, meets the needs of each person, stresses lifetime skills, is concerned with

health-related physical fitness, and is conducted by qualified faculty members. Courses such as wellness, jogging, weight-loss conditioning, cardiorespiratory conditioning, dance aerobics, and weight training are offered at most colleges. An important part of the instructional program is the teaching of skill-related activities. Instruction in activities such as tennis, dancing, swimming, badminton, archery, fencing, folk and square dance, modern dance, sailing, social dance, gymnastics, volleyball, golf, racquetball, aquatics, bowling, table tennis, skating, horseback riding, mountaineering, orienteering, snow skiing, judo, hiking, and camping is offered. Several colleges have introduced "foundations" courses that provide more background information about the activity in addition to the activity's skills. The trend is toward an emphasis on recreation and fitness activities and on coeducational classes.

Physical achievement tests are often used in college physical education programs to assess student needs and to better ensure progress. Special help and prescribed programs are provided for physically underdeveloped students. Many 2-year colleges require students to take physical education courses both years. Most programs require 2 hours of activity each week and stress the importance of the successful completion of the physical education program as a requirement for graduation.

Adapted Physical Education Programs

An adapted physical education program refers to that phase of physical education that meets the needs of a person who is temporarily or permanently unable to take part in the regular physical education program. This inability may be due to a physical inadequacy that might be improved through physical activity. In many cases, special provisions are made in regular physical education classes that enable handicapped students to participate in the activities. It also provides service to students who fail to meet the "average" or "normal" physical abilities for their age group. These students deviate from their peers in physical, mental, emotional, or social characteristics or in a combination of these traits.

All colleges have students who, because of heredity, environment, disease, or accident, have physical, mental, or emotional impairments. The responsibility of physical education programs is to help each person, even though a person may be handicapped. It is important for these individuals to enjoy the benefits of participating in physical education activities that have been adapted to meet their needs. The nationwide shortage of sound adapted physical education programs is a recognized problem. This is due to the lack of properly trained teachers, the financial cost of remedial instruction, and the tendency of physical educators to be unaware of their responsibility and potential contribution to this program. These obstacles are gradually being overcome as the public and educators become aware of the need to physically educate all persons in every phase of an education program.

Intramural and Club Activities

A program of various leisure-time activities for those students not competing in intercollegiate athletics is frequently provided for all enrolled students in a college or university. The program is usually financed by the central administration or student government. In many cases the students direct the programs. A wide variety of activities are commonly provided to accommodate varied student interests. Activities are also conducted on a men's, women's, or coeducational basis. The most common intramural activities are flag football, volleyball, basketball, water polo, darts, billiards, softball, bowling, swimming, hockey, racquetball, tennis, floor hockey, ultimate frisbee, canoeing, surfing, windsurfing, and soccer.

Recreational activities other than intramural sports may include clubs, common interest groups, and extramural sports. The extramural programs may include activities such as bowling, fencing, karate, chess, sailing, rugby, snow skiing, scuba diving, water skiing, and soccer. Club activities usually have a faculty advisor and should have qualified personnel to train and teach the activity.

Intercollegiate Athletics

The function of an intercollegiate athletic program is to provide student athletes with an environment in which they are able to pursue excellence in selected extracurricular, education-related athletic activities. The athletic department sponsors a number of activities for men such as baseball, basketball, cross-country running, football, golf, soccer, swimming and diving, tennis, wrestling, hockey, fencing, and track and field. Activities for women include basketball, gymnastics, field hockey, fencing, cross-country running, softball, tennis, swimming and diving, and volleyball. The objective of the intercollegiate athletic program is to pursue excellence of performance within the structure of the rules and within the budgetary framework imposed by the funding provided.

Student Health Center

The college and university student health center provides medical care on an outpatient and limited inpatient basis for students and their dependents. Admission to the college or university is usually contingent on receipt of a personal health history and a physical examination, and this information becomes part of the student's health record.

Student health centers are usually open 24 hours a day, and a medical professional is on duty at least during school hours. The staff may include physicians, physician assistants, and nurses. Supporting professionals and technical personnel such as x-ray technicians, pharmacists, social workers, dentists, or physical therapists may be on the clinic's staff. Facilities and clinics that were cited in a survey of representative student health centers are listed below:

Typical Student Health Service Clinics

Facility	Function
Outpatient clinic	Primarily emergency care
Inpatient	Minor surgery, sickness
Trauma	Students experiencing a disordered state resulting from mental or emotional stress or physical injury
General medical consultation	Students seeking medical advice concerning their health problems
Gynecology	Female students having problems involving sexual reproduction system
Dental	Prevention of dental problems and treatment in some cases
Pharmacy	Drugs provided on a limited basis
Emergency	Open for health problems that need immediate attention
X-ray	For problems such as bone fracture
Optometric clinic	Eye examinations for defects and prescriptions for corrective lenses
Sports medicine	Prevention, treatment, and rehabilitation of sport-clinic related injuries

Appendix B

Food Composition Table

This food composition table, developed by Positive Input Corp., lists foods in Mosby's NutriTrac software, which is available as a supplement to this text. You will find a number of additional foods in Mosby's NutriTrac that are not listed in this food composition table.

When using Mosby's NutriTrac software, the quickest way to find a food is to use the "Search For" feature. However, if you do not have access to a computer or your computer time is limited, you can easily find a food using this food composition table. The foods in the table are arranged alphabetically. Note, however, that in some cases foods are arranged alphabetically within groups, such as Beef, Bread, and Soup, rather than by name alone.

Food from restaurants, including fast food (quick service), is cataloged separately, starting on p. B-26. These foods are listed alphabetically by restaurant name. If the fast-food/quick-service restaurant you are looking for is not listed, use the generic "Fast Food" category within the "Restaurant" section.

The code number in the left-hand column corresponds to the food data bank in Mosby's NutriTrac software. When you enter your intake into the software program, you may choose to use code numbers. Alternatively, you may choose to enter your intake into Mosby's NutriTrac by typing a food's name or partial name and selecting the "Search For" option.

Modified from Wardlaw GM, Insel PM: *Perspectives in nutrition*, ed 3, St Louis, 1996, Mosby.

Code	Name	Amount	Unit	Grams	Kilocalories	Carbohydrates (g)	Protein (g)	Fat (g)
11001	ALFALFA SEEDS, SPROUTED, FRESH	½	CUP	16.5	5	1	1	0
12067	ALMONDS, TOASTED, UNBLANCHED	½	CUP	71.0	418	16	14	36
19294	APPLE BUTTER	1	TBSP.	18.0	33	9	0	0
9400	APPLE JUICE, UNSWEETENED	¾	CUP	185.8	87	22	0	0
9003	APPLES, FRESH, W/ SKIN	1	MEDIUM	138.0	81	21	0	0
9020	APPLESAUCE, SWEETENED	½	CUP	127.5	97	25	0	0
9019	APPLESAUCE, UNSWEETENED	½	CUP	122.0	52	14	0	0
9024	APRICOTS, CND, JUICE PACK	½	CUP	124.0	60	15	1	0
9022	APRICOTS, CND, WATER PACK	½	CUP	121.5	33	8	1	0
9032	APRICOTS, DRIED, SULFURED	¼	CUP	32.5	77	20	1	0
9021	APRICOTS, FRESH	3	MEDIUM	106.0	51	12	1	0
11015	ASPARAGUS, CND	½	CUP	121.0	23	3	3	1
11011	ASPARAGUS, FRESH	½	CUP	67.0	15	3	2	0
11019	ASPARAGUS, FRZ, CKD	½	CUP	100.0	28	5	3	0
9037	AVOCADOS, FRESH	1	MEDIUM	201.0	324	15	4	31
10124	BACON	1	SLICE	6.0	35	0	2	3
10131	BACON, CANADIAN-STYLE BACON, GRILLED	1	SLICE	21.0	39	0	5	2
62528	BACON, TURKEY	1	SLICE	14.0	25	0	3	2
18001	BAGELS, PLAIN	1	3½ IN.	71.0	195	38	7	1
19400	BANANA CHIPS	1	OUNCE	28.4	147	17	1	10
9040	BANANAS, FRESH	1	MEDIUM	114.0	105	27	1	1
6150	BARBECUE SAUCE	½	CUP	125.0	94	16	2	2
15187	BASS, FRESHWATER, CKD, DRY HEAT	3	OUNCE	85.1	124	0	21	4
16006	BEANS, BAKED, CND, VEGETARIAN	½	CUP	127.0	118	26	6	1
16007	BEANS, BAKED, CND, W/ BEEF	½	CUP	133.0	161	22	8	5
16008	BEANS, BAKED, CND, W/ FRANKS	½	CUP	128.5	182	20	9	8
16009	BEANS, BAKED, CND, W/ PORK	½	CUP	126.5	134	25	7	2
16315	BEANS, BLACK, CKD	½	CUP	86.0	114	20	8	0
11056	BEANS, GREEN, CND	½	CUP	68.0	14	3	1	0
11052	BEANS, GREEN, FRESH	½	CUP	55.0	17	4	1	0
11061	BEANS, GREEN, FZN	½	CUP	67.5	18	4	1	0
16029	BEANS, KIDNEY, CND	½	CUP	128.0	104	19	7	0
16073	BEANS, LIMA, CND	½	CUP	120.5	95	18	6	0
11040	BEANS, LIMA, FZN	½	CUP	90.0	95	18	6	0
16039	BEANS, NAVY, CND	½	CUP	131.0	148	27	10	1
16044	BEANS, PINTO, CND	½	CUP	120.0	94	17	5	0
16103	BEANS, REFRIED, CND	½	CUP	126.5	135	23	8	1
13347	BEEF, CORNED, BRISKET, CKD	3	OUNCE	85.1	213	0	15	16
13355	BEEF, CURED, PASTRAMI	3	OUNCE	85.1	297	3	15	25
13357	BEEF, CURED, SAUSAGE, SMOKED	3	OUNCE	85.1	265	2	12	23
13358	BEEF, CURED, SMOKED, CHOPPED BEEF	3	OUNCE	85.1	105	2	17	4
13360	BEEF, CURED, THIN-SLICED BEEF	3	OUNCE	85.1	151	5	24	3
13300	BEEF, GROUND, EXTRA LEAN, PAN-FRIED	3	OUNCE	85.1	217	0	21	14
13307	BEEF, GROUND, LEAN, PAN-FRIED	3	OUNCE	85.1	234	0	21	16
13312	BEEF, GROUND, REGULAR, BROILED	3	OUNCE	85.1	246	0	20	18
13314	BEEF, GROUND, REGULAR, PAN-FRIED	3	OUNCE	85.1	260	0	20	19
13327	BEEF, LIVER, CKD, PAN-FRIED	3	OUNCE	85.1	185	7	23	7
13004	BEEF, STEAKS AND ROASTS, CKD., ¼ IN. FAT	3	OUNCE	85.1	259	0	22	18
7043	BEEF, THIN SLICED	1	SLICE	4.2	7	0	1	0
11081	BEETS, CKD	½	CUP	85.0	37	8	1	0
18009	BISCUITS, PLAIN OR BUTTERMILK	1	EACH	35.0	127	17	2	6
9050	BLUEBERRIES, FRESH	½	CUP	72.5	41	10	0	0
9055	BLUEBERRIES, FROZEN, SWEETENED	½	CUP	115.0	93	25	0	0
10126	BOLOGNA	1	SLICE	23.0	57	0	4	5
12078	BRAZILNUTS, DRIED, UNBLANCHED	½	CUP	70.0	459	9	10	46
19167	BREAD PUDDING	1	CUP	252.0	423	62	13	15
18080	BREAD STICKS, PLAIN	1	STICK	10.0	41	7	1	1
18020	BREAD, BANANA	1	SLICE	60.0	203	33	3	7
18024	BREAD, CORNBREAD	1	PIECE	65.0	173	28	4	5
18025	BREAD, CRACKED-WHEAT	1	SLICE	25.0	65	12	2	1

Saturated fat (g)	Monounsaturated fat (g)	Polyunsaturated fat (g)	Fiber (g)	Cholesterol (g)	Folate (g)	Vitamin A (RE)	Vitamin B6 (mg)	Vitamin B12 (μg)	Vitamin C (mg)	Vitamin E (mg)	Riboflavin (mg)	Thiamin (mg)	Calcium (mg)	Iron (mg)	Magnesium (mg)	Niacin (mg)	Phosphorus (mg)	Potassium (mg)	Sodium (mg)	Zinc (mg)
0	0	0	0	0	6	3	0	0	1	-	0	0	5	.2	4	.1	12	13	1	.2
3	23	8	8	0	45	0	.1	0	0	-	.4	.1	201	3.5	216	2	390	549	8	3.5
-	-	-	0	0	0	0	0	0	0	-	0	0	1	0	1	0	1	16	0	0
0	0	0	-	0	0	0	.1	0	77	0	0	0	13	.7	6	-	13	221	6	.1
0	0	0	4	0	4	7	.1	0	8	.8	0	0	10	.2	7	.1	10	159	0	.1
0	0	0	2	0	1	1	0	0	2	-	0	0	5	.4	4	.2	9	78	4	.1
0	0	0	1	0	1	4	0	0	1	-	0	0	4	.1	4	.2	9	92	2	0
0	0	0	2	0	2	210	.1	0	6	-	0	0	15	.4	12	.4	25	205	5	.1
0	0	0	2	0	2	157	.1	0	4	-	0	0	10	.4	9	.5	16	233	4	.1
0	0	0	3	0	3	235	.1	0	1	-	0	0	15	1.5	15	1	38	448	3	.2
0	0	0	3	0	9	277	.1	0	11	-	0	0	15	.6	8	.6	20	314	1	.3
0	0	0	2	0	116	64	.1	0	22	-	.1	.1	19	2.2	12	1.2	52	208	472	.5
0	0	1	0	86	39	.1	0	9	-	26	.1	.1	14	.6	12	.8	38	183	.1	3
0	0	0	-	0	135	82	0	0	24	-	.1	.1	23	.6	13	1	55	218	4	.6
5	19	4	12	0	124	123	.6	0	16	-	.2	.2	22	2.1	78	3.9	82	1204	20	.8
1	1	0	0	5	0	0	0	.1	2	-	0	0	1	.1	1	.4	20	29	96	.2
1	1	0	0	12	1	0	.1	.2	5	-	0	.2	2	.2	4	1.5	62	82	325	.4
1	-	-	-	10	-	0	-	-	0	-	-	-	0	0	-	-	-	-	170	-
0	0	0	1	0	16	0	0	0	2	-	.2	.4	53	2.5	21	3.2	68	72	379	.6
8	1	0	2	0	4	2	.1	0	2	-	0	0	5	.4	22	.2	16	152	2	.2
0	0	0	3	0	22	9	.7	0	10	.3	.1	.1	7	.4	33	.6	23	451	1	.2
0	1	1	1	0	5	109	.1	0	9	-	0	0	24	1.1	22	1.1	25	217	1019	.2
1	2	1	0	74	14	30	.1	2	2	-	.1	.1	88	1.6	32	1.3	218	388	77	.7
0	0	0	6	0	30	22	.2	0	4	-	.1	.2	64	.4	41	.5	132	376	504	1.8
2	2	0	-	29	58	28	.1	0	4	-	.1	.1	60	2.1	33	1.3	108	426	632	1.6
3	4	1	9	8	39	19	.1	0	3	-	.1	.1	62	2.2	36	1.2	134	302	553	2.4
1	1	0	7	9	46	23	.1	0	3	-	0	.1	67	2.2	43	.6	137	391	524	1.8
0	0	0	-	0	128	1	.1	0	0	-	.1	.2	23	1.8	60	.4	120	305	204	1
0	0	0	1	0	22	24	0	0	3	-	0	0	18	.6	9	.1	13	74	171	.2
0	0	0	2	0	20	37	0	0	9	-	.1	0	20	.6	14	.4	21	115	3	.1
0	0	0	2	0	6	36	0	0	6	-	0	0	30	.6	14	.3	16	76	9	.4
0	0	0	-	0	63	0	.1	0	2	-	.1	.1	35	1.6	40	.6	134	329	444	.7
0	0	0	6	0	61	0	.1	0	0	-	0	.1	25	2.2	47	.3	89	265	405	.8
0	0	0	-	0	14	15	.1	0	5	-	0	.1	25	1.8	50	.7	101	370	26	.5
0	0	0	7	0	82	0	.1	0	1	-	.1	.2	62	2.4	62	.6	176	377	587	1
0	0	0	4	0	72	0	.1	0	1	-	.1	.1	44	1.9	32	.4	110	361	499	.8
1	1	0	7	0	106	0	.1	0	8	-	.1	.1	58	2.2	49	.6	106	497	536	1.7
5	8	1	0	83	5	0	.2	1.4	14	-	.1	0	7	1.6	10	2.6	106	123	964	3.9
9	12	1	0	79	6	0	.2	1.5	3	-	.1	.1	8	1.6	15	4.3	128	194	1044	3.6
10	11	1	0	57	3	0	.1	1.6	10	-	.1	0	6	1.5	11	2.7	89	150	962	2.4
2	2	0	0	39	7	0	.3	1.5	18	-	.1	.1	7	2.4	18	3.9	154	321	1070	3.3
1	1	0	0	35	9	0	.3	2.2	12	-	.2	.1	9	2.3	16	4.5	143	365	1224	3.4
5	6	1	0	69	8	0	.2	1.7	0	-	.2	.1	6	2	18	4	136	265	60	4.6
6	7	1	0	71	8	0	.2	1.9	0	-	.2	0	9	1.9	17	4.1	135	254	65	4.4
7	8	1	0	77	8	0	.2	2.5	0	-	.2	0	9	2.1	17	4.9	145	248	71	4.4
8	8	1	0	76	8	0	.2	2.3	0	-	.2	0	9	2.1	17	5	145	255	71	4.3
2	1	1	0	410	187	9125	1.2	95.1	20	-	3.5	.2	9	5.3	20	12.3	392	310	90	4.6
7	8	1	0	75	6	0	.3	2.1	0	-	.2	.1	9	2.2	19	3.1	173	266	53	5
0	0	0	0	2	0	0	0	.1	1	-	0	0	0	.1	1	.2	7	18	60	.2
0	0	0	1	0	68	3	.1	0	3	-	0	0	14	.7	20	.3	32	259	65	.3
1	2	2	-	0	2	0	0	0	0	-	.1	.1	17	1.2	6	1.2	151	78	368	.2
-	-	-	2	0	5	7	0	0	9	-	0	0	4	.1	4	.3	7	65	4	.1
0	0	0	2	0	8	5	.1	0	8	-	.1	0	7	.4	2	.3	8	69	1	.1
2	2	0	0	14	1	0	.1	.2	8	-	0	.1	3	.2	3	.9	32	65	272	.5
11	16	17	4	0	3	0	.2	0	0	-	.1	.7	123	2.4	158	1.1	420	420	1	3.2
6	5	2	-	166	33	164	.2	-	2	-	.6	.2	287	2.8	48	1.6	275	564	582	1.3
0	0	0	-	0	3	0	0	0	0	-	.1	.1	2	.4	3	.5	12	12	66	.1
2	3	2	-	26	7	14	.1	.1	1	-	.1	.1	11	.8	8	.9	34	79	119	.2
1	1	2	-	26	12	35	.1	.1	0	-	.2	.2	162	1.6	16	1.5	110	96	428	.4
0	0	0	1	0	10	0	.1	0	0	-	.1	.1	11	.7	13	.9	38	44	135	.3

Food Composition Table—cont'd

Code	Name	Amount	Unit	Grams	Kilocalories	Carbohydrates (g)	Protein (g)	Fat (g)
18342	BREAD, DINNER ROLL, PLAIN	1	EACH	35.0	105	18	3	3
18347	BREAD, DINNER ROLL, WHEAT	1	EACH	33.0	90	15	3	2
18029	BREAD, FRENCH OR VIENNA	1	SLICE	25.0	69	13	2	1
18033	BREAD, ITALIAN	1	SLICE	30.0	81	15	3	1
18035	BREAD, MIXED-GRAIN	1	SLICE	26.0	65	12	3	1
18037	BREAD, OAT BRAN	1	SLICE	30.0	71	12	3	1
18041	BREAD, PITA, WHITE, ENRICHED	1	PITA	60.0	165	33	5	1
18042	BREAD, PITA, WHOLE-WHEAT	1	PITA	64.0	170	35	6	2
18044	BREAD, PUMPERNICKEL	1	SLICE	32.0	80	15	3	1
18046	BREAD, PUMPKIN	1	SLICE	60.0	199	31	2	8
18047	BREAD, RAISIN	1	SLICE	26.0	71	14	2	1
18060	BREAD, RYE	1	SLICE	32.0	83	15	3	1
18064	BREAD, WHEAT (INCLUDES WHEAT BERRY)	1	SLICE	25.0	65	12	2	1
18069	BREAD, WHITE	1	SLICE	25.0	67	12	2	1
11091	BROCCOLI, CKD	½	CUP	78.0	22	4	2	0
11093	BROCCOLI, FRZ, CHOPPED, CKD	½	CUP	92.0	26	5	3	0
18151	BROWNIES	1	EACH	56.0	227	36	3	9
11099	BRUSSELS SPROUTS, CKD	½	CUP	78.0	30	7	2	0
62601	BUFFALO (CHICKEN) WINGS	4	EACH	91.0	190	2	18	12
18351	BUNS, HAMBURGER OR HOT DOG, MIXED-GRAIN	1	EACH	43.0	113	19	4	3
18350	BUNS, HAMBURGER OR HOT DOG, PLAIN	1	EACH	43.0	123	22	4	2
4136	BUTTER, W/ SALT	1	PAT	5.0	36	0	0	4
1145	BUTTER, W/O SALT	1	PAT	5.0	36	0	0	4
1002	BUTTER, WHIPPED	1	TBSP.	11.0	79	0	0	9
11110	CABBAGE, CKD	½	CUP	75.0	17	3	1	0
11749	CABBAGE, FRESH	1	CUP	70.0	17	4	1	0
18096	CAKE, CHOCOLATE, W/ CHOCOLATE FROSTING	1	SLICE	64.0	235	35	3	10
18110	CAKE, FRUITCAKE	1	PIECE	43.0	139	26	1	4
18113	CAKE, GERMAN CHOCOLATE, W/ FROSTING	1	SLICE	111.0	404	55	4	21
18119	CAKE, PINEAPPLE UPSIDE-DOWN	1	SLICE	115.0	367	58	4	14
18120	CAKE, POUND	1	SLICE	28.4	110	14	2	6
18133	CAKE, SPONGE	1	SLICE	38.0	110	23	2	1
18139	CAKE, WHITE, W/ FROSTING	1	SLICE	74.0	264	42	4	9
18140	CAKE, YELLOW, W/ CHOCOLATE FROSTING	1	SLICE	64.0	243	35	2	11
18141	CAKE, YELLOW, W/ VANILLA FROSTING	1	SLICE	64.0	239	38	2	9
11655	CARROT JUICE, CND	¾	CUP	184.5	74	17	2	0
11125	CARROTS, CKD	½	CUP	78.0	35	8	1	0
11124	CARROTS, FRESH	1	MEDIUM	60.0	26	6	1	0
11131	CARROTS, FRZ, CKD	½	CUP	73.0	26	6	1	0
12585	CASHEW, DRY ROASTED	½	CUP	68.5	393	22	10	32
15235	CATFISH, CHANNEL, FARMED, CKD, DRY HEAT	3	OUNCE	85.1	129	0	16	7
15011	CATFISH, FRIED	3	OUNCE	85.1	195	7	15	11
11935	CATSUP	1	TBSP.	15.0	16	4	0	0
11135	CAULIFLOWER, FRESH	½	CUP	50.0	13	3	1	0
11138	CAULIFLOWER, FRZ, CKD	½	CUP	90.0	17	3	1	0
11144	CELERY, CKD	½	CUP	75.0	14	3	1	0
11143	CELERY, FRESH	½	CUP	60.0	10	2	0	0
8183	CEREALS, WHOLE WHEAT HOT NATURAL CEREAL	1	CUP	242.0	150	33	5	1
1150	CHEESE SPREAD, PAST. PROCESSED, AMERICAN	2	OUNCE	56.7	165	5	9	12
1147	CHEESE, AMERICAN, PASTEURIZED PROCESSED	2	OUNCE	56.7	213	1	13	18
1004	CHEESE, BLUE	1½	OUNCE	42.5	150	1	9	12
1005	CHEESE, BRICK	1½	OUNCE	42.5	158	1	10	13
1006	CHEESE, BRIE	1½	OUNCE	42.5	142	0	9	12
1008	CHEESE, CARAWAY	1½	OUNCE	42.5	160	1	11	12
1009	CHEESE, CHEDDAR, AMERICAN DOMESTIC	1½	OUNCE	42.5	171	1	11	14
1011	CHEESE, COLBY	1½	OUNCE	42.5	167	1	10	14
1015	CHEESE, COTTAGE, LOWFAT, 2% FAT	1½	OUNCE	42.5	38	2	6	1
1017	CHEESE, CREAM	1½	OUNCE	42.5	148	1	1	15
62554	CHEESE, CREAM, FAT FREE	2	TBSP.	35.0	35	2	5	0
62553	CHEESE, CREAM, LIGHT	2	TBSP.	32.0	70	2	3	5

Saturated fat (g)	Monounsaturated fat (g)	Polyunsaturated fat (g)	Fiber (g)	Cholesterol (g)	Folate (g)	Vitamin A (RE)	Vitamin B6 (mg)	Vitamin B12 (µg)	Vitamin C (mg)	Vitamin E (mg)	Riboflavin (mg)	Thiamin (mg)	Calcium (mg)	Iron (mg)	Magnesium (mg)	Niacin (mg)	Phosphorus (mg)	Potassium (mg)	Sodium (mg)	Zinc (mg)
1	1	0	1	0	11	0	0	0	0	-	.1	.2	42	1.1	8	1.4	41	47	182	.3
1	1	0	-	0	5	0	0	0	0	-	.1	.1	58	1.2	14	1.3	39	44	112	.3
0	0	0	1	0	8	0	0	0	0	-	.1	.1	19	.6	7	1.2	26	28	152	.2
0	0	0	1	0	9	0	0	0	0	-	.1	.1	23	.9	8	1.3	31	33	175	.3
0	0	0	2	0	12	0	.1	0	0	-	.1	.1	24	.9	14	1.1	46	53	127	.3
0	0	1	1	0	8	0	0	0	0	-	.1	.2	20	.9	9	1.4	32	34	122	.3
0	0	0	1	0	14	0	0	0	0	-	.2	.4	52	1.6	16	2.8	58	72	322	.5
0	0	1	5	0	22	0	.1	0	0	-	.1	.2	10	1.8	44	1.8	115	109	340	1
0	0	0	2	0	11	0	0	0	0	-	.1	.1	22	.9	17	1	57	67	215	.5
1	2	4	-	26	7	334	0	0	1	-	.1	.1	11	1	8	.8	32	55	188	.2
0	1	0	1	0	9	0	0	0	0	-	.1	.1	17	.8	7	.9	28	59	101	.2
0	0	0	2	0	16	0	0	0	-	-	.1	.1	23	.9	13	1.2	40	53	211	.4
0	0	0	1	0	10	0	0	0	0	-	.1	.1	26	.8	12	1	38	50	133	.3
0	0	0	1	0	9	0	0	-	0	-	.1	.1	27	.8	6	1	24	30	135	.2
0	0	0	2	0	39	108	.1	0	58	-	.1	0	36	.7	19	.4	46	228	20	.3
0	0	0	3	0	52	174	.1	0	37	-	.1	.1	47	.6	18	.4	51	166	22	.3
2	5	1	1	10	7	11	0	.1	0	-	.1	.1	16	1.3	17	1	57	83	175	.4
0	0	0	3	0	47	56	.1	0	48	-	.1	.1	28	.9	16	.5	44	247	16	.3
	-	-	-	100	-	60	-	-	1	-	-	-	24	.4	-	-	-	-	900	-
	1	0	2	0	12	0	0	0	0	-	.1	.2	41	1.7	21	1.9	52	65	197	.5
	1	0	-	0	12	0	0	0	0	-	.1	.2	60	1.4	9	1.7	38	61	241	.3
3	1	0	0	11	0	38	0	0	0	.1	0		1	0	0	0	1	1	1	0
3	1	0	0	11	0	38	0	0	0	.1	0	0	1	0	0	0	1	1	41	0
6	3	0	0	24	0	83	0	0	0	-	0	0	3	0	0	0	3	3	91	0
0	0	0	2	0	15	10	.1	0	15	-	0	0	23	.1	6	.2	11	73	6	.1
0	0	0	-	0	40	9	.1	0	36	-	0	0	33	.4	11	.2	16	172	13	.1
3	6	1	2	29	5	18	-	.1	0	-	.1	0	28	1.4	22	.4	78	128	214	.4
0	2	1	2	2	1	8	0	0	0	-	0	0	14	.9	7	.3	22	66	116	.1
5	9	5	-	53	4	23	0	.1	0	-	.1	.1	53	1.2	19	1.1	173	151	369	.5
3	6	4	-	25	8	75	0	.1	1	-	.2	.2	138	1.7	15	1.4	94	129	367	.4
3	2	0	-	63	3	44	0	.1	0	-	.1	0	10	.4	3	.4	39	34	113	.1
0	0	0	-	39	5	17	0	.1	0	-	.1	1	27	1	4	.7	52	38	93	.2
2	4	2	-	1	5	12	0	.1	0	-	.2	.1	96	1.1	9	1.1	69	70	242	.2
3	6	1	1	35	5	17	0	.1	0	-	.1	.1	24	1.3	19	.8	103	114	216	.4
2	4	3	-	36	6	12	0	.1	0	-	0	.1	40	.7	4	.3	92	34	220	.2
0	0	0	1	0	7	4751	.4	0	16	-	.1	.2	44	.8	26	.7	77	539	54	.3
0	0	0	3	0	11	1915	.2	0	2	-	0	0	24	.5	10	.4	23	177	51	.2
0	0	0	2	0	8	1688	.1	0	6	-	0	.1	16	.3	9	.6	26	194	21	.1
0	0	0	3	0	8	1292	.1	0	2	-	0	0	20	.3	7	.3	19	115	43	.2
6	19	5	2	0	47	0	.2	0	0	-	.1	.1	31	4.1	178	1	336	387	438	3.8
2	4	1	0	54	6	13	.1	2.4	1	-	.1	.4	8	.7	22	2.1	208	273	68	.9
3	5	3	-	69	14	7	.2	1.6	0	-	.1	.1	37	1.2	23	1.9	184	289	238	.7
.0	0	0	0	0	2	15	0	0	2	-	0	0	3	.1	3	.2	6	72	178	0
0	0	0	1	0	29	1	.1	0	23	-	0	0	11	.2	8	.3	22	152	15	.1
0	0	0	2	0	37	2	.1	0	28	-	0	0	15	.4	8	.3	22	125	16	.1
0	0	0	1	0	17	10	.1	0	5	-	0	0	32	.3	9	.2	19	213	68	.1
0	0	0	1	0	17	8	.1	0	4	-	0	0	24	.2	7	.2	15	172	52	.1
-	-	-	-	0	27	0	.2	0	0	-	.1	.2	17	1.5	53	2.2	167	172	564	1.2
8	4	0	0	31	4	107	.1	.2	0	-	.2	0	319	.2	16	.1	496	137	921	1.5
11	5	1	0	54	4	164	0	.4	0	-	.2	0	349	.2	13	0	252	92	369	1.7
8	3	0	0	32	15	97	.1	.5	0	-	.2	0	224	.1	10	.4	165	109	592	1.1
8	4	0	0	40	9	128	0	.5	0	-	.1	0	286	.2	10	.1	192	58	238	1.1
7	3	0	0	43	28	77	.1	.7	0	-	.2	0	78	.2	9	.2	80	65	268	1
8	4	0	0	40	8	123	0	.1	0	-	.2	0	286	.3	9	.1	208	40	293	1.3
9	4	0	0	45	8	129	0	.4	0	-	.2	0	307	.3	12	0	218	42	264	1.3
9	4	0	0	40	8	117	0	.4	0	-	.2	0	291	.3	11	0	194	54	257	1.3
1	0	0	0	4	6	9	0	.3	0	-	.1	0	29	.1	3	.1	64	41	173	.2
9	4	1	0	47	6	186	0	.2	0	-	.1	0	34	.5	3	0	44	51	126	.2
0	-	-	-	5	-	100	-	-	0	-	-	-	120	0	-	-	-	-	180	-
4	-	-	-	15	-	80	-	-	0	-	-	-	48	8	-	-	-	-	150	

Food Composition Table—cont'd

Code	Name	Amount	Unit	Grams	Kilocalories	Carbohydrates (g)	Protein (g)	Fat (g)
62579	CHEESE, FAT FREE SLICES, WHITE	1	SLICE	21.3	30	2	5	0
62578	CHEESE, FAT FREE SLICES, YELLOW	1	SLICE	21.3	30	2	5	0
1019	CHEESE, FETA	1½	OUNCE	42.5	112	2	6	9
1156	CHEESE, GOAT, HARD TYPE	1½	OUNCE	42.5	192	1	13	15
1159	CHEESE, GOAT, SOFT TYPE	1½	OUNCE	42.5	114	0	8	9
1022	CHEESE, GOUDA	1½	OUNCE	42.5	152	1	11	12
1025	CHEESE, MONTEREY	1½	OUNCE	42.5	159	0	10	13
1028	CHEESE, MOZZARELLA, PART SKIM MILK	1½	OUNCE	42.5	108	1	10	7
1026	CHEESE, MOZZARELLA, WHOLE MILK	1½	OUNCE	42.5	120	1	8	9
1161	CHEESE, MOZZERELLA, SUBSTITUTE	1½	OUNCE	42.5	105	10	5	5
1032	CHEESE, PARMESAN, GRATED	1	TBSP.	5.0	23	0	2	2
1035	CHEESE, PROVOLONE	1½	OUNCE	42.5	149	1	11	11
1037	CHEESE, RICOTTA, PART SKIM MILK	1½	OUNCE	42.5	59	2	5	3
1036	CHEESE, RICOTTA, WHOLE MILK	1½	OUNCE	42.5	74	1	5	6
1038	CHEESE, ROMANO	1½	OUNCE	42.5	164	2	14	11
1040	CHEESE, SWISS, DOMESTIC	1½	OUNCE	42.5	160	1	12	12
1044	CHEESE, SWISS, PASTEURIZED PROCESSED	2	OUNCE	56.7	189	1	14	14
18148	CHEESECAKE, NO-BAKE TYPE	1	SLICE	80.0	219	28	4	10
9072	CHERRIES, SWEET, CND, JUICE PACK	½	CUP	125.0	67	17	1	0
9070	CHERRIES, SWEET, FRESH	½	CUP	72.5	52	12	1	1
9076	CHERRIES, SWEET, FROZEN, SWEETENED	½	CUP	129.5	115	29	1	0
18308	CHERRY PIE	1	SLICE	125.0	325	50	3	14
19033	CHEX MIX	1	CUP	42.5	181	28	5	7
5283	CHICKEN SALAD SANDWICH SPREAD	3	OUNCE	85.1	170	6	10	11
5054	CHICKEN, BACK, MEAT ONLY, CKD, FRIED	3	OUNCE	85.1	245	5	26	13
5055	CHICKEN, BACK, MEAT ONLY, CKD, ROASTED	3	OUNCE	85.1	203	0	24	11
5050	CHICKEN, BACK, MEAT&SKIN, CKD, FRIED,FLR	3	OUNCE	85.1	282	6	24	18
5051	CHICKEN, BACK, MEAT&SKIN, CKD, ROASTED	3	OUNCE	85.1	255	0	22	18
5063	CHICKEN, BREAST, MEAT ONLY, CKD, FRIED	3	OUNCE	85.1	159	0	28	4
5064	CHICKEN, BREAST, MEAT ONLY, CKD, ROASTED	3	OUNCE	85.1	140	0	26	3
5059	CHICKEN, BREAST, MEAT&SKIN, CKD, FRIED, FLR	3	OUNCE	85.1	189	1	27	8
5060	CHICKEN, BREAST, MEAT&SKIN, CKD, ROASTED	3	OUNCE	85.1	168	0	25	7
5044	CHICKEN, DARK MEAT, MEAT ONLY, CKD, FRIED	3	OUNCE	85.1	203	2	25	10
5045	CHICKEN, DARK MEAT, MEAT ONLY, CKD, ROASTED	3	OUNCE	85.1	174	0	23	8
5036	CHICKEN, DARK MEAT, MEAT&SKIN, CKD, FRIED, FLR	3	OUNCE	85.1	242	3	23	14
5037	CHICKEN, DARK MEAT, MEAT&SKIN, CKD, ROASTED	3	OUNCE	85.1	215	0	22	13
5072	CHICKEN, DRUMSTICK, MEAT ONLY, CKD, FRIED	3	OUNCE	85.1	166	0	24	7
5073	CHICKEN, DRUMSTICK, MEAT ONLY, CKD, ROASTED	3	OUNCE	85.1	146	0	24	5
5068	CHICKEN, DRUMSTICK, MEAT&SKIN, CKD, FRIED, FLR	3	OUNCE	85.1	208	1	23	12
5069	CHICKEN, DRUMSTICK, MEAT&SKIN, CKD, ROASTED	3	OUNCE	85.1	184	0	23	9
5081	CHICKEN, LEG, MEAT ONLY, CKD, FRIED	3	OUNCE	85.1	177	1	24	8
5082	CHICKEN, LEG, MEAT ONLY, CKD, ROASTED	3	OUNCE	85.1	162	0	23	7
5077	CHICKEN, LEG, MEAT&SKIN, CKD, FRIED, FLOUR	3	OUNCE	85.1	216	2	23	12
5078	CHICKEN, LEG, MEAT&SKIN, CKD, ROASTED	3	OUNCE	85.1	197	0	22	11
5097	CHICKEN, THIGH, MEAT ONLY, CKD, FRIED	3	OUNCE	85.1	185	1	24	9
5098	CHICKEN, THIGH, MEAT ONLY, CKD, ROASTED	3	OUNCE	85.1	178	0	22	9
5093	CHICKEN, THIGH, MEAT&SKIN, CKD, FRIED, FLR	3	OUNCE	85.1	223	3	23	13
5094	CHICKEN, THIGH, MEAT&SKIN, CKD, ROASTED	3	OUNCE	85.1	210	0	21	13
5106	CHICKEN, WING, MEAT ONLY, CKD, FRIED	3	OUNCE	85.1	179	0	26	8
5107	CHICKEN, WING, MEAT ONLY, CKD, ROASTED	3	OUNCE	85.1	173	0	26	7
5102	CHICKEN, WING, MEAT&SKIN, CKD, FRIED, FLR	3	OUNCE	85.1	273	2	22	19
5103	CHICKEN, WING, MEAT&SKIN, CKD, ROASTED	3	OUNCE	85.1	247	0	23	175
16058	CHICKPEAS, CND	½	CUP	120.0	143	27	6	1
16059	CHILI W/ BEANS, CND	½	CUP	127.5	143	15	7	7
19183	CHOCOLATE PUDDING	1	CUP	298.1	396	68	8	12
15158	CLAM, CKD, BREADED AND FRIED	3	OUNCE	85.1	172	9	12	9
15160	CLAM, CND, DRAINED SOLIDS	3	OUNCE	85.1	126	4	22	2
19219	COCONUT CREAM PUDDING	1	CUP	280.0	291	50	9	7
15016	COD, ATLANTIC, CKD, DRY HEAT	3	OUNCE	85.1	89	0	19	1
15017	COD, ATLANTIC, CND	3	OUNCE	85.1	89	0	19	1

Saturated fat (g)	Monounsaturated fat (g)	Polyunsaturated fat (g)	Fiber (g)	Cholesterol (g)	Folate (g)	Vitamin A (RE)	Vitamin B6 (mg)	Vitamin B12 (μg)	Vitamin C (mg)	Vitamin E (mg)	Riboflavin (mg)	Thiamin (mg)	Calcium (mg)	Iron (mg)	Magnesium (mg)	Niacin (mg)	Phosphorus (mg)	Potassium (mg)	Sodium (mg)	Zinc (mg)
0	-	-	0	0	-	40	-	-	0	-	-	-	120	0	-	-	-	18	310	-
0	-	-	0	0	-	40	-	-	0	-	-	-	120	0	-	-	-	18	310	-
0	-	-	0	0	-	40	-	-	0	-	-	-	120	0	-	-	-	18	310	-
10	3	0	-	45	2	663	0	.1	0	-	.5	.1	381	.8	23	1	310	20	147	.7
6	2	0	0	20	5	578	.1	.1	0	-	.2	0	60	.8	7	.2	109	11	156	.4
7	3	0	0	48	9	74	0	.7	0	-	.1	0	298	,1	12	0	232	51	348	1.7
8	4	0	0	38	8	108	0	.4	0	-	.2	0	317	.3	11	0	189	34	228	1.3
4	2	0	0	25	4	75	0	.3	0	-	.1	0	275	.1	10	0	197	36	198	1.2
6	3	0	0	33	3	102	0	.3	0	-	.1	0	220	.1	8	0	158	29	159	.9
2	3	1	0	0	5	186	0	.3	0	-	.2	0	259	.2	17	.1	248	193	291	.8
1	0	0	0	4	0	9	0	.1	0	-	0	0	69	0	3	0	40	5	93	.2
7	3	0	0	29	4	112	0	.6	0	-	.1	0	321	.2	12	.1	211	59	372	1.4
2	1	0	0	13	6	48	0	.1	0	-	.1	0	116	.2	6	0	78	53	53	.6
4	2	0	0	22	5	57	0	.1	0	-	.1	0	88	.2	5	0	67	44	36	.5
7	3	0	0	44	3	60	0	.5	0	-	.2	0	452	.3	17	0	323	37	510	1.1
8	3	0	0	39	3	108	0	.7	0	-	.2	0	409	.1	15	0	257	47	111	1.7
9	4	0	0	48	3	130	0	.7	0	-	.2	0	438	.3	17	0	432	122	777	2
6	3	1	2	34	14	79	0	.2	0	-	.2	.1	138	.4	15	.4	187	169	304	.4
0	0	0	1	0	5	16	0	0	3	-	0	0	17	.7	15	.5	27	164	4	.1
0	0	0	2	0	3	15	0	0	5	-	0	0	11	.3	8	.3	14	162	0	0
0	0	0	1	0	5	25	0	0	1	-	.1	0	16	.5	13	.2	21	258	1	.1
3	7	3	1	0	10	-	.1	0	1	-	0	0	15	.6	10	.3	36	101	308	.2
-	-	-	-	0	0	6	.7	5.3	20	-	.2	.7	15	10.5	27	7.2	80	114	432	.9
3	3	5	0	26	4	36	.1	.3	1	-	.1	0	9	.5	9	1.4	28	156	321	.9
4	5	3	0	79	8	25	.3	.3	0	-	.2	.1	22	1.4	21	6.5	150	213	84	2.4
3	4	3	0	77	6	24	.3	.3	0	-	.2	.1	20	1.2	19	6	140	202	82	2.3
5	7	4	-	76	7	31	.3	.2	0	-	.2	.1	20	1.4	20	6.2	141	192	77	2.1
5	7	4	0	75	5	84	.2	.2	0	-	.2	.1	18	1.2	17	5.7	131	179	74	1.9
1	1	1	0	77	3	6	.5	.3	0	-	.1	.1	14	1	26	12.6	209	235	67	.9
1	1	1	0	72	3	5	.5	.3	0	-	.1	.1	13	.9	25	11.7	194	218	63	.9
2	3	2	-	76	3	13	.5	.3	0	-	.1	.1	14	1	26	11.7	198	220	65	9
2	3	1	0	71	3	23	.5	.3	0	-	.1	.1	12	.9	23	10.8	182	208	60	.9
3	4	2	0	82	8	20	.3	.3	0	-	.2	.1	15	1.3	21	6	159	215	82	2.5
2	3	2	0	79	7	19	.3	.3	0	-	.2	.1	13	1.1	20	5.6	152	204	79	2.4
4	6	3	-	78	7	26	.3	.3	0	-	.2	.1	14	1.3	20	5.8	150	196	76	2.2
4	5	3	0	77	6	49	.3	.2	0	-	.2	.1	13	1.2	19	5.4	143	187	74	2.1
2	3	2	0	80	8	15	.3	.3	0	-	.2	.1	10	1.1	20	5.2	158	212	82	2.7
1	2	1	0	79	8	15	.3	.3	0	-	.2	.1	10	1.1	20	5.2	156	209	81	2.7
3	5	3	-	77	7	21	.3	.3	0	-	.2	.1	10	1.1	20	5.1	150	195	76	2.5
3	4	2	0	77	7	26	.3	.3	0	-	.2	.1	10	1.1	20	5.1	149	195	77	2.4
2	3	2	0	84	8	17	.3	.3	0	-	.2	.1	11	1.2	21	5.7	164	216	82	2.5
2	3	2	0	80	7	16	.3	.3	0	-	.2	.1	10	1.1	20	5.4	156	206	77	2.4
3	5	3	-	80	7	24	.3	.3	0	-	.2	.1	11	1.2	20	5.6	155	198	75	2.3
3	4	3	0	78	6	33	.3	.3	0	-	.2	.1	10	1.1	20	5.3	148	191	74	2.2
2	3	2	0	87	8	18	.3	.3	0	-	.2	.1	11	1.2	22	6.1	169	220	81	2.4
3	4	2	0	81	7	17	.3	.3	0	-	.2	.1	10	1.1	20	5.5	156	202	75	2.2
3	5	3	-	82	7	25	.3	.3	0	-	.2	.1	12	1.3	21	5.9	159	202	75	2.1
4	5	3	0	79	6	41	.3	.2	0	-	.2	.1	10	1.1	19	5.4	148	189	71	2
2	3	2	0	71	3	15	.5	.3	0	-	.1	0	13	1	18	6.2	139	177	77	1.8
2	2	2	0	72	3	15	.5	.3	0	-	.1	0	14	1	18	6.2	141	179	78	1.8
5	8	4	-	69	3	32	.3	.2	0	-	.1	0	13	1.1	16	5.7	128	151	65	1.5
5	6	4	0	71	3	40	.4	.2	0	-	.1	0	13	1.1	16	5.7	128	156	70	1.5
0	0	1	5	0	80	2	.6	0	5	-	0	0	38	1.6	35	.2	108	206	359	1.3
3	3	0	6	22	29	43	.2	0	2	-	.1	.1	60	4.4	57	.5	196	465	666	2.6
2	5	4	3	9	9	33	.1	0	5	-	.5	.1	268	1.5	63	1	238	537	385	1.3
2	4	2	-	52	15	77	.1	34.2	9	-	.2	.1	54	11.8	12	1.8	160	277	310	1.2
0	0	0	0	57	24	145	.1	84.1	19	-	.4	.1	78	23.8	15	2.9	287	534	95	2.3
5	1	0	-	20	11	140	.4	.7	2	-	.4	.1	316	.6	45	.3	249	445	456	1
0	0	0	0	47	7	12	.2	.9	1	-	1	.1	12	.4	36	2.1	117	208	66	.5
0	0	0	0	47	7	12	.2	.9	1	-	.1	.1	18	.4	35	2.1	221	449	185	.5

Food Composition Table—cont'd

Code	Name	Amount	Unit	Grams	Kilocalories	Carbohydrates (g)	Protein (g)	Fat (g)
18104	COFFEECAKE	1	SLICE	63.0	263	29	4	15
11159	COLESLAW	½	CUP	64.0	44	8	1	2
11162	COLLARDS, CKD	½	CUP	64.0	17	4	1	0
11161	COLLARDS, FRESH	1	CUP	36.0	11	3	1	0
11164	COLLARDS, FRZ, CHOPPED, CKD	½	CUP	85.0	31	6	3	0
20092	CORN, CKD	½	CUP	70.0	88	20	2	1
11901	CORN, SWEET, WHITE, CKD	½	CUP	82.0	89	21	3	1
11905	CORN, SWEET, WHITE, CND	½	CUP	82.0	66	15	2	1
11906	CORN, SWEET, WHITE, CND, CREAM STYLE	½	CUP	128.0	92	23	2	1
11900	CORN, SWEET, WHITE, FRESH	½	CUP	77.0	66	15	2	1
11168	CORN, SWEET, YELLOW, CKD	½	CUP	82.0	89	21	3	1
11174	CORN, SWEET, YELLOW, CND, CREAM STYLE	½	CUP	128.0	92	23	2	1
11167	CORN, SWEET, YELLOW, FRESH	½	CUP	77.0	66	15	2	1
15137	CRAB, ALASKA KING, CKD, MOIST HEAT	3	OUNCE	85.1	82	0	16	1
15138	CRAB, ALASKA KING, IMITATION	3	OUNCE	85.1	87	9	10	1
18216	CRACKERS, CRISPBREAD, RYE	1	EACH	10.0	37	8	1	0
18217	CRACKERS, MATZO, PLAIN	1	EACH	28.4	112	24	3	0
18219	CRACKERS, MATZO, WHOLE-WHEAT	1	EACH	28.4	100	22	4	0
18220	CRACKERS, MELBA TOAST, PLAIN	1	EACH	5.0	20	4	1	0
18229	CRACKERS, RITZ	1	EACH	3.0	15	2	0	1
18226	CRACKERS, RYE, WAFERS, PLAIN	1	EACH	25.0	84	20	2	0
18228	CRACKERS, SALTINES	1	EACH	3.0	13	2	0	0
18232	CRACKERS, WHEAT, REGULAR	1	EACH	2.0	9	1	0	0
9078	CRANBERRIES, FRESH	½	CUP	47.5	23	6	0	0
9080	CRANBERRY JUICE BOTTLED	¾	CUP	189.4	108	27	0	0
14240	CRANBERRY-APRICOT JUICE DRINK, BOTTLED	¾	CUP	183.4	117	30	0	0
15243	CRAYFISH, FARMED, CKD, MOIST HEAT	3	OUNCE	85.1	74	0	15	1
18238	CREAM PUFFS, SHELL, W/ CUSTARD FILLING	1	EACH	130.0	335	30	9	20
1067	CREAM SUBSTITUTE, NONDAIRY, LIQUID	1	TBSP.	15.0	20	2	0	1
1069	CREAM SUBSTITUTE, NONDAIRY, POWDERED	1	TSP.	2.0	11	1	0	1
1049	CREAM, HALF AND HALF, CREAM AND MILK	1	TBSP.	15.0	20	1	0	2
1053	CREAM, HEAVY WHIPPING	1	TBSP.	15.0	52	0	0	6
1052	CREAM, LIGHT WHIPPING	1	TBSP.	15.0	44	0	0	5
1050	CREAM, LIGHT, COFFEE OR TABLE	1	TBSP.	15.0	29	1	0	3
1054	CREAM, WHIPPED, PRESSURIZED	1	TBSP.	3.0	8	0	0	1
18239	CROISSANTS, BUTTER	1	MEDIUM	57.0	231	26	5	12
18242	CROUTONS, PLAIN	1	CUP	30.0	122	22	4	2
18243	CROUTONS, SEASONED	1	CUP	40.0	186	25	4	7
11205	CUCUMBER, FRESH	½	CUP	52.0	7	1	0	0
18245	DANISH PASTRY, CHEESE	1	EACH	71.0	266	26	6	16
18246	DANISH PASTRY, FRUIT	1	EACH	71.0	263	34	4	13
18247	DANISH PASTRY, NUT	1	EACH	65.0	280	30	5	16
9087	DATES, DOMESTIC, NATURAL AND DRY	½	CUP	89.0	245	65	2	0
18251	DOUGHNUTS, CHOCOLATE, SUGARED OR GLAZED	1	EACH	42.0	175	24	2	8
18253	DOUGHNUTS, FRENCH CRULLERS, GLAZED	1	EACH	41.0	169	24	1	8
18255	DOUGHNUTS, GLAZED	1	EACH	60.0	242	27	4	14
18248	DOUGHNUTS, PLAIN	1	EACH	47.0	198	23	2	11
18249	DOUGHNUTS, PLAIN, CHOCOLATE-COATED OR FROSTED	1	EACH	43.0	204	21	2	13
18250	DOUGHNUTS, PLAIN, SUGARED OR GLAZED	1	EACH	45.0	192	23	2	10
18254	DOUGHNUTS, W/ CREME FILLING	1	EACH	85.0	307	26	5	21
18256	DOUGHNUTS, W/ JELLY FILLING	1	EACH	85.0	289	33	5	16
18257	ECLAIRS, CUSTARD-FILLED W/ CHOCOLATE GLAZE	1	EACH	62.0	162	15	4	10
19168	EGG CUSTARDS	1	CUP	282.0	296	30	14	13
1142	EGG SUBSTITUTE, FROZEN	1	CUP	240.0	384	8	27	27
1143	EGG SUBSTITUTE, LIQUID	1	CUP	251.0	211	2	30	8
1057	EGGNOG	1	CUP	254.0	342	34	10	19
11210	EGGPLANT, CKD	½	CUP	48.0	13	3	0	0
11209	EGGPLANT, FRESH	½	CUP	41.0	11	2	0	0
1128	EGGS, CHICKEN, WHOLE, CKD, FRIED	1	LARGE	46.0	92	1	6	7
1129	EGGS, CHICKEN, WHOLE, CKD, HARD-BOILED	1	LARGE	50.0	78	1	6	5

Saturated fat (g)	Monounsaturated fat (g)	Polyunsaturated fat (g)	Fiber (g)	Cholesterol (g)	Folate (g)	Vitamin A (RE)	Vitamin B_6 (mg)	Vitamin B_{12} (µg)	Vitamin C (mg)	Vitamin E (mg)	Riboflavin (mg)	Thiamin (mg)	Calcium (mg)	Iron (mg)	Magnesium (mg)	Niacin (mg)	Phosphorus (mg)	Potassium (mg)	Sodium (mg)	Zinc (mg)
4	8	2	2	20	20	18	0	.1	0	-	.1	.1	34	1.2	14	1.1	68	77	221	.5
0	0	1	-	5	17	52	.1	0	21	-	0	0	29	.4	6	.2	20	116	15	.1
-	-	-	1	0	4	175	0	0	8	-	0	0	15	.1	4	.2	5	84	10	.1
-	-	-	1	0	4	120	0	0	8	-	0	0	10	.1	3	.1	4	61	7	0
-	-	-	-	0	65	508	.1	0	22	-	.1	0	179	1	26	.5	23	213	43	.2
0	0	0	3	0	4	4	0	0	0	-	0	0	1	.2	25	.4	53	22	0	.4
0	0	0	5	0	38	0	0	0	5	-	.1	.2	2	.5	26	1.3	84	204	14	.4
0	0	0	2	0	57	0	.1	0	6	-	.1	0	4	.5	22	1.2	65	172	365	.7
0	0	0	2	0	35	0	0	0	5	-	0	.2	2	.4	28	1.3	69	208	12	.3
0	0	0	2	0	38	18	0	0	5	-	.1	.2	2	.5	26	1.3	84	204	14	.4
0	0	0	2	0	40	13	0	0	7	-	.1	0	4	.7	16	1	53	160	265	.3
0	0	0	2	0	57	13	.1	0	6	-	.1	0	4	.5	22	1.2	65	172	365	.7
0	0	0	2	0	35	22	0	0	5	-	0	.2	2	.4	28	1.3	69	208	12	.3
0	0	0	0	45	43	8	.2	9.8	6	-	0	0	50	.6	54	1.1	238	223	912	6.5
0	0	1	0	17	1	17	0	1.4	0	-	0	0	11	.3	37	.2	240	77	715	.3
0	0	0	2	0	2	0	0	0	0	-	0	0	3	.2	8	.1	27	32	26	.2
0	0	0	1	0	4	0	0	0	0	-	.1	.1	4	.9	7	1.1	25	32	1	.2
0	0	0	3	0	10	0	0	0	0	-	.1	.1	7	1.3	38	1.5	86	90	1	.7
0	0	0	0	0	1	0	0	0	0	-	0	0	5	.2	3	.2	10	10	41	.1
0	0	0	0	0	0	0	0	0	0	-	0	0	4	.1	1	.1	7	4	25	0
0	0	0	-	0	11	1	.1	0	0	-	.1	.1	10	1.5	30	.4	84	124	199	.7
0	0	0	0	0	1	0	0	0	0	-	0	0	4	.2	1	.2	3	4	39	0
0	0	0	0	0	0	0	0	0	0	-	0	0	1	.1	1	.1	4	4	16	0
-	-	-	2	0	1	2	0	0	6	-	0	0	3	.1	2	0	4	34	0	.1
-	-	-	0	0	0	0	0	0	67	-	0	0	6	.3	4	.1	4	34	4	.1
0	-	-	0	0	1	84	0	0	0	-	0	0	17	.3	6	.2	9	112	4	,1
0	0	0	0	117	9	13	.1	2.6	0	-	.1	0	43	.9	28	1.4	205	202	82	1.3
5	8	5	-	174	20	259	.1	.5	0	-	.4	.2	86	1.5	16	1.1	142	150	443	.8
0	1	-	0	0	1	0	0	0	0	-	0	0	1	0	0	0	10	29	12	0
1	0	0	0-	0	0	0	0	0	0	-	0	0	0	0	0	0	8	16	4	0
1	0	0	0	6	0	16	0	0	0	-	0	0	16	0	2	0	14	19	6	.1
3	2	0	0	21	1	63	0	0	0	-	0-	0	10	0	1	0	9	11	6	0
3	1	0	0	17	1	44	0	0	0	-	0	0	10	0	1	0	9	15	5	0
2	1	0	0	10	0	27	0	0	0	-	0	0	14	0	1	0	12	18	6	0
0	0	0	0	2	0	6	0	0	0	-	0	0	3	0	0	0	3	4	4	0
7	3	1	2	43	16	78	0	.2	0	-	.1	.2	21	1.2	9	1.2	60	67	424	.4
0	1	0	2	0	7	0	0	0	0	-	.1	.2	23	1.2	9	1.6	34	37	209	.3
2	4	1	2	1	16	2	0	0	0	-	.2	.2	38	1.1	17	1.9	56	72	495	.4
0	0	0	0	0	7	11	0	0	3	-	0	0	7	.1	6	.1	10	75	1	.1
5	8	2	-	32	18	44	0	.2	0	-	.2	.1	25	1.1	11	1.4	77	70	320	.6
3	7	2	1	15	11	11	-	.1	3	-	.2	.2	33	1.3	11	1.4	63	59	251	.4
4	8	4	1	30	18	9	.1	.1	1	-	.2	.1	61	1.2	21	1.5	72	62	236	.6
-	-	-	7	0	11	4	.2	0	0	-	.1	.1	28	1	31	2	36	580	3	3
2	5	1	1	24	7	11	0	.1	0	-	0	0	89	1	14	.2	68	50	143	.2
2	4	1	-	5	3	-	0	0	0	-	.1	.1	11	.6	5	.6	50	32	141	.1
3	8	2	1	4	13	-	0	.1	0	-	.1	.2	26	1.2	13	1.7	56	65	205	.5
2	5	4	1	17	4	8	0	.1	0	-	.1	.1	21	.9	9	.9	126	60	257	.3
4	7	2	1	25	7	13	0	.2	0	-	0	.1	15	1.1	17	.6	87	49	184	.3
2	5	1	-	14	5	1	0	.1	0	-	.1	.1	27	.5	8	.7	53	46	181	.2
6	11	3	-	20	12	7	0	.1	0	-	.1	.3	21	1.6	17	1.9	65	68	263	.7
4	9	2	-	22	14	7	0	1	1	-	.1	.3	21	1.5	17	1.8	72	67	249	.6
3	4	2	-	79	9	118	0	.2	0	-	.2	.1	39	.7	9	.5	66	73	209	.4
7	4	1	-	245	28	169	.1	.9	1	-	.6	.1	316	.8	39	.2	319	431	217	1.5
5	6	15	0	5	39	324	.3	.8	1	-	.9	.3	175	4.8	36	.3	172	512	479	2.4
2	2	4	0	3	37	542	0	.7	0	-	.8	.3	133	5.3	22	.3	304	828	444	3.3
11	6	1	0	149	2	203	.1	1.1	4	-	.5	.1	330	.5	47	.3	278	420	138	1.2
0	0	0	1	0	7	3	0	0	1	-	0	0	3	.2	6	.3	11	119	1	1
0	0	0	1	0	8	3	0	0	1	-	0	0	3	.1	6	.2	9	89	1	.1
2	3	1	0	211	17	114	.1	.4	0	-	.2	0	25	.7	5	0	89	61	162	.5
2	2	1	0	212	22	84	.1	.6	0	-	.3	0	25	.6	5	0	86	63	62	.5

Food Composition Table—cont'd

Code	Name	Amount	Unit	Grams	Kilocalories	Carbohydrates (g)	Protein (g)	Fat (g)
1131	EGGS, CHICKEN, WHOLE, CKD, POACHED	1	LARGE	50.0	75	1	6	5
1132	EGGS, CHICKEN, WHOLE, CKD, SCRAMBLED	½	CUP	110.0	183	2	12	13
18260	ENGLISH MUFFINS, MIXED-GRAIN (INCLUDES GRANOLA)	1	EACH	66.0	155	31	6	1
18258	ENGLISH MUFFINS, PLAIN	1	EACH	57.0	134	26	4	1
18264	ENGLISH MUFFINS, WHEAT	1	EACH	57.0	127	26	5	1
18170	FIG BARS	1	EACH	16.0	56	11	1	1
15027	FISH FILLETS AND STICKS, FRIED	3	OUNCE	85.1	231	20	13	10
15029	FLOUNDER, CKD, DRY HEAT	3	OUNCE	85.1	100	0	21	1
18269	FRENCH TOAST, MADE W/ LOWFAT (2%) MILK	1	SLICE	65.0	149	16	5	7
9103	FRUIT SALAD, JUICE PACK	½	CUP	124.5	62	16	1	0
9102	FRUIT SALAD, WATER PACK	½	CUP	122.5	37	10	0	0
18173	GRAHAM CRACKERS, PLAIN OR HONEY	1	EACH	7.0	30	5	0	1
19015	GRANOLA BARS, HARD, PLAIN	1	EACH	28.4	134	18	3	6
19020	GRANOLA BARS, SOFT, PLAIN	1	EACH	28.4	126	19	2	5
9135	GRAPE JUICE, CND OR BOTTLED, UNSWEETENED	¾	CUP	189.4	116	28	1	0
9124	GRAPEFRUIT JUICE, CND, SWEETENED	¾	CUP	187.0	86	21	1	0
9123	GRAPEFRUIT JUICE, CND, UNSWEETENED	¾	CUP	185.2	70	17	1	0
9404	GRAPEFRUIT JUICE, PINK, FRESH	¾	CUP	185.3	72	17	1	0
9128	GRAPEFRUIT JUICE, WHITE, FRESH	¾	CUP	185.3	72	17	1	0
9116	GRAPEFRUIT, FRESH, WHITE	1	MEDIUM	136.0	45	11	1	0
9120	GRAPEFRUIT, SECTIONS, CND, JUICE PACK	½	CUP	124.5	46	11	1	0
9119	GRAPEFRUIT, SECTIONS, CND, WATER PACK	½	CUP	122.0	44	11	1	0
9131	GRAPES, AMERICAN TYPE, FRESH	½	CUP	46.0	29	8	0	0
6114	GRAVY, AU JUS, CND	¼	CUP	59.6	10	1	1	0
6527	GRAVY, UNSPECIFIED TYPE	¼	CUP	65.4	22	4	1	0
15032	GROUPER, CKD, DRY HEAT	3	OUNCE	85.1	100	0	21	1
15037	HALIBUT, CKD, DRY HEAT	3	OUNCE	85.1	119	0	23	3
15196	HALIBUT, GREENLAND, CKD, DRY HEAT	3	OUNCE	85.1	203	0	16	15
7032	HAM AND CHEESE LOAF (OR ROLL), LUNCH MEAT	1	SLICE	28.4	73	0	5	6
7031	HAM SALAD SPREAD	1	TBSP.	15.0	32	2	1	2
7028	HAM, EXTRA LEAN, APPX 5% FAT	1	SLICE	28.4	37	0	5	1
62626	HAMBURGER PATTY, MEATLESS	1	EACH	90.0	140	8	18	4
20030	HOMINY, CND, WHITE	½	CUP	80.0	58	11	1	1
20330	HOMINY, CND, YELLOW	½	CUP	80.0	58	11	1	1
19296	HONEY	1	TBSP.	21.0	64	17	0	0
7022	HOT DOG, BEEF	1	EACH	57.0	180	1	7	16
7024	HOT DOG, CHICKEN	1	EACH	45.0	116	3	6	9
62605	HOT DOG, FAT FREE	1	EACH	50.0	40	2	7	0
7025	HOT DOG, TURKEY	1	EACH	45.0	102	1	6	8
16137	HUMMUS, FRESH	½	CUP	123.0	210	25	6	10
18270	HUSH PUPPIES	1	EACH	22.0	74	10	2	3
19270	ICE CREAM, CHOCOLATE	½	CUP	66.0	143	19	3	7
19090	ICE CREAM, FRENCH VANILLA, SOFT-SERVE	½	CUP	66.5	143	15	3	9
19271	ICE CREAM, STRAWBERRY	½	CUP	66.0	127	18	2	6
19095	ICE CREAM, VANILLA	½	CUP	66.0	133	16	2	7
19088	ICE MILK, VANILLA	½	CUP	66.5	92	15	3	3
19096	ICE MILK, VANILLA, SOFT SERVE	½	CUP	66.5	84	14	3	2
62547	ICED TEA, BOTTLED, ALL FLAVORS	1	CUP	236.6	118	29	0	0
19297	JAMS AND PRESERVES	1	TBSP.	20.0	48	13	0	0
19300	JELLIES	1	TBSP.	19.0	51	13	0	0
9148	KIWIFRUIT, FRESH	1	MEDIUM	76.0	46	11	1	0
17225	LAMB, GROUND, CKD, BROILED	3	OUNCE	85.1	241	0	21	17
17002	LAMB, MEAT AND FAT, CKD	3	OUNCE	85.1	250	0	21	18
4002	LARD	¼	CUP	51.3	462	0	0	51
11247	LEEKS, CKD	½	CUP	52.0	16	4	0	0
11246	LEEKS, FRESH	½	CUP	52.0	32	7	1	0
19380	LEMON PUDDING	1	CUP	298.1	373	75	0	9
9150	LEMONS, FRESH, W/O PEEL	1	MEDIUM	58.0	17	5	1	0
11252	LETTUCE, ICEBERG, FRESH	1	CUP	56.0	7	1	1	0
11253	LETTUCE, LOOSELEAF, FRESH	1	CUP	56.0	10	2	1	0

Saturated fat (g)	Monounsaturated fat (g)	Polyunsaturated fat (g)	Fiber (g)	Cholesterol (g)	Folate (g)	Vitamin A (RE)	Vitamin B_6 (mg)	Vitamin B_{12} (ug)	Vitamin C (mg)	Vitamin E (mg)	Riboflavin (mg)	Thiamin (mg)	Calcium (mg)	Iron (mg)	Magnesium (mg)	Niacin (mg)	Phosphorus (mg)	Potassium (mg)	Sodium (mg)	Zinc (mg)
2	2	1	0	212	18	95	.1	.4	0	-	.2	0	25	.7	5	0	89	60	140	.6
4	5	2	0	387	33	215	.1	.8	0	-	.5	.1	78	1.3	13	.1	187	152	308	1.1
0	1	0	-	0	23	1	.1	0	0	-	.2	.3	129	2	29	2.4	98	103	275	.6
0	0	1	-	0	21	0	0	0	0	-	.2	.3	99	1.4	12	2.2	76	75	264	.4
0	0	0	-	0	22	0	.1	0	0	-	.2	.2	101	1.6	22	1.9	66	106	218	.6
0	1	0	1	0	2	1	0	0	0	-	0	0	10	.5	4	.3	10	33	56	.1
3	4	3	0	95	15	26	.1	1.5	0	-	.2	.1	17	.6	21	1.8	154	222	495	.6
0	0	0	0	58	8	9	.2	2.1	0	-	.1	.1	15	.3	49	1.9	246	293	89	.5
2	3	2	-	75	15	86	0	.2	0	-	.2	.1	65	1.1	11	1.1	76	87	311	.4
0	0	0	-	0	3	756	0	0	4	-	0	0	14	.3	10	.4	17	1454	6	.2
0	0	0	-	0	3	54	0	0-	2	-	0	0	9	.4	6	.5	11	96	4	.1
0	0	0	0	0	1	0	0	0	0	-	0	0	2	.3	2	.3	7		42	.1
1	1	3	2	0	7	4	0	0	0	-	0	.1	17	.8	27	.4	79	95	83	.6
2	1	2	1	0	7	0	0	.1	0	-	0	.1	30	.7	21	.1	65	92	79	.4
0	0	0	0	0	5	2	.1	0	0	-	.1	0	17	.5	19	.5	21	250	6	.1
0	0	0	0	0	19	0	0	0	50	-	0	.1	15	.7	19	.6	21	303	4	.1
0	0	0	0	0	19	2	0	0	54	.1	0	.1	13	.4	19	.4	20	283	2	.2
0	0	0	-	0	19	82	.1	0	70	-	0	.1	17	.4	22	.4	28	300	2	.1
0	0	0	0	0	19	2	.1	0	70	-	0	.1	17	.4	22	.4	28	300	2	.1
0	0	0	1	0	14	1	.1	0	45	-	0	.1	16	.1	12	.4	11	201	0	.1
0	0	0	0	0	11	0	0	0	42	-	0	0	19	.3	14	.3	15	210	9	.1
0	0	0	0	0	11	0	0	0	27	-	0	0	18	.5	12	.3	12	161	2	.1
0	0	0	1	0	2	5	.1	0	2	-	0	0	6	.1	2	.1	5	88	1	0
0	0	0	-	0	1	0	0	.1	1	-	0	0	2	.4	1	.5	18	48	30	.6
0	0	0	-	0	1	0	0	0	0	-	0	0	9	.1	3	.2	12	16	356	.1
0	0	0	0	40	9	43	.3	.6	0	-	0	.1	18	1	31	.3	122	404	45	.4
0	1	1	0	35	12	46	.3	1.2	0	-	.1	.1	51	.9	91	6.1	242	490	59	.5
3	9	1	0	50	1	15	.4	.8	0	-	.1	.1	3	.7	28	1.6	179	293	88	.4
2	3	1	0	16	1	7	.1	.2	7	-	.1	.2	16	.3	5	1	72	83	381	.6
1	1	0	0	6	0	0	0	.1	1	-	0	.1	1	.1	2	.3	18	22	137	.2
0	1	0	0	13	1	0	.1	.2	7	-	.1	.3	2	.2	5	1.4	62	99	405	.5
2	-	1	5	0	-	0	-	-	0	-	-	.3	96	1.5	-	4	-	-	380	7.5
0	0	0	2	0	1	0	0	0	0-	-	0	0	8	.5	13	0	28	7	168	.8
0	0	0	-	0	1	9	0	0	0	-	0	0	8	.5	13	0	28	7	168	.8
-	-	-	0	0	0	0	0	0	0	-	0	0	1	.1	0	0	1	11	1	0
7	8	1	0	35	2	0	.1	.9	14	-	.1	0	11	.8	2	1.4	50	95	585	1.2
2	4	2	0	45	2	17	.1	.1	0	-	.1	0	43	.9	5	1.4	48	38	617	.5
0	0	0	0	15	-	0	-	-	0	-	-	-	0	.2	-	-	-	-	460	-
3	3	2	0	48	4	0	.1	.1	0	-	.1	0	48	.8	6	1.9	60	81	642	1.4
2	4	4	6	0	73	2	.5	0	10	-	.1	.1	61	1.9	36	.5	138	214	300	1.4
0	1	2	1	10	4	9	0	0	0	-	.1	.1	61	.7	5	.6	42	32	147	.1
4	2	0	-	22	11	79	0	.2	0	-	.1	0	72	.6	19	.1	71	164	50	.4
5	2	0	-	61	6	102	0	.3	1	-	.1	0	87	.1	8	.1	77	118	41	.3
-	-	-	-	19	8	51	0	.2	5	-	.2	0	79	.1	9	.1	66	124	40	.2
4	2	0	0	29	3	77	0	.3	0	-	.2	0	84	.1	9	.1	69	131	53	.5
2	1	0	0	9	4	31	0	.4	1	-	.2	0	92	.1	10	.1	72	140	57	.3
1	1	0	0	8	4	19	0	.3	1	-	.1	0	104	0	9	.1	80	147	47	.4
0	-	-	0	0	-	0	-	-	0-	-	-	-	0	0	-	-	-	-	10	-
0	0	0	0	0	7	0	0	0	2	-	0	0	4	.1	1	0	2	15	8	0
-	-	-	0	0	0	0	0	0	0	-	0	0	2	0	1	0	1	12	7	0
-	-	-	3	0	-	14	-	0	74	-	0	0	20	.3	23	.4	30	252	4	-
7	7	1	0	82	16	0	.1	2.2	-	.1	.2	.1	19	1.5	20	5.7	171	288	69	4
8	8	1	0	82	15	0	.1	2.2	0	-	.2	.1	14	1.6	20	5.7	160	264	61	3.8
20	23	6	0	49	0	0	0	0	0	.6	0	0	0	0	0	0	0	0	0	.1
0	0	0	-	0	13	3	.1	0	2	-	0	0	16	.6	7	.1	9	45	5	0
0	0	0	1	0	33	5	.1	0	6	-	0	0	31	1.1	15	.2	18	94	10	.1
1	4	3	-	0	0	0	0	0	0	-	0	0	6	.2	3	0	15	3	417	.1
0	0	0	2	0	6	2	0	0	31	-	0	0	15	.3	5	.1	9	80	1	0
0	0	0	1	0	31	18	0	0	2	-	0	0	11	.3	5	1	11	88	5	.1
0	0	0	1	0	28	106	0	0	10	-	0	0	38	.8	6	.2	14	148	5	.2

Food Composition Table—cont'd

Code	Name	Amount	Unit	Grams	Kilocalories	Carbohydrates (g)	Protein (g)	Fat (g)
11251	LETTUCE, ROMAINE, FRESH	1	CUP	56.0	9	1	1	0
15148	LOBSTER, NORTHERN, CKD, MOIST HEAT	3	OUNCE	85.1	83	1	17	1
62533	MACARONI AND CHEESE	1	CUP	111.9	360	44	1	13
20100	MACARONI, CKD, ENRICHED	1	CUP	140.0	197	40	7	1
20400	MACARONI, CKD, UNENRICHED	1	CUP	140.0	197	40	7	1
20106	MACARONI, VEGETABLE, CKD, ENRICHED	1	CUP	134.0	172	36	6	0
20108	MACARONI, WHOLE-WHEAT, CKD	1	CUP	140.0	174	37	7	1
62535	MANGO JUICE	¾	CUP	179.9	66	16	-	0
9176	MANGOS, FRESH	½	CUP	82.5	54	14	0	0
4128	MARGARINE, IMITATION (APPX 40% FAT)	1	TSP.	4.8	17	0	0	2
4132	MARGARINE, REGULAR, W/ SALT ADDED	1	TSP.	4.7	34	0	0	4
4130	MARGARINE, SOFT, W/ SALT ADDED	1	TSP.	4.7	34	0	0	4
11256	MARINARA SAUCE	½	CUP	125.0	85	13	2	4
19303	MARMALADE, ORANGE	1	TBSP.	20.0	49	13	0	0
19116	MARSHMALLOWS	1	CUP	46.0	146	37	1	0
4018	MAYONNAISE	1	TBSP.	14.7	57	4	0	5
62610	MAYONNAISE, FAT FREE	1	TBSP.	15.0	10	3	0	0
62609	MAYONNAISE, LIGHT	1	TBSP.	15.0	25	1	0	2
9181	MELONS, CANTALOUP, FRESH	1	WEDGE	80.0	28	7	1	0
9183	MELONS, CASABA, FRESH	1	WEDGE	164.0	43	10	1	0
9184	MELONS, HONEYDEW, FRESH	1	WEDGE	129.0	45	12	1	0
19120	MILK CHOCOLATE	1	BAR	44.0	226	26	3	13
19126	MILK CHOCOLATE COATED PEANUTS	1	OUNCE	28.4	147	14	4	9
19127	MILK CHOCOLATE COATED RAISINS	1	OUNCE	28.4	111	19	1	4
19132	MILK CHOCOLATE W/ ALMONDS	1	BAR	41.0	216	22	4	14
1110	MILK SHAKES, THICK CHOCOLATE	1	CUP	345.4	410	73	11	9
1111	MILK SHAKES, THICK VANILLA	1	CUP	345.4	386	61	13	10
1088	MILK, BUTTERMILK	1	CUP	245.0	99	12	8	2
1103	MILK, CHOCOLATE DRINK, LOWFAT, 2% FAT	1	CUP	250.0	179	26	8	5
1102	MILK, CHOCOLATE DRINK, WHOLE	1	CUP	250.0	208	26	8	8
1095	MILK, CND, CONDENSED, SWEETENED	¼	CUP	76.3	245	42	6	7
1082	MILK, LOWFAT, 1% FAT	1	CUP	244.0	102	12	8	3
1079	MILK, LOWFAT, 2% FAT	1	CUP	244.0	121	12	8	5
1085	MILK, SKIM	1	CUP	245.0	86	12	8	0
1077	MILK, WHOLE, 3.3% FAT	1	CUP	244.0	150	11	8	8
1078	MILK, WHOLE, 3.7% FAT	1	CUP	244.0	157	11	8	9
18274	MUFFINS, BLUEBERRY	1	LARGE	65.0	180	31	4	4
18279	MUFFINS, CORN	1	LARGE	65.0	198	33	4	5
18283	MUFFINS, OAT BRAN	1	LARGE	65.0	176	31	5	5
18273	MUFFINS, PLAIN	1	LARGE	65.0	192	27	4	7
18287	MUFFINS, WHEAT BRAN	1	LARGE	65.0	184	27	5	8
11261	MUSHROOMS, CKD	½	CUP	78.0	21	4	2	0
11264	MUSHROOMS, CND, DRAINED SOLIDS	½	CUP	78.0	19	4	1	0
11260	MUSHROOMS, FRESH	½	CUP	35.0	9	2	1	0
20113	NOODLES, CHINESE, CHOW MEIN	½	CUP	22.5	119	13	2	7
20310	NOODLES, EGG, CKD, ENRICHED	½	CUP	80.0	106	20	4	1
20510	NOODLES, EGG, CKD, UNENRICHED	½	CUP	80.0	106	20	4	1
20112	NOODLES, EGG, SPINACH, CKD, ENRICHED	½	CUP	80.0	106	19	4	1
20115	NOODLES, JAPANESE, SOBA, CKD	½	CUP	57.0	56	12	3	0
15058	OCEAN PERCH, ATLANTIC, CKD, DRY HEAT	3	OUNCE	85.1	103	0	20	2
4053	OIL, OLIVE	1	TBSP.	13.5	119	0	0	14
4042	OIL, PEANUT	1	TBSP.	13.5	119	0	0	14
4058	OIL, SESAME	1	TBSP.	13.6	121	0	0	14
4044	OIL, SOYBEAN	1	TBSP.	13.6	121	0	0	14
4034	OIL, SOYBEAN, (HYDR)	1	TBSP.	13.6	121	0	0	14
4543	OIL, SOYBEAN, (HYDR)&CTTNSD	1	TBSP.	13.6	121	0	0	14
4518	OIL, VEGETABLE, CORN	1	TBSP.	13.6	121	0	0	14
4582	OIL, VEGETABLE, CANOLA	1	TBSP.	13.6	121	0	0	14
4501	OIL, VEGETABLE, COCOA BUTTER	1	TBSP.	13.6	121	0	0	14
4502	OIL, VEGETABLE, COTTONSEED	1	TBSP.	13.6	121	0	0	14

Saturated fat (g)	Monounsaturated fat (g)	Polyunsaturated fat (g)	Fiber (g)	Cholesterol (g)	Folate (g)	Vitamin A (RE)	Vitamin B$_6$ (mg)	Vitamin B$_{12}$ (µg)	Vitamin C (mg)	Vitamin E (mg)	Riboflavin (mg)	Thiamin (mg)	Calcium (mg)	Iron (mg)	Magnesium (mg)	Niacin (mg)	Phosphorus (mg)	Potassium (mg)	Sodium (mg)	Zinc (mg)
0	0	0	1	0	767	146	0	0	13	-	.1	.1	20	.6	3	.3	25	162	4	.1
0	0	0	0	61	9	22	.1	2.6	0	-	.1	0	52	.3	30	.9	157	299	323	2.5
8	-	-	16	40	-	100	-	-	0	-	-	-	240	1.5	-	-	-	-	1029	-
0	0	0	2	0	10	0	0	0	0	-	.1	.3	10	2	25	2.3	76	43	1	.7
0	0	0	2	0	10	-	0	0	0	-	0	0	10	.7	25	.6	76	43	1	.7
0	0	0	6	0	8	7	0	0	0	-	.1	.2	15	.7	25	1.4	67	42	8	.6
0	0	0	6	0	7	0	.1	0	0	-	.1	.2	21	1.5	42	1	125	62	4	1.1
-	-	-	-	0	-	0	-	-	30	-	-	-	0	0	-	-	-	-	18	-
0	0	0	1	0	-	321	.1	0	23	.9	0	0	8	.1	7	.5	9	129	2	0
0	1	1	0	0	0	48	0	0	0	.2	0	0	1	0	0	0	1	1	46	0
1	2	1	0	0	0	47	0	0	0	.4	0	0	1	0	0	0	1	2	44	0
1	1	2	0	0	0	47	0	0	0	.3	0	0	1	0	0	0	1	2	51	0
1	2	1	-	0	17	120	.3	0	16	-	.1	.1	22	1	30	2	44	530	786	.3
-	-	-	0	0	7	1	0	0	1	-	0	0	8	0	0	0	1	7	11	0
-	-	-	0	0	0	0	0	0	0	-	0	.1	1	.1	1	0	4	2	22	0
1	1	3	0	4	1	12	0	0	0	.6	0	0	2	0	0	0	4	1	104	0
0	-	-	0	0	0	0	-	-	0	-	-	-	0	0	-	-	-	1	105	-
0	-	-	-	5	-	0	-	-	0	-	-	-	0	0	-	-	-	5	130	-
-	-	-	1	0	14	258	.1	0	34	.1	0	0	9	.2	9	.5	14	247	7	.1
-	-	-	1	0-	-	5	-	0	26	-	0	.1	8	.7	13	.7	11	344	20	-
-	-	-	1	0	-	5	.1	0	32	-	0	.1	8	.1	9	8	13	350	13	-
8	4	0	2	10	3	21	0	.2	0	-	.1	0	84	.6	26	.1	95	169	36	.6
4	4	1	1	3	2	0	.1	.1	0	-	0	0	29	.4	26	1.2	60	142	12	.5
2	1	0	1	1	1	2	0	.1	0	-	0	0	24	.5	13	.1	41	146	10	.2
7	6	1	3	8	5	6	0	.2	0	-	.2	0	92	.7	37	.3	108	182	30	.5
6	3	0	1	36	17	73	.1	1.1	0	-	.8	.2	456	1.1	55	.4	435	774	383	1.7
7	3	0	0	41	23	97	.1	1.8	0	-	.7	.1	505	.3	41	.5	398	631	330	1.3
1	1	0	0	9	12	20	.1	.5	2	-	.4	.1	285	.1	27	.1	219	371	257	1
3	1	0	4	17	12	142	.1	.8	2	-	.4	.1	284	.6	33	.3	254	150		1
5	2	0	4	30	12	72	.1	.8	2	-	.4	.1	280	.6	33	.3	251	417	149	1
4	2	0	0	26	9	62	0	.3	2	-	.3	.1	216	.1	20	.2	193	284	97	.7
2	1	0	0	10	12	144	.1	.9	2	-	.4	.1	300	.1	34	.2	235	381	123	1
3	1	0	0	18	12	139	.1	.9	2	-	.4	.1	297	.1	33	.2	232	377	122	1
0	0	0	0	4	13	149	.1	.9	2	-	.3	.1	302	.1	28	.2	247	406	126	1
5	2	0	0	33	12	76	.1	.9	2	-	.4	.1	291	.1	33	.2	228	370	120	.9
6	3	0	0	35	12	83	.1	.9	4	-	.4	.1	290	.1	33	.2	227	368	119	.9
1	2	1	2	20	10	-	0	.4	1	-	.1	.1	37	1	10	.7	128	80	291	.3
1	2	2	-	33	22	23	.1	.1	0	-	.2	.2	48	1.8	24	1.3	185	45	339	.5
1	1	3	5	0	12	-	.1	0	0	-	.1	.2	41	2.7	102	.3	244	330	255	1.2
1	2	4	2	25	8	26	0	.1	0	-	.2	.2	130	1.6	11	1.5	99	79	304	.4
1	2	4	-	21	34	163	.2	.1	5	-	.3	.2	122	2.7	51	2.6	185	207	382	1.8
0	0	0	2	0	14	0	.1	0	3	-	.2	.1	5	1.4	9	3.5	68	278	2	.7
0	0	0	2	0	10	0	0	0	0	-	0	.1	9	.6	12	1.2	51	101	332	.6
0	0	0	0	0	7	0	0	0	1	-	.2	0	2	.4	4	1.4	36	130	1	.3
1	2	4	1	0	5	2	0	0	0	-	.1	.1	5	1.1	12	1.3	36	27	99	.3
0	0	0	-	26	6	5	0	.1	0	-	.1	.1	10	1.3	15	1.2	55	22	132	.5
0	0	0	-	26	6	5	0	.1	0	-	0	0	10	.5	15	.3	55	22	132	.5
0	0	0	2	26	17	11	.1	.1	0	-	.1	.2	15	.9	19	1.2	46	30	10	.5
0	0	0	-	0	4	0	0	0	0	-	0	.1	2	.3	5	.3	14	20	34	.1
0	1	0	0	46	9	12	.2	1	1	-	.1	.1	117	1	33	2.1	236	298	82	.5
2	10	1	0	0	0	0	0	0	0	1.6	0	0	0	.1	0	0	0	0	0	0
2	6	4	0	0	0	0	0	0	0	1.6	0	0	0	0	0	0	0	0	0	0
2	5	6	0	0	0	0	0	0	0	.2	0	0	0	0	0	0	0	0	0	0
2	3	8	0	0	0	0	0	0	0	1.5	0	0	0	0	0	0	0	0	0	0
2	6	5	0	0	0	0	0	0	0	1.1	0	0	0	0	0	0	0	0	0	0
2	4	7	0	0	0	0	0	0	0	1.7	0	0	0	0	0	0	0	0	0	0
2	3	8	0	0	0	0	0	0	0	2	0	0	0	0	0	0	0	0	0	0
1	8	4	0	-	0	0	0	0	0	0	0	0	0	0	0	0	0	0	0	0
8	4	0	0	0	0	0	0	0	0	.2	0	0	0	0	0	0	0	0	0	0
4	2	7	0	0	0	0	0	0	0	4.8	-	0	0	0	0	0	0	0	0	0

Food Composition Table—cont'd

Code	Name	Amount	Unit	Grams	Kilocalories	Carbohydrates (g)	Protein (g)	Fat (g)
4055	OIL, VEGETABLE, PALM	1	TBSP.	13.6	121	0	0	14
4513	OIL, VEGETABLE, PALM KERNEL	1	TBSP.	13.6	118	0	0	14
4510	OIL, VEGETABLE, SAFFLOWER, LINOLEIC	1	TBSP.	13.6	121	0	0	14
4511	OIL, VEGETABLE, SAFFLOWER, OLEIC	1	TBSP.	13.6	121	0	0	14
4584	OIL, VEGETABLE, SUNFLOWER	1	TBSP.	13.6	121	0	0	14
11279	OKRA, CKD	½	CUP	80.0	26	6	1	0
11278	OKRA, FRESH	½	CUP	50.0	19	4	1	0
11281	OKRA, FRZ, CKD	½	CUP	92.0	34	8	2	0
11280	OKRA, FRZ, UNPREPARED	½	CUP	71.3	21	5	1	0
10161	OLIVE LOAF, LUNCH MEAT	1	SLICE	28.4	67	3	3	5
9194	OLIVES, RIPE, CANNED (JUMBO-SUPER COLOSSAL)	1	JUMBO	8.3	7	0	0	1
9193	OLIVES, RIPE, CANNED (SMALL-EXTRA LARGE)	1	SMALL	3.2	4	0	0	0
11282	ONIONS, FRESH	½	CUP	79.9	30	7	1	0
9206	ORANGE JUICE, FRESH	¾	CUP	186.0	84	19	1	0
9215	ORANGE JUICE, FROM CONCENTRATE	¾	CUP	186.4	84	20	1	0
9200	ORANGES, FRESH	1	MEDIUM	131.0	62	15	1	0
15168	OYSTER, EASTERN, BREADED AND FRIED	3	OUNCE	85.1	168	10	7	11
15170	OYSTER, EASTERN, CND	3	OUNCE	85.1	59	3	6	2
18390	PANCAKES, BUTTERMILK	1	4 IN.	9.5	22	3	1	1
18293	PANCAKES, PLAIN	1	4 IN.	9.5	22	3	1	1
18300	PANCAKES, WHOLE-WHEAT	1	4 IN.	44.0	92	13	4	3
9226	PAPAYAS, FRESH	1	MEDIUM	304.0	119	30	2	0
11808	PARSNIPS, CKD, W/ SALT	½	CUP	78.0	63	15	1	0
11299	PARSNIPS, CKD, W/O SALT	½	CUP	78.0	63	15	1	0
11298	PARSNIPS, FRESH	½	CUP	66.5	50	12	1	0
20321	PASTA, CKD, ENRICHED, W/ ADDED SALT	½	CUP	70.0	99	20	3	0
20121	PASTA, CKD, ENRICHED, W/O ADDED SALT	½	CUP	70.0	99	20	3	0
20094	PASTA, FRESH-REFRIGERATED, PLAIN, CKD	½	CUP	73.0	96	18	4	1
20096	PASTA, FRESH-REFRIGERATED, SPINACH, CKD	½	CUP	73.0	95	18	4	1
20097	PASTA, HOMEMADE, MADE W/ EGG, CKD	½	CUP	73.6	96	17	4	1
20098	PASTA, HOMEMADE, MADE W/O EGG, CKD	½	CUP	73.6	91	18	3	1
20127	PASTA, SPINACH, CKD	½	CUP	70.0	91	18	3	0
20125	PASTA, WHOLE-WHEAT, CKD	½	CUP	70.0	87	19	4	0
9251	PEACH NECTAR, CND, W/O ADDED VIT C	¾	CUP	186.4	101	26	1	0
9238	PEACHES, CND, JUICE PACK	½	CUP	124.0	55	14	1	0
9240	PEACHES, CND, LIGHT SYRUP PACK	½	CUP	125.5	68	18	1	0
9237	PEACHES, CND, WATER PACK	½	CUP	122.0	29	7	1	0
9246	PEACHES, DRIED, SULFURED	¼	CUP	40.0	96	25	1	0
9236	PEACHES, FRESH	1	MEDIUM	87.0	37	10	1	0
9250	PEACHES, FROZEN, SLICED, SWEETENED	½	CUP	125.0	118	30	1	0
16097	PEANUT BUTTER, CHUNK STYLE, W/ SALT	2	TBSP.	32.3	190	7	8	16
16098	PEANUT BUTTER, SMOOTH STYLE, W/ SALT	2	TBSP.	32.3	190	7	8	16
16088	PEANUTS, ALL TYPES, CKD, BOILED, W/ SALT	½	CUP	31.5	100	7	4	7
16090	PEANUTS, ALL TYPES, DRY-ROASTED, W/ SALT	½	CUP	73.0	427	16	17	36
16390	PEANUTS, ALL TYPES, DRY-ROASTED, W/O SALT	½	CUP	73.0	427	16	17	36
16087	PEANUTS, ALL TYPES, FRESH	½	CUP	73.0	414	12	19	36
16089	PEANUTS, ALL TYPES, OIL-ROASTED, W/ SALT	½	CUP	72.0	418	14	19	35
16389	PEANUTS, ALL TYPES, OIL-ROASTED, W/O SALT	½	CUP	72.0	418	14	19	35
9340	PEARS, ASIAN, FRESH	1	MEDIUM	122.0	51	13	1	0
9254	PEARS, CND, JUICE PACK	½	CUP	124.0	62	16	0	0
9253	PEARS, CND, WATER PACK	½	CUP	122.0	35	10	0	0
9252	PEARS, FRESH	1	MEDIUM	166.0	98	25	1	1
11300	PEAS, EDIBLE-PODDED, FRESH	½	CUP	72.5	30	5	2	0
11305	PEAS, GREEN, CKD	½	CUP	80.0	67	13	4	0
11308	PEAS, GREEN, CND	½	CUP	85.0	59	11	4	0
11304	PEAS, GREEN, FRESH	½	CUP	72.5	59	10	4	0
11313	PEAS, GREEN, FRZ, CKD	½	CUP	80.0	62	11	4	0
12142	PECANS, DRIED	½	CUP	54.0	360	10	4	37
11329	PEPPERS, HOT CHILI, GREEN, CND	1	EACH	73.0	18	4	1	0
11670	PEPPERS, HOT CHILI, GREEN, FRESH	1	EACH	45.0	18	4	1	0

Saturated fat (g)	Monounsaturated fat (g)	Polyunsaturated fat (g)	Fiber (g)	Cholesterol (g)	Folate (g)	Vitamin A (RE)	Vitamin B6 (mg)	Vitamin B12 (µg)	Vitamin C (mg)	Vitamin E (mg)	Riboflavin (mg)	Thiamin (mg)	Calcium (mg)	Iron (mg)	Magnesium (mg)	Niacin (mg)	Phosphorus (mg)	Potassium (mg)	Sodium (mg)	Zinc (mg)
7	5	1	0	0	0	0	0	0	0	2.6	0	0	0	0	0	0	0	0	0	-
11	2	0	0	0	0	0	0	0	0	-	0	0	0	0	0	0	0	0	0	-
1	2	10	0	0	0	0	0	0	0	4.7	0	0	0	0	0	0	0	0	0	0
1	10	2	0	0	0	0	0	0	0	4.7	0	0	0	0	0	0	0	0	0	0
1	11	1	0	-	0	0	0	0	0	-	0	0	0	0	0	0	0	0	0	0
0	0	0	2	0	37	46	.1	0	13	-	0	.1	50	.4	46	.7	45	258	4	.4
0	0	0	1	0	44	33	.1	0	11	-	0	.1	41	.4	29	.5	32	152	4	.3
0	0	0	3	0	134	47	0	0	11	-	.1	.1	88	.6	47	.7	42	215	3	.6
0	0	0	2	0	105	33	0	0	9	-	.1	.1	58	.4	31	.5	30	150	2	.4
2	2	1	0	11	1	6	.1	.4	2	-	.1	.1	31	.2	5	.5	36	84	421	.4
0	0	0	-	0	0	3	0	0	0	-	0	0	8	.3	0	0	0	1	75	0
0	0	0	-	0	0	1	0	0	0	-	0	0	3	.1	0	0	0	0	28	0
0	0	0	1	0	15	0	.1	0	5	.2	0	0	16	.2	8	.1	26	125	2	.2
0	0	0	0	0	56	37	.1	0	93	.1	.1	.2	20	.4	20	.7	32	372	2	.1
0	0	0	0	0	82	15	.1	0	73	-	0	.1	17	.2	19	.4	30	354	2	.1
0	0	0	3	0	40	28	.1	0	70	.3	.1	.1	52	.1	13	.4	18	237	0	.1
3	4	3	-	69	12	77	.1	13.3	3	-	.2	.1	53	5.9	49	1.4	135	208	355	74.1
1	0	1	0	47	8	77	.1	16.3	4	-	.1	.1	38	5.7	46	1.1	118	195	95	77.4
0	0	0	-	6	1	3	0	0	0	-	0		15	.2	1	.1	13	14	50	.1
0	0	0	-	6	1	5	0	0	0	-	0	0	21	.2	2	.1	15	13	42	.1
1	1	1	-	27	9	28	-	.1	0	-	.2	.1	110	1.4	20	1	164	123	252	.5
0	0	0	5	0	116	85	.1	0	188	-	.1	.1	73	.3	30	1	15	781	9	.2
0	0	0	-	0	45	0	.1	0	10	-	0	.1	29	.5	23	.6	54	286	192	.2
0	0	0	-	0	45	0	.1	0	10	-	0	.1	29	.5	23	.6	54	286	8	.2
0	0	0	3	0	44	0	.1	0	11	-	0	.1	24	.4	19	.5	47	249	7	.4
0	0	0	-	0	5	-	0	0	0	-	.1	.1	5	1	13	1.2	38	22	70	.4
0	0	01	0	0	5	-	0	0	0	-	.1	.1	5	1	13	1.2	38	22	1	.4
0	0	0	-	24	5	4	0	.1	0	-	.1	.2	4	.8	13	.7	46	18	4	.4
0	0	0	-	24	13	10	.1	.1	0	-	.1	.1	13	.8	18	.7	42	27	4	.5
0	0	0	-	30	14	13	0	.1	0	-	.1	.1	7	.9	10	.9	38	15	61	.3
0	0	0	-	0	13	0	0	0	0	-	.1	.1	4	.8	10	1	29	14	54	.3
0	0	0	-	0	8	11	.1	0	0	-	.1	.1	21	.7	43	1.1	76	41	10	.8
0	0	0	3	0	4	0	.1	0	0	-	0	.1	11	.7	21	.5	62	31	2	.6
0	0	0	1	0	3	48	0	0	10	-	0	0	9	.4	7	.5	11	75	13	.1
0	0	0	1	0	4	47	0	0	4	-	0	0	7	.3	9	.7	21	159	5	.1
0	0	0	1	0	4	44	0	0	3	-	0	0	4	.5	6	.7	14	122	6	.1
0	0	0	1	0	4	65	0	0	4	-	0	0	2	.4	6	.6	12	121	4	.1
0	0	0	3	0	0	86	0	0	2	-	.1	0	11	1.6	17	1.8	48	398	3	.2
0	0	0	2	0	3	47	0	0	6	-	0	0	4	.1	6	.9	10	171	0	.1
0	0	0	2	0	4	35	0	0	118	-	0	0	4	.5	6	.8	14	162	7	.1
3	8	5	2	0	30	0	.1	0	0	-	0	0	13	.6	51	4.4	102	241	157	.9
3	8	5	2	0	25	0	.1	0	0	-	0	0	11	.5	51	4.2	104	233	154	.8
1	3	2	3	0	23	0	0	0	0	-	0	.1	17	.3	32	1.7	62	57	237	.6
5	18	11	6	0	106	0	.2	0	0	5.7	.1	.3	39	1.6	128	9.9	261	480	593	2.4
5	18	11	6	0	106	0	.2	0	0	-	.1	.3	39	1.6	128	9.9	261	480	4	2.4
5	18	11	6	0	175	0	.3	0	0	6.1	.1	.5	67	3.3	123	8.8	274	515	13	2.4
5	18	11	7	0	91	0	.2	0	0	5	.1	.2	63	1.3	133	10.3	372	491	312	4.8
5	18	11	7	0	91	0	.2	0	0	-	.1	.2	63	1.3	133	10.3	372	491	4	4.8
0	0	0	4	0	10	0	0	0	5	-	0	0	5	0	10	.3	13	148	0	0
0	0	0	2	0	1	1	0	0	2	-	0	0	11	.4	9	.2	15	119	5	.1
0	0	0	2	0	1	0	0	0	1	-	0	0	5	.3	5	.1	9	65	2	.1
0	0	0	4	0	12	3	0	0	7	-	.1	0	18	.4	10	.2	18	208	0	.2
0	0	0	2	0	30	10	.1	0	44	-	.1	.1	31	1.5	17	.4	38	145	3	.2
0	0	0	4	0	51	48	.2	0	11	-	.1	.2	22	1.2	31	1.6	94	217	2	1
0	0	0	3	0	38	65	.1	0	8	-	.1	.1	17	.8	14	.6	57	147	186	.6
0	0	0	4	0	47	46	.1	0	29	.1	.1	.2	18	1.1	24	1.5	78	177	4	.9
0	0	0	4	0	47	54	.1	0	8	-	.1	.2	19	1.3	23	1.2	72	134	70	.9
3	23	9	4	0	21	7	.1	0	1	-	.1	.5	19	1.2	69	.5	157	212	1	3
0	0	0	1	0	7	45	.1	0	50	-	0	0	5	.4	10	.6	12	137	856	.1
0	0	0	1	0	11	35	.1	0	109	-	0	0	8	.5	11	.4	21	153	3	.1

Food Composition Table—cont'd

Code	Name	Amount	Unit	Grams	Kilocalories	Carbohydrates (g)	Protein (g)	Fat (g)
11820	PEPPERS, HOT CHILI, RED, CND	1	EACH	73.0	18	4	1	0
11819	PEPPERS, HOT CHILI, RED, FRESH	1	EACH	45.0	18	4	1	0
11632	PEPPERS, JALAPEÑO, CND	¼	CUP	34.0	8	2	0	0
11333	PEPPERS, SWEET, GREEN, FRESH	1	MEDIUM	74.0	20	5	1	0
11821	PEPPERS, SWEET, RED, FRESH	1	MEDIUM	74.0	20	5	1	0
11951	PEPPERS, SWEET, YELLOW, FRESH	1	MEDIUM	74.0	20	5	1	0
11945	PICKLE RELISH, SWEET	1	TBSP.	15.0	19	5	0	0
11941	PICKLE, CUCUMBER, SOUR	1	SLICE	7.0	1	0	0	0
11937	PICKLE, CUCUMBER, DILL	1	SLICE	6.0	1	0	0	0
11940	PICKLE, CUCUMBER, SWEET	1	SLICE	6.0	7	2	0	0
9273	PINEAPPLE JUICE, CND	¾	CUP	187.6	105	26	1	0
9268	PINEAPPLE, CND, JUICE PACK	½	CUP	125.0	75	20	1	0
9267	PINEAPPLE, CND, WATER PACK	½	CUP	123.0	39	10	1	0
9266	PINEAPPLE, FRESH	1	SLICE	84.0	41	10	0	0
12652	PISTACHIO, DRY ROASTED	½	CUP	64.0	388	18	10	34
9282	PLUMS, CND, PURPLE, JUICE PACK	½	CUP	126.0	73	19	1	0
9281	PLUMS, CND, PURPLE, WATER PACK	½	CUP	124.5	51	14	0	0
9279	PLUMS, FRESH	1	MEDIUM	66.0	36	9	1	0
19034	POPCORN, AIR-POPPED	1	CUP	8.0	31	6	1	0
19036	POPCORN, CAKES	1	CAKE	10.0	38	8	1	0
19038	POPCORN, CARAMEL-COATED, W/ PEANUTS	1	CUP	35.2	141	28	2	3
19039	POPCORN, CARAMEL-COATED, W/O PEANUTS	1	CUP	35.2	152	28	1	5
19040	POPCORN, CHEESE-FLAVOR	1	CUP	11.0	58	6	1	4
19035	POPCORN, OIL-POPPED	1	CUP	11.0	55	6	1	3
19408	PORK SKINS, BARBECUE-FLAVOR	1	OUNCE	28.4	153	0	16	9
19041	PORK SKINS, PLAIN	1	OUNCE	28.4	155	0	17	9
10193	PORK, BACKRIBS	3	OUNCE	85.1	315	0	21	25
10127	PORK, BRAUNSCHWEIGER	3	OUNCE	85.1	305	3	11	27
10220	PORK, GROUND, CKD	3	OUNCE	85.1	253	0	22	18
10154	PORK, HAM AND CHEESE LOAF OR ROLL	3	OUNCE	85.1	220	1	14	17
10147	PORK, HAM PATTIES, GRILLED	3	OUNCE	85.1	291	1	11	26
10148	PORK, HAM SALAD SPREAD	3	OUNCE	85.1	184	9	7	13
10185	PORK, HAM, CND, EXTRA LEAN AND REG, ROASTED	3	OUNCE	85.1	142	0	18	7
10140	PORK, HAM, CND, REGULAR (APPROX 13% FAT), ROASTED	3	OUNCE	85.1	192	0	17	13
10134	PORK, HAM, EXTRA LEAN (5% FAT), ROASTED	3	OUNCE	85.1	123	1	18	5
10133	PORK, HAM, EXTRA LEAN (5% FAT), UNHEATED	3	OUNCE	85.1	111	1	16	4
10183	PORK, HAM, EXTRA LEAN AND REG, ROASTED	3	OUNCE	85.1	140	0	19	7
10182	PORK, HAM, EXTRA LEAN AND REG, UNHEATED	3	OUNCE	85.1	138	2	16	7
10151	PORK, HAM, MEAT AND FAT, ROASTED	3	OUNCE	85.1	207	0	18	14
10153	PORK, HAM, MEAT ONLY, ROASTED	3	OUNCE	85.1	134	0	21	5
10136	PORK, HAM, REGULAR (11% FAT), ROASTED	3	OUNCE	85.1	151	0	19	8
10135	PORK, HAM, REGULAR (11% FAT), UNHEATED	3	OUNCE	85.1	155	3	15	9
10172	PORK, SMOKED LINK SAUSAGE, GRILLED	3	OUNCE	85.1	331	2	19	27
10089	PORK, SPARERIBS, MEAT AND FAT, CKD, BRAISED	3	OUNCE	85.1	338	0	25	26
10221	PORK, TENDERLOIN, MEAT AND FAT, CKD, BROILED	3	OUNCE	85.1	171	0	25	7
10223	PORK, TENDERLOIN, MEAT ONLY, CKD, BROILED	3	OUNCE	85.1	159	0	26	5
19042	POTATO CHIPS, BARBECUE-FLAVOR	1	OUNCE	28.4	139	15	2	9
19421	POTATO CHIPS, CHEESE-FLAVOR	1	OUNCE	28.4	141	16	2	8
19422	POTATO CHIPS, LIGHT	1	OUNCE	28.4	134	19	2	6
19411	POTATO CHIPS, PLAIN, SALTED	1	OUNCE	28.4	152	15	2	10
19811	POTATO CHIPS, PLAIN, UNSALTED	1	OUNCE	28.4	152	15	2	10
19043	POTATO CHIPS, SOUR-CREAM-AND-ONION-FLAVOR	1	OUNCE	28.4	151	15	2	10
11672	POTATO PANCAKES, HOME-PREPARED	1	OUNCE	28.4	77	8	2	4
11414	POTATO SALAD	½	CUP	125.0	179	14	3	10
19415	POTATO STICKS	1	OUNCE	28.4	148	15	2	10
11843	POTATOES, AU GRATIN, HOME-PREPARED	½	CUP	122.5	162	14	6	9
11363	POTATOES, BAKED, W/O SKIN	1	MEDIUM	202.0	188	44	4	0
11674	POTATOES, BAKED, W/ SKIN	1	MEDIUM	202.0	220	51	5	0
11365	POTATOES, BOILED, CKD IN SKIN, W/O SKIN	1	MEDIUM	202.0	176	41	4	0
11367	POTATOES, BOILED, CKD, W/O SKIN	1	MEDIUM	202.0	174	40	3	0

Saturated fat (g)	Monounsaturated fat (g)	Polyunsaturated fat (g)	Fiber (g)	Cholesterol (g)	Folate (g)	Vitamin A (RE)	Vitamin B6 (mg)	Vitamin B12 (ug)	Vitamin C (mg)	Vitamin E (mg)	Riboflavin (mg)	Thiamin (mg)	Calcium (mg)	Iron (mg)	Magnesium (mg)	Niacin (mg)	Phosphorus (mg)	Potassium (mg)	Sodium (mg)	Zinc (mg)
0	0	0	1	0	7	868	.1	0	50	-	0	0	5	.4	10	.6	12	137	856	.1
0	0	0	1	0	11	484	.1	0	109	-	0	0	8	.5	11	.4	21	153	3	.1
0	0	0	-	0	5	58	.1	0	4	-	0	0	9	1	4	.2	6	46	497	.1
0	0	0	1	0	16	47	.2	0	66	.5	0	0	7	.3	7	.4	14	131	1	.1
0	0	0	2	0	16	422	.2	0	141	.5	0	0	7	.3	7	.4	14	131	1	.1
-	-	-	-	0	19	18	.1	0	136	-	0	0	8	.3	9	.7	18	157	1	.1
0	0	0	-	0	0	2	0	0	0	-	0	0	0	.1	1	0	2	4	122	0
0	0	0	0	0	0	1	0	0	0	-	0	0	0	0	0	0	1	2	85	0
0	0	0	0	0	0	2	0	0	0	-	0	0	1	0	1	0	1	7	77	0
0	0	0	0	0	0	1	0	0	0	-	0	0	0	0	0	0	1	2	56	0
0	0	0	0	0	43	0	.2	0	20	-	0	.1	32	.5	24	.5	15	251	2	.2
0	0	0	1	0	6	5	.1	0	12	-	0	.1	17	.3	17	.4	7	152	1	.1
0	0	0	1	0	6	1	.1	0	9	-	0	.1	18	.5	20	.4	9	132	1	.2
0	0	0	1	0	6	2	.1	0	9	-	0	.1	18	.5	22	.4	5	156	1	.1
4	23	5	7	0	38	15	.2	0	5	-	.2	.3	45	2	83	.9	305	621	499	.9
0	0	0	1	0	3	127	0	0	4	-	.1	0	13	.4	10	.6	19	194	1	.1
0	0	0	1	0	3	113	0	0	3	-	.1	0	9	.2	6	.5	16	157	1	.1
0	0	0	1	0	1	21	.1	0	6	-	.1	0	3	.1	5	.3	7	114	0	.1
0	0	0	1	0	2	2	0	0	0	-	0	0	1	.2	10	.2	24	24	0	.3
0	0	0	0	0	2	1	0	0	0	-	0	0	1	.2	16	.6	28	33	29	.4
0	1	1	1	0	6	2	.1	0	0	-	0	0	23	1.4	28	.7	45	125	104	.4
1	1	2	2	2	1	4	0	0	0	-	0	0	15	.6	12	.8	29	38	73	.2
1	1	2	1	1	1	5	0	.1	0	-	0	0	12	.2	10	.2	40	29	98	.2
1	1	1	1	0	2	2	0	0	0	-	0	0	1	.3	12	.2	27	25	97	.3
3	4	1	-	33	9	52	0	0	0	-	.1	0	12	.3	0	1	62	51	756	.2
3	4	1	-	27	0	11	0	.2	0	-	.1	0	9	.2	3	.4	24	36	521	.2
9	11	2	-	100	3	3	.3	.5	0	-	.2	.4	38	1.2	18	3	166	268	86	2.9
9	13	3	0	133	37	3589	.3	17.1	8	-	1.3	.2	8	8	9	7.1	143	169	972	2.4
7	8	2	0	80	5	2	.3	.5	1	-	.2	.6	19	1.1	20	3.6	192	308	62	2.7
6	8	2	0	48	3	20	.2	.7	21	-	.2	.5	49	.8	14	2.9	215	250	1142	1.7
9	12	34	0	61	3	0	.1	.6	0	-	.2	.3	8	1.4	9	2.8	86	208	904	1.6
4	6	2	0	31	1	0	.1	.6	5	-	.1	.4	7	.5	9	1.8	102	128	776	.9
2	3	1	0	35	4	0	.3	.7	19	-	.2	.8	6	.9	17	4.3	188	299	908	2
4	6	2	0	53	4	0	.3	.9	12	-	.2	.7	7	1.2	14	4.5	207	304	800	2.1
2	2	0	0	45	3	0	.3	.6	18	-	.2	.6	7	1.3	12	3.4	167	244	1023	2.4
1	2	0	0	40	3	0	.4	.6	22	-	.2	.8	6	.6	14	4.1	185	298	1215	1.6
2	3	1	0	48	3	0	.3	.6	19	-	.2	.6	7	1.2	16	4.5	211	308	1178	2.2
2	3	1	0	45	3	0	.3	.7	23	-	.2	.8	6	.8	15	4.3	201	253	1087	1.7
5	7	2	0	53	3	0	.3	.5	-	-	.2	.5	6	.7	16	3.8	182	243	1010	2
2	2	1	0	47	3	0	.4	.6	-	-	.2	.6	6	.8	19	4.3	193	269	1129	2.2
3	4	1	0	50	3	0	.3	.6	19	-	.3	.6	7	1.1	19	5.2	239	348	1276	2.1
3	4	1	0	48	3	0	.3	.7	24	-	.3	.7	6	.8	16	4.5	210	282	1120	1.8
10	12	3	0	58	4	0	.3	1.4	2	-	.2	.6	26	1	16	3.9	138	286	1276	2.4
9	11	2	0	103	3	3	.3	.9	-	-	.3	.3	40	1.6	20	4.7	222	272	79	3.9
2	3	1	-	80	5	2	.4	.8	1	-	.3	.8	4	1.2	30	4.3	247	378	54	2.5
2	2	0	-	80	5	2	.4	.9	1	-	.3	.8	4	1.2	31	4.4	251	384	55	2.5
2	2	5	1	0	24	6	.2	0	10	-	.1	.1	14	.5	21	1.3	53	357	213	.3
2	2	3	-	1	0	2	.1	0	15	-	0	0	20	.5	21	1.4	85	433	225	.3
1	1	3	-	0	8	0	.2	0	7	-	.1	.1	6	.4	25	2	55	494	139	0
3	3	3	1	0	13	0	.2	0	9	-	.1	0	7	.5	19	1.1	47	361	168	.3
3	3	3	-	0	13	0	.2	0	9	-	.1	0	7	.5	19	1.1	47	361	2	.3
3	2	5	1	2	18	6	.2	.3	11	-	.1	.1	20	.5	21	1.1	50	377	177	.3
1	1	2	1	27	7	4	.1	.1	6	-	0	0	7	.4	9	.6	31	223	144	.2
2	3	5	-	85	8	41	.2	0	12	-	.1	.1	24	.8	19	1.1	65	317	661	.4
3	2	5	1	0	11	0	.2	0	13	-	0	0	5	.6	18	1.4	49	351	71	.3
4	3	1	-	18	10	47	.2	0	12	-	.1	.1	146	.8	24	1.2	138	485	530	.8
0	0	0	3	0	18	0	.6	0	26	-	0	.2	10	.7	51	2.8	101	790	10	.6
0	0	0	5	0	22	0	.7	0	26	-	.1	.2	20	2.7	55	3.3	115	844	16	.6
0	0	0	4	0	20	0	.6	0	26	-	0	.2	10	.6	44	2.9	89	766	8	.6
0	0	0	4	0	18	0	.5	0	15	-	0	.2	16	.6	40	2.7	81	663	10	.5

Food Composition Table—cont'd

Code	Name	Amount	Unit	Grams	Kilocalories	Carbohydrates (g)	Protein (g)	Fat (g)
11370	POTATOES, HASHED BROWN	½	CUP	78.0	119	6	2	11
11657	POTATOES, MASHED, HOME-PREPARED	½	CUP	105.0	81	18	2	1
11671	POTATOES, O'BRIEN, HOME-PREPARED	½	CUP	97.0	79	15	2	1
11844	POTATOES, SCALLOPED	½	CUP	122.5	105	13	4	5
19047	PRETZELS, HARD, PLAIN, SALTED	1	OUNCE	28.4	108	22	3	1
19814	PRETZELS, HARD, PLAIN, UNSALTED	1	OUNCE	28.4	108	22	3	1
19050	PRETZELS, HARD, WHOLE-WHEAT	1	OUNCE	28.4	103	23	3	1
9294	PRUNE JUICE, CND	¾	CUP	191.8	136	33	1	0
9289	PRUNES, DEHYDRATED	¼	CUP	33.0	112	29	1	0
9293	PRUNES, DRIED, STEWED, W/ ADDED SUGAR	¼	CUP	59.5	74	20	1	0
9292	PRUNES, DRIED, STEWED, W/O ADDED SUGAR	¼	CUP	53.0	57	15	1	0
9291	PRUNES, DRIED, UNCOOKED	¼	CUP	40.3	96	25	1	0
11429	RADISHES, FRESH	½	CUP	58.0	10	2	0	0
11431	RADISHES, ORIENTAL, CKD	½	CUP	73.5	12	3	0	0
11432	RADISHES, ORIENTAL, DRIED	½	CUP	58.0	157	37	5	0
11430	RADISHES, ORIENTAL, FRESH	½	CUP	44.0	8	2	0	0
9297	RAISINS, GOLDEN SEEDLESS	½	CUP	72.5	219	58	2	0
9299	RAISINS, SEEDED	½	CUP	72.5	215	57	2	0
9298	RAISINS, SEEDLESS	½	CUP	72.5	218	57	2	0
9302	RASPBERRIES, FRESH	½	CUP	61.5	30	7	1	0
9306	RASPBERRIES, FROZEN, RED, SWEETENED	½	CUP	125.0	129	33	1	0
62536	RAVIOLI, BEEF	1	CUP	243.9	230	36	9	5
62537	RAVIOLI, CHEESE	1	CUP	243.9	220	38	9	3
62557	RED BEANS AND RICE	2	OUNCE	56.7	189	40	8	1
19051	RICE CAKES, BROWN RICE, PLAIN	1	CAKE	9.0	35	7	1	0
19816	RICE CAKES, BROWN RICE, PLAIN, UNSALTED	1	CAKE	9.0	35	7	1	0
19193	RICE PUDDING	1	CUP	298.1	486	66	6	22
20037	RICE, BROWN, LONG-GRAIN, CKD	½	CUP	97.5	108	22	3	1
20045	RICE, WHITE, LONG-GRAIN, CKD	½	CUP	79.0	103	22	2	0
20049	RICE, WHITE, LONG-GRAIN, INSTANT, ENRICHED	½	CUP	82.5	81	18	2	0
20053	RICE, WHITE, SHORT-GRAIN, CKD	½	CUP	93.0	121	27	2	0
20057	RICE, WHITE, W/ PASTA, CKD	½	CUP	101.0	123	22	3	3
15232	ROUGHY, ORANGE, CKD, DRY HEAT	3	OUNCE	85.1	76	0	16	1
62541	SALAD DRESSING, BLUE CHEESE	2	TBSP.	32.0	90	5	1	7
62542	SALAD DRESSING, BLUE CHEESE, FAT FREE	2	TBSP.	35.0	50	12	1	0
4120	SALAD DRESSING, FRENCH	2	TBSP.	31.3	134	5	0	13
62545	SALAD DRESSING, FRENCH, FAT FREE	2	TBSP.	35.0	50	12	0	0
4020	SALAD DRESSING, FRENCH, LO FAT	2	TBSP.	32.5	44	7	0	2
4114	SALAD DRESSING, ITALIAN	2	TBSP.	29.4	137	3	0	14
62543	SALAD DRESSING, ITALIAN, FAT FREE	2	TBSP.	31.0	10	2	0	0
4021	SALAD DRESSING, ITALIAN, LO CAL	2	TBSP.	30.0	32	1	0	3
62539	SALAD DRESSING, RANCH	2	TBSP.	29.0	170	2	0	18
62540	SALAD DRESSING, RANCH, FAT FREE	2	TBSP.	35.0	50	11	0	0
4015	SALAD DRESSING, RUSSIAN	2	TBSP.	30.7	151	3	0	16
4022	SALAD DRESSING, RUSSIAN, LOW CAL	2	TBSP.	32.5	46	9	0	1
4016	SALAD DRESSING, SESAME SEED	2	TBSP.	30.7	136	3	1	14
4017	SALAD DRESSING, THOUSAND ISLAND	2	TBSP.	31.3	118	5	0	11
4023	SALAD DRESSING, THOUSAND ISLAND, LO CAL	2	TBSP.	30.7	49	5	0	3
62544	SALAD DRESSING, THOUSAND ISLAND, FAT FREE	2	TBSP.	35.0	45	11	0	0
4135	SALAD DRESSING, VINEGAR AND OIL	2	TBSP.	31.3	140	1	0	16
15209	SALMON, ATLANTIC, WILD, CKD, DRY HEAT	3	OUNCE	85.1	155	0	22	7
15212	SALMON, PINK, CKD, DRY HEAT	3	OUNCE	85.1	127	0	22	4
62546	SALSA	2	TBSP.	33.0	20	5	0	0
15088	SARDINE, ATLANTIC, CND IN OIL	3	OUNCE	85.1	177	0	21	10
6313	SAUCE, WHITE	½	CUP	131.9	120	11	5	7
11439	SAUERKRAUT, CND, SOL&LIQ	½	CUP	118.0	22	5	1	0
7003	SAUSAGE, BEERWURST, PORK	1	SLICE	23.0	55	0	3	4
7006	SAUSAGE, BOCKWURST	1	LINK	65.0	200	0	9	18
7013	SAUSAGE, BRATWURST	1	LINK	85.0	256	2	12	22

Saturated fat (g)	Monounsaturated fat (g)	Polyunsaturated fat (g)	Fiber (g)	Cholesterol (g)	Folate (g)	Vitamin A (RE)	Vitamin B6 (mg)	Vitamin B12 (ug)	Vitamin C (mg)	Vitamin E (mg)	Riboflavin (mg)	Thiamin (mg)	Calcium (mg)	Iron (mg)	Magnesium (mg)	Niacin (mg)	Phosphorus (mg)	Potassium (mg)	Sodium (mg)	Zinc (mg)
4	5	1	2	-	6	0	.2	0	4	-	0	.1	6	.6	16	1.6	33	250	19	.2
0	0	0	2	2	9	20	.2	0	7	-	0	.1	27	.3	19	1.2	50	314	318	.3
1	0	0	-	4	8	55	.2	0	16	-	.1	.1	35	.5	17	1	49	258	210	.3
2	2	1	-	7	11	23	.2	0	13	-	.1	.1	70	.7	23	1.3	77	463	410	.5
0	0	0	1	0	24	0	0	0	0	-	.2	.1	10	1.2	10	1.5	32	41	486	.2
0	0	0	1	0	24	0	0	0	0	-	.2	.1	10	1.2	10	1.5	32	41	82	.2
0	0	0	-	0	15	-0	.1	0	0	-	.1	.1	8	.8	9	1.9	35	122	58	.2
0	0	0	2	0	1	0	.4	0	8	-	.1	0	23	2.3	27	1.5	48	529	8	.4
0	0	0	-	0	1	58	.2	0	0	-	.1	0	24	1.2	21	1	37	349	2	.2
0	0	0	2	0	0	17	.1	0	2	-	.1	0	12	.6	11	.4	20	186	1	.1
0	0	0	3	0	0	16	.1	0	2	-	.1	0	12	.6	11	.4	19	177	1	.1
0	0	0	3	0	1	80	.1	0	1	-	.1	0	21	1	18	.8	32	300	2	.2
0	0	0	1	0	16	1	0	0	13	-	0	0	12	.2	5	.2	10	135	14	.1
0	0	0	1	0	13	0	0	0	11	-	0	0	12	.1	7	.1	18	209	10	.1
0	0	0	-	0	171	0	.4	0	0	-	.4	.2	365	3.9	99	2	118	2027	161	1.2
0	0	0	1	0	12	0	0	0	10	-	0	0	12	.2	7	.1	10	100	9	.1
0	0	0	3	0	2	3	.2	0	2	-	.1	0	38	1.3	25	.8	83	541	9	.2
0	0	0	5	0	2	0	.1	0	4	-	.1	.1	20	1.9	22	.8	54	598	20	.1
0	0	0	3	0	2	1	.2	0	2	-	.1	.1	36	1.5	24	.6	70	544	9	.2
0	0	0	4	0	16	8	0	0	15	.2	.1	0	14	.4	11	.6	7	93	0	.3
0	0	0	5	0	32	7	0	0	21	-	.1	0	19	.8	16	.3	21	142	1	.2
2	-	-	4	20	-	150	-	-	2	-	-	-	0	1.5	-	-	-	-	1150	-
1	-	-	4	15	-	60	-	-	1	-	-	-	24	1.5	-	-	-	-	1280	-
0	-	-	7	0	-	99	-	-	6	-	-	.2	48	1.5	-	2.8	-	-	786	-
0	0	0	0	0	2	0	0	0	0	-	0	0	1	.1	12	.7	32	26	29	.3
0	0	0	0	0	2	0	0	0	0	-	0	0	1	.1	12	.7	32	26	2	.3
3	10	8	-	3	9	104	.1	.6	1	-	.2	.1	155	.9	24	.5	203	179	253	1.5
0	0	0	2	0	4	0	.1	0	0	-	0	.1	10	.4	42	1.5	81	42	5	.6
0	0	0	0	0	2	0	.1	0	0	-	0	.1	8	.9	9	1.2	34	28	1	.4
0	0	0	0	0	3	0	0	0	0	-	0	.1	7	.5	4	.7	12	3	2	.2
0	0	0	-	0	2	0	.1	0	0	-	0	.2	1	1.4	7	1.4	31	24	0	.4
1	1	1	4	1	7	0	.1	.1	0	-	.1	.1	8	.9	12	1.8	37	42	574	.3
0	1	0	0	22	7	20	.3	2	0	-	.2	-	-	-	-	-	-	-	30	-
4	-	0	10	-	0	-	-	-	0	-	-	-	24	0	-	-	-	-	470	-
0	-	0	0	0	-	0	-	-	0	.4	-	-	0	0	-	-	-	-	340	-
3	3	7	0	18	1	6	0	0	0	1.6	0	0	3	.1	0	0	4	25	428	0
0	-	-	0	0	-	100	-	-	0	-	-	-	0	0	-	-	-	-	300	-
0	0	1	0	2	0	0	0	0	0	.3	0	0	4	.1	0	0	5	26	256	.1
2	3	8	0	0	1	7	0	0	0	1.5	0	0	3	.1	0	0	1	4	231	0
0	-	-	0	0	-	0	-	-	0	-	-	-	0	0	-	-	-	-	290	-
0	1	2	0	0	0	0	0	0	0	.3	0	0	1	.1	0	0	2	5	236	0
3	-	-	0	5	-	0	-	-	0	-	-	-	0	0	-	-	-	-	270	-
0	-	-	0	0	-	0	-	-	0	.6	-	-	0	0	-	-	-	-	310	-
2	4	9	0	6	3	63	0	.1	2	1.8	0	0	6	.2	0	.2	11	48	266	.1
0	0	1	0	2	1	5	0	0	2	.1	0	0	6	.2	0	0	12	51	282	0
2	4	8	-	0	0	63	0	0	0	1.5	0	0	6	.2	0	0	11	48	307	0
2	3	6	1	8	2	30	0	.1	0	1.3	0	0	3	.2	1	0	5	35	219	0
0	1	2	0	5	2	29	0	.1	0	.3	0	0	3	.2	0	0	5	35	307	0
0	-	-	0	0	-	0	-	-	0	-	-	-	0	0	-	-	-	-	300	-
3	5	8	0	0	0	0	0	0	0	1.3	0	0	0	0	0	0	0	2	0	0
1	2	3	0	60	25	11	.8	2.6	0	-	.4	.2	13	.9	31	8.6	218	534	48	.7
1	1	1	0	57	4	35	.2	2.9	0	-	.1	.2	14	.8	28	7.3	251	352	73	.6
0	-	-	0	0	-	80	-	-	4	-	-	-	0	0	-	-	-	-	240	-
1	3	4	0	121	10	57	.1	7.6	0	-	.2	.1	325	2.5	33	4.5	417	338	430	1.1
3	2	1	-	17	8	46	0	.5	1	-	.2	0	212	.1	132	.3	128	222	398	.3
0	0	0	3	0	28	2	.2	0	17	-	0	0	35	1.7	15	.2	24	201	780	.2
1	2	1	0	14	1	0	.1	.2	7	-	0	.1	2	.2	3	.7	24	58	285	.4
7	8	2	0	38	4	4	.1	.5	0	-	.1	.3	10	.4	12	2.7	95	176	718	1
8	10	2	0	51	2	0	.2	.8	1	-	.2	.4	37	1.1	13	2.7	127	180	473	2

Food Composition Table—cont'd

Code	Name	Amount	Unit	Grams	Kilocalories	Carbohydrates (g)	Protein (g)	Fat (g)
7089	SAUSAGE, ITALIAN, CKD	1	LINK	83.0	268	1	17	21
7037	SAUSAGE, KIELBASA, KOLBASSY	1	LINK	85.0	264	2	11	23
7038	SAUSAGE, KNOCKWURST	1	LINK	68.0	209	1	8	19
7075	SAUSAGE, LINK, PORK AND BEEF	1	LINK	68.0	228	1	9	21
16107	SAUSAGE, MEATLESS	1	LINK	25.0	64	2	5	5
7057	SAUSAGE, PEPPERONI	1	SLICE	5.5	27	0	1	2
7059	SAUSAGE, POLISH-STYLE	1	EACH	227.0	740	4	32	65
7064	SAUSAGE, PORK, LINKS OR BULK, CKD	1	LINK	13.0	48	0	3	4
7072	SAUSAGE, SALAMI, BEEF AND PORK, DRY	1	SLICE	10.0	42	0	2	3
7068	SAUSAGE, SALAMI, BEEF, CKD	1	SLICE	23.0	60	1	3	5
7074	SAUSAGE, SMOKED LINK, PORK	1	LINK	68.0	265	1	15	22
15092	SEA BASS, CKD, DRY HEAT	3	OUNCE	85.1	105	0	20	2
12036	SEEDS, SUNFLOWER, DRIED	½	CUP	72.0	410	14	16	36
12537	SEEDS, SUNFLOWER, DRY ROASTED, W/ SALT ADDED	½	CUP	64.0	372	15	12	32
12538	SEEDS, SUNFLOWER, OIL ROASTED, W/ SALT ADDED	½	CUP	67.5	415	10	14	39
12539	SEEDS, SUNFLOWER, TOASTED, W/ SALT ADDED	½	CUP	67.0	415	14	12	38
14346	SHAKE, CHOCOLATE	1	CUP	226.4	288	46	8	8
14428	SHAKE, STRAWBERRY	1	CUP	226.4	256	43	8	6
14347	SHAKE, VANILLA	1	CUP	226.4	251	41	8	7
11640	SHALLOTS, FREEZE-DRIED	½	CUP	7.2	25	6	1	0
11677	SHALLOTS, FRESH	½	CUP	79.9	58	13	2	0
19097	SHERBET, ALL FLAVORS	1	CUP	192.0	265	58	2	4
15150	SHRIMP, CKD, BREADED AND FRIED	3	OUNCE	85.1	206	10	18	10
15151	SHRIMP, CKD, MOIST HEAT	3	OUNCE	85.1	84	0	18	1
15149	SHRIMP, FRESH	3	OUNCE	85.1	90	1	17	1
15102	SNAPPER, CKD, DRY HEAT	3	OUNCE	85.1	109	0	22	1
62599	SORBET, ALL FLAVORS	½	CUP	90.0	100	25	0	0
6474	SOUP, BEAN W/ BACON	1	CUP	264.9	106	16	5	2
6007	SOUP, BEAN W/ HAM	1	CUP	243.0	231	27	13	9
6406	SOUP, BEAN W/ HOT DOGS	1	CUP	250.0	187	22	10	7
6404	SOUP, BEAN W/ PORK	1	CUP	253.0	172	23	8	6
6008	SOUP, BEEF BROTH OR BOUILLON	1	CUP	240.0	17	0	3	1
6547	SOUP, BEEF MUSHROOM	1	CUP	244.0	73	6	6	3
6409	SOUP, BEEF NOODLE	1	CUP	244.0	83	9	5	3
6070	SOUP, BEEF, CHUNKY	1	CUP	240.0	170	20	12	5
6402	SOUP, BLACK BEAN	1	CUP	247.0	116	20	6	2
6478	SOUP, CAULIFLOWER	1	CUP	256.1	69	11	3	2
6411	SOUP, CHEESE	1	CUP	247.0	156	11	5	10
6480	SOUP, CHICKEN BROTH OR BOUILLON	1	CUP	244.0	22	1	1	1
6417	SOUP, CHICKEN GUMBO	1	CUP	244.0	56	8	3	1
6549	SOUP, CHICKEN MUSHROOM	1	CUP	244.0	132	9	4	9
6419	SOUP, CHICKEN NOODLE	1	CUP	241.0	75	9	4	2
6018	SOUP, CHICKEN NOODLE, CHUNKY	1	CUP	240.0	175	17	13	6
6485	SOUP, CHICKEN RICE	1	CUP	252.8	61	9	2	1
6022	SOUP, CHICKEN RICE, CHUNKY	1	CUP	240.0	127	13	12	3
6425	SOUP, CHICKEN VEGETABLE	1	CUP	241.0	75	9	4	3
6024	SOUP, CHICKEN VEGETABLE, CHUNKY	1	CUP	240.0	166	19	12	5
6412	SOUP, CHICKEN W/ DUMPLINGS	1	CUP	241.0	96	6	6	6
6423	SOUP, CHICKEN W/ RICE	1	CUP	241.0	60	7	4	2
6015	SOUP, CHICKEN, CHUNKY	1	CUP	251.0	178	17	13	7
6426	SOUP, CHILI BEEF	1	CUP	250.0	170	21	7	7
6027	SOUP, CLAM CHOWDER, MANHATTAN STYLE	1	CUP	240.0	134	19	7	3
6230	SOUP, CLAM CHOWDER, NEW ENGLAND	1	CUP	248.0	164	17	9	7
6034	SOUP, CRAB	1	CUP	244.0	76	10	5	2
6201	SOUP, CREAM OF ASPARAGUS	1	CUP	248.0	161	16	6	8
6210	SOUP, CREAM OF CELERY	1	CUP	248.0	164	15	6	10
6216	SOUP, CREAM OF CHICKEN	1	CUP	248.0	191	15	7	11
6243	SOUP, CREAM OF MUSHROOM	1	CUP	248.0	203	15	6	14
6246	SOUP, CREAM OF ONION	1	CUP	248.0	186	18	7	9
6253	SOUP, CREAM OF POTATO	1	CUP	248.0	149	17	6	6

Saturated fat (g)	Monounsaturated fat (g)	Polyunsaturated fat (g)	Fiber (g)	Cholesterol (g)	Folate (g)	Vitamin A (RE)	Vitamin B$_6$ (mg)	Vitamin B$_{12}$ (µg)	Vitamin C (mg)	Vitamin E (mg)	Riboflavin (mg)	Thiamin (mg)	Calcium (mg)	Iron (mg)	Magnesium (mg)	Niacin (mg)	Phosphorus (mg)	Potassium (mg)	Sodium (mg)	Zinc (mg)
8	10	3	0	65	4	0	.3	1.1	2	-	.2	.5	20	1.2	15	3.5	141	252	765	2
8	11	3	0	57	4	0	.2	1.4	18	-	.2	.2	37	1.2	14	2.4	126	230	915	1.7
7	9	2	0	39	1	0	.1	.8	18	-	.1	.2	7	.6	7	1.9	67	135	687	1.1
7	10	2	0	48	1	0	.1	1	13	-	.1	.2	7	1	8	2.2	73	129	643	1.4
1	1	2	1	0	7	16	.2	0	0	-	.1	.6	16	.9	9	2.8	56	58	222	.4
1	1	0	0	4	0	0	0	.1	0	-	0	0	1	.1	1	.3	7	19	112	.1
23	31	7	0	159	5	0	.4	2.2	2	-	.3	1.1	27	3.3	32	7.8	309	538	1989	4.4
1	2	0	0	11	0	0	0	.2	0	-	0	.1	4	.2	2	.6	24	47	168	.3
1	2	0	0	8	0	0	.1	.2	3	-	0	.1	1	.2	2	.5	14	38	186	.3
2	2	0	0	15	0	0	0	.7	4	-	0	0	2	.5	3	.7	26	52	270	.5
8	10	3	0	46	3	0	.2	1.1	1	-	.2	.5	20	.8	13	3.1	110	228	1020	1.9
1	0	1	0	45	5	54	.4	.3	0	-	.1	.1	11	.3	45	1.6	211	279	74	.4
4	7	24	8	0	164	4	.6	0	1	-	.2	1.6	84	4.9	255	3.2	508	496	2	3.6
3	6	21	4	0	152	0	.5	0	1	-	.2	.1	45	2.4	83	4.5	739	544	499	3.4
4	7	26	5	0	158	3	.5	0	1	-	.2	.2	38	4.5	86	2.8	769	326	407	3.5
4	7	25	-	0	159	0	.5	0	1	-	.2	.2	38	4.6	86	2.8	776	329	411	3.6
5	2	0	-	29	8	52	.1	.8	1	-	.6	.1	256	.7	38	.4	231	453	220	.9
4	-	-	-	25	7	66	.1	.7	2	-	.4	.1	256	.2	29	.4	226	412	188	.8
4	2	0	-	25	7	72	.1	.8	2	-	.4	.1	276	.2	27	.4	231	394	186	.8
0	0	0	-	0	8	404	0	0	3	-	0	0	13	.4	7	.1	21	119	4	.1
0	0	0	-	0	27	998	.3	0	6	-	0	0	30	1	17	.2	48	267	10	.3
2	1	0	-	10	8	27	.1	.2	8	-	.1	0	104	.3	15	.2	77	184	88	.9
2	3	4	-	151	7	48	.1	1.6	1	-	.1	.1	57	1.1	34	2.6	185	191	293	1.2
0	0	0	0	166	3	56	.1	1.3	2	-	0	0	33	2.6	29	2.2	117	155	191	1.3
0	0	1	0	129	3	46	.1	1	2	-	0	0	44	2	31	2.2	174	157	126	.9
0	0	1	0	40	5	30	.4	3	1	-	0	0	34	.2	31	.3	171	444	48	.4
0	-	-	1	0	-	0	-	-	12	-	-	-	0	0	-	-	-	-	10	-
1	1	0	9	3	8	5	0	0	0	-	.3	.1	56	1.3	29	.4	90	326	927	.7
3	4	1	11	22	29	396	.1	.1	4	-	.1	.1	78	3.2	46	1.7	143	425	972	1.1
2	3	2	-	12	30	87	.1	.1	1	-	.1	.1	87	2.3	47	1	165	477	1092	1.2
2	2	2	9	3	32	89	0	.1	2	-	0	.1	81	2	46	.6	132	402	951	1
0	0	0	0	0	5	0	0	.2	0	-	.1	0	14	.4	5	1.9	31	130	782	0
1	1	0	-	7	10	0	0	.2	5	-	.1	0	5	.9	10	1	34	154	942	1.5
1	1	0	1	5	4	63	0	.2	0	-	.1	.1	15	1.1	11	1.1	46	100	952	1.5
3	2	0	1	14	13	262	.1	.6	7	-	.2	.1	31	2.3	5	2.7	120	336	866	2.6
0	1	0	4	0	25	49	.1	0	1	-	.1	.1	44	2.1	42	.5	106	274	1198	1.4
0	1	1	-	0	3	0	0	.2	3	-	.1	.1	10	.5	3	.5	51	105	843	.3
7	3	0	-	30	5	109	0	0	0	-	.1	0	141	.7	5	.4	136	153	958	.6
0	0	0	0	0	2	12	0	0	0	-	0	0	15	.1	5	.2	12	24	1484	0
0	1	0	2	5	5	15	.1	0	5	-	0	0	24	.9	5	.7	24	76	954	.4
2	4	2	-	10	2	112	0	0	0	-	.1	0	29	.9	10	1.6	27	154	942	1
1	1	1	1	7	2	72	0	.1	0	-	.1	.1	17	.8	5	1.4	36	55	1106	.4
1	3	2	4	19	5	122	0	.3	0	-	.2	.1	24	1.4	10	4.3	72	108	850	1
0	1	0	1	3	1	0	0	.1	0	-	0	0	8	0	0	.4	10	10	981	.1
1	1	1	1	12	4	586	0	.3	4	-	.1	0	34	1.9	10	4.1	72	108	888	1
1	1	1	-	10	5	265	0	.1	1	-	.1	.1	17	.9	7	1.2	41	154	945	.4
1	2	1	-	17	12	600	.1	.2	6	-	.2	0	26	1.5	10	3.3	106	367	1068	2.2
1	3	1	1	34	2	53	0	.2	0	-	.1	0	14	.6	5	1.8	60	116	860	.4
0	1	0	1	7	1	65	0	.1	0	-	0	0	17	.7	0	1.1	22	101	815	.3
2	3	1	2	30	5	131	.1	.3	1	-	.2	.1	25	1.7	8	4.4	113	176	889	1
3	3	0	9	12	17	150	.2	.3	4	-	.1	.1	42	2.1	30	1.1	147	525	1035	1.4
2	1	0	3	14	9	329	.3	7.9	12	-	.1	.1	67	2.6	19	1.8	84	384	1001	1.7
3	2	1	1	22	10	40	.1	10.2	3	-	.2	.1	186	1.5	22	1	156	300	992	.8
0	1	0	1	10	15	51	.1	.2	0	-	.1	.2	66	1.2	15	1.3	88	327	1235	1.5
3	2	2	1	22	30	84	.1	.3	4	-	.3	.1	174	.9	20	.9	154	360	1042	.9
4	2	3	1	32	8	67	.1	.5	1	-	.2	.1	186	.7	22	.4	151	310	1009	.2
5	4	2	0	27	8	94	.1	.5	1	-	.3	.1	181	.7	17	.9	151	273	1047	.7
5	3	5	0	20	10	37	.1	.5	2	-	.3	.1	179	.6	20	.9	156	270	1076	.6
4	3	2	1	32	12	67	.1	.5	2	-	.3	.1	179	.7	22	.6	154	310	1004	.6
4	2	1	0	22	9	67	.1	.5	1	-	.2	.1	166	.5	17	.6	161	322	1061	.7

Food Composition Table—cont'd

Code	Name	Amount	Unit	Grams	Kilocalories	Carbohydrates (g)	Protein (g)	Fat (g)
6256	SOUP, CREAM OF SHRIMP	1	CUP	248.0	164	14	7	9
6501	SOUP, CREAM OF VEGETABLE	1	CUP	260.1	107	12	2	6
6036	SOUP, GAZPACHO	1	CUP	244.0	56	1	9	2
6037	SOUP, LENTIL W/ HAM	1	CUP	248.0	139	20	9	3
6440	SOUP, MINESTRONE	1	CUP	241.0	82	11	4	3
6039	SOUP, MINESTRONE, CHUNKY	1	CUP	240.0	127	21	5	3
6493	SOUP, MUSHROOM	1	CUP	253.0	96	11	2	5
6445	SOUP, ONION	1	CUP	241.0	58	8	4	2
6249	SOUP, PEA, GREEN	1	CUP	254.0	239	32	13	7
6451	SOUP, PEA, SPLIT W/ HAM	1	CUP	253.0	190	28	10	4
6050	SOUP, PEA, SPLIT W/ HAM, CHUNKY	1	CUP	240.0	185	27	11	4
6359	SOUP, TOMATO	1	CUP	248.0	161	22	6	6
6461	SOUP, TOMATO BEEF W/ NOODLE	1	CUP	244.0	139	21	4	4
6463	SOUP, TOMATO RICE	1	CUP	247.0	119	22	2	3
6499	SOUP, TOMATO VEGETABLE	1	CUP	253.0	56	10	2	1
6465	SOUP, TURKEY NOODLE	1	CUP	244.0	68	9	4	2
6466	SOUP, TURKEY VEGETABLE	1	CUP	241.0	72	9	3	3
6064	SOUP, TURKEY, CHUNKY	1	CUP	236.0	135	14	10	4
6500	SOUP, VEGETABLE BEEF	1	CUP	253.1	53	8	3	1
6067	SOUP, VEGETABLE, CHUNKY	1	CUP	240.0	122	19	4	4
6468	SOUP, VEGETARIAN VEGETABLE	1	CUP	241.0	72	12	2	2
1056	SOUR CREAM	1	TBSP.	12.0	26	1	0	3
62556	SOUR CREAM, FAT FREE	1	TBSP.	16.0	13	3	1	0
1074	SOUR CREAM, IMITATION, NONDAIRY, CULTURED	1	TBSP.	14.4	30	1	0	3
62555	SOUR CREAM, LIGHT	1	TBSP.	16.0	16	1	1	1
6134	SOY SAUCE	1	TBSP.	18.0	10	2	1	0
11455	SPAGHETTI SAUCE	½	CUP	124.5	136	20	2	6
11458	SPINACH, CKD	½	CUP	90.0	21	3	3	0
11461	SPINACH, CND, DRAINED SOLIDS	½	CUP	107.0	25	4	3	1
11457	SPINACH, FRESH	1	CUP	56.0	12	2	2	0
11464	SPINACH, FRZ, CKD	½	CUP	95.0	27	5	3	0
11642	SQUASH, SUMMER, CKD	½	CUP	90.0	18	4	1	0
11641	SQUASH, SUMMER, FRESH	½	CUP	65.0	13	3	1	0
11644	SQUASH, WINTER, BAKED	½	CUP	102.5	40	9	1	1
11643	SQUASH, WINTER, FRESH	½	CUP	58.0	21	5	1	0
11953	SQUASH, ZUCCHINI, BABY, FRESH	1	MEDIUM	11.0	2	0	0	0
9316	STRAWBERRIES, FRESH	½	CUP	74.5	22	5	0	0
9320	STRAWBERRIES, FROZEN, SWEETENED	½	CUP	127.5	122	33	1	0
9318	STRAWBERRIES, FROZEN, UNSWEETENED	½	CUP	74.5	26	7	0	0
11508	SWEET POTATOES, BAKED IN SKIN	½	CUP	100.0	103	24	2	0
11510	SWEET POTATOES, BOILED, W/O SKIN	½	CUP	164.0	172	40	3	0
11659	SWEET POTATOES, CANDIED	½	CUP	113.4	155	32	1	4
11514	SWEET POTATOES, MASHED	½	CUP	127.5	129	30	3	0
15111	SWORDFISH, CKD, DRY HEAT	3	OUNCE	85.1	132	0	22	4
19348	SYRUP, CHOCOLATE, FUDGE-TYPE	1	TBSP.	21.0	73	12	1	3
19349	SYRUP, CORN, DARK	1	TBSP.	20.0	56	15	0	0
19351	SYRUP, CORN, HIGH-FRUCTOSE	1	TBSP.	19.0	53	14	0	0
19350	SYRUP, CORN, LIGHT	1	TBSP.	20.0	56	15	0	0
19353	SYRUP, MAPLE	1	TBSP.	20.0	52	13	0	0
19128	SYRUP, PANCAKE, LO CAL	1	TBSP.	20.0	33	9	0	0
19360	SYRUP, PANCAKE, W/ 2% MAPLE	1	TBSP.	20.0	53	14	0	0
19113	SYRUP, PANCAKE, W/ BUTTER	1	TBSP.	20.0	59	15	0	0
18360	TACO SHELLS, BAKED	1	MEDIUM	13.0	61	8	1	3
9221	TANGERINE JUICE, FRESH	¾	CUP	185.2	80	19	1	0
9219	TANGERINES, CND, JUICE PACK	½	CUP	124.5	46	12	1	0
9220	TANGERINES, CND, LIGHT SYRUP PACK	½	CUP	126.0	77	20	1	0
9218	TANGERINES, FRESH	1	MEDIUM	84.0	37	9	1	0
19218	TAPIOCA PUDDING	1	CUP	298.1	355	58	6	11
6112	TERIYAKI SAUCE	1	TBSP.	18.0	15	3	1	0
16126	TOFU, FRESH, FIRM	1	OUNCE	28.4	41	1	4	2

Saturated fat (g)	Monounsaturated fat (g)	Polyunsaturated fat (g)	Fiber (g)	Cholesterol (g)	Folate (g)	Vitamin A (RE)	Vitamin B6 (mg)	Vitamin B12 (µg)	Vitamin C (mg)	Vitamin E (mg)	Riboflavin (mg)	Thiamin (mg)	Calcium (mg)	Iron (mg)	Magnesium (mg)	Niacin (mg)	Phosphorus (mg)	Potassium (mg)	Sodium (mg)	Zinc (mg)
6	3	0	0	35	10	55	.4	1	1	-	.2	.1	164	.6	22	.5	146	248	1037	.8
1	3	1	1	0	8	3	0	.1	4	-	.1	1.2	31	.5	10	.5	55	96	1170	.3
0	1	1	4	0	10	20	.1	0	3	-	0	0	24	1	7	.9	37	224	1183	.2
1	1	0	-	7	50	35	.2	.3	4	-	.1	.2	42	2.7	22	1.4	184	357	1319	.7
1	1	1	1	2	16	234	.1	0	1	-	0	.1	34	.9	7	.9	55	313	911	.7
1	1	0	2	5	31	434	.2	0	5	-	.1	.1	60	1.8	14	1.2	110	612	864	1.4
1	2	2	1	0	5	0	0	.3	1	-	.1	.3	66	.5	5	.5	76	200	1020	.1
0	1	1	1	0	15	0	0	0	1	-	0	0	27	.7	2	.6	12	67	1053	.6
4	2	1	3	18	8	58	.1	.4	3	-	.3	.2	173	2	56	1.3	239	376	1046	1.8
2	2	1	-	8	3	46	.1	.3	2	-	.1	.1	23	2.3	48	1.5	213	400	1007	1.3
2	2	1	4	7	5	487	.2	.2	7	-	.1	.1	34	2.1	38	2.5	178	305	965	3.1
3	2	1	0	17	21	109	.2	.4	68	-	.2	.1	159	1.8	22	1.5	149	449	932	.3
2	2	1	1	5	7	54	.1	.2	0	-	.1	.1	17	1.1	7	1.9	56	220	917	.8
1	1	1	1	2	14	77	.1	0	15	-	0	.1	22	.8	5	1.1	35	331	815	.5
0	0	0	1	0	10	20	.1	0	6	-	0	.1	8	.6	20	.8	30	104	1146	.2
1	1	0	1	5	2	29	0	.1	0	-	.1	.1	12	1	5	1.4	49	76	815	.6
1	1	1	0	2	5	243	0	.2	0	-	0	0	17	.8	5	1	41	176	906	.6
1	2	1	-	9	11	715	.3	2.1	6	-	.1	0	50	1.9	24	3.6	104	361	923	2.1
1	0	0	1	0	8	23	.1	.3	1	-	0	0	13	.9	23	.5	35	76	1002	.3
1	2	1	1	0	17	588	.2	0	6	-	.1	.1	55	1.6	7	1.2	72	396	1010	3.1
0	1	1	0	0	11	301	.1	0	1	-	0	.1	22	1.1	7	.9	34	210	822	.5
2	1	0	0	5	1	23	0	0	0	-	0	0	14	0	1	0	10	17	6	.6
0	-	-	3	-	30	-	-	-	0	-	-	-	36	0	-	-	-	-	18	-
3	0	0	0	0	0	0	0	0	0	-	0	0	0	.1	1	0	6	23	15	.2
1	-	-	5	-	18	-	-	-	0	-	-	-	22	0	-	-	-	27	9	-
0	0	0	0	0	3	0	0	0	0	-	0	0	3	.4	6	.6	20	32	1029	.1
1	3	2	4	0	27	153	.4	0	14	-	.1	.1	35	.8	30	1.9	45	478	618	.3
0	0	0	2	0	131	737	.2	0	9	-	.2	.1	122	3.2	78	.4	50	419	63	.7
0	0	0	-	0	105	939	.1	0	15	-	.1	0	136	2.5	81	.4	47	370	29	.5
0	0	0	2	0	109	376	.1	0	16	-	.1	0	55	1.5	44	.4	27	312	44	.3
0	0	0	3	0	102	739	.1	0	12	-	.2	.1	139	1.4	66	.4	46	283	82	.7
0	0	0	1	0	18	26	.1	0	5	-	0	0	24	.3	22	.5	35	173	1	.4
0	0	0	1	0	17	13	.1	0	10	-	0	0	13	.3	15	.4	23	127	1	.2
0	0	0	3	0	29	365	.1	0	10	-	0	.1	14	.3	8	.7	21	448	1	.3
0	0	0	1	0	13	235	0	0	7	-	0	.1	18	.3	12	.5	19	203	2	.1
0	0	0	-	0	2	5	0	0	4	-	0	0	2	.1	4	.1	10	50	0	.1
0	0	0	2	0	13	2	0	0	42	.1	0	0	10	.3	7	.2	14	124	1	.1
0	0	0	2	0	19	3	0	0	53	-	.1	0	14	.8	9	.5	17	125	4	.1
0	0	0	2	0	13	3	0	0	31	.2	0	0	12	.6	8	.3	10	110	1	.1
0	0	0	3	0	23	2182	.2	0	25	-	.1	.1	28	.4	20	.6	55	348	10	.3
0	0	0	4	0	18	2796	.4	0	28	-	.2	.1	34	.9	16	1	44	302	21	.4
2	1	0	-	9	13	475	0	0	8	-	0	0	29	1.3	12	.4	29	214	79	.2
0	0	0	-	0	14	1929	.3	0	7	-	.1	0	38	1.7	31	1.2	66	268	96	.3
1	2	1	0	43	2	35	.3	1.7	1	-	.1	0	5	.9	29	10	287	314	98	1.3
1	1	1	0	3	1	5	0	.1	0	-	0	0	21	.3	10	0	36	45	27	.2
-	-	-	0	0	0	0	0	0	0	-	0	0	4	.1	2	0	2	9	31	0
-	-	-	0	0	0	0	0	0	0	-	0	0	0	0	0	0	0	0	0	0
-	-	-	0	0	0	0	0	0	0	-	0	0	1	0	0	0	0	1	24	0
-	-	-	0	0	0	0	0	0	0	-	0	0	13	.2	3	0	0	41	2	.8
-	-	-	0	0	0	0	0	0	0	-	0	0	0	0	0	0	9	1	40	0
-	-	-	0	0	0	0	0	0	0	-	0	0	1	0	0	0	2	1	12	0
0	0	0	-	1	0	3	0	0	0	-	0	0	0	0	0	0	2	1	20	0
0	1	1	1	0	1	5	0	0	0	-	0	0	21	.3	14	.2	32	23	48	.2
0	0	0	0	0	9	78	.1	0	57	-	0	.1	33	.4	15	.2	26	330	2	.1
0	0	0	1	0	6	106	.1	0	43	-	0	.1	14	.3	14	.6	12	166	6	.6
0	0	0	1	0	6	106	.1	0	25	-	.1	.1	9	.5	10	.6	13	98	8	.3
0	0	0	2	0	17	77	.1	0	26	-	0	.1	12	.1	10	.1	8	132	1	.2
2	5	4	0	3	12	0	.3	.3	2	-	.3	.1	250	.7	24	.9	236	310	352	.8
0	0	0	0	0	4	0	0	0	0	-	0	0	5	.3	11	.2	28	41	690	0
0	1	1	1	0	8	5	0	0	0	-	0	0	58	3	27	.1	54	67	4	.4

Food Composition Table—cont'd

Code	Name	Amount	Unit	Grams	Kilocalories	Carbohydrates (g)	Protein (g)	Fat (g)
16127	TOFU, FRESH, REGULAR	1	OUNCE	28.4	22	1	2	1
16129	TOFU, FRIED	1	OUNCE	28.4	77	3	5	6
11954	TOMATILLOS, FRESH	1	MEDIUM	34.0	11	2	0	0
11540	TOMATO JUICE, CND, W/ SALT	¾	CUP	183.0	31	8	1	0
11886	TOMATO JUICE, CND, W/O SALT	¾	CUP	183.0	31	8	1	0
11533	TOMATOES, CND, STEWED	½	CUP	127.5	33	8	1	0
11537	TOMATOES, CND, W/ GREEN CHILIES	½	CUP	120.5	18	4	1	0
11531	TOMATOES, CND, WHOLE, REG PK	½	CUP	120.0	24	5	1	0
11529	TOMATOES, FRESH	1	MEDIUM	123.0	26	6	1	0
11527	TOMATOES, GREEN, FRESH	1	MEDIUM	123.0	30	6	1	0
11955	TOMATOES, SUN-DRIED	¼	CUP	13.5	35	8	2	0
11956	TOMATOES, SUN-DRIED, PACKED IN OIL	¼	CUP	27.5	59	6	1	4
62538	TORTELLINI, BEEF	1	CUP	257.9	230	46	5	1
19057	TORTILLA CHIPS, NACHO-FLAVOR	1	OUNCE	28.4	141	18	2	7
19424	TORTILLA CHIPS, NACHO-FLAVOR, LIGHT	1	OUNCE	28.4	126	20	2	4
19056	TORTILLA CHIPS, PLAIN	1	OUNCE	28.4	142	18	2	7
19058	TORTILLA CHIPS, RANCH-FLAVOR	1	OUNCE	28.4	139	18	2	7
18363	TORTILLAS, CORN	1	MEDIUM	25.0	56	12	1	1
18364	TORTILLAS, FLOUR	1	MEDIUM	35.0	114	19	3	2
15219	TROUT, CKD, DRY HEAT	3	OUNCE	85.1	162	0	23	7
15241	TROUT, RAINBOW, FARMED, CKD, DRY HEAT	3	OUNCE	85.1	144	0	21	6
15116	TROUT, RAINBOW, WILD, CKD, DRY HEAT	3	OUNCE	85.1	128	0	19	5
15128	TUNA SALAD	3	OUNCE	85.1	159	8	14	8
15183	TUNA, LIGHT MEAT, CND IN OIL	3	OUNCE	85.1	168	0	25	7
15184	TUNA, LIGHT MEAT, CND IN WATER	3	OUNCE	85.1	111	0	25	0
15185	TUNA, WHITE MEAT, CND IN OIL	3	OUNCE	85.1	158	0	23	7
15186	TUNA, WHITE MEAT, CND IN WATER	3	OUNCE	85.1	116	0	23	2
15221	TUNA, YELLOWFIN, CKD, DRY HEAT	3	OUNCE	85.1	118	0	25	1
5297	TURKEY BOLOGNA	1	SLICE	21.0	42	0	3	3
7079	TURKEY BREAST MEAT	1	SLICE	21.0	23	0	5	0
5287	TURKEY LUNCH MEAT	1	SLICE	28.4	36	0	5	1
5296	TURKEY ROAST, ROASTED	3	OUNCE	85.1	132	3	18	5
5291	TURKEY ROLL, LIGHT AND DARK MEAT	3	OUNCE	85.1	127	2	15	6
5290	TURKEY ROLL, LIGHT MEAT	3	OUNCE	85.1	125	0	16	6
5299	TURKEY SALAMI	1	SLICE	28.4	56	0	5	4
5294	TURKEY THIGH, PREBASTED, MEAT&SKIN, CKD, ROASTED	3	OUNCE	85.1	134	0	16	7
5190	TURKEY, BACK, MEAT&SKIN, CKD, ROASTED	3	OUNCE	85.1	207	0	23	12
5192	TURKEY, BREAST, MEAT&SKIN, CKD, ROASTED	3	OUNCE	85.1	161	0	24	6
5188	TURKEY, DARK MEAT, CKD, ROASTED	3	OUNCE	85.1	159	0	24	6
5184	TURKEY, DARK MEAT, MEAT&SKIN, CKD, ROASTED	3	OUNCE	85.1	188	0	23	10
5306	TURKEY, GROUND, CKD	3	OUNCE	85.1	200	0	23	11
5194	TURKEY, LEG, MEAT&SKIN, CKD, ROASTED	3	OUNCE	85.1	177	0	24	8
5186	TURKEY, LIGHT MEAT, CKD, ROASTED	3	OUNCE	85.1	134	0	25	3
5182	TURKEY, LIGHT MEAT, MEAT&SKIN, CKD, ROASTED	3	OUNCE	85.1	168	0	24	7
5168	TURKEY, MEAT ONLY, CKD, ROASTED	3	OUNCE	85.1	145	0	25	4
5166	TURKEY, MEAT&SKIN, CKD, ROASTED	3	OUNCE	85.1	177	0	24	8
5288	TURKEY, THIN SLICED	3	OUNCE	85.1	94	0	19	1
5196	TURKEY, WING, MEAT&SKIN, CKD, ROASTED	3	OUNCE	85.1	195	0	23	11
11565	TURNIPS, CKD	½	CUP	78.0	14	4	1	0
11564	TURNIPS, FRESH	½	CUP	65.0	18	4	1	0
18328	VANILLA CREAM PIE	1	SLICE	126.0	350	41	6	18
19201	VANILLA PUDDING	1	CUP	298.1	388	65	7	11
17089	VEAL, MEAT AND FAT, CKD	3	OUNCE	85.1	196	0	26	10
17091	VEAL, MEAT ONLY, CKD	3	OUNCE	85.1	167	0	27	6
11578	VEGETABLE JUICE CND	¾	CUP	181.5	34	8	1	0
11581	VEGETABLES, MIXED, CND	½	CUP	81.5	38	8	2	0
11584	VEGETABLES, MIXED, FRZ	½	CUP	91.0	54	12	3	0
18392	WAFFLES, BUTTERMILK	1	EACH	75.0	217	25	6	10
18367	WAFFLES, PLAIN	1	EACH	75.0	218	25	6	11
18403	WAFFLES, PLAIN, FROZEN, TOASTED	1	EACH	33.0	87	13	2	3

Saturated fat (g)	Monounsaturated fat (g)	Polyunsaturated fat (g)	Fiber (g)	Cholesterol (g)	Folate (g)	Vitamin A (RE)	Vitamin B6 (mg)	Vitamin B12 (µg)	Vitamin C (mg)	Vitamin E (mg)	Riboflavin (mg)	Thiamin (mg)	Calcium (mg)	Iron (mg)	Magnesium (mg)	Niacin (mg)	Phosphorus (mg)	Potassium (mg)	Sodium (mg)	Zinc (mg)
0	0	1	0	0	4	3	0	0	0	-	0	0	30	1.5	29	.1	27	34	2	.2
1	1	3	1	0	8	0	0	0	0	-	0	0	105	1.4	17	0	81	41	5	.6
-	-	-	1	0	2	4	0	0	4	-	0	0	2	.2	7	.6	13	91	0	.1
0	0	0	1	0	36	102	.2	0	33	-	.1	.1	16	1.1	20	1.2	35	403	661	.3
0	0	0	1	0	36	102	.2	0	33	-	.1	.1	16	1.1	20	1.2	35	403	18	.3
0	0	0	-	0	7	70	0	0	17	-	0	.1	42	.9	15	.9	26	305	324	.2
0	0	0	-	0	11	47	.1	0	7	-	0	0	24	.3	13	.8	17	129	483	.2
0	0	0	1	0	9	72	.1	0	18	-	0	.1	31	.7	14	.9	23	265	196	.2
0	0	0	1	0	18	76	.1	0	23	.4	.1	.1	6	.6	14	.8	30	273	11	.1
0	0	0	2	0	11	79	.1	0	29	-	0	.1	16	.6	12	.6	34	251	16	.1
0	0	0	2	0	9	12	0	0	5	-	.1	.1	15	1.2	26	1.2	48	463	283	.3
1	2	1	-	0	6	35	.1	0	28	-	.1	.1	13	.7	22	1	38	430	73	.2
0	-	-	9	15	-	150	-	-	4	-	-	-	96	1.5	-	-	-	-	770	-
1	4	1	2	1	4	12	.1	0	1	-	.1	0	42	.4	23	.4	69	61	201	.3
1	3	1	-	1	7	12	.1	0	0	-	.1	.1	45	.5	27	.1	90	77	284	-
1	4	1	2	0	3	6	.1	0	0	-	.1	0	44	.4	25	.4	58	56	150	.4
1	4	1	-	0	5	8	.1	0	0	-	.1	0	40	.4	25	.4	68	69	174	.4
0	0	0	1	0	4	6	.1	0	0	-	0	0	44	.4	16	.4	79	39	40	.2
0	1	1	1	0	4	0	0	0	0	-	.1	.2	44	1.2	9	1.3	43	46	167	.2
1	4	2	0	63	13	16	.2	6.4	0	-	.4	.4	47	1.6	24	4.9	267	394	57	.7
2	2	2	0	58	20	73	.3	4.2	3	-	.1	.2	-	.3	27	7.5	226	375	36	.4
1	1	2	0	59	16	13	.3	5.4	2	-	.1	.1	-	.3	26	4.9	229	381	48	.4
1	2	4	0	11	6	23	.1	1	2	-	.1	0	14	.9	16	5.7	151	151	342	.5
1	3	2	0	15	5	20	.1	1.9	0	-	.1	0	11	1.2	26	10.5	265	176	43	.8
0	0	0	0	15	4	20	.3	1.9	0	-	.1	0	10	2.7	25	10.5	158	267	43	.4
1	2	3	0	26	4	20	.4	1.9	0	-	.1	0	3	.6	29	9.9	227	283	43	.4
1	1	1	0	36	3	20	.4	1.9	0	-	0	0	3	.5	29	4.9	227	241	43	.4
0	0	0	0	49	2	17	.9	.5	1	-	0	.4	18	.8	54	10.2	208	484	40	.6
1	1	1	0	21	1	0	0	.1	0	-	0	0	18	.3	3	.7	28	42	184	.4
0	0	0	0	9	1	0	.1	.4	0	-	0	0	1	.1	4	1.7	48	58	301	.2
0	0	0	0	16	2	0	.1	.1	0	-	.1	0	3	.8	5	1	54	92	282	.8
2	1	1	0	45	4	0	.2	1.3	-	-	.1	0	4	1.4	19	5.3	208	253	578	2.2
2	2	2	0	47	4	0	.2	.2	0	-	.2	.1	27	1.1	15	4.1	143	230	498	1.7
2	2	1	0	37	3	0	.3	.2	0	-	.2	.1	34	1.1	14	6	156	213	416	1.3
1	1	1	0	23	1	0	.1	.1	0	-	0	0	6	.5	4	1	30	69	285	.5
2	2	2	0	53	5	0	.2	.2	0	-	.2	.1	7	1.3	14	2	145	205	372	3.5
4	4	3	0	77	7	0	.3	.3	0	-	.2	0	28	1.9	19	2.9	161	221	62	3.3
2	2	2	0	63	5	0	.4	.3	0	-	.1	0	18	1.2	23	5.4	179	245	54	1.7
2	1	2	0	72	8	0	.3	.3	0	-	.2	.1	27	2	20	3.1	174	247	67	3.8
3	3	3	0	76	8	0	.3	.3	0	-	.2	0	28	1.9	20	3	167	233	65	3.5
3	4	3	0	87	6	0	.3	.3	0	-	.1	0	21	1.6	20	4.1	167	230	91	2.4
3	2	2	0	72	8	0	.3	.3	0	-	.2	.1	27	2	20	3	169	238	65	3.6
1	0	1	0	59	5	0	.5	.3	0	-	.1	.1	16	1.1	24	5.8	186	259	54	1.7
2	2	2	0	65	5	0	.4	.3	0	-	.1	.1	16	1.1	24	5.8	186	259	54	1.7
1	1	1	0	65	6	0	.4	.3	0	-	.2	0	18	1.2	22	5.3	177	242	54	1.7
2	3	2	0	70	6	0	.3	.3	0	-	.2	.1	21	1.5	22	4.6	181	253	60	2.6
0	0	0	0	35	3	0	.3	1.7	0	-	.1	0	22	1.5	21	4.3	173	238	58	2.5
3	4	3	0	69	5	0	.4	.3	0	-	.1	0	6	.3	17	7.1	195	236	1217	1
0	0	0	2	0	7	0	.1	0	9	-	0	0	20	1.2	21	4.9	168	226	52	1.8
0	0	0	1	0	9	0	.1	0	14	-	0	0	17	.2	6	.2	15	105	39	.2
5	8	4	-	78	14	107	.1	.4	1	-	.3	0	25	.4	4	.1	220	45	197	.1
2	5	4	0	21	0	18	0	.3	0	-	.4	.2	113	1.3	16	1.2	131	159	328	.7
4	4	1	0	97	13	0	.3	1.3	0	.3	.3	.1	19	1	22	6.8	203	276	74	4
2	2	1	0	100	14	0	.3	1.4	0	.4	.3	.1	20	1	24	7.2	213	287	76	4.3
0	0	0	1	0	38	212	.3	0	50	-	.1	.1	20	.8	20	1.3	31	350	662	.4
0	0	0	-	0	19	949	.1	0	4	-	0	0	22	.9	13	.5	34	237	121	.3
0	0	0	5	0	17	389	.1	0	3	-	.1	.1	23	.7	20	.8	46	154	32	.4
2	3	5	-	50	11	26	0	.2	0	-	.3	.2	137	1.6	14	1.5	124	128	451	.6
2	3	5	-	52	11	49	0	.2	0	-	.3	.2	191	1.7	14	1.6	143	119	383	.5
0	1	1	-	8	12	120	.3	.8	0	-	.2	.1	77	1.5	7	1.5	139	42	260	.2

Food Composition Table—cont'd

Code	Name	Amount	Unit	Grams	Kilocalories	Carbohydrates (g)	Protein (g)	Fat (g)
15223	WHITEFISH, CKD, DRY HEAT	3	OUNCE	85.1	146	0	21	6
15131	WHITEFISH, SMOKED	3	OUNCE	85.1	92	0	20	1
20089	WILD RICE, CKD	½	CUP	82.0	83	17	3	0
62552	YOGURT, FROZEN, FAT FREE	½	CUP	67.0	100	22	4	0
62604	YOGURT, FRUIT, FAT FREE	1	CUP	248.0	233	48	10	0
62627	YOGURT, FRUIT, FAT FREE, LIGHT	1	CUP	248.0	110	19	10	0
1121	YOGURT, FRUIT, LOWFAT, 10 G PROTEIN PER 8 OZ	1	CUP	227.0	231	43	10	2
62603	YOGURT, PLAIN, FAT FREE	1	CUP	248.0	120	17	13	0
1119	YOGURT, VANILLA, LOWFAT, 11 G PROTEIN PER 8 OZ	1	CUP	227.0	194	31	11	3

Restaurants, Including Fast Food (Quick Service)

Code	Name	Amount	Unit	Grams	Kilocalories	Carbohydrates (g)	Protein (g)	Fat (g)
32391	ARBY'S-BEEF'N CHEDDAR SANDWICH	1	EACH	194.0	443	30	35	20
32400	ARBY'S-CHICKEN BREAST FILLET SANDWICH	1	EACH	204.0	547	53	26	28
32413	ARBY'S-CURLY FRIES	1	EACH	99.2	337	43	4	18
32405	ARBY'S-FISH FILLET SANDWICH	1	EACH	221.0	526	50	23	27
32411	ARBY'S-FRENCH FRIES	1	EACH	70.9	246	30	2	13
32406	ARBY'S-HAM'N CHEESE SANDWICH	1	EACH	170.1	411	38	24	19
32390	ARBY'S-REGULAR ROAST BEEF	1	EACH	155.9	388	38	25	16
32393	ARBY'S-SUPER ROAST BEEF	1	EACH	241.0	516	51	26	23
32410	ARBY'S-TURKEY SUB	1	EACH	277.0	599	54	33	28
34858	BURGER KING-BACON DOUBLE CHEESEBURGER	1	EACH	202.0	613	29	34	40
34856	BURGER KING-CHEESEBURGER	1	EACH	134.7	360	35	18	16
34857	BURGER KING-DOUBLE CHEESEBURGER	1	EACH	191.4	537	32	33	30
34855	BURGER KING-HAMBURGER	1	EACH	122.9	310	35	16	12
34841	BURGER KING-SALAD W/ HOUSE DRESSING	1	EACH	176.0	159	8	3	13
34846	BURGER KING-SALAD W/ REDUCED-CALORIE ITALIAN	1	EACH	176.0	42	7	2	1
34859	BURGER KING-WHOPPER	1	EACH	283.5	684	54	28	39
21002	FAST FOOD-BISCUIT W/ EGG	1	EACH	136.0	316	24	11	20
21003	FAST FOOD-BISCUIT W/ EGG AND BACON	1	EACH	150.0	458	29	17	31
21004	FAST FOOD-BISCUIT W/ EGG AND HAM	1	EACH	192.0	442	30	20	27
21005	FAST FOOD-BISCUIT W/ EGG AND SAUSAGE	1	EACH	180.0	581	41	19	39
21007	FAST FOOD-BISCUIT W/ EGG, CHEESE, AND BACON	1	EACH	144.0	477	33	16	31
21008	FAST FOOD-BISCUIT W/ HAM	1	EACH	113.0	386	44	13	18
21009	FAST FOOD-BISCUIT W/ SAUSAGE	1	EACH	124.0	485	40	12	32
21010	FAST FOOD-BISCUIT W/ STEAK	1	EACH	141.0	455	44	13	26
21001	FAST FOOD-BISCUIT, PLAIN	1	EACH	74.0	276	34	4	13
21027	FAST FOOD-BROWNIE	1	EACH	60.0	243	39	3	10
21060	FAST FOOD-BURRITO W/ BEANS	1	EACH	108.5	224	36	7	7
21061	FAST FOOD-BURRITO W/ BEANS AND CHEESE	1	EACH	93.0	189	27	8	6
21062	FAST FOOD-BURRITO W/ BEANS AND CHILI PEPPERS	1	EACH	102.0	206	29	8	7
21063	FAST FOOD-BURRITO W/ BEANS AND MEAT	1	EACH	115.5	254	33	11	9
21064	FAST FOOD-BURRITO W/ BEANS, CHEESE, AND BEEF	1	EACH	101.5	165	20	7	7
21065	FAST FOOD-BURRITO W/ BEANS, CHEESE, AND CHILI PEPPERS	1	EACH	167.0	329	42	17	11
21066	FAST FOOD-BURRITO W/ BEEF	1	EACH	110.0	262	29	13	10
21067	FAST FOOD-BURRITO W/ BEEF AND CHILI PEPPERS	1	EACH	100.5	213	25	11	8
21068	FAST FOOD-BURRITO W/ BEEF, CHEESE, AND CHILI PEPPERS	1	EACH	152.0	316	32	20	12
21069	FAST FOOD-BURRITO W/ FRUIT (APPLE OR CHERRY)	1	EACH	74.0	231	35	3	10
21100	FAST FOOD-CHEESEBURGER, LARGE, DOUBLE PATTY	1	EACH	258.0	704	40	38	44
21098	FAST FOOD-CHEESEBURGER, LARGE, SINGLE PATTY	1	EACH	219.0	563	38	28	33
21097	FAST FOOD-CHEESEBURGER, LARGE, SINGLE PATTY W/ BCN&COND	1	EACH	195.0	608	37	32	37
21096	FAST FOOD-CHEESEBURGER, LARGE, SINGLE PATTY, PLAIN	1	EACH	185.0	609	47	30	33
21095	FAST FOOD-CHEESEBURGER, REGULAR, DOUBLE PATTY	1	EACH	228.0	650	53	30	35
21091	FAST FOOD-CHEESEBURGER, REGULAR, SINGLE PATTY	1	EACH	154.0	359	28	18	20
21089	FAST FOOD-CHEESEBURGER, REGULAR, SINGLE PATTY, PLAIN	1	EACH	102.0	319	32	15	15
21101	FAST FOOD-CHEESEBURGER, TRIPLE PATTY, PLAIN	1	EACH	304.0	796	27	56	51
21103	FAST FOOD-CHICKEN FILLET SANDWICH W/ CHEESE	1	EACH	228.0	632	42	29	39

Saturated fat (g)	Monounsaturated fat (g)	Polyunsaturated fat (g)	Fiber (g)	Cholesterol (g)	Folate (g)	Vitamin A (RE)	Vitamin B6 (mg)	Vitamin B12 (μg)	Vitamin C (mg)	Vitamin E (mg)	Riboflavin (mg)	Thiamin (mg)	Calcium (mg)	Iron (mg)	Magnesium (mg)	Niacin (mg)	Phosphorus (mg)	Potassium (mg)	Sodium (mg)	Zinc (mg)
1	2	2	0	65	14	33	.3	.8	0	-	.1	.1	28	.4	36	3.3	294	345	55	1.1
0	0	0	0	28	6	48	.3	2.8	0	-	.1	0	15	.4	20	2	112	360	867	.4
0	0	0	1	0	21	0	.1	0	0	-	.1	0	2	.5	26	1.1	67	83	2	1.1
0	-	-	-	0	-	20	-	-	0	-	-	-	96	0	-	-	-	-	70	-
0	0	0	0	7	-	0	-	-	0	-	-	-	438	0	-	-	-	423	153	-
0	0	0	0	5	-	0	-	-	15	-	-	-	420	.2	-	-	-	510	160	-
2	1	0	0	10	21	25	.1	1.1	1	-	.4	.1	345	.2	33	.2	271	442	133	1.7
0	0	0	0	5	-	0	-	-	4	-	.2	-	480	0	-	-	0	600	170	-
2	1	0	0	11	24	30	.1	1.2	2	-	.5	.1	389	.2	37	.2	306	498	149	1.9

Saturated fat (g)	Monounsaturated fat (g)	Polyunsaturated fat (g)	Fiber (g)	Cholesterol (g)	Folate (g)	Vitamin A (RE)	Vitamin B6 (mg)	Vitamin B12 (μg)	Vitamin C (mg)	Vitamin E (mg)	Riboflavin (mg)	Thiamin (mg)	Calcium (mg)	Iron (mg)	Magnesium (mg)	Niacin (mg)	Phosphorus (mg)	Potassium (mg)	Sodium (mg)	Zinc (mg)
10	4	4	1	85	45	64	.4	2.3	1	.4	.5	.4	202	5.6	44	6.5	442	380	1801	6
6	11	11	2	101	35	17	.7	.4	0	2.9	.4	.5	123	3.9	51	16.4	322	366	1130	1.9
7	8	2	-	0	-	-	-	-	-	-	.1	.1	16	.8	-	1.9	-	724	167	-
7	9	11	-	44	-	-	-	-	1	-	.3	.3	72	2.1	-	5.3	-	450	872	-
3	6	5	-	0	-	-	-	-	4	-	-	.1	-	.6	-	1.9	-	240	114	-
7	8	2	1	68	83	112	.2	.6	3	1.3	.6	.4	151	3.8	19	3.1	177	338	899	1.6
4	8	2	1	58	45	71	.3	1.4	2	.2	.3	.4	61	4.7	35	6.6	268	354	888	3.8
9	8	6	2	41	42	0	.5	4.4	0	.4	.6	.6	118	6.6	60	9.7	414	518	822	11
6	7	8	-	82	-	-	-	-	-	-	.4	.5	94	3.2	-	9.4	-	-	1432	-
17	15	6	1	115	32	74	.4	3.4	8	1.6	.4	.3	162	4.1	39	8.4	386	480	833	6.6
-	-	-	-	-	-	-	-	-	-	-	-	-	-	-	-	-	-	-	705	-
14	12	2	2	111	34	111	.3	2	7	2	.3	.2	210	3.3	34	5.5	339	383	947	4.5
-	-	-	-	-	-	-	-	-	-	-	-	-	-	-	-	-	-	-	560	-
-	-	-	-	11	-	-	-	-	25	-	0	0	352	.1	95	.2	592	402	293	.1
-	-	-	-	0	-	-	-	-	25	-	0	0	320	.1	105	.2	472	390	430	.1
18	15	2	3	113	34	209	.3	3.1	14	4.2	0	0	113	6.5	54	5.6	339	565	1075	5.8
6	8	4	-	233	30	178	.1	.7	0	-	.3	.3	154	3.1	20	.7	185	160	654	1.1
10	13	6	-	353	30	53	.1	1	3	-	.2	.1	189	3.7	24	2.4	239	251	999	1.6
8	11	5	-	300	33	240	.3	1.2	0	-	.6	.7	221	4.6	31	2	317	319	1382	2.2
15	16	4	-	302	40	164	.2	1.4	0	-	.5	.5	155	4	25	3.6	490	320	1141	2.2
11	14	3	-	261	37	166	.1	1.1	2	-	.4	.3	164	2.5	20	2.3	459	230	1260	1.5
11	5	1	-	25	8	34	.1	0	0	-	.3	.5	160	2.7	23	3.5	554	197	1433	1.6
14	13	3	1	35	9	14	.1	.5	0	-	.3	.4	128	2.6	20	3.3	446	198	1071	1.6
7	11	6	-	25	11	16	.2	.9	0	-	.4	.4	116	4.3	27	4.2	204	234	795	2.7
9	3	1	-	5	6	24	0	.1	0	-	.2	.3	90	1.6	9	1.6	260	87	584	.3
3	4	4	-	10	4	2	0	.2	3	-	.1	.1	25	1.3	16	.6	88	83	153	.6
3	2	1	-	2	59	16	.2	.5	1	-	.3	.3	56	2.3	43	2	49	327	493	.8
3	1	1	-	14	41	119	.1	.4	1	-	.4	.1	107	1.1	40	1.8	90	248	583	.8
4	3	0	-	16	59	10	.1	.6	1	-	.4	.2	50	2.3	36	2.2	57	290	522	1.7
4	4	1	-	24	37	32	.2	.9	1	-	.4	.3	53	2.4	42	2.7	70	328	668	1.9
4	2	1	-	62	30	75	.1	.5	3	-	.4	.2	65	1.9	25	1.9	70	205	495	1.2
6	4	1	-	78	72	190	.2	1	3	-	.6	.3	144	3.8	48	3.8	142	402	1024	3
5	4	0	-	32	20	14	.2	1	1	-	.5	.1	42	3	41	3.2	87	370	746	2.4
4	3	0	-	27	18	23	.2	.6	1	-	.4	.2	43	2.2	30	2.5	70	249	558	2.2
5	5	1	-	85	29	56	.2	1	2	-	.6	.3	111	3.9	35	4.2	158	333	1046	4
5	3	1	-	4	4	37	.1	.5	1	-	.2	.2	16	1.1	7	1.9	15	104	212	.4
18	17	5	-	142	49	54	.4	3.4	1	-	.5	.4	240	5.9	52	7.2	395	596	1148	6.7
15	13	2	-	88	28	129	.3	2.6	8	1.2	.5	.4	206	4.7	44	7.4	311	445	1108	4.6
16	14	3	-	111	33	80	.3	2.3	2	-	.4	.3	162	4.7	45	6.6	400	332	1043	6.8
15	13	2	-	96	39	148	.3	2.5	0	-	.6	.5	91	5.5	39	11.2	422	644	1589	5.6
13	13	6	-	93	34	84	.3	2.1	3	2	.4	.6	169	4.7	36	8.3	349	390	921	4.1
9	7	1	-	52	22	71	.2	1.2	2	-	.2	.3	182	2.6	26	6.4	216	229	976	2.6
6	6	2	-	50	27	37	.1	1	0	-	.4	.4	141	2.4	21	3.7	196	164	500	2.4
22	22	3	-	161	52	85	.6	5.9	3	-	.6	.6	283	8.3	61	11.5	541	821	1213	10.9
12	14	10	-	78	46	128	.4	.5	3	-	.5	.4	258	3.6	43	9.1	406	333	1238	2.9

Restaurants, Including Fast Food (Quick Service)—cont'd

Code	Name	Amount	Unit	Grams	Kilocalories	Carbohydrates (g)	Protein (g)	Fat (g)
21102	FAST FOOD-CHICKEN FILLET SANDWICH, PLAIN	1	EACH	182.0	515	39	24	29
21037	FAST FOOD-CHICKEN NUGGETS, PLAIN	1	EACH	17.0	48	3	3	3
21038	FAST FOOD-CHICKEN NUGGETS, W/ BARB. SAUCE	1	EACH	17.0	43	3	2	2
21039	FAST FOOD-CHICKEN NUGGETS, W/ HONEY	1	EACH	17.0	49	4	2	3
21040	FAST FOOD-CHICKEN NUGGETS, W/ MUST. SAUCE	1	EACH	17.0	42	3	2	2
21041	FAST FOOD-CHICKEN NUGGETS, W/ SWEET AND SOUR	1	EACH	17.0	45	4	2	2
21042	FAST FOOD-CHILI CON CARNE	1	CUP	253.0	256	22	25	8
21070	FAST FOOD-CHIMICHANGA, W/ BEEF	1	EACH	174.0	425	43	20	20
21071	FAST FOOD-CHIMICHANGA, W/ BEEF AND CHEESE	1	EACH	183.0	443	39	20	23
21030	FAST FOOD-CHOCOLATE CHIP COOKIES	1	BOX	55.0	233	36	3	12
21043	FAST FOOD-CLAMS, BREADED AND FRIED	3	OUNCE	85.1	333	29	9	20
21128	FAST FOOD-CORN ON THE COB W/ BUTTER	1	EACH	146.0	155	32	4	3
21045	FAST FOOD-CRAB, SOFT-SHELL, FRIED	1	EACH	125.0	334	31	11	18
21011	FAST FOOD-CROISSANT W/ EGG AND CHEESE	1	EACH	127.0	368	24	13	25
21012	FAST FOOD-CROISSANT W/ EGG, CHEESE, AND BACON	1	EACH	129.0	413	24	16	28
21013	FAST FOOD-CROISSANT W/ EGG, CHEESE, AND HAM	1	EACH	152.0	474	24	19	34
21014	FAST FOOD-CROISSANT W/ EGG, CHEESE, AND SAUSAGE	1	EACH	160.0	523	25	20	38
21015	FAST FOOD-DANISH PASTRY, CHEESE	1	EACH	91.0	353	29	6	25
21016	FAST FOOD-DANISH PASTRY, CINNAMON	1	EACH	88.0	349	47	5	17
21017	FAST FOOD-DANISH PASTRY, FRUIT	1	EACH	94.0	335	45	5	16
21104	FAST FOOD-EGG AND CHEESE SANDWICH	1	EACH	146.0	340	26	16	19
21018	FAST FOOD-EGG, SCRAMBLED	2	EGGS	94.0	199	2	13	15
21074	FAST FOOD-ENCHILADA W/ CHEESE	1	EACH	163.0	319	29	10	19
21075	FAST FOOD-ENCHILADA W/ CHEESE AND BEEF	1	EACH	192.0	323	30	12	18
21076	FAST FOOD-ENCHIRITO W/ CHEESE, BEEF, AND BEANS	1	EACH	193.0	344	34	18	16
21019	FAST FOOD-ENG. MUFFIN W/ BUTTER	1	EACH	63.0	189	30	5	6
21020	FAST FOOD-ENG. MUFFIN W/ CHEESE AND SAUSAGE	1	EACH	115.0	393	29	15	24
21021	FAST FOOD-ENG. MUFFIN W/ EGG, CHEESE, AND CAN. BACON	1	EACH	146.0	383	31	20	20
21022	FAST FOOD-ENG. MUFFIN W/ EGG, CHEESE, AND SAUSAGE	1	EACH	165.0	487	31	22	31
21047	FAST FOOD-FISH FILLET, BATTERED AND FRIED	1	EACH	91.0	211	15	13	11
21105	FAST FOOD-FISH SANDWICH W/ TARTAR SAUCE	1	EACH	158.0	431	41	17	23
21106	FAST FOOD-FISH SANDWICH W/ TARTAR SAUCE AND CHEESE	1	EACH	183.0	523	48	21	29
21023	FAST FOOD-FRENCH TOAST W/ BUTTER	1	SLICE	67.5	178	18	5	9
21031	FAST FOOD-FRIED PIE, FRUIT (APPLE, CHERRY, OR LEMON)	1	EACH	85.0	266	33	2	14
21077	FAST FOOD-FRIJOLES W/ CHEESE	3	OUNCE	85.1	115	15	6	4
21116	FAST FOOD-HAM AND CHEESE SANDWICH	1	EACH	146.0	352	33	21	15
21117	FAST FOOD-HAM, EGG, AND CHEESE SANDWICH	1	EACH	143.0	347	31	19	16
21114	FAST FOOD-HAMBURGER, DOUBLE PATTY W/ COND AND VEG	1	EACH	226.0	540	40	34	27
21111	FAST FOOD-HAMBURGER, DOUBLE PATTY W/ CONDIMENTS	1	EACH	215.0	576	39	32	32
21110	FAST FOOD-HAMBURGER, DOUBLE PATTY, PLAIN	1	EACH	176.0	544	43	30	28
21113	FAST FOOD-HAMBURGER, LARGE, SINGLE PATTY W/ COND&VEG	1	EACH	218.0	512	40	26	27
21112	FAST FOOD-HAMBURGER, LARGE, SINGLE PATTY, PLAIN	1	EACH	137.0	426	32	23	23
21108	FAST FOOD-HAMBURGER, SINGLE PATTY W/ CONDIMENTS	1	EACH	107.0	275	33	14	10
21107	FAST FOOD-HAMBURGER, SINGLE PATTY, PLAIN	1	EACH	90.0	275	31	12	12
21115	FAST FOOD-HAMBURGER, TRIPLE PATTY W/ CONDIMENTS	1	EACH	259.0	692	29	50	41
21119	FAST FOOD-HOT DOG W/ CHILI	1	EACH	114.0	296	31	14	13
21120	FAST FOOD-HOT DOG W/ CORN FLOUR COATING (CORNDOG)	1	EACH	175.0	460	56	17	19
21118	FAST FOOD-HOT DOG, PLAIN	1	EACH	98.0	242	18	10	15
21028	FAST FOOD-ICE MILK, VANILLA, SOFT-SERVE W/ CONE	1	EACH	103.0	164	24	4	6
21078	FAST FOOD-NACHOS W/ CHEESE	3	OUNCE	85.1	260	27	7	14
21079	FAST FOOD-NACHOS W/ CHEESE AND JALAPENO PEPPERS	3	OUNCE	85.1	253	25	7	14
21080	FAST FOOD-NACHOS W/ CHEESE, BEANS, GROUND BEEF	3	OUNCE	85.1	190	19	7	10
21081	FAST FOOD-NACHOS W/ CINNAMON AND SUGAR	3	OUNCE	85.1	462	49	6	28
21130	FAST FOOD-ONION RINGS, BREADED AND FRIED	1	EACH	10.0	33	4	0	2
21048	FAST FOOD-OYSTERS, BATTERED OR BREADED, AND FRIED	3	OUNCE	85.1	225	24	8	11
21025	FAST FOOD-PANCAKES W/ BUTTER AND SYRUP	1	EACH	74.0	166	29	3	4
21049	FAST FOOD-PIZZA W/ CHEESE	1	SLICE	63.0	140	21	8	3
21050	FAST FOOD-PIZZA W/ CHEESE, SAUSAGE, AND VEGETABLES	1	SLICE	79.0	184	21	13	5
21051	FAST FOOD-PIZZA W/ PEPPERONI	1	SLICE	71.0	181	20	10	7
21131	FAST FOOD-POTATO, BAKED W/ CHEESE SAUCE	1	EACH	296.0	474	47	15	29

Saturated fat (g)	Monounsaturated fat (g)	Polyunsaturated fat (g)	Fiber (g)	Cholesterol (g)	Folate (g)	Vitamin A (RE)	Vitamin B₆ (mg)	Vitamin B₁₂ (µg)	Vitamin C (mg)	Vitamin E (mg)	Riboflavin (mg)	Thiamin (mg)	Calcium (mg)	Iron (mg)	Magnesium (mg)	Niacin (mg)	Phosphorus (mg)	Potassium (mg)	Sodium (mg)	Zinc (mg)
9	10	8	-	60	29	31	.2	.4	9	-	.2	.3	60	4.7	35	6.8	233	353	957	1.9
1	1	0	0	10	2	5	.1	.1	0	-	0	0	3	.2	3	1.1	34	42	90	.2
1	1	0	-	8	4	6	0	0	0	-	0	0	3	.2	3	.9	28	42	108	.1
1	1	0	-	9	2	4	0	0	0	-	0	0	3	.2	3	1	30	38	79	.2
1	1	0	-	8	2	4	0	0	0	-	0	0	3	.2	3	.9	29	37	103	.1
1	1	0	-	8	2	10	0	0	0	-	0	0	3	.2	3	.9	28	36	89	.1
3	3	1	-	134	30	167	.3	1.1	2	-	1.1	.1	68	5.2	46	2.5	197	691	1007	3.6
9	8	1	-	9	31	16	.3	1.5	5	-	.6	.5	63	4.5	63	5.8	124	586	910	5
11	9	1	-	51	33	126	.2	1.3	3	-	.9	.4	238	3.8	60	4.7	187	203	957	3.4
5	5	1	-	12	16	15	0	.1	1	.4	.2	.1	20	1.5	17	1.4	52	82	188	.3
5	8	5	-	65	7	27	0	.8	0	-	.2	.2	15	2.3	23	2.1	176	196	617	1.2
2	1	1	-	6	44	96	.3	0	7	-	.1	.2	4	.9	41	2.2	108	359	29	.9
4	8	5	-	45	20	4	.2	4.5	1	-	.1	.1	55	1.8	25	1.8	131	163	1118	1.1
14	8	1	-	216	37	255	.1	.8	0	-	.4	.2	244	2.2	22	1.5	348	174	551	1.8
15	9	2	-	215	35	120	.1	.9	2	-	.3	.3	151	2.2	23	2.2	276	201	889	1.9
17	11	2	-	213	36	117	.2	1	11	-	.3	.5	144	2.1	26	3.2	336	272	1081	2.2
18	14	3	-	216	38	109	.1	.9	0	-	.3	1	144	3	24	4	290	283	1115	2.1
5	16	2	-	20	15	43	.1	.2	3	-	.2	.3	70	1.8	15	2.5	80	116	319	.6
3	11	2	-	27	14	5	.1	.2	3	-	.2	.3	37	1.8	14	2.2	74	96	326	.5
3	10	2	-	19	15	24	.1	.2	2	-	.2	.3	22	1.4	14	1.8	69	110	333	.5
7	8	3	-	291	37	181	.1	1.1	1	-	.6	.3	225	3	22	2.1	302	188	804	1.6
6	6	2	0	400	53	252	.2	.9	3	.9	.5	.1	54	2.4	13	.2	227	138	211	1.6
11	6	1	-	44	34	186	.4	.7	1	-	.4	.1	324	1.3	51	1.9	134	240	784	2.5
9	6	1	-	40	192	142	.3	1	1	-	.4	.1	228	3.1	83	2.5	167	574	1319	2.7
8	7	0	-	50	253	133	.2	1.6	5	-	.7	.2	218	2.4	71	3	224	560	1251	2.8
2	2	1	-	13	17	33	0	0	1	.1	.3	.3	103	1.6	13	2.6	85	69	386	.4
10	10	3	-	59	18	86	.1	.7	1	-	.3	.7	168	2.3	24	4.1	186	215	1036	1.7
9	7	2	-	234	44	158	.2	.8	1	.6	.5	.5	207	3.3	34	3.9	320	213	784	1.8
12	13	3	-	274	54	172	.2	1.4	1	-	.5	.8	196	3.5	30	4.5	287	294	1135	2.4
3	2	6	-	31	51	11	.1	1	0	-	.1	.1	16	1.9	22	1.9	156	291	484	.4
5	8	8	-	55	44	30	.1	1.1	3	.9	.2	.3	84	2.6	33	3.4	212	340	615	1
8	9	9	-	68	31	97	.1	1.1	3	1.8	.4	.5	185	3.5	37	4.2	311	353	939	1.2
-	-	-	-	58	15	73	0	.2	0	-	.2	.3	36	.9	8	2	73	88	257	.3
7	6	1	-	13	4	33	0	.1	1	.4	.1	.1	13	.9	8	1	37	51	325	.2
2	1	0	-	19	57	36	.1	.3	1	-	.2	.1	96	1.1	43	4	89	308	449	.9
6	7	1	-	58	72	76	.2	.5	3	.3	.5	.3	130	3.2	16	2.7	152	291	771	1.4
7	6	2	-	246	43	149	.2	1.2	3	-	.6	.4	212	3.1	26	4.2	346	210	1005	1.8
11	10	3	-	122	27	11	.5	4.1	1	-	.4	.4	102	5.9	50	7.6	314	570	791	5.7
12	14	3	-	103	45	4	.4	3.3	1	-	.4	.3	92	5.5	45	6.7	284	527	742	5.8
10	12	2	-	99	37	0	.3	2.9	0	1.3	.4	.3	86	4.6	37	8.3	234	363	554	5.7
10	11	2	-	87	37	33	.3	2.4	3	-	.4	.4	96	4.9	44	7.3	233	480	824	4.9
8	10	2	-	71	32	0	.2	2.1	0	-	.3	.3	74	3.6	27	6.2	175	267	474	4.1
4	4	2	-	43	17	13	.1	.8	3	.4	.3	.3	51	2.5	22	4.7	110	215	564	2.1
4	5	1	-	35	25	0	.1	.9	0	.5	.3	.3	63	2.4	19	3.7	103	145	387	2
16	18	3	-	142	31	16	.6	4.9	1	-	.5	.3	65	8.3	54	11	394	785	712	10.7
5	7	1	-	51	50	6	0	.3	3	-	.4	.2	19	3.3	10	3.7	192	166	480	.8
5	9	3	-	79	60	37	.1	.4	0	-	.7	.3	102	6.2	18	4.2	166	263	973	1.3
5	7	2	-	44	29	0	0	.5	0	-	.3	.2	24	2.3	13	3.6	97	143	670	2
4	2	0	-	28	5	52	.1	.2	1	.4	.3	.1	153	1	15	.3	139	169	92	.6
6	6	2	-	14	8	69	.2	.6	1	-	.3	.1	205	1	42	1.2	208	129	614	1.3
6	6	2	-	35	8	196	.2	.4	0	-	.2	.1	259	1	45	1.2	164	122	724	1.2
4	4	2	-	7	13	156	.1	.3	2	-	.2	.1	128	.9	32	1.1	129	151	600	1.2
14	9	2	-	31	6	9	.1	1.3	6	-	.3	.1	66	2.3	15	3.1	26	61	343	.5
1	1	0	-	2	1	0	0	0	0	0	0	0	9	.1	2	.1	10	16	52	0
3	4	3	-	66	8	66	0	.6	3	-	.2	.2	17	2.7	14	2.7	120	111	414	9.6
2	2	1	-	19	11	22	0	.1	3	.4	.2	.1	41	.8	16	1.1	152	80	352	.3
2	1	0	-	9	59	74	0	.3	1	-	.2	.2	117	.6	16	2.5	113	110	336	.8
2	3	1	-	21	27	101	.1	.4	2	-	.2	.2	101	1.5	18	2	131	179	382	1.1
2	3	1	-	14	53	55	.1	.2	2	-	.2	.1	65	.9	9	3	75	153	267	.5
11	11	6	-	18	27	228	.7	.2	26	-	.2	.2	311	3	65	3.3	320	1166	382	1.9

Restaurants, Including Fast Food (Quick Service)—cont'd

Code	Name	Amount	Unit	Grams	Kilocalories	Carbohydrates (g)	Protein (g)	Fat (g)
21132	FAST FOOD-POTATO, BAKED W/ CHEESE SAUCE AND BACON	1	EACH	299.0	451	44	18	26
21133	FAST FOOD-POTATO, BAKED W/ CHEESE SAUCE AND BROCCOLI	1	EACH	339.0	403	47	14	21
21134	FAST FOOD-POTATO, BAKED W/ CHEESE SAUCE AND CHILI	1	EACH	395.0	482	56	23	22
21135	FAST FOOD-POTATO, BAKED W/ SOUR CREAM AND CHIVES	1	EACH	302.0	393	50	7	22
21136	FAST FOOD-POTATO, FRENCH FRIED IN BEEF TALLOW	1	LARGE	115.0	359	44	5	19
21137	FAST FOOD-POTATO, FRENCH FRIED IN BEEF TALLOW AND VEG OIL	1	LARGE	115.0	358	44	5	19
21138	FAST FOOD-POTATO, FRENCH FRIED IN VEGETABLE OIL	1	LARGE	115.0	355	44	5	19
21139	FAST FOOD-POTATOES, MASHED	½	CUP	120.0	100	19	3	1
21026	FAST FOOD-POTATOES, HASHED BROWN	½	CUP	72.0	151	16	2	9
21122	FAST FOOD-ROAST BEEF SANDWICH W/ CHEESE	1	EACH	176.0	473	45	32	18
21121	FAST FOOD-ROAST BEEF SANDWICH, PLAIN	1	EACH	139.0	346	33	22	14
21052	FAST FOOD-SALAD, W/O DRESSING	½	CUP	69.3	11	2	1	0
21053	FAST FOOD-SALAD, W/O DRESSING, W/ CHEESE AND EGG	½	CUP	72.3	34	2	3	2
21054	FAST FOOD-SALAD, W/O DRESSING, W/ CHICKEN	½	CUP	72.7	35	1	6	1
21055	FAST FOOD-SALAD, W/O DRESSING, W/ PASTA AND SEAFOOD	½	CUP	139.0	126	11	5	7
21056	FAST FOOD-SALAD, W/O DRESSING, W/ SHRIMP	½	CUP	78.7	35	2	5	1
21058	FAST FOOD-SCALLOPS, BREADED AND FRIED	1	EACH	24.0	64	6	3	3
21059	FAST FOOD-SHRIMP, BREADED AND FRIED	1	OUNCE	28.4	79	7	3	4
21123	FAST FOOD-STEAK SANDWICH	1	EACH	140.0	315	36	21	10
21124	FAST FOOD-SUBMARINE SANDWICH W/ COLDCUTS	1	EACH	228.0	456	51	22	19
21125	FAST FOOD-SUBMARINE SANDWICH W/ ROAST BEEF	1	EACH	216.0	410	44	29	13
21126	FAST FOOD-SUBMARINE SANDWICH W/ TUNA SALAD	1	EACH	256.0	584	55	30	28
21032	FAST FOOD-SUNDAE, CARAMEL	1	EACH	155.0	304	49	7	9
21033	FAST FOOD-SUNDAE, HOT FUDGE	1	EACH	158.0	284	48	6	9
21034	FAST FOOD-SUNDAE, STRAWBERRY	1	EACH	153.0	268	45	6	8
21082	FAST FOOD-TACO	1	LARGE	263.0	568	41	32	32
21083	FAST FOOD-TACO SALAD	½	CUP	66.0	93	8	4	5
21084	FAST FOOD-TACO SALAD W/ CHILI CON CARNE	½	CUP	87.0	97	9	6	4
21088	FAST FOOD-TOSTADA W/ GUACAMOLE	1	OUNCE	28.4	39	3	1	3
21085	FAST FOOD-TOSTADA, W/ BEANS AND CHEESE	1	EACH	144.0	223	27	10	10
21086	FAST FOOD-TOSTADA, W/ BEANS, BEEF, AND CHEESE	1	EACH	225.0	333	30	16	17
21087	FAST FOOD-TOSTADA, W/ BEEF AND CHEESE	1	EACH	163.0	315	23	19	16
40349	HARDEE'S-BIG CHEESE	1	EACH	141.8	495	28	30	30
40350	HARDEE'S-BIG DELUXE	1	EACH	248.1	675	46	31	41
40356	HARDEE'S-BIG FISH SANDWICH	1	EACH	191.4	514	49	20	26
40353	HARDEE'S-BIG ROAST BEEF	1	EACH	163.0	365	39	22	13
40351	HARDEE'S-BIG TWIN	1	EACH	141.8	369	28	19	20
40358	HARDEE'S-BISCUIT	1	EACH	78.0	275	35	5	13
40348	HARDEE'S-CHEESEBURGER	1	EACH	100.6	335	29	17	17
40357	HARDEE'S-CHICKEN FILLET	1	EACH	191.4	510	42	27	26
40347	HARDEE'S-HAMBURGER	1	EACH	100.1	305	29	17	13
40354	HARDEE'S-HOT DOG	1	EACH	50.0	346	26	11	22
40355	HARDEE'S-HOT HAM & CHEESE	1	EACH	141.8	376	37	23	15
40352	HARDEE'S-ROAST BEEF SANDWICH	1	EACH	141.8	323	39	19	11
44118	JACK IN THE BOX-BACON CHEESEBURGER	1	EACH	242.0	705	41	35	45
44101	JACK IN THE BOX-BREAKFAST JACK	1	EACH	126.0	313	29	19	14
44141	JACK IN THE BOX-CHEESECAKE	1	EACH	99.0	309	29	8	18
44115	JACK IN THE BOX-JUMBO JACK	1	EACH	222.0	497	41	25	26
44116	JACK IN THE BOX-JUMBO JACK W/ CHEESE	1	EACH	242.0	559	40	28	31
44136	JACK IN THE BOX-REGULAR FRENCH FRIES	1	EACH	109.0	351	45	4	17
44135	JACK IN THE BOX-SMALL FRENCH FRIES	1	EACH	68.0	219	28	3	11
47265	K.F.C.-COLONEL'S CHICKEN SANDWICH	1	EACH	166.0	482	39	21	27
47261	K.F.C.-FRENCH FRIES	1	EACH	77.0	244	31	3	12
47260	K.F.C.-MASHED POTATOES AND GRAVY	1	EACH	98.0	71	12	2	2
47239	K.F.C.-ORIGINAL RECIPE CENTER BREAST	1	EACH	103.0	261	9	25	15
47240	K.F.C.-ORIGINAL RECIPE DRUMSTICK	1	EACH	57.0	169	5	12	12
47241	K.F.C.-ORIGINAL RECIPE THIGH	1	EACH	95.0	324	11	16	24
47237	K.F.C.-ORIGINAL RECIPE WING	1	EACH	53.0	172	5	12	11
48204	MCDONALD'S-BACON, EGG AND CHEESE BISCUIT	1	EACH	153.0	432	32	18	26
48174	MCDONALD'S-BIG MAC	1	EACH	215.0	560	43	25	32

Saturated fat (g)	Monounsaturated fat (g)	Polyunsaturated fat (g)	Fiber (g)	Cholesterol (g)	Folate (g)	Vitamin A (RE)	Vitamin B₆ (mg)	Vitamin B₁₂ (µg)	Vitamin C (mg)	Vitamin E (mg)	Riboflavin (mg)	Thiamin (mg)	Calcium (mg)	Iron (mg)	Magnesium (mg)	Niacin (mg)	Phosphorus (mg)	Potassium (mg)	Sodium (mg)	Zinc (mg)
10	10	5	-	30	30	173	.7	.3	29	-	.2	.3	308	3.1	69	4	347	1178	972	2.2
9	8	4	-	20	61	278	.8	.3	48	-	.3	.3	336	3.3	78	3.6	346	1441	485	2
13	7	1	-	32	51	174	.9	.2	32	-	.4	.3	411	6.1	111	4.2	498	1572	699	3.8
10	8	3	-	24	33	278	.8	.2	34	-	.2	.3	106	3.1	69	3.7	184	1383	181	.9
9	8	1	-	21	38	3	.3	.1	6	-	0	.2	18	1.6	38	2.6	153	819	187	.6
8	8	2	-	16	38	3	.3	.1	6	-	0	.2	18	1.6	38	2.6	153	819	187	.6
6	9	3	-	0	38	3	.3	.1	6	-	0	.2	18	1.6	38	2.6	153	819	187	.6
1	0	0	-	2	10	12	.3	.1	0	-	.1	.1	25	.6	22	1.4	66	353	272	.4
4	4	0	-	9	8	3	.2	0	5	.1	0	.1	7	.5	16	1.1	69	267	290	.2
9	4	4	-	77	40	46	.3	2.1	0	-	.5	.4	183	5.1	40	5.9	401	345	1633	5.4
4	7	2	-	51	40	21	.3	1.2	2	-	.3	.4	54	4.2	31	5.9	239	316	792	3.4
0	0	0	-	0	26	79	.1	0	16	-	0	0	9	.4	8	.4	27	119	18	.1
1	1	0	-	33	28	38	0	.1	3	-	.1	0	33	.2	8	.3	44	124	40	.3
0	0	0	-	24	23	32	.1	.1	6	-	0	0	12	.4	11	2	57	149	70	.3
1	2	3	-	17	33	213	.1	.6	13	-	.1	.1	24	1.1	17	1.2	68	200	524	.6
0	0	0	-	60	29	26	0	1.3	3	-	.1	0	20	.3	13	.4	53	135	163	.4
1	2	0	-	18	7	7	0	.1	0	-	.1	0	3	.3	5	0	49	49	153	.2
1	3	0	-	35	8	6	0	0	0	-	.2	0	14	.5	7	0	60	32	250	.2
3	4	2	-	50	62	31	.3	1.1	4	-	.3	.3	63	3.5	34	5	204	360	547	3.1
7	8	2	-	36	55	80	.1	1.1	12	-	.8	1	189	2.5	68	5.5	287	394	1651	2.6
7	2	3	-	73	45	50	.3	1.8	6	-	.4	.4	41	2.8	67	6	192	330	845	4.4
5	13	7	-	49	56	41	.2	1.6	4	-	.3	.5	74	2.6	79	11.3	220	335	1293	1.9
5	3	1	0	25	12	68	0	.6	3	.9	.3	.1	189	.2	28	.9	217	318	195	.8
5	2	1	0	21	9	57	.1	.6	2	.7	.3	.1	207	.6	33	1.1	228	395	182	.9
4	3	1	0	21	18	58	.1	.6	2	.8	.3	.1	161	.3	24	.9	155	271	92	.7
17	10	1	-	87	37	226	.4	1.6	3	-	.7	.2	339	3.7	108	4.9	313	729	1233	6
2	2	1	-	15	13	26	.1	.2	1	-	.1	0	64	.8	17	.8	48	139	254	.9
2	2	1	-	2	21	71	.2	.2	1	-	.2	.1	82	.9	17	.8	51	130	295	1.1
1	1	0	-	4	12	24	0	.1	0	-	.1	0	46	.2	8	.2	25	71	87	.4
5	3	1	-	30	75	85	.2	.7	1	-	.3	.1	210	1.9	59	1.3	117	403	543	1.9
11	4	1	-	74	97	173	.2	1.1	4	-	.5	.1	189	2.5	68	2.9	173	491	871	3.2
10	3	1	-	41	15	96	.2	1.2	3	-	.6	.1	217	2.9	64	3.1	179	572	897	3.7
-	-	-	-	-	-	-	-	-	-	-	-	-	-	-	-	-	-	-	1251	-
-	-	-	-	-	-	-	-	-	-	-	-	-	-	-	-	-	-	-	1063	-
-	-	-	-	-	-	-	-	-	-	-	-	-	-	-	-	-	-	-	314	-
6	6	2	1	55	29	0	.3	3	0	.2	.4	.4	80	4.5	40	6.6	280	389	1071	7.4
9	7	4	1	45	28	14	.2	1.9	2	.7	.3	.2	66	3.3	29	5.5	161	229	475	3.8
-	-	-	-	-	-	-	-	-	-	-	-	-	-	-	-	-	-	-	650	-
-	-	-	-	-	-	-	-	-	2	-	.3	.5	-	-	-	5.5	-	-	789	-
-	-	-	-	-	-	-	-	-	-	-	-	-	-	-	-	-	-	-	360	-
-	-	-	-	-	-	-	-	-	2	-	.6	.6	-	-	-	6.4	-	-	682	-
-	-	-	-	-	-	-	-	-	-	-	-	-	-	-	-	-	-	-	744	-
-	-	-	-	-	-	-	-	-	-	-	-	-	-	-	-	-	-	-	1067	-
5	5	2	1	44	25	0	.3	2.6	0	.2	.4	.3	70	3.9	35	5.7	244	323	908	6.5
15	16	9	-	113	-	70	-	-	8	-	.5	.2	200	2.8	-	8.4	-	-	1240	-
5	5	3	-	190	-	138	.1	1.1	3	-	.5	4	184	2.6	25	5.3	323	198	1080	1.9
9	7	2	-	63	-	-	-	-	-	-	.2	0	88	.3	-	1.9	-	-	208	-
10	11	2	-	72	-	67	.3	2.4	4	-	.3	.4	121	4.1	40	10.5	236	444	1023	3.8
13	11	2	-	98	-	196	.3	2.7	4	-	.3	.5	243	4.1	44	10.1	366	444	1482	4.3
4	7	-	-	0	-	-	-	-	26	-	0	.2	-	.7	-	3.6	-	-	194	-
3	7	-	-	0	-	-	-	-	16	-	-	.1	-	.4	-	2.3	-	-	121	-
6	4	9	1	47	29	14	.6	.3	0	2.3	.3	.4	100	3.1	41	10.6	261	297	1060	1.5
3	7	1	-	2	-	-	-	-	16	-	.1	.2	-	.3	-	1.9	-	-	139	-
1	0	0	-	-	-	-	-	-	-	-	0	-	16	.2	-	1.1	-	-	339	-
4	4	2	0	87	4	15	.6	.4	0	.5	.1	.1	16	1.2	31	14	238	265	603	1.1
2	3	2	-	59	5	14	.2	.2	0	.4	.1	0	7	.7	13	3.4	99	130	268	1.7
6	6	3	0	103	8	28	.3	.3	0	.5	.2	.1	13	1.4	23	6.5	176	224	549	2.4
3	6	2	-	59	-	-	-	-	-	-	.1	0	24	.3	-	2.9	-	-	383	-
8	16	2	1	248	18	157	.2	.6	0	1.5	.3	.4	181	2.6	30	2.5	442	232	1206	1.7
10	20	2	-	103	21	106	.3	1.8	2	-	.4	.5	256	4	38	6.8	314	237	950	4.7

Restaurants, Including Fast Food (Quick Service)—cont'd

Code	Name	Amount	Unit	Grams	Kilocalories	Carbohydrates (g)	Protein (g)	Fat (g)
48205	MCDONALD'S-BISCUIT W/ SPREAD	1	EACH	75.0	260	32	5	13
48170	MCDONALD'S-CHEESEBURGER	1	EACH	116.0	310	30	15	13
48187	MCDONALD'S-CHEF SALAD	1	EACH	265.0	215	7	20	12
48181	MCDONALD'S-CHICKEN MCNUGGETS	1	EACH	18.5	45	3	3	3
48226	MCDONALD'S-CHOCOLATE LOWFAT MILK SHAKE	1	EACH	294.1	321	66	11	2
48189	MCDONALD'S-CHUNKY CHICKEN SALAD	1	EACH	255.0	143	5	23	3
48198	MCDONALD'S-EGG MCMUFFIN	1	EACH	135.0	284	27	18	11
48201	MCDONALD'S-ENGLISH MUFFIN W/ SPREAD	1	EACH	58.0	170	26	5	4
48175	MCDONALD'S-FILET O' FISH	1	EACH	141.0	437	38	14	26
48188	MCDONALD'S-GARDEN SALAD	1	EACH	189.0	50	6	4	2
48169	MCDONALD'S-HAMBURGER	1	EACH	102.0	255	30	12	9
48209	MCDONALD'S-HASH BROWN POTATOES	1	EACH	53.0	130	15	1	7
48210	MCDONALD'S-HOTCAKES W/ MARGARINE AND SYRUP	1	EACH	174.0	440	74	8	12
48180	MCDONALD'S-LARGE FRENCH FRIES	1	EACH	122.0	400	46	6	22
48176	MCDONALD'S-MCCHICKEN	1	EACH	187.0	415	39	19	20
48223	MCDONALD'S-MCDONALDLAND COOKIES	1	EACH	56.7	290	47	4	9
48179	MCDONALD'S-MEDIUM FRENCH FRIES	1	EACH	97.0	320	36	4	17
48171	MCDONALD'S-QUARTER POUNDER	1	EACH	166.0	410	34	23	20
48207	MCDONALD'S-SAUSAGE BISCUIT	1	EACH	118.0	420	32	12	28
48203	MCDONALD'S-SAUSAGE BISCUIT W/ EGG	1	EACH	175.0	505	33	19	33
48199	MCDONALD'S-SAUSAGE MCMUFFIN	1	EACH	135.0	345	27	15	20
48200	MCDONALD'S-SAUSAGE MCMUFFIN W/ EGG	1	EACH	159.0	430	27	21	25
48208	MCDONALD'S-SCRAMBLED EGGS	1	EACH	100.0	140	1	12	10
48190	MCDONALD'S-SIDE SALAD	1	EACH	106.0	30	4	2	1
48178	MCDONALD'S-SMALL FRENCH FRIES	1	EACH	68.0	220	26	3	12
48227	MCDONALD'S-STRAWBERRY LOWFAT MILK SHAKE	1	EACH	294.1	320	67	11	1
48225	MCDONALD'S-VANILLA LOWFAT MILK SHAKE	1	EACH	294.1	290	60	11	1
52366	PIZZA HUT-CHEESE PIZZA, HAND TOSSED	1	SLICE	70.0	259	28	17	10
52359	PIZZA HUT-CHEESE PIZZA, PAN	1	SLICE	70.0	246	29	15	9
53322	PIZZA HUT-CHEESE PIZZA, THIN'N CRISPY	1	SLICE	70.0	199	19	14	9
52363	PIZZA HUT-PEPPERONI PIZZA, THIN'N CRISPY	1	SLICE	70.0	207	18	13	10
52370	PIZZA HUT-PEPPERONI PERSONAL PAN PIZZA	1	EACH	250.0	675	76	37	29
52367	PIZZA HUT-PEPPERONI PIZZA, HAND TOSSED	1	SLICE	70.0	250	25	14	12
52360	PIZZA HUT-PEPPERONI PIZZA, PAN	1	SLICE	70.0	270	31	15	11
52365	PIZZA HUT-SUPER SPRM PIZZA, THIN'N CRISPY	1	SLICE	70.0	232	22	15	11
52362	PIZZA HUT-SUPER SUPREME PIZZA, PAN	1	SLICE	70.0	282	27	17	13
52369	PIZZA HUT-SUPER SUPREME, HAND TOSSED	1	SLICE	70.0	278	27	17	13
52371	PIZZA HUT-SUPREME PERSONAL PAN PIZZA	1	EACH	250.0	647	76	33	28
52368	PIZZA HUT-SUPREME PIZZA, HAND TOSSED	1	SLICE	70.0	270	25	16	13
52361	PIZZA HUT-SUPREME PIZZA, PAN	1	SLICE	70.0	295	27	16	15
52364	PIZZA HUT-SUPREME PIZZA, THIN'N CRISPY	1	SLICE	70.0	230	21	14	11
62559	SUBWAY-BMT, ON ITALIAN ROLL	1	12 IN.	213.0	982	83	44	55
62561	SUBWAY-CLUB SANDWICH, ON ITALIAN ROLL	1	12 IN.	213.0	693	83	46	22
62562	SUBWAY-COLD CUT COMBO, ON ITALIAN ROLL	1	12 IN.	184.0	853	83	46	40
62564	SUBWAY-HAM AND CHEESE, ON ITALIAN ROLL	1	12 IN.	184.0	643	81	38	18
62565	SUBWAY-MEAT BALL SANDWICH, ON ITALIAN ROLL	1	12 IN.	215.0	918	96	42	44
62567	SUBWAY-ROAST BEEF, ON ITALIAN ROLL	1	12 IN.	184.0	689	84	42	23
62569	SUBWAY-SEAFOOD, ON ITALIAN ROLL	1	12 IN.	210.0	986	94	29	57
62571	SUBWAY-SPICY ITALIAN, ON ITALIAN ROLL	1	12 IN.	213.0	1043	83	42	63
62572	SUBWAY-STEAK AND CHEESE, ON ITALIAN ROLL	1	12 IN.	213.0	765	83	43	32
58318	TACO BELL-BEAN BURRITO	1	EACH	206.0	387	63	15	14
58319	TACO BELL-BEEF BURRITO	1	EACH	206.0	431	48	25	21
58321	TACO BELL-BURRITO SUPREME	1	EACH	198.0	440	55	20	22
62585	TACO BELL-LIGHT 7-LAYER BURRITO	1	EACH	276.0	440	67	19	9
62583	TACO BELL-LIGHT BEAN BURRITO	1	EACH	198.0	330	55	14	6
62586	TACO BELL-LIGHT BURRITO SUPREME	1	EACH	248.0	350	50	20	8
62584	TACO BELL-LIGHT CHICKEN BURRITO	1	EACH	170.0	290	45	12	6
62587	TACO BELL-LIGHT CHICKEN BURRITO SUPREME	1	EACH	248.0	410	62	18	10
62582	TACO BELL-LIGHT CHICKEN SOFT TACO	1	EACH	120.0	180	26	9	5
62575	TACO BELL-LIGHT SOFT TACO	1	EACH	99.0	180	19	13	5

Saturated fat (g)	Monounsaturated fat (g)	Polyunsaturated fat (g)	Fiber (g)	Cholesterol (g)	Folate (g)	Vitamin A (RE)	Vitamin B6 (mg)	Vitamin B12 (μg)	Vitamin C (mg)	Vitamin E (mg)	Riboflavin (mg)	Thiamin (mg)	Calcium (mg)	Iron (mg)	Magnesium (mg)	Niacin (mg)	Phosphorus (mg)	Potassium (mg)	Sodium (mg)	Zinc (mg)
3	9	1	1	1	6	0	0	.1	0	1.8	.1	.2	75	1.3	14	1.5	168	100	730	.7
5	8	1	-	50	18	118	.1	.9	2	.5	.2	.3	199	2.3	21	3.9	177	223	750	2.1
6	6	1	-	120	-	385	-	-	13	-	.3	.3	240	1.4	-	3.4	-	-	459	-
1	2	0	-	9	-	-	-	-	-	-	0	0	-	.1	-	1.3	-	-	97	-
1	1	0	-	10	-	92	-	-	0	-	.5	.1	333	.8	-	.4	-	-	241	-
1	2	1	1	80	28	373	.6	.6	20	11	.2	.2	35	1	38	8.7	262	445	235	3
4	6	1	1	221	43	147	.2	.8	1	1.8	.3	.5	250	2.7	32	3.6	312	208	724	1.8
2	2	1	2	9	51	37	.1	-	0	.1	.1	.3	151	1.6	12	2.5	60	74	285	.4
5	10	11	1	50	20	44	.1	.8	-	-	.1	.3	164	1.8	27	2.7	227	149	1023	.9
1	1	0	-	65	-	900	-	-	21	-	.1	.1	32	.8	-	.4	-	-	70	-
3	5	1	-	37	-	40	-	-	2	-	.2	.3	80	1.5	-	3.8	-	-	490	-
1	4	2	-	0	-	-	-	-	1	-	-	.1	-	-	-	.8	-	-	330	-
2	5	5	-	8	-	40	-	-	-	-	.3	.3	80	1	-	2.9	-	-	685	-
5	15	2	-	0	-	-	-	-	15	-	-	.2	-	.6	-	2.9	-	-	20	-
4	9	7	-	50	-	20	-	-	2	-	.2	.9	120	1.5	-	8.6	-	-	830	-
1	7	1	-	0	-	-	-	-	-	-	.2	.2	-	1	-	1.9	-	-	300	-
4	12	2	-	0	-	-	-	-	12	-	-	.2	-	.4	-	2.9	-	-	150	-
8	11	1	-	85	-	40	-	-	4	-	.3	.4	120	2	-	6.7	-	-	645	-
8	17	3	-	44	-	-	-	-	-	-	.2	.5	64	1	-	3.8	-	-	1040	-
10	20	3	-	260	-	60	-	-	-	-	.3	.5	80	2	-	3.8	-	-	1210	-
7	11	2	-	57	-	40	-	-	-	-	.3	.5	160	1.5	-	4.8	-	-	770	-
8	14	3	-	270	-	100	-	-	-	-	.4	.5	200	2	-	4.8	-	-	920	-
3	5	2	-	425	-	100	-	-	-	-	.3	.1	48	1	-	-	-	-	290	-
0	1	0	-	33	-	800	-	-	12	-	.1	.1	16	.4	-	-	-	-	35	-
3	8	1	-	0	-	-	-	-	9	-	-	.2	-	.2	-	1.9	-	-	110	-
1	1	0	-	10	-	60	-	-	-	-	.5	.1	280	-	-	.4	-	-	170	-
1	1	0	-	10	-	60	-	-	-	-	.5	.1	280	-	-	-	-	-	170	-
7	3	-	-	28	-	50	-	.3	5	-	.2	.2	300	1.5	32	2.6	220	198	638	2.3
5	5	-	-	17	-	45	-	.3	4	-	.3	.3	252	1.5	26	2.5	188	160	470	2
5	3	-	-	17	-	35	-	.3	2	-	.2	.2	264	.9	21	2.3	188	131	434	1.8
5	5	-	-	23	-	35	-	.3	3	-	.2	.2	180	.9	19	2.5	148	144	493	1.7
13	17	-	-	53	-	120	-	.4	10	-	.7	.6	584	3.2	53	7.8	360	408	1335	3.8
6	5	-	-	25	-	50	-	.3	4	-	.3	.3	176	1.4	26	2.7	156	208	634	1.9
5	7	-	-	21	-	50	-	.3	4	-	.2	.3	208	1.8	25	2.6	176	203	564	2.1
5	5	-	-	28	-	50	-	.4	4	-	.2	.3	184	1.4	26	2.6	168	232	668	2.3
6	7	-	-	28	-	60	-	.4	5	-	.3	.4	216	1.9	32	3	188	266	724	2.7
7	6	-	-	27	-	55	-	.4	6	-	.3	.4	176	1.9	33	3.5	168	258	824	2.4
11	17	-	-	49	-	120	-	.5	11	-	.7	.6	416	3.7	53	7.6	320	487	1313	3.8
6	7	-	-	28	-	55	-	.4	6	-	.3	.3	192	2.3	35	3.4	184	289	735	2.9
5	8	-	-	24	-	60	-	.4	5	-	.4	.4	200	1.4	33	2.9	184	290	832	2.8
6	6	-	-	21	-	50	-	.3	-	-	.2	.3	172	1.7	30	2.6	160	272	664	2.3
20	24	7	5	133	63	67	.5	2.3	5	5.1	.3	.3	64	4.3	66	5.1	308	917	3139	6.1
7	8	4	5	84	47	74	.6	1	20	1.3	.3	.5	58	3.1	66	12.5	384	971	2717	2.5
12	15	10	5	166	39	87	.2	1.2	17	.9	.3	.4	227	2.9	28	3.8	315	876	2218	2.7
7	8	4	5	73	45	174	.3	.8	17	3.8	.4	.5	304	2.2	50	3.6	527	834	1710	2.8
17	17	4	3	88	35	72	.4	3.2	19	1	.4	3	78	5	47	9.4	263	1210	2022	6.2
8	9	4	5	83	54	58	.4	2	5	4.4	.3	.2	55	3.7	57	4.4	266	910	2288	5.3
11	15	28	-	56	91	107	.3	6.5	5	2.5	.4	.5	230	4.4	32	7	336	641	2027	5.3
23	28	7	5	137	-	-	-	-	-	-	-	-	-	-	-	-	-	880	2282	-
12	12	4	6	82	36	119	.4	2.5	6	.8	.5	.3	231	4.2	43	5.1	456	909	1556	6.8
4	-	2	3	9	-	-	-	-	53	-	2	.4	190	4	-	2.8	-	495	1148	-
8	-	2	2	57	-	-	-	-	2	-	.3	.4	150	3	-	3.2	-	380	1311	-
8	-	2	3	33	-	-	-	-	26	-	2.1	.4	190	4	-	3.6	-	501	1181	-
-	-	-	-	5	-	350	-	-	5	-	-	-	300	2.5	-	-	-	-	1130	-
-	-	-	-	5	-	300	-	-	2	-	-	-	120	2	-	-	-	-	1340	-
-	-	-	-	25	-	600	-	-	9	-	-	-	96	1.5	-	-	-	-	1160	-
-	-	-	-	30	-	200	-	-	4	-	-	-	72	1.5	-	-	-	-	900	-
-	-	-	-	65	-	250	-	-	5	-	-	-	72	1.5	-	-	-	-	1190	-
-	-	-	-	30	-	150	-	-	5	-	-	-	48	.8	-	-	-	-	570	-
4	-	1	2	25	-	40	-	-	0	-	.2	.4	48	.6	-	2.8	-	196	554	-

Restaurants, Including Fast Food (Quick Service)—cont'd

Code	Name	Amount	Unit	Grams	Kilocalories	Carbohydrates (g)	Protein (g)	Fat (g)
62581	TACO BELL-LIGHT SOFT TACO SUPREME	1	EACH	128.0	200	23	14	5
62574	TACO BELL-LIGHT TACO	1	EACH	78.0	140	11	11	5
62588	TACO BELL-LIGHT TACO SALAD	1	EACH	464.0	330	35	30	9
62580	TACO BELL-LIGHT TACO SUPREME	1	EACH	106.0	160	23	14	5
58328	TACO BELL-MEXICAN PIZZA	1	EACH	223.0	575	40	21	37
58325	TACO BELL-NACHOS	1	EACH	106.0	346	37	7	18
58323	TACO BELL-NACHOS BELL GRANDE	1	EACH	287.0	649	61	22	35
58329	TACO BELL-PINTOS 'N CHEESE	1	EACH	128.0	190	19	9	9
58337	TACO BELL-SALSA	1	EACH	10.0	18	4	1	0
58314	TACO BELL-SOFT TACO	1	EACH	92.0	225	18	12	12
58313	TACO BELL-TACO	1	EACH	78.0	183	11	10	11
58332	TACO BELL-TACO SALAD	1	EACH	575.0	905	55	34	61
58333	TACO BELL-TACO SALAD W/O SHELL	1	EACH	520.0	484	22	28	31
58316	TACO BELL-TOSTADA	1	EACH	156.0	243	27	9	11
61273	WENDY'S-BIG CLASSIC	1	EACH	251.0	480	44	27	23
62322	WENDY'S-BKD POTATO W/ BACON AND CHEESE	1	EACH	380.0	510	75	17	17
61287	WENDY'S-BKD POTATO W/ BROCCOLI AND CHEESE	1	EACH	411.0	450	77	9	14
62524	WENDY'S-BKD POTATO W/ CHEESE	1	EACH	383.0	550	74	14	24
61281	WENDY'S-CHICKEN CLUB SANDWICH	1	EACH	220.0	520	44	30	25
61285	WENDY'S-FRENCH FRIES, BIGGIE	1	EACH	170.0	450	62	6	22
61284	WENDY'S-FRENCH FRIES, MEDIUM	1	EACH	136.0	360	50	5	17
61283	WENDY'S-FRENCH FRIES, SMALL	1	EACH	91.0	240	33	3	12
61301	WENDY'S-FROSTY DAIRY DESSERT, MEDIUM	1	EACH	321.8	460	76	12	13
61271	WENDY'S-PLAIN SINGLE	1	EACH	133.0	350	31	25	15
61272	WENDY'S-SINGLE W/ EVERYTHING	1	EACH	219.0	440	36	26	23

Saturated fat (g)	Monounsaturated fat (g)	Polyunsaturated fat (g)	Fiber (g)	Cholesterol (g)	Folate (g)	Vitamin A (RE)	Vitamin B6 (mg)	Vitamin B12 (µg)	Vitamin C (mg)	Vitamin E (mg)	Riboflavin (mg)	Thiamin (mg)	Calcium (mg)	Iron (mg)	Magnesium (mg)	Niacin (mg)	Phosphorus (mg)	Potassium (mg)	Sodium (mg)	Zinc (mg)
-	-	-	-	25	-	100	-	-	2	-	-	.-	48	.6	-	-	-	-	610	-
4	-	1	1	20	-	40	-	-	0	-	.1	.1	0	0	-	1.2	-	159	276	-
-	-	-	-	50	-	1200	-	-	27	-	-	-	120	1.5	-	-	-	-	1610	-
-	-	-	-	20	-	100	-	-	2	-	-	-	0	0	-	-	-	-	340	-
11	-	10	3	52	-	-	-	-	31	-	.3	.3	257	4	-	3	-	408	1031	-
6	-	2	1	9	-	-	-	-	2	-	.2	-	191	1	-	.6	-	159	399	-
12	-	3	4	36	-	-	-	-	58	-	.3	.1	297	3	-	2.2	-	674	997	-
4	-	1	2	16	-	-	-	-	52	-	.2	.1	156	1	-	.4	-	384	642	-
0	-	0	0	0	-	-	-	-	-	-	.1	-	36	1	-	-	-	376	376	-
5	-	1	2	32	-	-	-	-	1	-	.2	.4	116	2	-	2.8	-	196	554	-
5	-	1	1	32	-	-	-	-	1	-	.1	.1	84	1	-	1.2	-	159	276	-
19	-	12	4	80	-	-	-	-	75	-	.6	.5	320	6	-	4.8	-	673	910	-
14	-	2	3	80	-	-	-	-	74	-	.4	.2	290	4	-	3.2	-	612	680	-
4	-	1	2	16	-	-	-	-	45	-	.2	.1	180	2	-	.6	-	401	596	-
7	8	7	-	75	-	60	-	-	12	-	.3	.5	120	3.5	-	6.7	-	500	850	-
4	3	8	-	15	-	100	-	-	36	-	.2	.5	80	2.5	-	6.7	-	1370	1170	-
2	3	7	-	0	-	200	-	-	60	-	.1	.3	80	2.5	-	4.8	-	1310	450	-
8	6	7	-	30	-	150	-	-	36	-	.2	.3	240	2	-	3.8	-	1210	640	-
6	7	9	-	75	-	20	-	-	9	-	.4	.6	80	8	-	15.2	-	470	980	-
5	15	1	-	0	-	-	-	-	12	-	.1	.3	16	.8	-	3.8	-	950	280	-
4	12	1	-	0	-	-	-	-	9	-	0	.2	16	.6	-	2.9	-	760	220	-
2	8	1	-	0	-	-	-	-	6	-	0	.2	-	.4	-	1.9	-	510	150	-
7	3	1	-	55	-	100	-	-	-	-	1	.2	320	.8	-	.8	-	830	260	-
6	7	2	-	70	-	-	-	-	-	-	.2	.4	80	3	-	5.7	-	280	510	-
7	7	7	-	75	-	60	-	-	9	-	.2	.4	80	3	-	6.7	-	430	850	-

Index